2010
YEAR BOOK OF
DERMATOLOGY
AND
DERMATOLOGIC
SURGERY™

The 2010 Year Book Series

Year Book of Anesthesiology and Pain Management™: Drs Chestnut, Abram, Black, Gravlee, Lien, Mathru and Roizen

Year Book of Cardiology®: Drs Gersh, Cheitlin, Elliott, Gold, Graham, and Suri

Year Book of Critical Care Medicine®: Drs Dellinger, Parrillo, Balk, Dorman, Dries, and Zanotti-Cavazzoni

Year Book of Dermatology and Dermatologic Surgery™: Dr Del Rosso

Year Book of Diagnostic Radiology®: Drs Osborn, Abbara, Birdwell, Elster, Manaster, Oestreich, Offiah, Rosado de Christenson, and Walker

Year Book of Emergency Medicine®: Drs Hamilton, Bruno, Handly, Mullin, Quintana, and Ramoska

Year Book of Endocrinology®: Drs Schott, Apovian, Clarke, Eugster, Ludlam, Meikle, Ovalle, Schinner, Schteingart, and Toth

Year Book of Gastroenterology™: Drs Talley, Dempsey, Harnois, Lange, Pearson, Picco, Rombeau, and Scolapio

Year Book of Hand and Upper Limb Surgery®: Drs Yao and Steinmann

Year Book of Medicine®: Drs Barker, Berney, Garrick, Gersh, Khardori, LeRoith, Talley, and Thigpen

Year Book of Neonatal and Perinatal Medicine®: Drs Fanaroff, Benitz, Donn, Neu, and Papile

Year Book of Neurology and Neurosurgery®: Drs Klimo and Rabinstein

Year Book of Obstetrics, Gynecology, and Women's Health®: Drs Dungan and Shulman

Year Book of Oncology®: Drs Thigpen, Arceci, Bauer, Byhardt, Gordon, and Lawton

Year Book of Ophthalmology®: Drs Rapuano, Cohen, Flanders, Hammersmith, Milman, Myers, Nelson, Penne, Pyfer, Sergott, Shields, and Vander

Year Book of Orthopedics®: Drs Morrey, Beauchamp, Huddleston, Swiontkowski, and Trigg

Year Book of Otolaryngology-Head and Neck Surgery®: Drs Sindwani, Balough, Franco, Gapany, and Mitchell

Year Book of Pathology and Laboratory Medicine®: Drs Raab, Parwani, Bejarano, and Bissell

Year Book of Pediatrics®: Dr Stockman

2010

The Year Book of DERMATOLOGY AND DERMATOLOGIC SURGERY™

Editor-in-Chief

James Q. Del Rosso, DO, FAOCD

Dermatology Residency Director, Valley Hospital Medical Center, Las Vegas, Nevada; Dermatology and Cutaneous Surgery, Las Vegas Skin and Cancer Clinics, Las Vegas and Henderson, Nevada

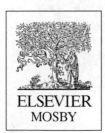

ELSEVIER
MOSBY

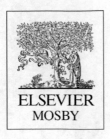

ELSEVIER
MOSBY

Vice President, Continuity: Kimberly Murphy
Editor: Carla Holloway
Supervisor, Electronic Year Books: Donna M. Skelton
Electronic Article Manager: Jennifer C. Pitts
Illustrations and Permissions Coordinator: Dawn Vohsen

Printed in the United States of America
Composition by TNQ Books and Journals Pvt Ltd, India
Printing/binding by Sheridan Books, Inc.

Editorial Office:
Elsevier
Suite 1800
1600 John F. Kennedy Blvd
Philadelphia, PA 19103-2899

International Standard Serial Number: 0093-3619
International Standard Book Number: 978-0-323-06827-7

Editorial Board

Martin A. Weinstock, MD, PhD

Professor of Dermatology and Community Health, Brown University; Chief of Dermatology, VA Medical Center; Director, Pigmented Lesion Unit and Photomedicine, Rhode Island Hospital, Providence, Rhode Island

Table of Contents

Journals Represented

Journals represented in this YEAR BOOK are listed below.

Allergy
American Journal of Obstetrics and Gynecology
American Journal of Clinical Nutrition
American Journal of Emergency Medicine
American Journal of Epidemiology
American Journal of Infection Control
American Journal of Ophthalmology
American Journal of Otolaryngology
American Journal of Pathology
American Journal of Preventive Medicine
American Journal of Surgical Pathology
American Surgeon
Anaesthesia
Annals of Plastic Surgery
Annals of Surgery
Annals of Surgical Oncology
Annals of the Rheumatic Diseases
Archives of Dermatology
Archives of Disease in Childhood
Arthritis & Rheumatism
Aesthetic Surgery Journal
BJU International
British Journal of Cancer
British Journal of Dermatology
Cancer
Cancer Epidemiology, Biomarkers & Prevention
Clinical Cancer Research
Clinical Infectious Diseases
Clinical Pediatrics Clinical Radiology
Contact Dermatitis
Contraception
Dermatologic surgery
Dermatology
European Journal of Internal Medicine
European Journal of Plastic Surgery
International Journal of Cancer
International Journal of Radiation Oncology Biology Physics
Journal of Allergy and Clinical Immunology
Journal of Clinical Microbiology
Journal of Clinical Oncology
Journal of Clinical Rheumatology
Journal of Cranio-Maxillo-Facial Surgery
Journal of Cutaneous Pathology
Journal of Immunology
Journal of Infectious Diseases
Journal of Oral and Maxillofacial Surgery
Journal of Pathology

Journal of Pediatric Surgery
Journal of Plastic, Reconstructive & Aesthetic Surgery
Journal of Rheumatology
Journal of the American Academy of Dermatology
Journal of the American Board of Family Medicine
Journal of the European Academy of Dermatology and Venereology
Journal of the National Cancer Institute
Journal of Vascular Surgery
Lancet
Modern Pathology
Ophthalmology
Oral Surgery Oral Medicine Oral Pathology Oral Radiology and Endodontics
Pediatric Dermatology
Pediatric Infectious Disease Journal
Pediatrics
Pharmacotherapy
Plastic and Reconstructive Surgery
Scandinavian Journal of Rheumatology
Skeletal Radiology
The Journal of Investigative Dermatology
Transplantation

STANDARD ABBREVIATIONS

The following terms are abbreviated in this edition: acquired immunodeficiency syndrome (AIDS), cardiopulmonary resuscitation (CPR), central nervous system (CNS), cerebrospinal fluid (CSF), computed tomography (CT), deoxyribonucleic acid (DNA), electrocardiography (ECG), health maintenance organization (HMO), human immunodeficiency virus (HIV), intensive care unit (ICU), intramuscular (IM), intravenous (IV), magnetic resonance (MR) imaging (MRI), ribonucleic acid (RNA), ultrasound (US), and ultraviolet (UV).

NOTE

The YEAR BOOK OF DERMATOLOGY AND DERMATOLOGIC SURGERY™ is a literature survey service providing abstracts of articles published in the professional literature. Every effort is made to ensure the accuracy of the information presented in these pages. Neither the editors nor the publisher of the YEAR BOOK OF DERMATOLOGY AND DERMATOLOGIC SURGERY™ can be responsible for errors in the original materials. The editors' comments are their own opinions. Mention of specific products within this publication does not constitute endorsement.

To facilitate the use of the YEAR BOOK OF DERMATOLOGY AND DERMATOLOGIC SURGERY™ as a reference tool, all illustrations and tables included in this publication are now identified as they appear in the original article. This change is meant to help the reader recognize that any illustration or table appearing in the YEAR BOOK OF DERMATOLOGY AND DERMATOLOGIC SURGERY™ may be only one of many in the original article. For this reason, figure and table numbers will often appear to be out of sequence within the YEAR BOOK OF DERMATOLOGY AND DERMATOLOGIC SURGERY™.

COLOR PLATE I

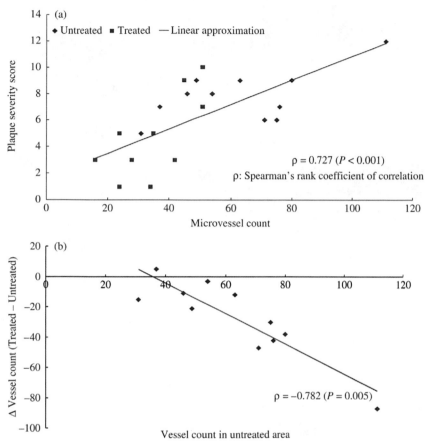

$\rho = 0.727$ ($P < 0.001$)

ρ: Spearman's rank coefficient of correlation

$\rho = -0.782$ ($P = 0.005$)

Fig 3, page 150

COLOR PLATE II

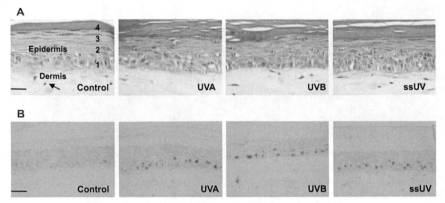

Fig 2 (A & B), page 229

COLOR PLATE III

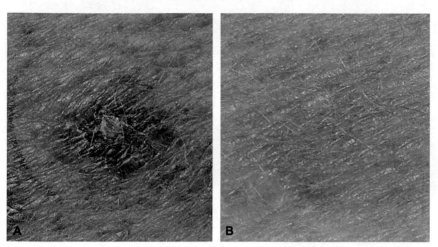

Fig 2, page 242

COLOR PLATE IV

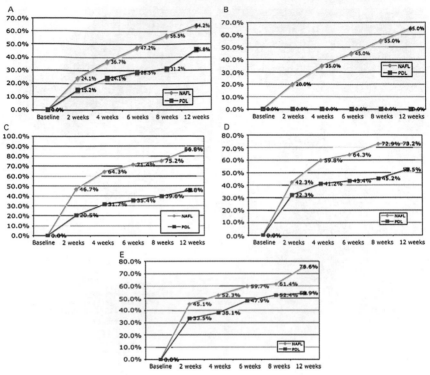

Fig 1, page 467

COLOR PLATE V

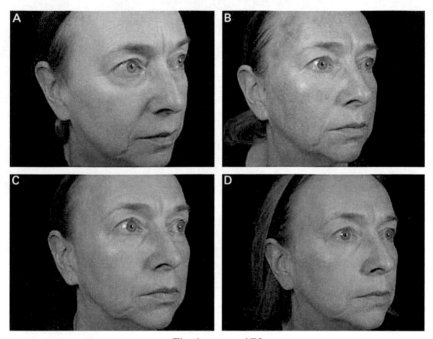

Fig 1, page 473

T Cell Receptor Gene Rearrangement Assays: A Review of Basic Science, Methodology, Clinical Applications, Potential Pitfalls, and Interpretation of Results for the Clinical Dermatologist

JACQUELYN LEVIN, DO, AND JAMES Q. DEL ROSSO, DO

Valley Hospital Medical Center, Las Vegas, Nevada

ABSTRACT

T cell receptor (TCR) gene rearrangement assays are mostly used by clinical dermatologists to differentiate benign T cell lymphoproliferations from malignant T cell lymphoproliferations such as lymphoma. In this article, we review the basics of TCR structure and the process of gene rearrangement, explain the latest methods used to detect TCR gene rearrangements, review the many clinical applications and potential pitfalls of TCR gene rearrangement assays, and finally discuss how to interpret the results of these assays in a clinical context.

Polymerase chain reaction (PCR) of the TCR gamma (G) loci and subsequent amplicon separation for the detection of a monoclonal T cell lymphoproliferation demonstrate significant sensitivity in cases of histologically diagnostic cutaneous T cell lymphoma (CTCL), as reported by other authors. We review studies that investigated the usefulness of monoclonal detection for the diagnosis of histologically nondiagnostic yet clinically suspicious CTCL and for CTCL staging. We also discuss briefly how TCR gene rearrangement assays can be used to differentiate disease with similar histology, detect the transformation of a benign disease to malignancy, detect minimal residual disease in a patient undergoing treatment, and design clone-specific probes.

Additionally, this article discusses many of the pitfalls of relying on this technology as an adjuvant diagnostic tool. These pitfalls stem from the fact that monoclonality is not always found in malignancy just as polyclonality is not always found in benign disease.

We conclude the review by presenting specific scenarios that the clinical physician may face when diagnosing clinically suspicious CTCL and discuss management considerations in each case that are supported by literature.

It is our conclusion that the detection of monoclonality in any scenario warrants further investigation and close monitoring. While the detection of polyclonality makes the diagnosis of malignancy less likely, gene rearrangement assay results should not be used as an independent diagnostic tool and should be interpreted in the context of the clinical and histologic picture with immunophenotypic evaluation.

INTRODUCTION

T cell receptor (TCR) gene rearrangement assays are mostly used by clinical dermatologists to differentiate benign T cell lymphoproliferations from malignant T cell lymphoproliferations such as lymphoma. In this article, we review the basics of TCR structure and the process of gene rearrangement, explain the latest methods used to detect TCR gene rearrangements, review the many clinical applications and potential pitfalls of TCR gene rearrangement assays, and finally discuss how to interpret the results of these assays in a clinical context.

1. WHAT IS THE TCR STRUCTURE AND HOW IS T CELL GENE REARRANGEMENT RESPONSIBLE FOR THE UNIQUE SPECIFICITY OF TCRs?

Before discussing the clinical applications of detecting clonal T cell lymphoproliferations, it is first worth reviewing the TCR structure and the properties of TCR rearrangements that lend themselves to the identification of T-cell clonality through gene rearrangement assays.

T lymphocytes (T cells) recognize foreign antigens through the TCR. Two types of TCRs have been identified on the surface of the T cells: TCR alpha/beta and TCR gamma/delta. TCR alpha/beta and TCR gamma/delta are each composed of 2 disulfide-linked polypeptide chains designated alpha (A) and beta (B) and gamma (G) and delta respectively.[1]

Each polypeptide chain of the TCR consists of a variable (V), joining (J), and constant (C) region; additionally, the beta and delta chains posses a diversity (D) region between the V and J regions. The extensive repertoire of immune recognition is achieved by these receptor genes undergoing variable somatic rearrangements. This process involves the V region of each protein chain coming into close proximity to the J region and, in the case of TCR beta and delta chains, a D gene segment becoming inter-collated between the V and J segments. The resulting V-J and V-D-J regions, together with a C region, encode the functional TCR. The unique sequences within the V-J and V-D-J regions account for the specificity of each TCR and its ability to recognize specific epitopes on foreign antigens.[1,2] In addition, during the above rearrangement process, a variable number of nucleotides (N) are inserted between the V, D, and J segments. The generation of these N regions provides an additional mechanism for generating specificity to each V-D-J junctional region of the TCR. It is estimated that 10^{15} unique TCRs can be produced in this way.[3]

During T lymphocyte maturation, when the genes coding for the TCR undergo rearrangement, TCR delta is the first gene rearranged followed by the rearrangement of the TCR genes coding for G, B, and A. Regardless of the ultimate phenotype of a mature T lymphocyte (TCRA/B or TCRG/delta), the G locus is more commonly rearranged than the B locus because of the ordered hierarchy of the TCR loci rearrangement. So despite the fact that the vast majority of T cells that pass through the skin express TCRA/B, understanding the ordered hierarchy of gene rearrangement tells us that the TCRG gene rearrangement can still be used a marker of clonality for T cell expressing TCRA/B. Restated, TCRG gene rearrangements can be used as markers of clonality not only in TCRG/delta positive malignancies (where rearrangements are functional) but also in TCRA/B malignancies (where TCRG rearrangements are nonfunctional).[4]

Another advantage of using the TCRG locus to detect clonality is that the TCRG locus is less complex than the other loci. The TCRG locus contains only 11 V regions, subdivided into 4 major V groups (V1-8, V9, V10, V11) and 5 joining segments (JP1, JP2, JP, J1, J2). The limited complexity of the TCRG locus is important when designing the primers used to amplify DNA in polymerase chain reaction (PCR) and adds to the sensitivity of this technique.[4]

Throughout T cell development and proliferation, the progeny of a single T cell will express the identical TCR and contain the identical TCR gene rearrangement that serves as a molecular marker of clonality.[1]

TCR gene rearrangement and subsequent T cell proliferation are important events in T cell ontogeny, and any dysregulation in these complex yet highly regulated processes may result in a malignant clonal T cell proliferation. Most normal inflammatory or reactive infiltrates of the skin are polyclonal without evidence of a monoclonal population of T cells. Hence, conducting a TCR gene rearrangement assay, to determine if a T cell proliferation is monoclonal or polyclonal, can be valuable information in the diagnosis of disease (by differentiating malignant versus reactive T cell proliferations).[5]

2. What are the current methods used to detect TCR gene rearrangements? What are their individual advantages and pitfalls?

Southern blot nalysis (SBA) was the initial method used to detect clonal lymphocyte populations. Familiarity with the technical aspects of SBA provides insight into the technique, the limits of sensitivity and specificity, and the importance of these limits in developing accurate clinical and diagnostic data. In SBA, DNA is extracted from the tissue sample and then digested and cleaved by specific restriction endonucleases. Then the resulting mixture of DNA fragments is separated by size using gel electrophoresis. In SBA, DNA from all skin components of the biopsy specimen (ie, keratinocytes, fibroblasts, endothelium, etc) are extracted and digested together with the lymphoid DNA and subsequently analyzed together. Restriction enzyme digestion results in the production of fragments of DNA whose sizes (restriction fragment length) depend on the distance between restriction enzyme sites. As TCR genes recombine and juxtapose V-D-J segments, intervening DNA is deleted, hence changing the size of the restriction fragments. It is the change in restriction fragment length resulting from such gene rearrangements that is detected by TCR probes on SBA. With radioactive labeling, fragments bearing the targeted genes appear as discreet bands on autoradiograph. The presence of 1 or 2 discrete bands signifies a probable monoclonal proliferation resulting from the rearrangement of one or both alleles of the TCR gene. In a polyclonal population of lymphocytes no one rearrangement is dominant or prevalent over another therefore on autoradiograph no distinct band is detected.[6,7]

The limit of detection sensitivity for SBA is 1%; therefore, when at least 1 in 100 cells carries a unique rearrangement, it will be detected. SBA has largely been replaced by PCR techniques due to its limits in detection sensitivity, its time consuming hybridization steps (2 weeks), and the need for fresh or frozen tissue.[8-12]

PCR amplification provides approximately 10 to 1000 times greater detection sensitivity than SBA in detecting clonal gene rearrangements.[13,14] The technique overcomes the sensitivity limitations of the SBA, in part by targeting the analysis to DNA from the lymphoid tissue within a skin biopsy, and having the ability to amplify target sequences of DNA.

PCR amplification uses oligonucleotide primers that recognize DNA sequences flanking each side of a targeted gene and initiate in vitro polymerization, resulting in multiple copies of the targeted gene. The process commences with a high temperature denaturization of double stranded DNA. This is followed by the annealing (alignment) and hybridization of the two specific oligonucleotides specifically chosen to be complimentary to the sequences flanking the target DNA. Finally, complimentary DNA strands are synthesized using a thermostable DNA polymerase as a catalyst. PCR can achieve amplification in the order of 10^9 to 10^{12} and therefore permits the use of very small amount of DNA; as, for example, the small amount of DNA present in a single paraffin section.[5]

TCR PCR fragments may be detected in variety of ways to discriminate between polyclonal and clonal populations. These methods include fluorescent gene scanning, heteroduplex analysis, single strand conformation polymorphism (SSCP), denaturing gradient gel electrophoresis (DGGE), temperature gradient gel electrophoresis (TGGE), and cloning and sequencing.

Fluorescent gene scanning (GS) involves the PCR amplification of specific TCR genes using fluorescently labeled primers. Such analysis is used in the routine clonality assessment of TCRG and TCRB genes and in minimal residual disease studies. The resulting PCR products are run on a gene sequencer and analyzed using Gene Scan software. Polyclonal populations with varying PCR fragment lengths demonstrate normal Gaussian distribution visualized by a series of peaks. Clonal populations are seen as discreet peaks. The resolution of this method allows the separation of PCR products differing in length by as little as one base pair.[11] Because of its enhanced speed, accuracy, and interpretation, GS analysis is slightly favored over HD analysis.[15] In addition, Cozzio et al[16] suggest that GS allows a more accurate comparisons of amplicons from different tissue samples in the same patient because GS allows discrimination by size and V family usage while, other techniques such as DGGE, HD, and SSCP depend on the conformation of nucleic acids.

Heteroduplex (HD) analysis relies on conformational changes caused by alignment and hybridization mismatch at the junctional region. True clonal PCR products give rise to homoduplexes (PCR products with identical junctional regions from clonal populations), where as polyclonal PCR products form heteroduplexes (PCR products with heterogeneous junctional regions) upon renaturization. Because of the differences in conformation, the clonal homoduplexes migrate rapidly through the gel and are seen as intense clonal bands, whereas heteroduplexes with their less perfectly matched sequences appear as ill defined smears running behind the homoduplex.[7]

Single strand conformation polymorphism (SSCP) is another technique used to evaluate sequence differences in PCR products. It relies on the fact that single stranded DNA will assume a uniquely folded conformation based on their primary sequences and that these differences in conformation will alter their mobility through a nondenaturing gel.[17]

Denaturing gradient gel electrophoresis (DGGE) and temperature gradient gel electrophoresis (TGGE) of PCR products will also separate amplification products based on their sequence rather than their size. Based on the base composition of a particular sequence, small regions within double stranded DNA fragments will denature or melt at differing positions creating different single stranded domains. When the PCR products are run through a gel with an increasing concentration denaturing gradient, the single stranded domains within a fragment reduce the mobility of the fragment at various positions within the gel. Fragments of identical sequences, such as those of a clonal TCR rearrangement, will migrate to a precise position within the gel and will be detected as a single band.[13,18,19]

Sequencing is the best method of assessing clonality within T cell populations. This technique allows a detailed analysis of the CDR3 region, including V, D, and J gene identification in addition to the identification of non template encoded nucleotides. However, this technique is both costly and labor intensive.[2,16,17,20-23]

Based on the fact that SSCP, HD, DGGE, and TGGE are all based on conformational changes in the PCR amplicon, it would seems likely that the results of using these methods would be broadly similar. However, some inconsistencies between these methods will invariably occur and a formal comparison should be considered.

PCR techniques have largely replaced SBA for clonality studies because PCR offers several advantages. PCR takes only 48 hours to complete (versus the 2-week time frame for SBA), is less labor intensive, and requires much less high-molecular weight DNA. SBA analysis often cannot be performed on paraffin-embedded tissue because the isolated DNA is often degraded and this presents a problem because paraffin wax embedded material is often the only material available in routine diagnostic pathology laboratories.[10,11]

As discussed previously, PCR analysis of TCRG genes is the protocol most widely applied to clonality studies because of the limited complexity of the TCRG genes which limits the number of required PCR primers resulting in an increased the sensitivity of this technique. However the limited repertoire of the TCRG locus can result in high background amplification of similar rearrangements in normal T cells resulting in an obscuring of the monoclonal TCRG rearrangement and increased false-negative (FN) results.[9] Most laboratories use TCRG PCR due to its early rearrangement during T cell maturation, whereas TCRB PCR is rarely applied, due to its locus complexity.[24,25]

The relative sensitivity of detecting monoclonality in malignancy using PCR versus SBA is controversial, with some authors suggesting comparable,[26,27] heightened PCR[28,30] or reduced sensitivity of PCR.[31,32] A likely source for the variability of PCR sensitively reported may be due to the late advent of standard PCR protocols and primers. Varying the method of PCR detection in turn varies the sensitivity of the assay for the detection of clonality. For example, using HD analysis, after PCR only has a 5% detection limit for clonality while GS can reach sensitivities of 0.5-1%. Therefore, if a laboratory uses HD analysis they have a higher likelihood of obtaining FN results. Also many studies have reported different sensitivities depending on the TCRG primers used. Table 1 lists the sensitivity for detecting monoclonality in cutaneous T cell lymphoma (CTCL) based on the method and specific primers used. As seen in Table 1, depending on the method and primers used the sensitivity for monoclonal detection can vary from 2-100%.[33] Hence, PCR analysis can yield more FN results than SB analysis in the cases when the applied PCR primer sets are inappropriate for recognizing each rearranged TCR gene segment. However, many believe that the efficiency of the PCR technique compensates for these disadvantages and may be particularly important for detecting small numbers of malignant cells.[34,35]

A European project (BIOMED-2) is trying to deal with the problem of false negativity common to all PCR protocols (Table 2). There is a well defined and fully standardized set of oligonucleotide primers and PCR protocols published by the BIOMED-2 Concerted action.[67] The project has involved the design of new and specific primers for all TCR loci and protocols for the standardized testing of all patients. The BIOMED-2 multiplex PCR approach is a rapid and reliable procedure that reports more sensitivity than SB analysis in detecting clonality in suspect lymphoproliferations.[63] In fact, in the results of their study, SBA showed a much higher FN rate than PCR technique in cases of true malignancy.

Based on BIOMED-2 concerted actions current results and extensive experience with TCR gene studies in gene rearrangements, they developed a flowchart that they feel demonstrates the most efficient strategy in detecting T cell clonality. This strategy holds true for fresh or frozen tissue samples and may be applicable to paraffin embedded tissue samples, provided that DNA quality is such that PCR products of <300 base pairs can be amplified.[63]

Standardization of PCR techniques and primers used to detect malignancy is very important when comparing studies and collating data. There are many studies published about the efficacy of PCR for diagnosing malignant lymphoproliferations in skin but unfortunately each study differs in their methods as well as their choice in primers. It would be very valuable to have multiple studies using the same PCR protocol, such as the BIOMED-2 protocol, investigating the detection of malignancy.

TABLE 1.—This Table Lists the Sensitivity for Detecting Monoclonality in CTCL Based on the Method and Specific Primers Used. As Seen in this Table, Depending on the Method and Primers Used the Sensitivity for Monoclonal Detection can Vary From 2% to 100%

Reference	Stage of Disease	PCR Primers	Method	Sensitivity
9[a]	CTCL	v1-v8, v9, v10, v11, v12, jg1/2	PCR/DGGE	87.10%
36[b]	SS/MF	v1-v8, v9, jg1, jg2	PCR/DGGE	90.00%
36	SS/MF	v9, jg1, jg2	PCR/DGGE	80.00%
36	SS/MF	v9, jg1, jg2	PCR/DGGE	35.00%
37	CTCL	v1-v8, v9, jg1/2	PCR/SSCP	90.00%
37	CTCL	v1-v8, jg1/2	PCR/SSCP	83.30%
37	CTCL	v9, jg1/2	PCR/SSCP	4.20%
37	CTCL	v10, jg1/2	PCR/SSCP	8.30%
37	CTCL	v11, jg1/2	PCR/SSCP	0.00%
37	CTCL	v1-v8, v9-11, jg1/2	PCR/SSCP	95.00%
33	CTCL	v1-v8, v9, jg	PCR/DGGE	100.00%
33	CTCL	v1-v8	PCR/DGGE	79.60%
33	CTCL	v1-v8, v9	PCR/DGGE	18.40%
33	CTCL	v10-v11, jg1/jg2	PCR/DGGE	2.00%
38[c]	CTCL	v1-v8, v9, v10/v11, jg1/2, jp1/2	PCR/HD	83.50%
38	MF-T1 score	v1-v8, v9, v10/v11, jg1/2, jp1/2	PCR/HD	71.40%
38	MF-T2 score	v1-v8, v9, v10/v11, jg1/2, jp1/2	PCR/HD	76.10%
38	MF-T3/T4 score	v1-v8, v9, v10/v11, jg1/2, jp1/2	PCR/HD	100%
38	CTCL - Histologic score <5	v1-v8, v9, v10/v11, jg1/2, jp1/2	PCR/HD	51.30%
38	CTCL - Histologic score >5	v1-v8, v9, v10/v11, jg1/2, jp1/2	PCR/HD	92.00%
39[d]	Advanced stage CTCL	v1-v8, v9-v11, j1, j2, jp, jp1, jp2	PCR/GS	76.00%
40[e]	CTCL	v1-v8, v9-v11, j1, jp, jp1, jp2	PCR/DGGE	79.00%
40	MF	v1-v8, v9-v11, j1, jp, jp1, jp2	PCR/DGGE	53.00%
41[d]	Tumor stage MF	v1-v8, v9-v11, j1, j2, jp, jp1, jp2	PCR/PAGE	100.00%
41	Plaque stage MF	v1-v8, v9-v11, j1, j2, jp, jp1, jp2	PCR/PAGE	73.00%
41	Patch stage MF	v1-v8, v9-v11, j1, j2, jp, jp1, jp2	PCR/PAGE	57.00%
41	Erythroderma	v1-v8, v9-v11, j1, j2, jp, jp1, jp2	PCR/PAGE	81.00%
42	Tumor stage MF	v1-v8, v9, j1/j2	PCR/DGGE	100.00%
42	Plaque/patch stage MF	v1-v8, v9, j1/j2	PCR/DGGE	66.00%
43[d]	Early stage MF	v1-v8, v9-v11, j1, j2, jp, jp1, jp2	PCR/GS	66.00%
44	CTCL	v1-v8, v9, jg1, jg2	PCR/DGGE TCRG	26.67%
44	CTCL	v1-v8, v9, jg1, jg2	PCR/DGGE TCRG&B	80.00%

(Continued)

TABLE 1. (continued)

Reference	Stage of Disease	PCR Primers	Method	Sensitivity
44	CTCL	v1–v8, v9, jg1, jg2	PCR/DDGE TCR B	13.33%
45[f]	MF	v1–v8, v10/v11, jg1/2, jp1/2	PCR/PAGE	59.00%
46[f]	T cell lymphoma (all types)	v1–v8, v10/v11, jg1/2, jp1/2	PCR/DGGE	87.50%
47	MF	v1–v8, v9–v11, j1/j2		77.00%
48[g]	CTCL	v1–8, v9–v11, j2, jp, jp1, jp2	PCR/DGGE	74.00%
27	CTCL	v1–v8, j1, j2, jp, jp1, jp2	PCR/DGGE	75.00%
27	CTCL	v9, j1, j2, jp, jp1, jp2	PCR/DGGE	44.44%
49[h]	Patch stage MF	v1–v8, v9–v11, j1, j2, jp, jp1, jp2	PCR/DGGE	53.00%
49	plaque/tumor stage MF	v1–v8, v9–v11, j1, j2, jp, jp1, jp2	PCR/DGGE	94.00%
49[i]	Erythroderma	v1–v8, v9–v11, j1, j2, jp, jp1, jp2	PCR/DGGE	75.00%
49[j]	Nodules/tumors (nonMF CTCL)	v1–v8, v9–v11, j1, j2, jp, jp1, jp2	PCR/DGGE	100.00%
50[k]	CTCL	v1–8, v9–v11, j2, jp, jp1/jp2	PCR/PAGE	69.00%
51[l]	CTCL	v1–v8, v9–v11, j1, jp, jp1, jp2	PCR/PAGE	40.40%
52[l]	CTCL	v1–v8, v9–v11, j1, jp, jp1, jp2	PCR/PAGE	62.00%
53[m]	CTCL	v1–v8, v9–v11, j1, jp, jp1, jp2	PCR/DGGE	70.0%
54	CTCL	v1–v8, j1/2	PCR/HD	72.5%
55[l]	CTCL	v1–v8, v9–v11, j1, jp, jp1, jp2	PCR/DGGE	69.4%
56	CTCL	v1–v8, j1/2	PCR/HD	42.8%

[a] 92% specificity, 93.1% PPV, 85.2% NPV
[b] In this study 6% clonality was detected in benign inflammatory disease (BID)
[c] Methods described by Bottero et al,[57] 2.3% clonality was detected in BID, 97.7% specificity, PPV 95.3%, NPV 91.5%
[d] Methods described by Trainer et al[31]
[e] Methods described by Lefranc et al[58]
[f] Methods described by Slack et al[59]
[g] Methods described by Greiner et al[60]
[h] 76% specificity
[i] 100% specificity
[j] 75% specificity
[k] Modified methods based on those described by Greiner et al[60]
[l] Methods described by Theodorou et al[40]
[m] 24% clonality detected in BID

TABLE 2.—This Table Summarizes Additional Possible Sources for False-Negative and False-Positive Results Using PCR Methods to Detect Clonality, Hence Affecting the Method Sensitivity, Specificity, PPV, and NPV

	Potential Causes of False-Negative PCR Results	Reference
1	DNA might not be amplified due to partial rearrangements	61
2	DNA might not be amplified due to chromosomal translocations inhibiting the juxtaposition of the VJ regions	61
3	Some tumors display somatic hypermutations which can prevent primers from annealing to the DNA	61
4	Sampling error	62
5	Inhibition of the reaction due to contaminants	13
6	Poor selection of oligonucleotide primers	63
	Potential Causes of False-Positive PCR Results	**Reference**
1	Detection of a low locally reactive lymphocyte clone	57, 64-66
2	Low starting population of polyclonal lymphocytes	57, 64-65

3. How is the detection of clonality via TCR gene rearrangement assay useful to the clinical dermatologist?

In clinical dermatology, TCR gene rearrangement studies are used as a diagnostic aid in the evaluation of lymphoproliferative skin diseases. In theory, the detection of TCR clonality allows the clinical physician to distinguish benign polyclonal T cell proliferations (ie, "reactive" lymphoproliferations) from monoclonal proliferations (ie, "malignant" lymphoproliferations).

By characterizing the type of clonal proliferation present (ie, reactive versus malignant), clinical physicians are, in theory, able to diagnose, stage, prognose, and monitor the treatment effectiveness of malignancy. Clonality studies have the potential to be particularly helpful in 5% to 10% of patients where other methods of diagnosis such as histology and immunophenotype are inconclusive or nondiagnostic.[63]

Unfortunately, monoclonality does not always equate to malignancy just as the absence of monoclonality does not always rule out malignancy. There are some specific benign conditions that demonstrate monoclonality and some cases of malignancy that demonstrate oligoclonality or polyclonality (Table 1, Table 3).

In the next sections, we review some specific clinical applications of TCR gene rearrangement assays and later we review situations where the detection of monoclonality fail to help clinically (ie, the pitfalls of TCR gene rearrangement).

TABLE 3.—This Table Contains a List of Benign Clonal Proliferations that have Monoclonal Lymphoproliferations Detected by TCR Gene rearrangement and their Risk for Malignant Transformation

Disease[A]	Studies Demonstrating a Monoclonal Proliferation	Risk of Malignant Transformation
Dermatitis	39, 131	25%[E]
Parapsoriasis lichenoides[B]	132-136	20%[F]
PLEVA	132, 136-139	10-20%[G]
Pityriasis lichenoides chronica (PLC)	136, 137, 139, 140	-
Large plaque parapsoriasis (LPP)	43, 136, 139-143, 145	10-46%[H]
Small plaque parapsoriasis (SPP)[C]	43, 45, 146	1 case[I]
Lichen planus	147-149	-
Lichen sclerosis et atrophicus	150	-
Primary pigmented purpuric dermatosis	139, 151, 152	-
Cutaneous lymphoid hyperplasia	153-157	unknown[J]
Erythroderma of uncertain etiology	53	-
Pseudolymphoma[D]	30, 31, 40, 96, 158-161	-
Drug-associated lymphomatoid hypersenistivtity	152, 158, 162	-

[A]Lymphomatoid papulosis, follicular mucinosis, and granulomatous slack skin were not included in this table because of their recent classification by the ECRTC and WHO as an indolent lymphomas.
[B]Parapsoriasis Lichenoides includes data for both PLEVA and PLC.
[C]SPP is considered by the WHO not to be malignant precursor for CTCL and despite earlier studies showing monoclonality. The general consensus is that SPP is not a monoclonal proliferation.[107,145]
[D]Pseudolymphoma includes lymphomatoid drug eruptions, lymphomatoid contact dermatitis, persistent arthropod bit reaction, actinic reticuloid, and idiopathic pseudolymphoma.
[E]63, 131
[F]163
[G]164, 165
[H]141, 163
[I]166
[J]153

A. TCR Gene rearrangement assays aid in the diagnosis and staging of CTCL

CTCL is a form of post-thymic T cell lymphoma that includes mycosis fungoides (MF) and its leukemic variant, Sézary syndrome (SS).[68] MF is the most common form of cutaneous lymphoma. It has a protracted clinical course and presents with cutaneous patches that can progress to plaques, tumor nodules, and lymphadenopathy with visceral involvement.[69] SS patients classically exhibit total body erythema, leukemia, and lymphadenopathy and histologically show the presence of Sézary cells.[5] Since its original description by Alibert in 1806, our understanding of CTCL has progressed through many important stages including: the recognition that MF and SS are variants of the same disease, the discovery that CTCL is almost always a disorder of CD4+ (helper) T cells, and the demonstration that, like most other lymphoid neoplasms, CTCL is a monoclonal disorder.[68,70]

The first step in diagnosing patients with the clinical suspicion for CTCL consists of histomorphology, immunophenotyping, and cytological analysis on various tissue samples involved such as skin, lymph nodes (LN), and peripheral blood (PB). Generally, these standard diagnostic tests come back as diagnostic, suggestive, inconclusive, or non-diagnostic for CTCL. In cases that are only suggestive or inconclusive for CTCL, the demonstration of a predominant T cell clone by analysis of the TCR gene rearrangement pattern has the potential to be extremely helpful in differentiating the diagnosis.[34,45,71]

The detection of monoclonality in cases of **diagnostic** CTCL has been extensively studied and reviewed. In general, the sensitivity for monoclonal detection in patients with diagnostic CTCL can range anywhere from 2% to 100% (Table 1) depending on the method of detection. As previously noted, much of the variation in the sensitivity has to do with the choice of TCRG primers used in PCR analysis while a slight variation results from the type of tissue sample (ie, frozen or paraffin embedded). Table 1 reports the sensitivities from many studies that investigated the detection of monoclonality in diagnostic CTCL samples using PCR methodology and different sets of primers.

Yet, testing for monoclonality in histological and immunophenotypical **diagnostic** CTCL via histology and immunophenotype is not necessary and not cost effective in the clinical setting. TCR gene rearrangement studies could be most useful in early and less defined cases of CTCL where clinical, histologic, and immunophenotype are only suggestive or inconclusive.

1) Diagnosing CTCL in cases of indeterminate histology and immunophenotype

It is often difficult to reach a definitive diagnosis of CTCL, especially in the early stages of the disease where histologic characteristics for malignancy are less well defined or inconclusive. TCR gene rearrangement assays using PCR based methods present the unique opportunity to detect clonal T cells even in early stages of CTCL, where clonal tumor cells represent only a small minority of the entire lymphoid infiltrate.[36,71]

In this section, we present studies that investigate the usefulness of TCR gene rearrangement assays in situations where histology and immunophenotype are indeterminate (ie, suggestive or inconclusive but not diagnostic). It is important to remember that within those cases that are inconclusive or suggestive for CTCL, a variable of number cases are not true malignancy. Therefore studies that report the sensitivity of monoclonal detection in inconclusive or suggestive cases without longitudinal follow up for the progression to malignancy does not help determine the effectiveness of TCR gene rearrangements. It is helpful when studies conduct long-term follow up of inconclusive cases to see if those cases with detected monoclonal proliferations develop malignancy and those with polyclonal proliferations remain benign.

In a study by Nagasawa et al,[10] PCR/DGGE was performed on fresh frozen biopsies from 16 patients with cutaneous T cell lymphoproliferative diseases in whom a diagnosis was difficult to make on morphological and immunohistochemical grounds alone. Monoclonal rearrangement of TCR was observed in 3 of 16 patients tested using four sets of primers designated for V families and four sets of primers designated for the different J genes. Clinical diagnosis of these three cases were MF, cutaneous invasion of adult

T cell leukemia (ATL), and large granular lymphocytic leukemia (LGL) of T type respectively, but they were all histologically difficult to differentiate from reactive cutaneous T cell proliferation and thereby categorized as "suggestive" for malignancy. The clinical course for these patients over time was as follows: the skin lesions of LGL patient worsened and died 2 years after biopsy, the patient with suspected plaque stage MF died due to dissemination of tumors 22 months after the biopsy, the patient with ATL survived with cutaneous lesions for over 4 years, and the remaining 13 patients, where clonality was not demonstrated, had favorable clinical courses. These findings demonstrated that clonal TCR gamma gene rearrangement using the PCR-DGGE method is very helpful for differentiating cutaneous T cell neoplasms from benign lymphoproliferations.[10]

In another study,[50] clonality was detected in 69% of cases of MF with classic histology, 16% of cases with inconclusive histologic evidence, and in none of the control cases using the TCRG gene primers (V1-8, V9, V10, V11, j1/j2, jp, jp1, and jp2) in a method described by Greiner et al.[60] In this study, classic MF histologic evidence was closely associated with clonality, whereas histologic evidence for benign inflammatory dermatoses was associated with no clonality. In the group with histologically inconclusive evidence 16% of cases had detected monoclonality. However, no longitudinal studies were performed to see if those inconclusive cases of MF with clonality ever progressed to malignancy. Thus, it is difficult to say with certainty that clonality was a useful predictor of the clinical course or malignancy.[50]

Ashton-Key et al[45] investigated the use of PCR in a series of borderline biopsy samples from patients who subsequently developed cutaneous lymphoma. In this study, formalin fixed paraffin-embedded tissue was collected from 27 patients with clinically and histologically diagnostic MF, 10 histologically borderline patients who subsequently developed MF (pre-MF), 32 clinically suspicious and histologically borderline patients (borderline), and 31 patients with chronic dermatitis. PCR amplification of TCRG was performed using methods described by McCarthy et al[72] using 2 reactions with primer mixes V1-8, V10/V11, J1/2 and V1-V8, V10/V11, JP1/JP2. Products were then separated by size on 10% acrylamide gels. Monoclonality was demonstrated in 16 of 27 (59%) patients with MF, 6 of 10 (60%) pre-MF patients, and 6 of 32 (19%) borderline patients while all the 31 patients with dermatitis gave rise to polyclonal PCR products.

While this study detected monoclonality in 59% of diagnostic MF, which is in the range reported by others, it should be noted that many studies have reported higher detection of monoclonality (Table 1). This lower detection rate may have been due to their choice of primers, the method used to analyze the PCR amplicons (they choose gel electrophoresis which separates by size and is not as sensitive as other methods such as GS or DGGE), and/or use of paraffin versus frozen tissue (they used paraffin which has decreased sensitivity compared to frozen tissue). However, it should be noted that they did not see any FP results in their control patients.

Taking a closer look at the results obtained in the 10 pre-MF patients, 7 patients had detectable monoclonality with diagnostic MF histology at the later time period and 6 of those 7 patients had detectable monoclonality with borderline histology at the earlier time period. Therefore, 6 of 7 patients could have been diagnosed with MF before the detection of malignant histologic changes using TCR gene rearrangement analysis. In addition, it should be noted that the same size monoclonal band was detected in earlier and later time periods using TCR gene rearrangement assays. The 3 cases of pre-MF that demonstrated polyclonality in both borderline and diagnostic histologic stages may once again be a result of decreased method sensitivity in this experimental design. Even so, it can be inferred from these results that the demonstration of a dominant clone in a skin biopsy showing borderline histologic features provides strong evidence of an evolving CTCL.

Unfortunately, no long-term follow-up was conducted on the borderline histologic cases with detected monoclonality (6 of 32 patients); therefore, it is impossible to interpret the significance of monoclonal proliferation in these cases.

Fucich et al[44] analyzed a total of 90 cases by PCR for the presence of TCR monoclonality. Of the 45 histologically **diagnostic** CTCL cases analyzed, 36 (80%) showed the presence of monoclonal T-cell expansion. Eighteen cases showed both TCR B and G gene rearrangements, 6 cases showed rearranged bands in TCR B region only, and the remaining 12 showed TCR G only. Nine (20%) malignant cases failed to demonstrate clonality and are assumed to be FN results. Of the 24 histologically **indeterminate** cases, 18 (75%) cases demonstrated monoclonality in the TCR gene; 10 in TCRG, 7 in TCR G and B, and 1 in the TCR B region. Fifteen of the 24 indeterminate cases were later reclassified as CTCL after immunophenotypic assessment and clinical development. Of those 15 reclassified cases, 13 had monoclonal TCR gene rearrangement studies and 2 were polyclonal FN. Hence, within the indeterminate histologic group, TCR gene rearrange studies had a sensitivity, specificity, PPV and NPV of 13/15 (86.7%), 4/9 (44.4%), 13/18 (72.2%), and 4/6 (66.7%), respectively. Within the inflammatory dermatoses, 2 of 11 samples also showed monoclonal proliferation of the TCR B and G genes. However, these 2 samples were clinically suspicious for lymphomatoid papulosis (LyP) and parapsoriasis, and it is now known that LyP is a malignant condition and parapsoriasis can have benign monoclonal proliferation and has the capacity for malignant transformation. As evidenced by this study, the detection of a monoclonal proliferation should be interpreted with high suspicion for malignancy.

Dadej et al[46] completed a small study to determine whether histologic grade (benign or borderline) or monoclonal detection most closely correlated with malignant transformation to CTCL. This was done by comparing the histologic grade and monoclonality of two groups of 22 patients using SBA and PCR of both TCR G and B. Group 1 consisted of 22 patients that later progressed to CTCL and group 2 consisted of

22 patients that did not progress to malignancy. Interestingly the same histologic entities were found in both groups; chronic dermatitis, atypical lymphocytic skin infiltrates, cutaneous lymphoid hyperplasia, actinic reticuloid and psoriasis. Clonal gene rearrangements were only found in lesions in group 1 that progressed to malignancy. Six of 7 chronic dermatitis, 4 of 7 atypical lymphocytic infiltrates, 5 of 5 cutaneous lymphoid hyperplasias, 2 of 2 actinic reticuloids, and 1 of 1 cases of psoriasis were shown to be clonal. Remarkably, in the group of patients with a benign clinical outcome (group 2), none of 22 lymphocytic infiltrates displayed evidence of T cell clonality, in spite of the fact that their histologic diagnoses were similar to the group that demonstrated malignant transformation (group 1). This study confirms that histologic grade alone is often insufficient to distinguish between genuinely malignant or benign lesions, and that detection of monoclonal infiltrates either by PCR or SBA can be helpful for their proper classification.

Taken together, the data suggest that there are two distinct categories of histologically borderline lymphoproliferations; those that are monoclonal and those that are polyclonal. Monoclonal infiltrates are associated with the development of CTCL, whereas polyclonal infiltrates are more likely associated with a benign course. These results give additional evidence supporting the earlier hypothesis of Wood et al,[36,73] Algara et al,[74] and others[2,75] who claim that clonal lesions are potentially malignant and should be classified separately from their non-clonal counterparts.

Unfortunately, few long-term large studies have been conducted to confirm the usefulness of clonality in these inconclusive scenarios. Those studies presented above show promise for using TCR gene rearrangement to detect CTCL earlier and in cases of indeterminate histology although further research is needed.

2) Staging CTCL to determine prognosis and appropriate treatment

After having made the diagnosis of CTCL, the next important step is to stage the disease. Staging of CTCL is important because patients who present with early stage disease (ie, disease confined to the skin) typically have an indolent course with a 5 year survival rate of approximately 87%[76,77] while patients with advanced stage CTCL (with disseminated extracutaneous progression involving the lymph nodes, blood, and visceral organs[78-80] have a poorer prognosis, with a 5-year survival rate of nearly 40%.[81-83] Therefore, accurate staging is crucial for determining patient prognosis and appropriate treatment.

The initial staging of CTCL (ie, TNM scoring 87) involves assessment of the extent of cutaneous disease (cutaneous T score) and the palpation for lymph node enlargement (N score). LN enlargement is defined as palpable induration and diameter >1 cm. Current recommendations state that only those patients with detectable lymph node enlargement warrant subsequent LN biopsy and further histologic evaluation.[84]

The histology of the biopsied LN is evaluated using a lymph node grading system proposed by Sausville et al.[85] In this system, LN1 nodes have single infrequent atypical lymphocytes in paracortical T cell regions, LN2 nodes have small clusters of paracortical atypical cells, LN3 nodes have large clusters of atypical cells, and LN4 nodes are partially or totally effaced by atypical cells. (Note: LN1 and LN2 are sometimes referred as dermatopathic lymph nodes, characterized by reactive lymphoid hyperplasia with expansion of the paracortical T cell domain by macrophages containing melanin and by variable numbers of atypical lymphoid cells.)[86-89] Both the CTCL TNM stage and LN grade system inversely correlate with survival; meaning the higher the stage or grade the worse the patient prognosis.[88]

However, the neoplastic character of lymph node involvement is difficult to assess by histologic examination alone and is considered by many to be a subjective assessment. TCR gene rearrangement assays offer an objective diagnostic tool that could be very useful to assess cancer progression via detecting the presence of a monoclonal proliferation in a patient's LN or PB. Unfortunately, as discussed below, studies investigating the usefulness of TCR gene rearrangement assays in staging CTCL have conflicting results.

Juarez et al[90] studied the prognostic value of LN clonality studies in CTCL. They found that the predictive value of T cell clonality in the LN by any assessment method was inferior to that of a simple clinical cutaneous assessment (T score). They also found that clinical detection of lymphadenopathy (N score) was pragmatically more relevant than finding a T cell clone by PCR. Furthermore, they concluded that the old SBA clonality test, which has been broadly replaced by more practical and sensitive PCR methods, was more effective than PCR in predicting poor clinical outcome. But as noted by Guitart et al[91] the poorer prognosis noted in patients with T cell clonality by SBA is consistent with the lower sensitivity of the method. In other words, a substantial tumor burden is required for a positive test, which by itself tends to correlate with a poor outcome.[91] This study demonstrates the inability of T cell clonality by PCR methodology to accurately stage malignancy and predict patient prognosis.

Although Juarez[90] did not find a predictive value of T cell clonality detected by PCR, a recent report from by Assaf,[92] using a more sensitive and comprehensive PCR method, identified a subset of patient's LN with positive monoclonality and negative histologic findings with a poor prognosis. The study conducted by Assaf et al[92] differs from the study by Juarez et al[90] in that all the study patients had palpable lymphadenopathy, probes for both TCR G and B gene were used, a highly sensitive method of PCR product analysis (gene scan analysis) was used, and clonal results were confirmed by the detection of the identical clone in skin. Using this highly sensitive experimental design, Assaf et al demonstrated a poor prognosis associated with the presence of clonal T cells in the LN of CTCL patients regardless of histology. These results are consistent with other previous studies using SBA to examine LN T cell clonality in patients with CTCL.[93-95] Using SBA technique, Lynch et al[94] found T cell clonality in 47% of dermatopathic LN (LN1 and 2) and 90% of histologically clearly effaced LN (LN 4), indicating the correlation between T cell clonality and palpable LN. Moreover, a poorer prognosis was associated with the presence of clonality (versus the absence of clonality) detected in patients with dermatopathic LN. These results demonstrate that TCR-B and TCR-G PCR analysis is an important adjunct for early diagnosis of lymph node involvement in CTCL before the disturbance of lymph node architecture, and is therefore an important additional step in achieving an accurate clinical staging.[96]

Considering clonal T cells can be detected via TCR gene rearrangement assay before the visualization of histologic changes and are associated with a poor prognosis raises the question, "When should the clinical physician order TCR gene rearrangement studies on LN and PB?" The only recommendations to date that we are aware of are made by Kern et al.[14] Their recommendations for when to order TCR gene rearrangement assays are based on the histologic grade of the lymph node. Kern et al[14] argue that patients with histopathologic grade LN0 or LN1 do not need clonality testing because there is likely no additional information to be gained from testing. Yet patients with an intermediate LN grade LN2 (and LN3 in some studies[94]) warrant doing clonality studies of their LN DNA because there is the potential to gain additional information regarding the prognosis of the patient and could be considered for more aggressive treatment options. The utility of TCR gene rearrangement studies on LN DNA for patients with CTCL with an advanced histopathologic classification (LN3 or LN4) is less clear because patients with an LN3 or LN4 classification generally are already known to have a poor clinical outcome. However, in the study by Kern et al,[14] TCR clonality analysis would have incorrectly predicted a good outcome for 1 patient with histologic grade LN3 at the time of initial staging. More data are necessary to determine whether TCR analysis with minimally or advanced node classification is sufficiently instructive to be cost-effective. As with any clonality test, a positive result with the presence of clonality must be interpreted in the context of each patient as once again, clonality does not always equal malignancy. Furthermore, a negative result with TCR analysis shares the same problem as histologic examination (ie, the problem of sampling error, as well as the possibility of a lymphoma that has lost the TCRG gene).

The recommendations by Kern et al[14] were based on their findings by SBA and not PCR detection of clonality. As mentioned earlier, PCR detection methods may lead to even earlier discovery of malignant spread to the lymph nodes therefore new considerations should be made. It is our recommendation that LN detection by PCR methods be conducted on all patients with LN0-LN2 (or LN3) due to the proven poor prognosis associated with clonal detection by Assaf et al[51] in LN and the effect this finding would have on a patients treatment plan. However, further studies are needed to confirm the cost effectiveness of this strategy.

Despite the fact that the above study focused on the detection of clonality in lymph nodes, it should be mentioned that the same poor prognosis applies to those patients with clonality detected in the PB.[95] In addition, there have been studies demonstrating the higher sensitivity of clonal analysis of PB versus morphologic analysis for malignancy.[95] It is our recommendation to test those with early to intermediate stage CTCL for PB spread as well as lymph node spread. Once again, it must be realized that in advanced disease the prognosis and treatment are less likely to be affected by the detection of clonality.

B. TCR Gene rearrangement assays help differentiate disease with similar histology

In addition to using TCR gene rearrangement assays as a diagnostic tool for CTCL, it can also be used to differentiate disease with similar histology, particularly in a category of diseases known as pseudolymphomas. Pseudolymphomas are a benign group of diseases that resemble lymphoma clinically and histologically. This group includes lymphomatoid drug eruptions,[96,97] lymphomatoid contact dermatitis,[98,99] persistent arthropod bite reaction,[100] actinic reticuloid,[101,102] and idiopathic pseudolymphoma.[103] Presented in this section are studies that demonstrate the usefulness of TCR gene rearrangement assays in differentiating two types of pseudolymphomas from CTCL.

Phenytoin-induced pseudolymphoma:

Phenytoin hypersensitivity syndrome (PHS) (also known as phenytoin-induced pseudolymphoma) is characterized by fever, rash, lymphadenopathy, and hepatitis associated with leukocytosis and eosinophilia. Several reports in the literature discuss the similarity between the cutaneous manifestations of PHS and CTCL, hence the name "pseudolymphoma."[96,97,104,105] The progression of manifestations in PHS is usually benign, with complete resolution after discontinuation of the phenytoin treatment. Histologically, the dermal infiltrates of these cases of PHS appear malignant, making differentiation from lymphoma difficult. Only the detection of monoclonality via PCR and SBA techniques has proven to be reliable in differentiating this pseudolymphoma from actual lymphoma by demonstrating the presence of a polyclonal T cell proliferation in PHS and a monoclonal proliferation in CTCL.

One case report presented by Weinberg et al[7] describes a patient taking phenytoin with the clinical, pathologic, and immunologic findings of SS.[96] Yet on further evaluation, the TCR gene rearrangement assay demonstrated a polyclonal T cell lymphoproliferation hence suggesting the diagnosis of a drug-induced pseudolymphoma. True to form, after the discontinuation of the drug, the eruption completely resolved, confirming the diagnosis. From TCR gene rearrangement studies, lymphoma-like reactions associated with phenytoin therapy appear to be reactive in nature and hence clonality studies can be useful in differentiating them from CTCL when other parameters are equivocal.[7]

Actinic reticuloid:

Actinic reticuloid (AR) is a severe, chronic photosensitivity disorder that has been described as another pseudolymphoma. The clinical picture is characterized by an eczematous, pruritic eruption predominately present on light exposed areas of the skin. Frequently lesions spread to covered areas, leading to erythroderma. This erythrodermic variant of actinic reticuloid can resemble Sezary syndrome, not only in clinical picture but also due to the presence of atypical lymphocytes in the blood. Detection of monoclonal proliferation by gene rearrangement assay has been suggested as a potential diagnostic criterion to distinguish these two diseases. In a study by Bakels et al[106] clonal T cell populations were detected in 19 of 20 patients with SS but were not detected in any of the 12 patients with AR using TCRG PCR/DGGE. The results of this study demonstrate that gene rearrangement analysis can be an important adjunct in differentiating between AR and CTCL.

C. TCR gene rearrangement assays can detect the transformation of a benign disease to malignancy

There are some benign inflammatory dermatoses that have the capability to transform to malignancy.[107] Detection of a monoclonal T cell proliferation can aid in the diagnosis of malignant transformation of a benign disease when histology is equivocal. Examples of well studied benign dermatoses which have the capacity to transform into malignancy include: erythroderma of uncertain etiology, large plaque parapsoriasis, cutaneous lymphoid hyperplasia, primary follicular mucinosis, and clonal dermatitis (Table 3). But only erythroderma of uncertain etiology can be differentiated from malignant transformation via monoclonal analysis and hence is discussed here in this section. The other diseases are presented later in this review as examples of the pitfalls of TCR gene rearrangement assays.

Erythroderma of uncertain etiology:

Erythroderma of uncertain etiology refers to a diagnosis of exclusion for a generalized exfoliative erythroderma that does not fit into any one specific diagnostic category. These patients with diffuse erythema are difficult to differentiate from those with the leukemic variant of CTCL–Sszary Syndrome (SS), and some cases can progress to malignancy.[105] In one study, a series of 18 patients with erythroderma of uncertain etiology were followed for a mean time of 5 years, and none of these patients developed a systemic lymphoma.[108] Yet another study reported a series of 38 patients with chronic exfoliative erythroderma of uncertain etiology, and during a follow-up period of 15 years, 13 developed CTCL lymphoma.[109]

Erythema of uncertain etiology, as documented by both of the series described above, represents a relatively benign disease that can progress into a lethal lymphoma.[110] To better identify such patients developing a malignant transformation, TCR gene rearrangement assay may be well suited as an adjunct test.[5] A study by Cordel et al[49] confirmed the usefulness of TCR gene rearrangement in the setting of erythroderma by showing how the combined histologic and clonality detection increases CTCL diagnostic sensitivity (87%) compared with the sensitivity of using histologic diagnosis alone (62%). Ponti et al[38] obtained similar results when using TCR gene rearrangement assays to differentiate erythrodermic CTCL and benign erythroderma, showing a sensitivity of 91.9%. Also, both studies by Cordel et al[49] and Ponti et al[38] showed no clonal T cell rearrangements in any patient with inflammatory erythroderma, resulting in 100% specificity for both studies. Thus in the clinical setting of erythroderma of uncertain etiology, TCR gene rearrangement is a useful diagnostic tool for differentiation of erythrodermic CTCL and inflammatory erythroderma and hence will lead to more effective therapy in a subset of patients.

D. TCR gene rearrangement assays can be used to detect minimal residual disease

In addition to the use of TCR gene rearrangement assays for the diagnosis and staging of CTCL patients, these techniques have also been used to monitor the response of the disease to treatment.[111,112] During the treatment of malignancy, tumor cells may become undetectable in blood, bone marrow, and skin by conventional methodology. However many cases still relapse, indicating that biological remission has not been achieved. Minimal residual disease describes the presence of tumor cells at a level below that detectable by conventional methodology. TCR gene rearrangements can be utilized to monitor the response of T cell lymphomas to therapy[75] by detecting residual disease during treatment of malignancy providing more sensitive information about the efficacy of treatment.[113-115]

E. TCR gene rearrangement assays are used to design clone specific probes

Another application of TCR gene rearrangements has been the development of clone specific molecular probes.[21-23,116] As with other types of T cell neoplasia, the same tumor clone is typically present in all sites of disease involvement. Isolating and sequencing the monoclonal TCR gene rearrangement from a diagnostic CTCL specimen and then using this tumor specific dominant sequence to generate probes or PCR primers constitutes a unique method for the early diagnosis and staging of cutaneous lymphoma, and detecting minimal residual disease in patients undergoing treatment. This method has already been applied successfully to MF and SS.[22,23,117]

4. WHAT ARE THE PITFALLS OF TCR GENE REARRANGEMENT ASSAYS?

The pitfalls of using TCR gene rearrangement assays stem from the fact that monoclonality does not always equate to malignancy. In this section, we discuss possible theories as to why polyclonality can be detected in overt cases of malignancy and gives specific scenarios where monoclonality can be detected nonmalignant conditions. In addition, we show how even with the detection of specific clone in a patient does not allow us to predict disease as many of the same TCR gene rearrangements have been detected in many different types of malignancies.

A. Polyclonal proliferations are detected by TCR gene rearrangement assays in cases of overt malignancy

One of the many pitfalls of using monoclonality to diagnose malignancy is that not all malignancies have shown to be monoclonal. In other words, some malignancies have demonstrated polyclonal proliferations via TCR gene rearrangement assay. Three explanations should be considered for the absence of a predominant TCR rearrangement.

1) TCR gene rearrangement assays are not 100% sensitive or specific

The pitfalls in the methodology used to detect monoclonal T cell proliferations are discussed in a previous section.

2) Early stage malignancy may be polyclonal or oligoclonal

Patients with certain lymphoproliferative disorders are at increased risk for malignant lymphoproliferative diseases, including CTCL. It has been suggested that monoclonal T cell malignancy arises from the polyclonal inflammatory T cells via acquisition of mutations that may alter its clinical, histologic, immunophenotypic characteristics. In this report, we have termed this theory the "polyclonal progression theory of malignancy."

This theory arises from the fact that malignant disease is seen to develop from polyclonal inflammatory conditions[118-120] and oligoclonal T cells has been detected in early cases of malignancy.[41]

The significance of the oligoclonal T cell population in lymphoproliferative disorders is uncertain because oligoclonality has been detected both in malignant disease and other nonmalignant unique conditions.

One study by Hodges et al[2] demonstrated that up to 30% of cases of CTCL demonstrate oligoclonal T cell populations.

Another study[121] presented a specific case of a patient diagnosed clinically and histologically with plaque stage CTCL and an oligoclonal T cell proliferation detected by gene rearrangement assay. This patient's oligoclonal proliferation progressed to a monoclonal proliferation as the patients clinical disease progressed to advanced tumor stage CTCL. It was also observed that within the oligoclonal bands from the clinical plaque stage lesion there was a band matching the position of the monoclonal band from the late-tumor stage lesion. Thus, a progression of monoclonality from oligoclonality was implied as the patient's malignancy progressed to the tumor stage.

These studies suggest that CTCL might involve a polyclonal progression to oligoclonality and then eventual monoclonality. If this statement is true then the value of not detecting a monoclonal proliferation in a patient with suggestive malignancy will be of limited value as the patient at anytime could progress to an oligoclonal and then monoclonal state.

In contrast, the finding of oligoclonality is not always clinically relevant. Oligoclonal T cell populations have been detected in PB of the elderly,[53,122] in patients diagnosed with autoimmune diseases, and in patients with viral infections.[2]

3) There are no TCR gene rearrangements to detect

The third explanation for why monoclonal TCR gene rearrangements may not be detected in cases of malignancy is that the TCRG locus could be in germline configuration.[39,43,123,124]

This statement is supported by the fact that some T cell lymphomas do not regularly demonstrate rearrangement of the TCR. Namely, natural killer/T cell lymphomas[125] and extranodal peripheral T cell lymphomas.[126] In addition, newer cytogenic studies have demonstrated the deletion, mutation, and translocation of the TCR loci in malignancy.[123] In conclusion, the detection of polyclonality by TCR gene rearrangement in some cases of CTCL does not exclude a diagnosis of malignancy.[123,124,127]

As discussed above, a T cell monoclonal proliferation may NOT be detected in malignancy due to the limitations in technology and methodologies, the possibility of a polyclonal progression to malignancy, and finally because there really is no TCR gene rearrangement and monoclonal proliferation to detect.

B. Monoclonality does not always mean malignancy

1) Pseudomonoclonality leads to false positive results

One of the pitfalls of TCR gene rearrangement assays and one of the many supporting arguments for why monoclonality does not always mean malignancy is the concept of pseudomonoclonality. Pseudomonoclonality can be explained by the high sensitivity of TCR PCR methods such as GS for detecting small T cell clones within low density inflammatory infiltrates. Although repeated TCRG gene rearrangement analysis in these scenarios will confirm clonal dominance, which is a characteristic feature of pseudomonoclonality, the dominant PCR amplicon will be a different clone and have differing size and sequence on repeated assays and separation. In contrast, repeated determinations of the same lesion in a truly monoclonal lesion such as CTCL would result in an identical clone in each repeated assay. Hence, in order to distinguish pseudomonoclonal lesions from monoclonal lesions, repeated PCR determinations of the same lesions are necessary. Monoclonality therefore should be defined as the occurrence of 1 or 2 dominant peaks (monoallelic/biallelic) that are reproducibly detected by repeated amplification and separation. The same precautions are necessary towards apparently oligoclonal profiles as some infiltrates that are seemingly oligoclonal are not reproducible.[39,43,128,129]

2) Benign conditions can demonstrate monoclonal proliferations

It is now realized that monoclonality at times can also occur in benign cutaneous inflammatory disorders, autoimmune disease, in association with certain viral infections, and in the peripheral blood of the elderly.[5,7,120]

Table 3 displays the specific benign conditions in which monoclonality has been detected.

In addition to demonstrating clonality, several of these benign inflammatory disorders can be difficult to differentiate from CTCL by histology or immunophenotype and/or can undergo malignant transformation. Some of these disorders include clonal dermatitis, PLEVA, primary follicular mucinosis, and LPP. Also, many of these diseases are incompletely characterized in terms of their own clonality which makes the detection of malignancies or malignant transformation even more difficult.[7,130]

The significance of these benign clonal lymphoproliferations is unknown and is not correlated with increased rates of malignant transformation. The presence of such proliferation could lead to increased False Positive TCR gene rearrangement results and are a major pitfall for using clonality methods as an adjuvant in the diagnosis of malignancy.

C. Manifestations of disease vary among individuals with identical TCR gene rearrangements

While TCR gene rearrangement is a marker of lymphoid clonality, it is only one property of the lymphoid population and does not necessarily reflect the full biologic behavior of the cells. This can be demonstrated by the fact that the same T cell clone can be associated with variable disease manifestations. For example, in one study the same TCR rearrangement was present in different biopsy specimens displaying, at different times, Hodgkin's disease, LyP, and CTCL.[167] Similarly in another study, one patient was found to have the same TCR gene rearrangement in different biopsy specimens showing LyP and lymphomatoid granulomatosis (nasal lethal midline granuloma.[168] As apparently different diseases can be associated with identical molecular abnormalities, it would seem likely that the different clinical and histopathological manifestations may reflect unrecognized or undetected genetic changes and host response. This means that what may be detected as monoclonal and identical TCR gene rearrangements may actually have genetic changes that we are not able to detect with current methodologies, and this is the reason that seemingly identical genetic rearrangements lead to multiple diseases with differing histology and host responses such as those illustrated in the cases above.

To accommodate these new concepts, it has been proposed that cutaneous lymphoproliferative disease should be assessed by a multifaceted approach and the detection of monoclonality should never been interpreted as an independent variable in the diagnosis of disease.[119] Considering the above, it seems reasonable for the diagnostic gold standard to remain that of clinical assessment, light microscopy, clinicopathological correlation, and follow-up. However, when available, the results of modern investigative techniques should be taken into account for each disease and individual patient.[6]

5. AS A CLINICAL PHYSICIAN, HOW DO I INTERPRET THE RESULTS OF TCR GENE REARRANGEMENT ASSAYS?

The following scenarios help illustrate real-world situations that the clinical physician may face in differentiating malignancy from benign dermatoses using TCR gene rearrangement as a diagnostic tool.

Scenario A: Clinically suspicious, histology and immunophenotype benign, and monoclonality present by TCR gene rearrangement

In this scenario it is important to consider any benign inflammatory diseases that can present with monoclonal proliferations and especially those benign inflammatory conditions that can progress to malignancy (see Table 3). In addition, it is important to consider other variables in a case by case basis that that may lead to oligoclonal/monoclonal proliferations such as advanced age, certain viral infections, or autoimmune diseases.

If the possibility of benign monoclonal proliferation seems unlikely, it is suggested by many authors[34,63,106] that clonality be taken seriously even in cases of benign histology and immunophenotype. Based on the high sensitivity and PPV for monoclonality in malignancy and its value in detecting malignant transformation of a benign disease, it is generally recommended that a patient with this scenario be monitored closely with additional biopsies taken immediately and at regularly scheduled intervals.

Scenario B: Clinically suspicious, histology and immunophenotype suggestive (but non-diagnostic), and monoclonality present by TCR gene rearrangement

Similar to the above scenario, this scenario should be taken seriously.[63,106] Perhaps even more serious given the clinical, histologic, and immunophenotypic suspicion for malignancy. In this scenario, the patient should be watched very closely and have repeated biopsies taken immediately and at regular short intervals to watch for disease progression.[123]

Some studies have even recommended starting to treat these patients as you would a diagnostic early CTCL. This is specially the case if clinical suspicion is high for advanced disease, the patient has identical clones at different biopsy sites, or repetitive dominant T cell clones persist over time. Starting treatment early benefits patient prognosis.[33,139]

Scenario C: Clinically suspicious, histology and immunophenotype diagnostic for malignancy, and polyclonal proliferation detected by TCR gene rearrangement

TCR gene rearrangement assays have not yet proven to be an independent diagnostic tool for malignancy and should always be interpreted together with clinical, histologic, and immunologic data. In this scenario, there is high suspicion for malignancy based on 3 out of 4 tests, which implies that this polyclonal proliferation may be a result of the limitations of technique's sensitivity, a malignancy that may not be monoclonal de novo (ie, polyclonal progression theory), or due to a sampling error on biopsy.[2,38]

It would be prudent to also consider benign causes that mimic malignancy histologically such as pseudolymphoma and erythroderma as discussed earlier in this review. In these scenarios demonstration of polyclonality has demonstrated high specificity for ruling out malignancy.[38]

Taken together, it is generally recommended to treat this scenario as a malignancy. Clonality is an adjuvant diagnostic tool and the failure to detect monoclonality should NOT exclude a diagnosis of malignancy.[2,39,124,169]

Scenario D: Clinically suspicious, histology and immunophenotype suggestive (but non-diagnostic), and polyclonal proliferation detected by TCR gene rearrangement

Unlike the above scenario, this patient most likely does not need immediate treatment and likely does not have an overt malignancy. Yet given the clinical suspicion for malignancy, it would be appropriate to monitor this patient at regularly scheduled intervals and take repeated biopsies if the disease should progress.

CONCLUSION

Molecular clonality analysis is based on the fact that, in principle, all cells of a malignancy have a common clonal origin and show clonally (identically) rearranged TCR genes. The diagnosis of malignant T cell proliferations is therefore supported by the finding of TCR gene clonality, whereas reactive lymphoproliferations are supported by the finding of polyclonally rearranged TCR genes.

In patients with suspected lymphoproliferative disorders, discrimination between reactive (polyclonal) and malignant (monoclonal) cell populations can be assessed by histomorphology, cytomorphology, and supplemented with immunophenotyping. However, in 5% to 10% of patients, diagnosis is more complicated and less straightforward.[63]

It was the hope of many physicians that TCR gene rearrangement analysis would be an objective diagnostic tool to rule in or rule out malignancy in cases with nondiagnostic histology and immunophenotype. Unfortunately, our understanding of the biologic significance of a monoclonal population of lymphocytes appearing in the skin is not complete. This is demonstrated by the fact that monoclonal proliferations are seen in some benign inflammatory conditions and the fact that oligoclonal or polyclonal proliferations are seen in cases of malignancy. Because of this, the detection of TCR gene rearrangement has limited clinical application in terms of diagnostic and prognostic information and basing clinical decisions on this single laboratory parameter is not recommended or appropriate. It is recommended that the results of TCR gene rearrangement assays and the assessment of clonality be interpreted along with the clinical picture as well as histologic and immunophenotype findings.

Although clonality studies may not be sufficient as an independent diagnostic tool, our recommendation, which is in agreement with many others,[34,38,63,106,139] is that any positive monoclonal proliferation, even in the absence of histologic/immunophenotype correlation, be taken seriously. Therefore, any patient with clinical suspicion for CTCL, nondiagnostic histology and immunology, and detectable monoclonal proliferation should be closely monitored for the development of malignancy, and in cases where clinical suspicion is high, treatment may be the best course of action.[34,63,106]

Despite the relatively high sensitivity for monoclonality in malignancy, it is unsure if the absence of monoclonal gene rearrangement can be used to rule out malignancy because the population of malignant cells may be at a level below the sensitivity of the technique and there is always the possibility of a sampling error. In addition, according to the polyclonal progression theory of malignancy, some CTCL might not be monoclonal de novo but oligoclonal instead, and the malignant clone may develop eventually from one of the oligoclonal populations during disease progression.

Therefore, a lot of clinical judgment is still required by the physician to interpret all the combination of possible results, and further studies still need to be conducted as to how (and if) the detection of clonality can sway the diagnosis of suggestive or inconclusive tests.

References

1. Moss PAH, Rosenberg WMC, Bell JI. The human T-cell receptor in health and disease. *Annu Rev Immunol.* 1992;10:71-96.
2. Hodges E, Krishna MT, Pickard C, Smith JL. Diagnostic role of tests for T cell receptor (TCR) genes. *J Clin Pathol.* 2003;56:1-11.
3. Davis MM, Bjorkman PJ. T cell antigen receptor genes and T cell recognition. *Nature.* 1988;344:395-402.
4. Blom B, Verschuren MCM, Heemskerk MHM, et al. TCR gene rearrangements and expression of the pre-T cell receptor complex during T-cell differentiation. *Blood.* 1999;93:3033-3043.
5. Lessin SR, Rook AH. T-cell receptor gene rearrangement studies as a diagnostic tool in lymphoproliferative skin diseases. *Exp Dermatol.* 1993;2:53-62.
6. Slater DN. Review of investigative diagnostic techniques for cutaneous lymphoma. *Semin Dermatol.* 1994;13:166-171.
7. Weinberg JM, Rook AH, Lessin SR. Molecular diagnosis of lymphocytic infiltrates of the skin. *Arch Dermatol.* 1993;129:1491-1500.
8. Weiss LM, Hu E, Wood GS, et al. Clonal rearrangements of the T cell receptor gene in mycosis fungoides and dermatopathic lymphadenopathy. *N Engl J Med.* 1985;313:539-544.
9. Khalil SH, Hamadah IR. The applicability of T-cell receptor gamma gene rearrangement as an adjuvant diagnostic tool in skin biopsies for cutaneous T-cell lymphoma. *Saudi Med J.* 2006;27:951-954.
10. Nagasawa T, Nakatsuka S, Miwa H, et al. Analysis of T-cell antigen receptor gamma chain gene rearrangement by polymerase chain reaction in combination with denaturing gradient gel electrophoresis in the differential diagnosis of cutaneous T-lymphoproliferative diseases. *J Dermatol.* 2000;27:238-243.
11. Flaig MJ, Schuhmann K, Sander CA. Impact of molecular analysis in the diagnosis of cutaneous lymphoid infiltrates. *Semin Cutan Med Surg.* 2000;19:87-90.
12. Medeiroes JL, Bagg A, Cossman J. Application of molecular genetics to the diagnosis of hematopoietic neoplasms. In: Knowles DM, ed. *Neoplastic Hematopathology.* Baltimore, MD: Williams & Wilkins; 1992:263-298.
13. Bourguin A, Tung R, Galili N, Sklar J. Rapid, nonradioactive detection of clonal T-cell receptor gene rearrangements in lymphoid neoplasms. *Proc Natl Acad Sci U S A.* 1990;87:8536-8540.
14. Kern DE, Kidd PG, Moe R, Hanke D, Olerud JE. Analysis of T-cell receptor gene rearrangement in lymph nodes of patients with mycosis fungoides. Prognostic implications. *Arch Dermatol.* 1998;134:158-164.
15. van Dongen JJ, Langerak AW, Bruggemann M, et al. Design and standardization of PCR primers for detection of clonal immunoglobulin and T-cell receptor gene recombinations in suspect lymphoproliferations: report of the BIOMED-2 Concerted Action BMH4-CT98-3936. *Leukemia.* 2003;17:2257-2317.

16. Cozzio A, French LE. T-cell clonality assays: how do they compare? *J Invest Dermatol.* 2008;128:771-773.

17. Orita M, Suzuki Y, Sekiya T, Hayashi K. Rapid and sensitive detection of point mutations and DNA polymorphisms using the polymerase chain. *Genomics.* 1989;5:874-879.

18. Abrams ES, Murdaugh SE, Lerman LS. Comprehensive detection of single base changes in human genomic DNA using denaturing gradient gel electrophoresis and a GC clamp. *Genomics.* 1990;7:463-475.

19. Fodde R, Losekoot M. Mutation detection by denaturing gradient gel electrophoresis (DGGE). *Hum Mutat.* 1994;3:83-94.

20. Danenberg PV, Horikoshi T, Volkenandt M, et al. Detection of point mutations in human DNA by analysis of RNA conformation polymorphism(s). *Nucleic Acid Res.* 1992;20:573-579.

21. Yamada M, Hudson S, Tournay O, et al. Detection of minimal residual disease in hematopoietic malignancies of the B-cell lineage by using third complementarily determining region (CDR-III)-specific probes. *Proc Natl Acad Sci U S A.* 1989;86:5123-5127.

22. Volkenandt M, Soyer HP, Kerl H, Bertino JR. Development of a highly specific and sensitive molecular probe for detection of cutaneous lymphoma. *J Invest Dermatol.* 1991;97:137-140.

23. Lessin SR, Rook AH, Rovera G. Molecular diagnosis of cutaneous T-cell lymphoma: polymerase chain reaction amplification of T-cell antigen receptor beta-chain gene rearrangements. *J Invest Dermatol.* 1991;96:299-302.

24. Lukowsky A, Richter S, Dijkstal K, Sterry W, Muche JM. A T-cell receptor gamma polymerase chain reaction assay using capillary electrophoresis for the diagnosis of cutaneous T-cell lymphomas. *Diagn Mol Pathol.* 2002;11:59-66.

25. Witzens M, Möhler T, Willhauck M, Scheibenbogen C, Lee KH, Keilholz U. Detection of clonally rearranged T-cell-receptor gamma chain genes from T-cell malignancies and acute inflammatory rheumatic disease using PCR amplification, PAGE, and automated analysis. *Ann Hematol.* 1997;74:123-130.

26. Wan JH, Sykes PJ, Orell SR, Morley AA. Rapid method for detecting monoclonality in B cell lymphoma in lymph node aspirates using the polymerase chain reaction. *J Clin Pathol.* 1992;45:420-423.

27. Anderson WK, Li N, Bhawan J. Polymerase chain reaction-denaturing gradient gel electrophoresis (PCR/DGGE)-based detection of clonal T-cell receptor gamma gene rearrangements in paraffin-embedded cutaneous biopsies in cutaneous T-cell lymphoproliferative diseases. *J Cutan Pathol.* 1999;26:176-182.

28. Sioutos N, Bagg A, Michaud GY, et al. Polymerase chain reaction versus Southern blot hybridization. Detection of immunoglobulin heavy-chain gene rearrangements. *Diag Mol Pathol.* 1995;4:8-13.

29. Whittaker S, Woolford A, Russell-Jones R, Fraser-Andrews E. Analysis of gamma T-cell receptor genes in cutaneous T-cell lymphoma. *Br J Dermatol.* 1999;140:766-767.

30. Curcó N, Servitje O, Llucià M, et al. Genotypic analysis of cutaneous T-cell lymphoma: a comparative study of Southern blot analysis with polymerase chain reaction amplification of the T-cell receptor-gamma gene. *Br J Dermatol.* 1997;137:673-679.

31. Trainor KJ, Brisco MJ, Wan JH, Neoh S, Grist S, Morley AA. Gene rearrangement in B and T-lymphoproliferative disease detected by the polymerase chain reaction. *Blood.* 1991;78:192-196.

32. Porter-Jordan K, Keiser J, Garrett C. Interfering substances that cause inhibition in polymerase chain reaction PCR assays. *J Anal Chem.* 1990;337:119-120.

33. Li N, Bhawan J. New insights into the applicability of T-cell receptor gamma gene rearrangement analysis in cutaneous T-cell lymphoma. *J Cutan Pathol.* 2001;28:412-418.

34. Sandberg Y, Heule F, Lam K, et al. Molecular immunoglobulin/T-cell receptor clonality analysis in cutaneous lymphoproliferations. Experience with the

BIOMED-2 standardized polymerase chain reaction protocol. *Haematologica.* 2003;88:659-670.

35. Derksen PW, Langerak AW, Kerkhof E, et al. Comparison of different polymerase chain reaction-based approaches for clonality assessment of immunoglobulin heavy-gene rearrangements in B-cell neoplasia. *Mod Pathol.* 1999; 12:794-805.

36. Wood GS, Tung RM, Haeffner AC, et al. Detection of clonal T-cell receptor gamma gene rearrangement in early mycosis fungoides/Sezary syndrome by polymerase chain reaction and denaturing gradient gel electrophoresis (PCR/DGGE). *J Invest Dermatol.* 1994;103:34-41.

37. Signoretti S, Murphy M, Cangi MG, Puddu P, Kadin ME, Loda M. Detection of clonal T-cell receptor gamma gene rearrangements in paraffin-embedded tissue by polymerase chain reaction and nonradioactive single-strand conformation polymorphism analysis. *Am J Pathol.* 1999;154:67-75.

38. Ponti R, Quaglino P, Novelli M, et al. T-cell receptor gamma gene rearrangement by multiplex polymerase chain reaction/heteroduplex analysis in patients with cutaneous T-cell lymphoma (mycosis fungoides/Sézary syndrome) and benign inflammatory disease: correlation with clinical, histological, and immunophenotypical findings. *Br J Dermatol.* 2005;153:565-573.

39. Dippel E, Assaf C, Hummel M, et al. Clonal T-cell receptor gamma-chain gene rearrangement by PCR-based GeneScan analysis in advanced cutaneous T-cell lymphoma: a critical evaluation. *J Pathol.* 1999;188:146-154.

40. Theodorou I, Delfau-Larue MH, Bigorgne C, et al. Cutaneous T-cell infiltrates: analysis of T-cell receptor gamma gene rearrangement by polymerase chain reaction and denaturing gradient gel electrophoresis. *Blood.* 1995;86:305-310.

41. Bachelez H, Bioul L, Flageul B, et al. Detection of clonal T-cell receptor gamma gene rearrangements with the use of the polymerase chain reaction in cutaneous lesions of mycosis fungoides and Sézary syndrome. *Arch Dermatol.* 1995;131: 1027-1031.

42. Bakels V, van Oostveen JW, van der Putte SC, Meijer CJ, Willemze R. Immunophenotyping and gene rearrangement analysis provide additional criteria to differentiate between cutaneous T-cell lymphomas and pseudo-T-cell lymphomas. *Am J Pathol.* 1997;150:1941-1949.

43. Klemke CD, Dippel E, Dembinski A, et al. Clonal T cell receptor gamma-chain gene rearrangement by PCR-based GeneScan analysis in skin and blood of patients with parapsoriasis and early-stage mycosis fungoides. *J Pathol.* 2002; 197:348-354.

44. Fucich LF, Freeman SF, Boh EE, McBurney E, Marrogi AJ. Atypical cutaneous lymphocytic infiltrate and a role for quantitative immunohistochemistry and gene rearrangement studies. *Intl J Dermatol.* 1999;38:749-756.

45. Ashton-Key M, Diss TC, Du MQ, Kirkham N, Wotherpoon A, Issacson PG. The value of the polymerase chain reaction in the diagnosis of cutaneous T-cell infiltrates. *Am J Surg Pathol.* 1997;21:743-747.

46. Dadej K, Gaboury L, Lamarre L, et al. The value of clonality in the diagnosis and follow-up of patients with cutaneous T-cell infiltrates. *Diagn Mol Pathol.* 2001;10:78-88.

47. Murphy M, Signoretti S, Kadin ME, Loda M. Detection of TCR-gamma gene rearrangements in early mycosis fungoides by non-radioactive PCR-SSCP. *J Cutan Pathol.* 2000;27:228-234.

48. Tok J, Szabolcs M, Silvers DN, Zhong J, Matsushima AY. Detection of clonal T-cell receptor gamma chain gene rearrangements by polymerase chain reaction and denaturing gradient gel electrophoresis (PCR/DGGE) in archival specimens from patients with early cutaneous T-cell lymphoma: correlation of histologic findings with PCR/DGGE. *J Am Acad Dermatol.* 1998;38:453-460.

49. Cordel N, Lenormand B, Courville P, Helot MF, Benichou J, Joly P. Usefulness of cutaneous T-cell clonality analysis for the diagnosis of cutaneous T-cell lymphoma in patients with erythroderma. *Arch Pathol Lab Med.* 2005;129: 372-376.

50. Bergman R, Faclieru D, Sahar D, et al. Immunophenotyping and T-cell receptor gamma gene rearrangement analysis as an adjunct to the histopathologic diagnosis of mycosis fungoides. *J Am Acad Dermatol.* 1998;39:554-559.
51. Delfau-Larue MH, Petrella T, Lahet C, et al. Value of clonality studies of cutaneous T lymphocytes in the diagnosis and follow-up of patients with mycosis fungoides. *J Pathol.* 1998;184:185-190.
52. Delfau-Larue MH, Dalac S, Lepage E, et al. Prognostic significance of a polymerase chain reaction-detectable dominant T-lymphocyte clone in cutaneous lesions of patients with mycosis fungoides. *Blood.* 1998;92:3376-3380.
53. Delfau-Larue MH, Laroche L, Wechsler J, et al. Diagnostic value of dominant T-cell clones in peripheral blood in 363 patients presenting consecutively with a clinical suspicion of cutaneous lymphoma. *Blood.* 2000;96:2987-2992.
54. Kohler S, Jones CD, Warnke RA, Zehnder JL. PCR-heteroduplex analysis of T-cell receptor gamma gene rearrangement in paraffin-embedded skin biopsies. *Am J Dermatopathol.* 2000;22:321-327.
55. Beylot-Barry M, Sibaud V, Thiebaut R, et al. Evidence that an identical T cell clone in skin and peripheral blood lymphocytes is an independent prognostic factor in primary cutaneous T cell lymphomas. *J Invest Dermatol.* 2001;117:920-926.
56. Cherny S, Mraz S, Su L, Harvell J, Kohler S. Heteroduplex analysis of T-cell receptor gamma gene rearrangement as an adjuvant diagnostic tool in skin biopsies for erythroderma. *J Cutan Pathol.* 2001;28:351-355.
57. Bottaro M, Berti E, Biondi A, Migone N, Crosti L. Heteroduplex analysis of T-cell receptor gamma gene rearrangements for diagnosis and monitoring of cutaneous T-cell lymphomas. *Blood.* 1994;83:3271-3278.
58. Lefranc MP, Chuchana P, Dariavach P, et al. Molecular mapping of the human T cell gamma (TRG) genes and linkage of the variable and constant regions. *Eur J Immunol.* 1989;19:989-994.
59. Slack DN, McCarthy KP, Wiedemann LM, Sloane JP. Evaluation of sensitivity, specificity, reproducibility of an optimized method for detecting clonal rearrangements of immunoglobulin and T-cell receptor genes in formalin-fixed, paraffin-embedded sections. *Diagn Mol Pathol.* 1993;2:223-232.
60. Greiner TC, Raffeld M, Lutz C, Dick F, Jaffe ES. Analysis of T cell receptor-gamma gene rearrangements by denaturing gradient gel electrophoresis of GC-clamped polymerase chain reaction products: Correlation with tumor-specific sequences. *Am J Pathol.* 1995;146:46-55.
61. Letwin BW, Wallace PK, Muirhead KA, Hensler GL, Katshatus WH, Horan PK. An improved clonal excess assay using flow cytometry and B cell gating. *Blood.* 1990;75:1178-1185.
62. Davis TH, Yockey CE, Balk SP. Detection of clonal immunoglobulin gene rearrangements by polymerase chain reaction amplification and single strand conformation polymorphism analysis. *Am J Pathol.* 1993;142:1841-1847.
63. Sandberg Y, van Gastel-Mol EJ, Verhaaf B, Lam KH, van Dongen JJ, Langerak AW. BIOMED-2 multiplex immunoglobulin/T-cell receptor polymerase chain reaction protocols can reliably replace Southern blot analysis in routine clonality diagnostics. *J Mol Diagn.* 2005;7:495-503.
64. Szczepański T, Pongers-Willemse MJ, Langerak AW, van Dongen JJ. Unusual immunoglobulin and T-cell receptor gene rearrangement patterns in acute lymphoblastic leukemias. *Curr Top Microbiol Immunol.* 1999;246:205-215.
65. Beishuizen A, Verhoeven MA, Mol EJ, van Dongen JJ. Detection of immunoglobulin kappa light-chain gene rearrangement patterns by Southern blot analysis. *Leukemia.* 1994;8:2228-2236.
66. Mahalingam M. Atypical cutaneous lymphocytic infiltrates—paucicellularity and 'pseudo'clonality. *J Cutan Pathol.* 2003;30:521.
67. Brugnoni D, Airó P, Rossi G, et al. A case of hypereosinophillic syndrome is associated with the expansion of CD3-CD4+ T-cell population able to secrete large amount of interleukin-5. *Blood.* 1996;87:1416-1422.

68. Zelickson BD, Peters MS, Muller SA, et al. T-cell receptor gene rearrangement analysis: cutaneous T cell lymphoma, peripheral T cell lymphoma, and premalignant and benign cutaneous lymphoproliferative disorders. *J Am Acad Dermatol.* 1991;25:787-796.
69. Barcos M. Mycosis fungoides: Diagnosis and pathogenesis. *Am J Clin Pathol.* 1993;99:452-458.
70. Greisser J, Palmedo G, Sander C, et al. Detection of clonal rearrangement of T-cell receptor genes in the diagnosis of primary cutaneous CD30+ lymphoproliferative disorders. *J Cutan Pathol.* 2006;33:711-715.
71. Terhune MH, Cooper KD. Gene rearrangements and T-cell lymphomas. *Arch Dermatol.* 1993;129:1484-1490.
72. McCarthy KP, Sloane JP, Kabarowski JH, Matutes E, Wiedemann LM. A simplified method of detection of clonal rearrangements of the T-cell receptor-gamma chain gene. *Diagn Mol Pathol.* 1992;1:173-179.
73. Wood GS. Lymphocyte activation in cutaneous T-cell lymphoma. *J Invest Dermatol.* 1995;105:105S-109S.
74. Algara P, Sonia C, Matinez P, et al. Value of PCR detection of TCR gamma gene rearrangement in the diagnosis of cutaneous lymphocytic infiltrates. *Diagn Mol Pathol.* 1994;3:275-282.
75. Waldmann TA, Davis MM, Bongiovanni KF, Korsmeyer SJ. Rearrangements of genes for the antigen receptor on T cells as markers of lineage and clonality in human lymphoid neoplasms. *N Engl J Med.* 1985;313:776-783.
76. Zackheim HS, Amin S, Kashani-Sabet M, Mcmillan A. Prognosis in cutaneous T-cell lymphoma by skin stage: long term survival in 489 patients. *J Am Acad Dermatol.* 1999;40:418-425.
77. Diamandidou E, Colome M, Fayad L, Duvic M, Kurzrock R. Prognostic factor analysis in mycosis fungoides/Sézary syndrome. *J Am Acad Dermatol.* 1999;40: 914-924.
78. Lorincz AL. Cutaneous T-cell lymphoma (mycosis fungoides). *Lancet.* 1996; 347:871-876.
79. Siegel RS, Pandolfino T, Guitart J, Rosen S, Kuzel TM. Primary cutaneous T-cell lymphoma: review and current concepts. *J Clin Oncol.* 2000;18:2908-2925.
80. Asssaf C, Hummel M, Zemlin M, et al. Transition of Sézary syndrome into mycosis fungoides after complete clinical and molecular remission under extracorporeal photophoresis. *J Clin Pathol.* 2004;57:1325-1328.
81. Diamandidou E, Cohen PR, Kurzrock R. Mycosis fungoides and Sezary syndrome. *Blood.* 1996;88:2385-2409.
82. van Doorn R, Van Haselen CW, van Voorst Vader PC, et al. Myscosis fungoides: disease evolution and prognosis of 309 Dutch patients. *Arch Dermatol.* 2000; 136:504-510.
83. de Coninck EC, Kim YH, Varghese A, Hoppe RT. Clinical characteristics and outcome of patients with extracutaneous mycosis fungoides. *J Clin Oncol.* 2001;19:779-784.
84. Keehn CA, Belongie IP, Shistik G, Fenske NA, Glass F. The diagnosis, staging, and treatment options for mycosis fungoides. *Cancer Control.* 2007;14: 102-111.
85. Sausville EA, Worsham GF, Matthews MJ, et al. Histologic assessment of lymph nodes in mycosis fungoides/Sézary syndrome (cutaneous T-cell lymphoma): clinical correlations and prognostic import of a new classification system. *Hum Pathol.* 1985;16:1098-1109.
86. Colby TV, Burke JS, Hoppe RT. Lymph node biopsy in mycosis fungoides. *Cancer.* 1981;47:351-359.
87. Galindo LM, Garcia FU, Hanau CA, et al. Fine needle aspiration biopsy in the evaluation of lymphadenopathy associated with cutaneous T-cell lymphoma (mycosis fungoides/Sézary syndrome). *Am J Clin Pathol.* 2000;113:865-871.
88. van der Valk P, Meijer CJ. The histology of reactive lymph nodes. *Am J Surg Pathol.* 1987;11:866-882.

89. Geissman F, Dieu-Nosjean MC, Dezutter C, et al. Accumulation of immature Langerhans cells in human lymph nodes draining chronically inflamed skin. *J Exp Med*. 2002;196:417-430.

90. Juarez T, Isenhath SN, Polissar NL, et al. Analysis of T-cell receptor gene rearrangement for predicting clinical outcome in patients with cutaneous T-cell lymphoma: a comparison of Southern blot and polymerase chain reaction methods. *Arch Dermatol*. 2005;141:1107-1113.

91. Guitart J, Camisa C, Ehrlich M, Bergfeld WF. Long-term implications of T-cell receptor gene rearrangement analysis by Southern blot in patients with cutaneous T-cell lymphoma. *J Am Acad Dermatol*. 2003;48:775-779.

92. Assaf C, Hummel M, Steinhoff M, et al. Early TCR-beta and TCR-gamma PCR detection of T-cell clonality indicates minimal tumor disease in lymph nodes of cutaneous T-cell lymphoma: diagnostic and prognostic implications. *Blood*. 2005;105:503-510.

93. Bakels V, Van Oostveen JW, Geerts ML, et al. Diagnostic and prognostic significance of clonal T-cell receptor beta gene rearrangements in lymph nodes of patients with mycosis fungoides. *J Pathol*. 1993;170:249-255.

94. Lynch JW Jr, Linoilla I, Sausville EA, et al. Prognostic implications of evaluation for lymph node involvement by T-cell antigen receptor gene rearrangement in mycosis fungoides. *Blood*. 1992;79:3293-3299.

95. Muche JM, Lukowsky A, Hein J, Friedrich M, Audring H, Sterry W. Demonstration of frequent occurrence of clonal T cells in the peripheral blood but not in the skin of patients with small plaque parapsoriasis. *Blood*. 1999;94:1409-1417.

96. D'Incan M, Souteyrand P, Bignon YJ, Fonck Y, Roger H. Hydantoin-induced cutaneous pseudolymphoma with clinical, pathologic, and immunologic aspects of Sézary syndrome. *Arch Dermatol*. 1992;128:1371-1374.

97. Rijlaarsdam U, Scheffer E, Meijer CJ, Kruyswijk MR, Willemze R. Mycosis fungoides-like lesions associated with phenytoin and carbamazepine therapy. *J Am Acad Dermatol*. 1991;24:216-220.

98. Orbaneja JG, Diez LI, Lozano JL, Salazar LC. Lymphomatoid contact dermatitis: a syndrome produced by epicutaneous hypersensitivtity with clinical features and a histopathologic picture similar to that of mycosis fungoides. *Contact Dermatitis*. 1976;2:139-143.

99. Fisher AA. Allergic contact dermatitis mimicking mycosis fungoides. *Cutis*. 1987;40:19-21.

100. Ackerman AB, Breza TS, Capland L. Spongiotic stimulants of mycosis fungoides. *Arch Dermatol*. 1974;109:218-220.

101. Toonstra J, Henquet CJ, van Weelden H, van der Putte SC, van Vloten WA. Actinic reticuloid. A clinical photobiologic, histopathologic, and follow-up study of 16 patients. *J Am Dermatol*. 1989;21:205-214.

102. Toonstra J, van Weelden H, Gmelig Meyling FH, van der Putte SC, Baart de la Faille H. Actinic reticuloid simulating Sézary syndrome. Report of two cases. *Arch Dermatol Res.*. 1985;277:159-166.

103. Rijlaarsdam JU, Scheffer E, Meijer CJ, Willemze R. Cutaneous pseudo-T-cell lymphomas. A clinicopathologic study of 20 patients. *Cancer*. 1992;69:717-724.

104. Souteyrand P, d'Incan M. Drug-induced mycosis fungoides-like lesions. *Curr Probl Dermatol*. 1990;19:176-182.

105. Vonderheid EC, Sobel EL, Nowell PC, Finan JB, Helfrich MK, Whipple DS. Diagnostic and prognostic significance of Sézary cells in peripheral blood smears from patients with cutaneous T cell lymphoma. *Blood*. 1985;66:358-366.

106. Bakels V, van Oostveen JW, Preesman AH, Meijer CJ, Willemze R. Differentiation between actinic reticuloid and cutaneous T cell lymphoma by T cell receptor gamma gene rearrangement analysis and immunophenotyping. *J Clin Pathol*. 1998;51:154-158.

107. Willemze E, Jaffe ES, Burg G, et al. WHO-EORTC classification for cutaneous lymphomas. *Blood*. 2005;105:3768-3785.

108. Winklemann RK, Buechner SA, Diaz-Perez JL. Pre-Sézary syndrome. *J Am Acad Dermatol.* 1984;10:992-999.
109. Thestrup-Pederson K, Halkier-Sørensen L, Sogaard H, Zachariae H. The red man syndrome. Exfoliative dermatitis of unknown etiology: a description and follow-up of 38 patients. *J Am Acad Dermatol.* 1988;18:1307-1312.
110. Zelickson BD, Peters MS, Pittelkow MR. Gene rearrangement analysis in lymphoid neoplasia. *Clin Dermatol.* 1991;9:119-128.
111. Wood GS, Haeffner A, Dummer R, Crooks CF. Molecular biology techniques for the diagnosis of cutaneous T-cell lymphoma. *Dermatol Clin.* 1994;12: 231-241.
112. Lessin SR, Benoit BM, Jaworsky C, et al. Skin as a reservoir of minimal residual disease in cutaneous T-cell lymphoma after complete clinical response to biological response modifier therapy. *J Invest Dermatol.* 1993;100:507.
113. van Dongen JJ, Wolvers-Tettero LM. Analysis of immunoglobulin and T cell receptor genes. Part II: Possibilities and limitations in the diagnosis and management of lymphoproliferative diseases and related disorders. *Clin Chim Acta.* 1991;198:93-174.
114. Campana D, Pui CH. Detection of minimal residual disease in acute leukemia: methodologic advances and clinical significance. *Blood.* 1995;85:1416-1434.
115. Fodinger M, Buchmayer H, Schwarzinger I, et al. Multiplex PCR for rapid detection of T-cell receptor-gamma chain gene rearrangements in patients with lymphoproliferative diseases. *Br J Haematol.* 1996;94:136-139.
116. Sklar J. Antigen receptor genes: structure, function, and techniques for analysis of their rearrangements. In: Knowles DM, ed. *Neoplastic Hematopathology.* Baltimore, MD: Williams & Wilkins; 1992:215.
117. Kono DH, Baccala R, Balderas RS, et al. Application of a multiprobe RNase protection assay and junctional sequences to define V beta gene diversity in Sezary syndrome. *Am J Pathol.* 1992;140:823-830.
118. Slater DN. Cutaneous lymphoproliferative disorders: an assessment of recent investigative techniques. *Br J Dermatol.* 1991;124:309-323.
119. Slater DN. Diagnostic difficulties in 'non-mycotic' cutaneous lymphoproliferative diseases. *Histopathology.* 1992;21:203-213.
120. Slater DN. Clonal dermatoses: a conceptual and diagnostic dilemma. *J Pathol.* 1990;162:1-3.
121. Wood GS, Crooks CF, Uluer AZ. Lymphomatoid papulosis and associated cutaneous lymphoproliferative disorders exhibit a common clonal origin. *J Invest Dermatol.* 1995;105:51-55.
122. Posnett DN, Sinha R, Kabak S, Russo C. Clonal populations of T cells in normal elderly humans: the T cell equivalent to "benign monoclonal gammapathy". *J Exp Med.* 1994;179:609-618.
123. Bachelez H. The clinical use of molecular analysis of clonality in cutaneous lymphocytic infiltrates. *Arch Dermatol.* 1999;135:200-202.
124. Weiss LM, Picker LJ, Grogan TM, Warnke RA, Sklar J. Absence of clonal beta and gamma T-cell receptor gene rearrangement in a subset of peripheral T cell lymphomas. *Am J Pathol.* 1988;130:436-442.
125. Jaffe ES, Chan JK, Su IJ, et al. Report of the Workshop on Nasal and Related Extranodal Angiocentric T/Natural Killer Cell Lymphomas. Definitions, differential diagnosis, and epidemiology. *Am J Surg Pathol.* 1996;20:103-111.
126. Sander CA, Kaudewitz P, Kutzner H, et al. T-cell-rich B-cell lymphoma presenting in the skin. A clinicopathologic analysis of six cases. *J Cutan Pathol.* 1996; 23:101-108.
127. Yoshikai T, Toyonaga B, Koga Y, Kimura N, Griesser H, Mak TW. Repertoire of the human T cell gamma genes: high frequency of nonfunctional transcripts in thymus and mature T cells. *Eur J Immunol.* 1987;17:119-126.
128. Ponti R, Fierro MT, Quaglino P, et al. TCRgamma-chain gene rearrangement by PCR-based GeneScan: diagnostic accuracy improvement and clonal heterogeneity analysis in multiple cutaneous T-cell lymphoma samples. *J Invest Dermatol.* 2008;128:1030-1038.

129. Vega F, Luthra R, Medeiros LJ, et al. Clonal heterogeneity in mycosis fungoides and its relationship to clinical course. *Blood.* 2002;100:3369-3373.
130. Wood GS. The benign and malignant cutaneous lymphoproliferative disorders including mycosis fungoides. In: Knowles DM, ed. *Neoplastic Hematopathology.* Baltimore, MD: Williams & Wilkins; 1992:917.
131. Wood GS. Analysis of clonality in cutaneous T cell lymphoma and associated diseases. *Ann N Y Acad Sci.* 2001;941:26-30.
132. Dereure O, Levi E, Kadin ME. T-cell clonality in pityriasis lichenoides et varioloformis acuta: a heteroduplex analysis of 20 cases. *Arch Dermatol.* 2000; 136:1483-1486.
133. Kikuchi A, Naka W, Nishikawa T. Cutaneous T-cell lymphoma arising from parakeratosis variegate: long-term observation with monitoring of T-cell receptor gene rearrangements. *Dermatology.* 1995;190:124-127.
134. Kiene P, Fölster-Holst R, Mielke V. [Parakeratosis variegata after pityriasis lichenoides et varioliformis acuta] [article in German]. *Hautarzt.* 1995;46:498-501.
135. Popp C, Bacharach-Buhles M, Sterry W, Greisser H, Altmeyer P. [Considerations of the pathogenesis of parakeratosis variegate based on morphologic and molecular findings] [in German]. *Hautarzt.* 1992;43:634-639.
136. Weiss LM, Wood GS, Ellisen LW, Reynolds TC, Sklar J. Clonal T-cell populations in pityriasis lichenoides et varioloformis acuta (Mucha-Habermann disease). *Am J Pathol.* 1987;126:417-421.
137. Weinberg JM, Kristal L, Chooback L, Honig PJ, Kramer M, Lessin SR. The clonal nature of pityriasis lichenoides. *Arch Dermatol.* 2002;138:1063-1067.
138. Magro C, Crowson AN, Kovatich AL, Burns F. Pityriasis lichenoides: a clonal T-cell lymphoproliferative disorder. *Hum Pathol.* 2002;33:788-795.
139. Plaza JA, Morrison C, Magro CM. Assessment of TCR-beta clonality in a diverse group of cutaneous T-cell infiltrates. *J Cutan Pathol.* 2008;35: 358-365.
140. Shieh S, Mikkola DL, Wood GS. Differentiation and clonality of lesional lymphocytes in pityriasis lichenoides chronica. *Arch Dermatol.* 2001;137: 305-308.
141. Kikuchi A, Naka W, Harada T, Sakuraoka K, Harada R, Nishikawa T. Parapsoriasis en plaque: its potential for progression to malignant lymphoma. *J Am Acad Dermatol.* 1993;29:419-422.
142. Simon M, Flaig MF, Kind P, Sander CA, Kuadewitz P. Large plaque parapsoriasis: clinical and genotypic correlations. *J Cutan Pathol.* 2000;27:57-60.
143. Staib G, Sterry W. Use of polymerase chain reaction in the detection of clones in lymphoproliferative diseases of the skin. *Recent Results Cancer Res.* 1995;139: 239-247.
144. Jaffe ES, Harris NL, Stein H, et al. *World Health Organization Classification of Tumors of Haematopoietic and Lymphoid Tissue.* Lyon: IARC Press; 2001.
145. Bernier C, Nguyen JM, Quéreux G, Renault JJ, Bureau B, Dreno B. CD 13 and TCR clonal markers of early mycosis fungoides. *Acta Derm Venerol.* 2007;87: 155-159.
146. Haeffner AC, Smoller BR, Zepter K, Wood GS. Differentiation and clonality of lesional lymphocytes in small plaque parapsoriasi. *Arch Dermatol.* 1995;131: 321-324.
147. Sander CA, Kind P, Flaig M, et al. Genotypic analysis in cutaneous lymphoproliferative disease – a reliable test? *J Cutan Pathol.* 1998;25:511.
148. Schiller PI, Flaig MJ, Puchta U, Kind P, Sander CA. Detection of clonal T cells in lichen planus. *Arch Dermatol Res.* 2000;292:568-569.
149. Holm N, Flaig MJ, Yazdi AS, Sander CA. The value of molecular analysis by PCR in the diagnosis of cutaneous lymphocytic infiltrates. *J Cutan Pathol.* 2002;29:447-452.
150. Lukowsky A, Muche JM, Sterry W, Audring H. Detection of expanded T cell clones in skin biopsy samples of patients with lichen sclerosis et atrophicus by T cell receptor gamma polymerase chain reaction assays. *J Invest Dermatol.* 2000;115:254-259.

151. Toro JR, Sander CA, Le Boit PE. Persistent pigmented purpuric dermatitis and mycosis fungoides: stimulant, precursor, or both? A study by light microscopy and molecular methods. *Am J Dermatopathol.* 1997;19:108-118.
152. Crowson AN, Magro CM, Zahorchak R. Atypical pigmentary purpura: a clinical, histopathologic, and genotypic study. *Hum Pathol.* 1999;30:1004-1012.
153. Nihal M, Mikkola D, Horvath N, et al. Cutaneous lymphoid hyperplasia: a lymphoproliferative continuum with lymphomatous potential. *Hum Pathol.* 2003;34:617-622.
154. Wood GS, Nygan BY, Tung R, et al. Clonal rearrangements of immunoglobulin genes and progression to B cell lymphoma in cutaneous lymphoid hyperplasia. *Am J Pathol.* 1989;135:13-19.
155. Landa N, Zelickson BD, Peters MS, Muller SA, Pittelkow MR. Cutaneous lymphoma versus pseudolymphoma: gene rearrangement study of 21 cases with clinicopathologic correlation. *J Invest Dermatol.* 1991;96:749-754.
156. Rijlarrsdam U, Bakels V, van Oostveen JW, et al. Demonstration of clonal immunoglobulin gene rearrangements in cutaneous B-cell lymphomas and pseudo B-cell lymphomas: differential diagnostic and pathogenic aspects. *J Invest Dermatol.* 1992;99:749-754.
157. Hammer E, Sangueza O, Suwanjindar P, White CR Jr, Braziel RM. Immunophenotypic and genotypic analysis in cutaneous lymphoid hyperplasia. *J Am Acad Dermatol.* 1993;28:426-433.
158. Magro CM, Crowson NA, Kovatich AJ, Burns F. Drug-induced reversible lymphoid dyscrasia: a clonal lymphomatoid dermatitis of memory and activated T cells. *Human Pathol.* 2003;34:119-129.
159. Guitart J, Kaul K. A new polymerase chain reaction-based method for the detection of T-cell clonality in patients with possible cutaneous T-cell lymphoma. *Arch Dermatol.* 1999;135:158-162.
160. Farber E. Clonal adaptation during carcinogenesis. *Biochem Pharmacol.* 1990; 39:1837-1846.
161. Gordon KB, Guitart J, Kuzel T, et al. Pseudo-mycosis fungoides in patients taking clonazepam and fluoxetine. *J Am Acad Dermatol.* 1996;34:304-306.
162. Brady SP, Magro CM, Diaz-Cano SJ, Wolfe HJ. Analysis of clonality of atypical cutaneous infiltrates associated with drug therapy by PCR/DGGE. *Hum Pathol.* 1999;30:130-136.
163. Bonvalet D, Colau-Gohm K, Belaïch S, Civatte J, Degos R. Les differentes forms du parapsoriasis en plaque: a propos de 90 cas. *Ann Dermatol Venereal.* 1977; 104:18-25.
164. Macaulay WL. Lymphomatoid papulosis update: a historical perspective. *Arch Dermatol.* 1989;125:1387-1389.
165. Thomsen K, Wantzin GL. Lymphomatoid papulosis. A follow-up study of 30 patients. *J Am Acad Dermatol.* 1987;17:632-636.
166. Belousova IE, Vaneck T, Samtsov AV, Michal M, Kazakov DV. A patient with clinicopathologic features of small plaque parapsoriasis presenting later with plaque-stage mycosis fungoides: report of a case and comparative retrospective study of 27 cases of "nonprogressive" small plaque parapsoriasis. *J Am Acad Dermatol.* 2008;59:474-482.
167. Davis TH, Morton CC, Miller-Cassman R, Balk SP, Kadin ME. Hodgkin's disease, lymphomatoid papulosis, and cutaneous T-cell lymphoma derived from a common T-cell clone. *N Engl J Med.* 1992;326:1115-1122.
168. Harabuchi Y, Kataura A, Kobayashi K, et al. Lethal midline granuloma (peripheral T-cell lymphoma) after lymphomatoid papulosis. *Cancer.* 1992;70: 835-839.
169. Dippel E, Goerdt S, Assaf C, Stein H, Orfanos CE. Cutaneous T-cell lymphoma severity index and T-cell gene rearrangement. *Lancet.* 1997;35:1776-1777.

Statistics of Interest to the Dermatologist

Martin A. Weinstock, MD, PhD, and Margaret M. Boyle, BS
Brown University Dermatoepidemiology Unit, Providence, Rhode Island

Morbidity and Mortality

Health Care Delivery in the United States

Miscellaneous

TABLE 1.—New Cases of Selected Reportable Infectious Diseases in the United States

	1940	1950	1960	1970	1980	1990	2000	2009*
AIDS	***	***	***	***	***	41,595	40,758	39,202**
Anthrax	76	49	23	2	1	0	1	~
Congenital Rubella	***	***	***	77	50	11	9	257
Congenital Syphilis	***	***	***	***	***	3,865	529	~
Diphtheria	15,536	5,796	918	435	3	4	1	~
Gonorrhea	175,841	286,746	258,933	600,072	1,004,029	690,169	358,995	260,530
Hansen's Disease	0	44	54	129	223	198	91	59
Lyme Disease	0	0	0	0	0	0	17,730	29,780
Measles	291,162	319,124	441,703	47,351	13,506	27,786	86	61
Plague	1	3	2	13	18	2	6	7
Rocky Mountain Spotted Fever	457	464	204	390	1,163	651	495	1,393
Syphilis (primary and secondary)	***	23,939	16,145	21,982	27,204	50,223	5,979	12,833
Toxic Shock Syndrome	***	***	***	***	***	322	135	76
Tuberculosis#	102,984###	121,742##	55,494	37,137	27,749	25,701	16,377	11,540
U.S. Population (millions)	132	151	179	203	227	249	281	307

Key:
*For 52 weeks ending January 2, 2010. Incidence data for reporting year 2009 is provisional.
**Total number of acquired immunodeficiency syndrome (AIDS) cases reported to the Division of HIV/AIDS Prevention, National Center for HIV/AIDS, Viral Hepatitis, STD, and TB Prevention (NCHHSTP), through December 31, 2008. Includes 672 cases of AIDS in persons with unknown state of area of residence that were reported in 2008.
***Data not available.
~No reported cases.
#Reporting criteria changed in 1975.
##Data include newly reported active and inactive cases.
###Of 62 cases reported, 51 were indigenous, and 11 were imported from another country.

Source:
Centers for Disease Control and Prevention: Summary of Notifiable Diseases, United States, 2009. *Morbidity and Mortality Weekly Report* 58(51&52):1458-1467, 2010.
Centers for Disease Control and Prevention: Reported cases of notifiable diseases by geographic division and area - United States, 2008. *Morbidity and Mortality Weekly Report* 58(31):856-857;859-869, 2009.
Centers for Disease Control and Prevention: Summary of Notifiable Diseases, United States, 2000. *Morbidity and Mortality Weekly Report* 49(51&52):1167-1174,2001.
Centers for Disease Control and Prevention: Annual Summary 1994:Reported morbidity and mortality. *Morbidity and Mortality Weekly Report* 1994;43(53):[70-71].
Centers for Disease Control and Prevention: Annual Summary 1984:Reported morbidity and mortality. *Morbidity and Mortality Weekly Report* 33:124-129, 1986.

TABLE 2.—Estimates of HIV/AIDS, 2008

Region	Adults and Children Living with HIV	Adults and Children Newly Infected with HIV	Adult Prevalence (%)	Adult and Child Deaths Due to AIDS
Sub-Saharan Africa	20.8-24.1 million	1.6-2.2 million	4.9-5.4	1.1-1.7 million
Middle East and North Africa	250,000-380,000	24,000-46,000	<0.2-0.3	15,000-25,000
South and South-East Asia	3.4-4.3 million	240,000-320,000	0.2-0.3	220,000-310,000
East Asia	700,000-1.0 million	58,000-88,000	<0.1	46,000-71,000
Oceania	51,000-68,000	2,900-5,100	<0.3-0.4	1,100-31,000
Latin America	1.8-2.2 million	150,000-200,000	0.5-0.6	66,000-89,000
Caribbean	220,000-260,000	16,000-24,000	0.9-1.1	9,300-14,000
Eastern Europe and Central Asia	1.4-1.7 million	100,000-130,000	0.6-0.8	72,000-110,000
Western and Central Europe	710,000-970,000	23,000-35,000	0.2-0.3	10,000-15,000
North America	1.2-1.6 million	36,000-61,000	0.5-0.7	20,000-31,000
Total	33.4 million	2.7 million	0.80%	2.0 million
	31.1-35.8 million	2.4-3.0 million	<0.8-0.8	1.7-2.4 million

Source: AIDS Epidemic Update, Joint United Nations Programme on HIV/AIDS (UNAIDS) World Health Organization (WHO), December 2009.

TABLE 3.—AIDS Cases by Age Group and Exposure Category, and Cumulative Totals Through 2007, United States

	2007		Totals Cumulative Total*	
	No	(%)	No.	(%)
Adult/adolescent exposure category				
Male-to-male sexual contact	14,383	(38%)	445,645	(44%)
Injection drug use	4,736	(12%)	235,842	(23%)
Male-to-male sexual contact and injection drug use	1,514	(4%)	67,797	(7%)
Hemophilia/coagulation disorder	46	(0%)	5,567	(1%)
Heterosexual contact	7,504	(20%)	142,852	(14%)
Receipt of blood transfusion, blood components, or tissue***	109	(0%)	9,315	(1%)
Other/risk factor not reported or identified****	10,005	(26%)	114,224	(11%)
Adult/adolescent SUBTOTAL	38,297	(100%)	1,021,242	(100%)
Pediatric exposure category (<13 years at diagnosis)				
Hemophilia/coagulation disorder	0	(0%)	229	(2%)
Mother with/at risk for HIV infection	73	(84%)	8,797	(92%)
Receipt of blood transfusion blood components, or tissue+	1	(1%)	383	(4%)
Other/risk not reported or identified++	13	(15%)	181	(2%)
Pediatric SUBTOTAL	87	(100%)	9,590	(100%)
TOTAL	38,384	(100%)	1,030,832**	(100%)

*From the beginning of the epidemic through 2007.

**Includes two persons of unknown sex.

***AIDS developed in 43 adults/adolescents after they received transfusion of HIV-infected that had tested negative for HIV antibodies. AIDS developed in 13 additional adults after they received tissue, organs, or artificial insemination from HIV-infected donors.

****Includes 37 adults/adolescents who were exposed to HIV-infected blood, body fluids, or concentrated virus in health care, laboratory, or household settings, as supported by seroconversion, epidemiologic, or laboratory evidence. One person was infected after intentional inoculation with HIV- infected blood. Includes an additional 908 persons who acquired HIV infection perinatally but who were more than 12 years of age when AIDS was diagnosed. These 908 persons are not counted in the values for the pediatric transmission category.

+AIDS developed in 3 children after they received transfusion of HIV-infected blood that had tested negative for HIV antibodies.

++Includes 25 children who had sexual contact with an HIV-infected man, and an additional 4 children who were exposed to HIV-infected blood in household, health care, or other settings as supported by seroconversion, epidemiologic, or laboratory evidence.

Source:

Centers for Disease Control and Prevention: *HIV/AIDS Surveillance Report, 2007* Vol.19. Atlanta: U.S. Department of Health and Human Services, Centers for Disease Control and Prevention; 2009:40. Also available at: http://www.cdc.gov/hiv/topics/surveillance/resources/reports/.

TABLE 4.—Selected Causes of Death, United States, 1997 and 2007

| | Number of Deaths | |
Cause of Death	1997	2007
Malignant melanoma	7,238	8,461
Infections of the skin	870	1,834
Motor vehicle traffic accidents	42,340	42,031
Accident involving animal being ridden	76	101
Accidental drowning and submersion	3,561	3,443
Victim of lightning	58	46
Homicide and legal intervention	19,846	18,773
All cancer	539,577	562,875
All causes	2,314,245	2,423,712

Source:
National Center for Health Statistics, Division of Vital Statistics. personal communication, May 2010.

TABLE 5.—Annual Percent Change in Cancer Incidence in the United States

| | Average Annual Percent Change | |
Top 20 Highest Incidence Sites	1992-2007	1975-1991
Thyroid	5.4	0.8
Liver and Intrahepatic Bile Duct	3.2	3.0
Melanoma of the skin	2.5	3.7
Kidney and Renal Pelvis	2.2	2.4
Pancreas	0.5	−0.2
Non-Hodgkin Lymphoma	0.4	3.6
Hodgkin Lymphoma	0.4	0.4
Esophagus	0.2	0.7
Urinary Bladder	0.0	0.6
Myeloma	−0.2	1.2
Leukemia	−0.3	0.1
Brain and Other Nervous System	−0.3	1.2
Corpus Uteri	−0.4	−2.1
Breast	−0.7	2.2
Lung and Bronchus	−0.9	1.5
Oral Cavity and Pharynx	−1.1	−0.6
Ovary	−1.2	0.0
Colon and Rectum	−1.5	−0.1
Prostate	−1.5	4.9
Stomach	−1.6	−1.5
All sites	−0.5	1.3

Note:
SEER 9 registries and NCHS public use data file for the total US. Rates are per 100,000 and age-adjusted to the 2000 US Standard Population (19 age groups–Census P25-1130) standard.
Rates are for invasive cancers only.
Source:
Surveillance Research Program, National Cancer Institute SEER*Stat Software (www.seer.cancer.gov/seerstat) version 6.6.2.
Surveillance, Epidemiology, and End-Results (SEER) Program (www.seer.cancer.gov) SEER*Stat Database: Incidence-SEER 17 Regs Limited-Use+Hurricane Katrina impacted Louisiana Cases, Nov. 2009 Sub (1973–2007 varying)– Linked to County Attributes–Total U.S., 1969-2007 Counties, National Cancer Institute DCCPS, Surveillance Research Program, Cancer Statistics Branch, released April, 2010, based on the November 2009 submission.
Altekruse SF, Kosary, CL, Krapcho M, Neyman N, Aminou R, Waldron W, Ruhl J, Howlader N, Tatalovich Z, Cho H, Mariotto A, Eisner MP, Lewis DR, Cronin K, Chen HS, Feuer EJ, Stinchcomb DG, Edwards BK (eds). *SEER Cancer Statistics Review: 1975-2007*, National Cancer Institute. Bethesda, MD, http://seer.cancer.gov/csr/1975-2007/, based on November, 2009 SEER data submission posted to the SEER website, 2010.

TABLE 6.—Melanoma Incidence and Mortality Rates, United States

Year	Incidence*	Mortality**
1975	7.9	2.1
1976	8.2	2.2
1977	8.9	2.3
1978	8.9	2.3
1979	9.5	2.4
1980	10.5	2.3
1981	11.1	2.4
1982	11.2	2.5
1983	11.1	2.5
1984	11.4	2.5
1985	12.7	2.6
1986	13.3	2.6
1987	13.7	2.6
1988	12.9	2.6
1989	13.7	2.7
1990	13.8	2.8
1991	14.6	2.7
1992	14.8	2.7
1993	14.6	2.7
1994	15.6	2.7
1995	16.4	2.7
1996	17.3	2.8
1997	17.7	2.7
1998	17.9	2.8
1999	18.2	2.6
2000	18.8	2.7
2001	19.6	2.7
2002	19.1	2.6
2003	19.3	2.7
2004	20.2	2.7
2005	21.7	2.7
2006	21.1	—

Note:
—Data not available
*SEER 9 areas. Rates are per 100,000 and are age-adjusted to the 2000 US Standard population (19 age groups- Census P25-1130) standard.
**National Center for Health Statistics public use data file for the total US. Rates per 100,000 and age-adjusted to the 2000 U.S. standard population. (19 age groups – Census P25-1130) standard.
Source:
Surveillance Research Program, National Cancer Institute SEER*stat (www.seer.cancer.gov/seerstat) version 6.4.4.
Surveillance, Epidemiology, and End-Results (SEER) Program, (www.seer.cancer.gov) SEER*Stat Database: Incidence-SEER 17 Regs Limited-Use+Hurricane Katrina impacted Louisiana Cases, Nov. 2008 Sub (1973–2006 varying)– Linked to County Attributes–Total U.S., 1969-2006 Counties, National Cancer Institute DCCPS, Surveillance Research Program, Cancer Statistics Branch, released April 2009, based on the November 2008 submission.
Surveillance, Epidemiology, and End-Results (SEER) Program, SEER* Stat Database:Mortality-All COD, Total US (1969-2005) Linked to County Attributes – Total U.S., 1969-2005 Counties. National Cancer Institute DCCPS, Surveillance Research Program, Cancer Statistics Branch, released January 2008. Underlying mortality data provided by the National Center for Health Statistics (www.cdc.gov/nchs).
Horner MJ, Ries LAG, Krapcho M, Nayman N, Aminou R, Howlader N, Altekruse SF, Feuer EJ, Huang L, Mariotto A, Miller BA, Lewis DR, Eisner MP, Stinchcomb DG, Edwards BK (eds). *SEER Cancer Statistics Review: 1975-2006*, National Cancer Institute. Bethesda, MD, http://seer.cancer.gov/csr/1975-2006/, based on November 2008 SEER data submission posted to the SEER website, 2009.

TABLE 7.—Melanoma Five-Year Relative Survival

Year	Whites	Blacks
	By Year at Diagnosis	
1960-63*	60%	—
1970-73*	68%	—
1975-77+	82%	60%
1978-80+	83%	60%
1981-83+	83%	61%
1984-86+	87%	70%
1987-89+	88%	80%
1990-92+	90%	60%
1993-95+	90%	67%
1996-98+	91%	75%
1999-2006+	93%	78%
	By Stage at Diagnosis (1999-2005)**	
Local	98%	93%
Regional	62%	45%
Distant	15%	33%

Key:
—Insufficient data.
*Rates are based on the End Results data from a series of hospital registries and one population-based registry.
+Rates are from the SEER 9 registries. Rates are based on follow-up of patients into 2007.
**Rates are from the SEER 17 registries. Rates are based on follow-up of patients into 2007.
Notes:
Relative survival is the observed survival divided by the survival expected in a demographically similar subgroup of the general population.
Survival estimates among blacks are imprecise due to small numbers of cases observed.
Source:
Surveillance, Epidemiology, and End-Results (SEER) Program, (www.seer.cancer.gov) SEER*Stat Database: Incidence-SEER 17 Regs Limited-Use + Hurricane Katrina impacted Louisiana Cases, Nov. 2009 Sub (1973-2006 varying) - Linked to County Attributes—Total U.S., 1969-2007 Counties, National Cancer Institute DCCPS, Surveillance Research Program, Cancer Statistics Branch, released April 2010, based on the November 2009 submission.
Altekruse SF, Kosary CL, Krapcho M, Neyman N, Aminou R, Waldron W, Ruhl J, Howlader N, Tatalovich Z, Cho H, Mariotto A, Eisner MP, Lewis DR, Cronin K, Chen HS, Feuer EJ, Stinchcomb DG, Edwards BK (eds). *SEER Cancer Statistics Review: 1975-2007*, National Cancer Institute, Bethesda, MD, http://seer.cancer.gov/csr/1975-2007/, based on November, 2009 SEER data submission posted to the SEER website, 2010.

TABLE 8.—Contact Dermatitis in Belgium: Proportion of Positive Patch Tests to Standard Chemicals in 281 Patients With at Least 1 Positive Reaction (Among 494 Patients Tested in 2009)

1.	Nickel sulphate	31.2%
2.	Fragrance mix I	21.0%
3.	Fragrance mix II	14.1%
4.	Cobalt chloride	13.6%
5.	Paraphenylenediamine	11.6%
6.	Balsam of Peru	11.2%
7.	Potassium dichromate	7.9%
8.	Formaldehyde	4.4%
9.	Neomycin sulphate	4.4%
10.	Colophonium	4.0%
11.	Methyl(chloro)isothiazolinone	3.6%
12.	Wool alcohols	3.6%
13.	Hydroxyisohexyl-3-cyclohexene carboxaldehyde	2.9%
14.	Tixocortol pivalate	2.9%
15.	Methyldibromo glutaronitrile	2.6%
16.	Budesonide	2.2%
17.	Epoxy resin	1.8%
18.	Isopropyl-phenylparaphenylenediamine	1.8%
19.	Benzocaine	1.8%
20.	Thiuram mix	1.8%
21.	Sesquiterpene lactone mix	1.1%
22.	Paratertiarybutylphenol-formaldehyde resin	1.1%
23.	Quaternium-15	0.7%
24.	Mercaptobenzothiazole	0.7%
25.	Mercapto mix	0.7%
26.	Clioquinol	0.4%
27.	Primin	0.4%
28.	Paraben mix	0.4%

(From Goossens A., University Hospital, Katholieke Universiteit Leuven, Belgium, personal communication, January 2010.)

TABLE 9.—Dermatology Trainees in the United States

Year Residency to be Completed	Male Residents	Female Residents	Unknown	Total
MD Programs				
2010	139	232		371
2011	142	253		395
2012	148	245		393
2013	8	9		17
2014	1	2		3
DO Programs				
2010	13	19		32
2011	11	25		36
2012	13	17	2	32

Source:
American Academy of Dermatology. personal communication, January 2010.

TABLE 10.—Diplomates Certified by the American Board of Dermatology from 1933-2009

Decade Totals (Inclusive Dates)	Average Number Certified per Year
1933-1940	69
1941-1950	74
1951-1960	76
1961-1970	112
1971-1980	247
1981-1990	271
1991-2000	295
2001-2009	336
TOTAL 1933 through 2009	14,340

Individual Year Totals	Actual Number Certified
1999	286
2000	283
2001	305
2002	309
2003	307
2004	329
2005	352
2006	319
2007	342
2008	377
2009	385

Source:
The American Board of Dermatology, Inc. personal communication, January 2010.

TABLE 11.—Physicians Certified in Dermatologic Subspecialties

A. Physicians Certified for Special Qualification in Dermatopathology, 1974-2009

Year	Average Number Certified Per Year		Total
	Dermatologists	Pathologists	
1974-75	108	44	302
1976-80	54	49	515
1981-85	37	34	351
1986-90	11	14	125
1991-95	20	20	196
1996-00	14	32	227
2001-05	15	46	306
Actual Number Certified			
2006	32	37	69
2007	26	50	76
2008	27	54	81
2009	28	51	79
Total Number Certified 1974 through 2009	1083	1247	2330

B. Dermatologists Certified for Special Qualification in Clinical and Laboratory Dermatological Immunology, 1985-2009

Year	Number Certified
1985	52
1987	16
1989	22
1991	15
1993	5
1997	5
2001	6
Total 1985 through 2009	121

C. Dermatologists Certified for Special Qualification in Pediatric Dermatology, 2004, 2006 and 2008

Year	Number Certified
2004	90
2006	41
2008	31
Total 2004 through 2009	162

Note:
–No special qualification examination for Dermatopathology was administered in 1992, 1994, and 1996.
–No special qualification examination in Clinical and Laboratory Dermatological Immunology was administered in 1986, 1988, 1990, 1992, 1994, 1995, 1996, 1998, 1999, 2000, 2002, 2003, 2004, 2005, 2006, 2007, 2008 or 2009.
–Special qualification in Pediatric Dermatology began in 2004. No special qualification examination in Pediatric Dermatology was administered in 2005, 2007, or 2009.
Source:
American Board of Dermatology and American Board of Pathology, personal communication, January 2010.

TABLE 12.—Visits to Non-Federal Office-Based Physicians in the United States, 2007

	Type of Physician					
	Dermatologist		Other		All Physicians	
	Number of		Number of		Number of	
Diagnosis	Visits (1000's)	Percent	Visits (1000's)	Percent	Visits (1000's)	Percent
Acne vulgaris	4,482	10.0	*	*	5,201	0.5
Eczematous dermatitis	4,059	9.1	7,411	0.8	11,470	1.2
Warts	1,318	2.9	1,373	0.1	2,691	0.3
Skin cancer	4,348	9.7	1,100	0.1	5,448	0.6
Psoriasis	1,526	3.4	*	*	1,740	0.2
Fungal infections	*	*	2,032	0.2	2,897	0.3
Hair disorders	*	*	*	*	1,264	0.1
Actinic keratosis	4,539	10.1	*	*	4,963	0.5
Benign neoplasm of the skin	2,666	5.9	804	0.1	3,470	0.4
All disorders	44,874	100.0	949,447	100.0	994,321	100.0

*Figure suppressed due to small sample size.
Figures may not add to totals because of rounding.
Source: Centers for Disease Control and Prevention, National Center for Health Statistics, 2007 National Ambulatory Medical Care Survey, personal communication, March 2010.

TABLE 13.—Health Insurance Coverage of the United States Population, 2008

	Children 1-17 Years	Adults 18-64 Years	Adults 65 Years and Over
Individually Purchased Insurance	5%	6%	27%
Employment-based-Coverage	56%	61%	35%
Public Insurance, All types	33%	19%	94%
Medicaid	30%	15%	9%
No Health Insurance	10%	17%	2%

Note: Some individuals have both public and private insurance, so the numbers will not add to 100%.
Source:
Employee Benefit Research Institute, *Issue Brief No. 334*, "Sources of Health Insurance and Characteristics of the Uninsured: Analysis of the March 2009 Current Population Survey," September 2009, Washington, DC, personal communication, March 2009.
DeNavas-Walt, Carmen, Bernadette D. Proctor, and Jessica C. Smith. "Income, Poverty, and Health Insurance Coverage in the United States: 2008." *Current Population Reports*. P60-236. Washington, DC: U.S. Department of Commerce, Economics and Statistics Administration, September 2009.
U.S. Census Bureau, Current Population Survey, 2000 to 2009 Annual Social and Economic Supplements.

TABLE 14.—Nonelderly Population With Selected Sources of Health Insurance, by Family Income, 2009

Yearly Family Income Level	Employment-Based Coverage %	Individually Purchased %	Public %	Uninsured %	Total %
under $10,000	11	5	49	35	100
$10,000-$19,999	19	5	44	33	100
$20,000-$29,999	36	6	31	30	100
$30,000-$39,999	50	6	23	25	100
$40,000-$49,999	61	6	19	19	100
$50,000-$74,000	74	7	12	13	100
$75,000 and over	85	7	7	7	100
Total	61	6	19	17	100

Note: Details may not add to totals because individuals may receive coverage from more than one source.
Source:
Fronstin P, "Sources of Health Insurance and Characteristics of the Uninsured: Analysis of the March 2009 Current Population Survey." *EBRI Issue Brief*, No. 334 (Washington, DC. Employee Benefit Research Institute), September 2009.

TABLE 15.—Health Maintenance Organization (HMO) Market Penetration in the United States, July 1, 2009

HMO Penetration in Region

Pacific	40%
Northeast	32%
Mid-Atlantic	30%
Mountain	23%
East North Central	21%
South Atlantic	20%
West North Central	15%
East South Central	13%
West South Central	13%

HMO Penetration Top Ten Most Highly Penetrated Metropolitan Statistical Areas

Vallejo-Fairfield, CA	73%
Leominster-Fitchburg-Gardner, MA	60%
Napa, CA	59%
Sacramento-Arden-Arcade–Roseville, CA	58%
Worcester, MA-CT	58%
Oakland-Fremont-Hayward, CA	58%
Madison, WI	56%
Stockton, CA	54%
Springfield, MA	52%
Fresno, CA	51%

Source: 2009 HealthLeaders-Interstudy Publications, *Managed Care Census*, Nashville, TN. personal communication, April 2010.

TABLE 16.—National Health Expenditure Amounts: Selected Calendar Years

| Spending Category | 1980 | 1990 | (Billions of Dollars) | | | |
			2000	2005	2008	2019*
Total National Health Expenditures	246	696	1,310	1,983	2,339	4,483
Health Services and Supplies	234	670	1,262	1,852	2,181	4,170
Personal Health Care	215	609	1,138	1,655	1,952	3,709
Hospital Care	102	254	417	608	718	1,375
Professional Services	67	217	425	622	731	1,371
Physician and Clinical Services	47	158	289	422	496	882
Other Professional Services	4	18	39	56	66	124
Dental Services	13	32	61	86	101	180
Other Personal Health Care	3	10	37	62	68	185
Nursing Home and Home Health	20	65	126	178	203	400
Home Health Care	2	13	32	53	65	154
Nursing Home Care	18	53	94	125	138	246
Retail Outlet Sale of Medical Products	26	73	171	276	300	564
Prescription Drugs	12	40	122	217	234	458
Other Medical Products	14	33	49	59	66	106
Durable Medical Equipment	4	11	18	24	27	43
Other Non-Durable Medical Products	10	23	31	36	39	63
Program Administration and Net Cost of Private Health Insurance	12	40	81	145	160	320
Government Public Health Activities	7	20	44	59	69	140
Investment	12	26	48	139	158	313
Research+	6	13	29	42	44	91
Structures and Equipment	7	14	19	98	114	222

Note: Numbers may not add to totals because of rounding.

*Projected values. The health spending projections were based on the 2008 version of the National Health Expenditures (NHE) released in January 2010.

+Research and development expenditures of drug companies and other manufacturers and providers of medical equipment and supplies are excluded from research expenditures. These research expenditures are implicitly included in the expenditure class in which the product falls, in that they are covered by the payment received for that product.

Source:
Centers for Medicare and Medicaid Services, Office of the Actuary, March 2010.

TABLE 17.—Spending on Consumer Advertising of Prescription Products, United States

Year	(Annual Dollars in Millions)
2009	4,571
2008	4,412
2007	4,905
2006	4,745
2005	4,132
2004	4,084
2003	3,082
2002	2,514
2001	2,479
2000	2,150*
1999	1,590
1998	1,173
1997	844
1996	595
1995	313
1994	242
1993	165
1992	156
1991	56
1990	48
1989	12

*Estimated.
Source: Kantar Media, Copyright 2010. Magazine Publishers of America, Inc: personal communication, March 2010.

TABLE 18.—Results of the American Academy of Dermatology Skin Cancer Screening Program, 1985-2009

Year	Number Screened	Suspected Diagnosis		
		Basal Cell Carcinoma	Squamous Cell Carcinoma	Malignant Melanoma
1985	32000	1056	163	97
1986	41486	3049	398	262
1987	41649	2798	302	257
1988	67124	4457	474	435
1989	78486	6266	761	593
1990	98060	7959	1069	872
1991	102485	8110	1193	1062
1992	98440	8403	1280	1054
1993	97553	7067	1068	2465+
1994	86895	6908	1235	1010
1995	88934	7503	1317	1353
1996	94363	8713	1656	1399
1997	99554	8730	1685	1469
1998	89536	6687	1308	1078
1999	89916	5790	1136	635
2000	65854	5074	1053	653
2001	70562	5192	1102	642
2002	64492	4733	1009	692
2003	70692	4481	1032	489
2004	71243	4891	1165	760
2005	82532	5659	1411	794
2006	85272	6354	1649	876
2007	90484	6193	1852	883
2008	88249	5746	1739	749
2009	92977	6179	1928	906
Total	1,988,838	147,998	28,985	21,485

Key:
+Number of cases included melanoma, "rule out melanoma," and lentigo maligna.
Source:
American Academy of Dermatology: *2009 Skin Cancer Screening Program Statistical Summary Report*, March 2010.

TABLE 19.—Leading Dermatology Journals

Journal	Total Citations in 2008	Number of Articles Published in 2008	Impact Factor
Journal of Investigative Dermatology	19395	297	5.3
Journal of the American Academy of Dermatology	17616	296	4.1
British Journal of Dermatology	16437	330	3.5
Archives of Dermatology	12138	121	3.4
Contact Dermatitis	5399	92	3.5
Dermatologic Surgery	4895	221	2.1
Dermatology	4806	113	2.2
International Journal of Dermatology	4774	262	1.4
Acta Dermato-Venereologica	3545	74	2.5
Clinical and Experimental Dermatology	3376	155	1.8
Burns	3285	185	1.6
Journal of Cutaneous Pathology	2707	202	1.6
Journal of the European Academy of Dermatology	2563	165	2.3
American Journal of Dermatopathology	2541	123	1.5
Experimental Dermatology	2160	120	3.3
Pediatric Dermatology	2145	173	1.0
Archives of Dermatological Research	2132	86	1.9
Pigment Cell Melanoma Research	2114	52	4.6
Wound Repair and Regeneration	2018	94	2.2
Cutis	1968	124	0.8
Mycoses	1879	118	1.5
Journal of Dermatology	1831	110	1.2
Journal of Dermatological Science	1756	72	3.0

Source:
  Journal Citation Reports Web Version 2008:JCR, Science Edition. Philadelphia: Thomson Reuters. March 2010.

CLINICAL DERMATOLOGY

1 Urticarial and Eczematous Disorders

Safety and efficacy of desloratadine in chronic idiopathic urticaria in clinical practice: an observational study of 9246 patients
Augustin M, Ehrle S (Univ Hosp Eppendorf, Hamburg, Germany; Essex Pharma, GmbH, Munich, Germany)
J Eur Acad Dermatol Venereol 23:292-299, 2009

Background.—Post-marketing surveillance studies (PMSS) of medications are often mandated by authorities, provide crucial insights for health services and are useful to define the clinical profiles of therapies. Desloratadine, a non-sedating, second-generation H1-receptor antagonist, is an effective and well-tolerated treatment for chronic idiopathic urticaria (CIU).

Methods.—A PMSS in CIU patients evaluated the tolerability and efficacy of desloratadine in clinical practice. At Visit 1 (baseline), demographic and CIU history were recorded and patients/physicians rated the severity of CIU symptoms, interference with sleep/daily activities and the general state of urticaria. Patients also noted the use and effectiveness of previous antihistamine therapy. At the end of treatment (Visit 2), CIU symptom severity and other disease criteria were re-assessed. Adverse events reported during or ≤ 30 days after treatment were collected.

Results.—A total of 9246 patients with CIU participated (63% female). Itching, number of wheals and the size of the largest wheal decreased significantly from baseline with desloratadine therapy $(P < 0.0001)$. Improvements in CIU-impaired sleep and daily activities were reported by 67% and 71% of patients, respectively $(P < 0.0001)$. In patients that received previous therapy with cetirizine, loratadine or fexofenadine alone, patients rated the onset of efficacy of desloratadine as faster in 55.5%, 54.7% and 57.6% of cases, respectively. The incidence of adverse events was low (0.5% of patients) and no serious adverse events were reported.

Conclusions.—This large PMSS confirms evidence from multiple placebo-controlled trials that desloratadine is effective and well tolerated in the treatment of CIU.

▶ This study reviews chronic idiopathic urticaria (CIU) and notes patient discomfort and a decrease in the quality of life in patients with this common condition. Although much is known about the symptoms and discomfort, there is still no clear etiology for causes of CIU. The introduction of additional therapeutic regime to treat CIU is shown to be beneficial in patients by decreasing the size of the wheal as well as the itching and associated discomfort. Desloratadine has been shown in this observational study of 9246 patients to be effective with a low side-effect rate. This study shows desloratadine treatment decreases the signs and symptoms of itching, wheal size, number, and overall response to treatment, and was rated high by patients and physicians.

L. Cleaver, DO

Comparison of the efficacy of levocetirizine 5 mg and desloratadine 5 mg in chronic idiopathic urticaria patients
Potter PC, Kapp A, Maurer M, et al (Univ of Cape Town Lung Inst, South Africa; Hannover Med School, Germany; Charité- Universitätsmedizin, Berlin, Germany; et al)
Allergy 64:596-604, 2009

Background.—Nonsedating H1-antihistamines are recommended for the treatment of urticaria by the recent EAACI/GA^{2}LEN/EDF guidelines. The aim of this study was to compare the efficacy, after 4 weeks of treatment, with levocetirizine 5 mg and desloratadine 5 mg, both once daily in the morning, in symptomatic chronic idiopathic urticaria (CIU) patients.

Methods.—This multi-center, randomized, double-blind study involved 886 patients (438 on levocetirizine and 448 on desloratadine). The primary objective was to compare their efficacy on the mean pruritus severity score after 1 week of treatment. Mean pruritus severity score over 4 weeks and pruritus duration score, number and size of wheals, mean CIU composite score (sum of the scores for pruritus severity and numbers of wheals), quality of life, and the patient's and investigator's global satisfaction with treatment, were secondary efficacy measures.

Results.—Levocetirizine led to a significantly greater decrease in pruritus severity than desloratadine over the first treatment week; mean pruritus severity scores of 1.02 and 1.18 for levocetirizine and desloratadine, respectively $(P < 0.001)$. The result was similar for the entire 4-week treatment period $(P = 0.004)$. In addition, levocetirizine decreased pruritus duration and the mean CIU composite scores to a significantly greater extent than desloratadine during the first week $(P = 0.002$ and 0.005, respectively) and over the entire study $(P = 0.009$ and $P < 0.05$, respectively). Similarly, levocetirizine increased the patients' global satisfaction after one and 4 weeks $(P = 0.012$ and 0.021, respectively), compared with desloratadine. Safety and tolerability were similar in both groups.

Conclusions.—Levocetirizine 5 mg was significantly more efficacious than desloratadine 5 mg in the treatment of CIU symptoms.

▶ This is one of the first head-to-head studies in the new generation of modern nonsedating antihistamines for chronic idiopathic urticaria. This study looks at several useful end points and evaluation of this common disorder. In this double-blind study, levocetirizine 5 mg and desloratadine 5 mg were used. It was found that both drugs were safe and efficacious in the treatment of chronic idiopathic utricaria. It reviewed the disorder and shows that both medications are safe and well tolerated. The end points in addition to the pruritus scores, and the quality of life evaluation, demonstrated favorable results for both medications. It did indicate that there was a slightly higher incidence of adverse effects with levocetirizine. The time to first improvement in the study drugs shows a slight advantage in the levocetirizine group compared with subjects in the desloratadine study arm. Possible mechanisms also included the higher receptor occupancies for levocetirizine, 54% compared with desloratadine 34% at 24 hours, which may be the cause of the consequence of higher receptor occupancy and the edge of levocetirizine over desloratadine. The study reviews previous studies that both drugs showed positive clinical improvement in the quality of life index and the pruritus scores. This study demonstrates that both drugs are efficacious in idiopathic chronic urticaria and that levocetirizine is slightly more advantageous and possibly faster than desloratadine. Both drugs were well tolerated with only minimal side effects.

L. Cleaver, DO

Chronic urticaria: do urticaria nonexperts implement treatment guidelines? A survey of adherence to published guidelines by nonexperts
Ferrer M, Jáuregui I, Bartra J, et al (Hosp de Basurto, Bilbao, Spain; Hosp Clínic, Barcelona, Spain; Hosp Clínico, Salamanca, Spain; et al)
Br J Dermatol 160:823-827, 2009

Background.—Guidelines including level of evidence and grade of recommendation were recently published for chronic urticaria (CU).

Objectives.—To describe the therapeutic approach in patients with CU, and to depict how recent guidelines are implemented in the daily practice of management of CU.

Methods.—We performed a cross-sectional multicentre study through a questionnaire answered by 139 specialists. In total, 695 patients were evaluated, mean ± SD age $42·3 ± 15$ years, $62·1\%$ women. Of the patients, 168 were treated by an allergist, 473 by a dermatologist and in 54 cases the specialist was not stated. The drug prescribed was the main variable, and χ^2 and Fisher's tests were utilized for the statistical analysis.

Results.—Nonsedating anti-H1 antihistamines taken regularly were the most common drugs prescribed, followed by nonsedating anti-H1 antihistamines taken as needed, corticosteroids, sedating antihistamines taken regularly, sedating antihistamines taken as needed, anti-H2 antihistamines, leukotriene antagonists, ciclosporin and doxepin. Nonsedating antihistamines plus corticosteroids was the most frequent drug combination prescribed. When comparing between allergists and dermatologists we found a positive and significant correlation only between prescription of cetirizine, dexchlorfeniramine, leukotriene antagonists and anti-H2 antihistamines and being treated by an allergist. A positive correlation was found with desloratadine and being seen by a dermatologist. We did not find any difference in CU management in the rest of the treatments studied.

Conclusions.—It is surprising that a large amount of sedating antihistamines was prescribed. In many instances these were prescribed as needed. This fact could have a negative impact on urticaria control and patient satisfaction. It seems difficult for the nonexpert to differentiate between CU and any kind of physical urticaria.

▶ This is an interesting article calling to light the need to revisit the management and treatment of chronic urticaria among nonurticarial expert dermatologists and allergists. The study acknowledges that despite recently published guidelines, dermatologists and allergists alike are finding difficulty in managing chronic urticaria. It should be noted that the study was limited to dermatologists and allergists in Spain, and thus, may not be representative of other geographic locations. Regardless, the notable contribution of this article is a well-founded pronouncement to the medical community on the lack of clinically meaningful clinic trials on the management of chronic urticaria and a need to expand and distribute information in this area, thereby providing better consistency in not only the management and treatment of chronic urticaria, but also ultimately, patient satisfaction.

B. D. Michaels, DO
J. Q. Del Rosso, DO

Chronic urticaria: a patient survey on quality-of-life, treatment usage and doctor-patient relation

Maurer M, Ortonne J-P, Zuberbier T (Charité–Universitätsmedizin, Berlin, Germany; Hôpital de L'Archet 2, Nice, France)
Allergy 64:581-588, 2009

Background.—Chronic urticaria (CU) is a common skin disorder characterized by recurrent spontaneous outbreaks of itchy wheals and/or angioedema. It has been shown to have substantial impact on patient quality-of-life, but little else is known about patient perspectives on CU and its treatment.

Methods.—An internet survey was conducted with 321 randomly selected, representative adults in Germany and France who were diagnosed with CU. The survey included the Skindex-29 questionnaire on quality-of-life and questions about treatment usage and patients' relation to their physician. Regression analyses were used to identify predictors of quality-of-life, use of prescription medication and various aspects of the doctor–patient relation.

Results.—The survey confirmed that CU has substantial impact on quality-of-life, with median Skindex scores of 68 for symptoms, 50 for functioning and 53 for emotions. Only two in three respondents were taking prescription medication for their CU. Older respondents, French respondents and fully employed respondents were significantly ($P < 0.01$) more likely to be taking prescription medication. Only three in five respondents under a physician's care reported that their physician had discussed the emotional impact of CU on them. Patients whose physicians had discussed this emotional impact were significantly ($P < 0.001$) more satisfied with treatment and more trusting of their physician.

Conclusions.—CU has a heavy impact on quality-of-life. Physicians need to be aware that many patients are not taking second generation anti-histamines and counsel them better on this point. Physicians should also discuss the emotional impact of CU with patients, because it improves their satisfaction and trust.

▶ Urticaria is a common condition frequently encountered in outpatient clinics. The goal of this study was to see how chronic urticaria affects the quality of life (QoL) of patients. An Internet survey was conducted in France and Germany and focused on QoL as well as other topics such as duration, frequency and timing, and previous and present treatments. The final study size was small ($N = 321$) with 83.5% of patients seeking care from a physician. Authors were able to show that chronic urticaria has a substantial effect on QoL. The article also portrays inadequate patient education by physicians. Pharmacologic treatment with second-generation antihistamines along with other nonpharmacologic options such as lotions, OTC products, and soothing baths may be beneficial. I agree with the authors' summary that patient education is very important and should be an integral part of any physician's practice. Patient education raises patient satisfaction and increases treatment compliance.

S. Bhambri, DO
J. Q. Del Rosso, DO

Experience with Cyclosporine in Children with Chronic Idiopathic Urticaria
Doshi DR, Weinberger MM (Univ of Iowa College of Medicine, Iowa City)
Pediatr Dermatol 26:409-413, 2009

Background.—The identification of an autoimmune mechanism for many patients with chronic idiopathic urticaria (CIU) was used as a rational for a controlled clinical trial of cyclosporine for adults with CIU not responsive to usual measures. That randomized placebo controlled clinical trial demonstrated clinical efficacy, acceptable safety, and a suggestion of inducing remission in such patients.

Objective.—To report our experience with cyclosporine in pediatric patients with CIU.

Methods.—Fifty-four patients with CIU were referred to us during the period from 2000 through June of 2005. Seven of those, aged 9–16, failed therapy with high dose antihistamines even with the addition of alternate morning prednisone. Neoral brand of cyclosporine, 3 mg/kg/day divided b.i.d., was initiated in these patients. Cyclosporine serum concentrations, blood urea nitrogen (BUN), creatinine, and blood pressure were routinely monitored.

Results.—All had cessation of hives. This occurred after 1–4 weeks for six of the seven and 8 weeks for one. While some experienced relapses, all were eventually off of all medications and free of hives. None of the seven experienced any adverse effects.

Conclusions.—Our experience in children is consistent with a previous controlled clinical trial in adults and supports the efficacy and safety of cyclosporine for CIU. However, we recommend that it be reserved for those whose CIU that is resistant to conventional measures and that patients be carefully monitored with cyclosporine serum concentrations and measures of renal function.

▶ Chronic idiopathic urticaria (CIU) is an autoimmune disease characterized by pruritic wheals that can be refractory to treatment. In the past, there have been studies documenting the safety and efficacy of cyclosporine for CIU in adults. This is a study of 54 pediatric patients with CIU referred to a tertiary center from 2000 to 2005. Of the 54 patients, 7 pediatric patients between 9 to 16 years of age failed resolution of hives with high dose antihistamines with alternating prednisone. Patients were given microemulsion formulation brand of cyclosporine (Neoral) 3 mg/kg/day twice a day, monitored with blood cyclosporine concentration, blood urea nitrogen (BUN), creatinine, and blood pressure monitored weekly then monthly. Patients had no other systemic disease except for CIU. Once there was cessation of hives for 1 month, cyclosporine was tapered at 2 to 4 weeks intervals until completely discontinued. Some patients experienced relapses, but all children were eventually off of all medications and free of hives varying from several months to years. There were no adverse effects or lab abnormalities observed in these 7 patients. Authors in this study concluded that low dose cyclosporine is a safe and effective alternative for pediatric patients with CIU resistant to conventional treatment. Limitations to this study included small study size, nonrandomized patients, and short follow-up period. Although authors claim that cyclosporine is safe in pediatric patients, those less than 9 years of age and neonates were not included in this study. To assure the safety profile in pediatric patients, there needs to be randomized placebo-controlled clinical trials with efficacy data for pediatric patients with CIU.

G. K. Kim, DO
J. Q. Del Rosso, DO

Hand eczema classification: a cross-sectional, multicentre study of the aetiology and morphology of hand eczema

Diepgen TL, on behalf of the European Environmental and Contact Dermatitis Research Group (Univ Hosp Heidelberg, Germany; et al)
Br J Dermatol 160:353-358, 2009

Background.—Hand eczema is a long-lasting disease with a high prevalence in the background population. The disease has severe, negative effects on quality of life and sometimes on social status. Epidemiological studies have identified risk factors for onset and prognosis, but treatment of the disease is rarely evidence based, and a classification system for different subdiagnoses of hand eczema is not agreed upon. Randomized controlled trials investigating the treatment of hand eczema are called for. For this, as well as for clinical purposes, a generally accepted classification system for hand eczema is needed.

TABLE 1.—Subdiagnoses Given for the 319 Patients Included in the Diagnostic Subgroups, and for 77 Patients not Included in the Diagnostic Subgroups

	Frequency	Percentage
ACD	60	15·2
ACD + ICD	60	15·2
ICD	85	21·5
AHE	23	5·8
AHE + ICD	31	7·8
Vesicular	37	9·3
Hyperkeratotic	21	5·3
Total 319 patients in the seven most frequent subdiagnostic groups		
ACD + AHE	9	2·3
ACD + AHE + protein contact dermatitis	1	0·3
ACD + AHE + vesicular eczema	1	0·3
ACD + hyperkeratotic eczema	2	0·5
ACD + ICD + AHE	6	1·5
ACD + ICD + AHE + hyperkeratotic eczema	1	0·3
ACD + ICD + AHE + vesicular eczema	1	0·3
ACD + ICD + AHE + vesicular eczema + hyperkeratotic eczema	1	0·3
ACD + ICD + hyperkeratotic eczema	4	1·0
ACD + vesicular eczema + hyperkeratotic eczema	1	0·3
AHE + hyperkeratotic eczema	1	0·3
AHE + vesicular eczema	8	2·0
AHE + vesicular eczema + hyperkeratotic eczema	1	0·3
Discoid eczema	3	0·8
Discoid eczema + other diagnosis	1	0·3
ICD + AHE + vesicular eczema	1	0·3
ICD + discoid eczema	4	1·0
ICD + hyperkeratotic eczema	9	2·3
ICD + vesicular eczema	15	3·8
ICD + vesicular eczema + discoid eczema	1	0·3
Other diagnosis	6	1·5
Total 77 patients outside the seven most frequent diagnostic subgroups		

ACD, allergic contact dermatitis; ICD, irritant contact dermatitis; AHE, atopic hand eczema.

TABLE 4.—Characteristics for the Various Subdiagnostic Groups

	Demographics	Medical History	Most Frequent Clinical Signs	Most Frequent Locations	Definition
ACD	Predominance of men	Relevant contact allergy; highest HECSI	Erythema, scaling, infiltration	Finger, palm, fingertip	Relevant contact allergy
ACD+ICD		Relevant contact allergy and relevant irritant exposure	Erythema, scaling, infiltration	Finger, fingertip/palm	Relevant contact sensitization and relevant irritant exposure
ICD	Most frequent diagnosis for women	Relevant irritant exposure; lowest HECSI	Erythema, scaling, infiltration	Finger, fingertip/palm	Relevant irritant exposure
AHE (endogenous)	Affects young age groups	Atopic dermatitis	Infiltration, erythema, scaling	Finger, palm	Atopic skin disease
AHE+ICD		Atopic dermatitis and relevant irritant exposure	Erythema, scaling	Finger, dorsal hand	Atopic skin disease and relevant irritant exposure
Vesicular (endogenous)	Predominance of men		Vesicles, erythema, scaling	Palm, finger	Vesicular morphology and no relevant contact sensitization, no relevant irritant exposure, no atopic disease
Hyperkeratotic (endogenous)	Affects older age groups	High HECSI	Infiltration, fissures, scaling	Palm, finger	Hyperkeratotic morphology in the palms and no relevant contact sensitization, no relevant irritant exposure, no atopic disease

ACD, allergic contact dermatitis; ICD, irritant contact dermatitis; AHE, atopic hand eczema; HECSI, Hand Eczema Severity Index.

Objectives.—The present study attempts to characterize subdiagnoses of hand eczema with respect to basic demographics, medical history and morphology.

Methods.—Clinical data from 416 patients with hand eczema from 10 European patch test clinics were assessed.

Results.—A classification system for hand eczema is proposed.

Conclusions.—It is suggested that this classification be used in clinical work and in clinical trials (Tables 1 and 4).

▶ This comprehensive report comes from many of the pre-eminent contact dermatitis centers in Europe. As such, it represents a collaboration of some of the leaders in the field. About 400 patients with all types of hand eczema were evaluated extensively. Over half had irritant contact dermatitis (ICD) as the sole or partial diagnosis. Allergic contact dermatitis (ACD) was found in about one third. Endogenous dermatitis, including vesicular, hyperkeratotic, atopic, etc, was also present in about one third. About 40% of the patients were given more than one diagnosis, with ICD as the most common exogenous factor.

This article is a fine, detailed analysis of the complex issue of diagnosis of hand eczema. Several excellent points should be useful for all clinical dermatologists.

(1) Patch testing is essential for diagnosis of chronic hand eczema. In this report 40% of hyperkeratotic hand eczema cases and 60% of vesicular cases had a component of ACD.

(2) Most cases of hand eczema are multifactorial. ICD is a frequent complicating factor, especially in patients who have atopic or other endogenous eczema.

(3) Variations in the etiology of hand eczema relate somewhat with age, occupation, and gender. ICD, for instance, was more common in women.

In summary, a brief review of this article is essential for practicing dermatologists and more serious reading will be useful for those working in the subspeciality of contact dermatitis.

J. F. Fowler, Jr, MD

Nickel allergy as risk factor for hand eczema: a population-based study
Josefson A, Färm G, Magnuson A, et al (Örebro Univ Hosp, Sweden; et al)
Br J Dermatol 160:828-834, 2009

Background.—In population-based studies using self-reported nickel allergy, a hand eczema prevalence of 30–43% has been reported in individuals with nickel allergy. In a previous Swedish study, 958 schoolgirls were patch tested for nickel. In a questionnaire follow up 20 years later no association was found between nickel allergy and hand eczema.

Objectives.—To investigate further the relation between nickel allergy and hand eczema.

Methods.—Three hundred and sixty-nine women, still living in the same geographical area, now aged 30–40 years, were patch tested and clinically investigated regarding hand eczema.

Results.—Patch testing showed 30·1% nickel-positive individuals. The adjusted prevalence proportion ratio (PPR) for hand eczema after age 15 years in relation to nickel patch test results was 1·03 (95% confidence interval, CI 0·71–1·50). A history of childhood eczema was reported by 35·9%, and the PPR for hand eczema in relation to childhood eczema was 3·68 (95% CI 2·45–5·54). When analyzing the relation separately in women with and without a history of childhood eczema a statistical interaction was found. The hand eczema risk was doubled in nickel-positive women without a history of childhood eczema, with a PPR of 2·23 (95% CI 1·10–4·49) for hand eczema after age 15 years.

Conclusions.—A doubled risk for hand eczema was found in nickel-positive women without a history of childhood eczema. When analysing all participants, there was no statistically significant difference between nickel-positive and nickel-negative women regarding occurrence of hand eczema. The most important risk factor for hand eczema was childhood eczema. The risk for hand eczema in nickel-positive women may previously have been overestimated.

▶ Hand eczema represents a difficult clinical scenario with regard to diagnosis and treatment. Not only are moderate to severe cases often recalcitrant to topical therapies, but also their etiologies are equally vexing to discover. Contact dermatitis, endogenous eczematous dermatitis such as atopic dermatitis and dyshidrosis, and psoriasis may represent some of the myriad causes of this common complaint. While patch testing is an invaluable component in the evaluation of these patients, a history of other inflammatory disorders is critical to clarify. Many studies have evaluated risk factors associated with hand eczema, including occupation, chronicity of wet work, history of atopy, and hypersensitivity to specific allergens. Studies are conflicting regarding the risk of hand eczema as it relates to metal allergy and history of childhood eczema. In this study, the latter was found to be most important. In occupational causes, rubber allergens along with preservatives, fragrances, and topical antibiotics tend to predominate in the United States. Other studies have demonstrated more significant clinical disease with allergy to metals such as nickel and chromate; the latter associated with a poorer prognosis and lower likelihood of improvement even with allergen avoidance.[1-2]

D. E. Cohen, MD, MPH

References

1. Hald M, Agner T, Blands J, Ravn H, Johansen JD. Allergens associated with severe symptoms of hand eczema and a poor prognosis. *Contact Dermatitis.* 2009;61: 101-108.

2. Warshaw EM, Ahmed RL, Belsito DV, et al. North American Contact Dermatitis Group. Contact dermatitis of the hands: cross-sectional analyses of North American Contact Dermatitis Group Data, 1994-2004. *J Am Acad Dermatol.* 2007; 57:301-314.

Allergens associated with severe symptoms of hand eczema and a poor prognosis

Hald M, Agner T, Blands J, et al (Natl Allergy Res Centre, Denmark; Univ of Copenhagen, Hellerup, Denmark; Natl Board of Health and Statens Serum Inst, Copenhagen, Denmark)
Contact Dermatitis 61:101-108, 2009

Background.—Contact allergy is frequent among persons with hand eczema and may be associated with a poor prognosis.

Objectives.—To identify allergens associated with the most severe initial clinical symptoms and the worst prognosis in a cohort of hand eczema patients followed for 6 months.

Methods.—The study population comprised 799 consecutive hand eczema patients enrolled during January 2006–February 2007. All patients were patch tested with the European baseline series. Severity assessment of the hand eczema was performed initially and at the 6-month follow-up using a validated scoring system (HECSI). With logistic regression analyses, associations of severe hand eczema or a poor prognosis with 15 individual allergens were analysed and adjusted for by sex, age, atopic dermatitis and other allergens.

Results.—At baseline, greater severity of hand eczema was associated with a positive patch test to formaldehyde, methyldibromo glutaronitrile, sesquiterpene lactone mix, nickel sulfate and potassium dichromate. A poor prognosis was associated with chromate allergy, odds ratio: 4.18 (95% CI: 1.42–12.28).

Conclusions.—Nickel, chromate, formaldehyde, methyldibromo glutaronitrile and sesquiterpene lactone mix were allergens associated with the greatest severity of hand eczema. Patients with chromate allergy had the worst prognosis.

▶ Some individuals that develop hand eczema may also have contact allergy coupled with an atopic history. Symptoms of hand eczema can progress to exhibit a chronic course initiated by exposure to irritants. The aim of this study was to identify allergens associated with the greatest initial severity of clinical symptoms and the worst prognosis in 799 hand eczema patients who were followed for 6 months. Patients were also patch tested with 15 different allergens and analyzed with adjustment for sex, age, atopic dermatitis, and other allergens. Nine dermatology clinics participated in this study and assessed patients according to the hand eczema severity index (HECSI) by a dermatologist, and a self-rated severity assessment was done by patients using a photographic guide. The prevalence of atopic dermatitis was 28.7%. Nickel was the most common allergen with a frequency of 19.4% and was generally not associated with severe hand eczema. The allergens causing the highest number of positive results among women were nickel sulfate, fragrance, and cobalt chloride, whereas in men it was fragrance, nickel sulfate, and chromate. Clinical status of patients after 6 months of initial evaluation revealed that chromate contact allergy demonstrated the worst prognosis. Other factors along with poor prognosis showed no interaction for chromate contact allergy and sex ($P = .875$), age ($P = .912$), or socioeconomic groups (0.998). This study revealed that the severity of symptoms of hand eczema at baseline were associated with a positive patch test to formaldehyde, methyldibromo glutaronitrile, sesquiterpene lactone mix, and chromate. One limitation of this study was the short follow-up period. Another limitation was that only 15 allergens were tested, and no other previous history of allergies was mentioned. The long-term implications of chromate allergy were also not discussed. It was also unknown whether those with chromate contact allergy and hand eczema were at an increased risk for treatment resistance and persistent eczema beyond 6 months. There were also patients that did not follow-up after the initial visit and others that did not complete the questionnaires, which could have also influenced the data.

G. K. Kim, DO

J. Q. Del Rosso, DO

Filaggrin mutations may confer susceptibility to chronic hand eczema characterized by combined allergic and irritant contact dermatitis
Molin S, Vollmer S, Weiss EH, et al (Ludwig-Maximilians-Univ, Munich, Germany)
Br J Dermatol 161:801-807, 2009

Background.—The pathogenesis of chronic hand eczema (CHE) is multifactorial and involves both endogenous predisposition and environmental triggers.

Objectives.—Filaggrin is a structural protein of the cornified envelope and important for the formation of the epidermal skin barrier. The aim of this investigation was to evaluate the role of mutations in the filaggrin gene (*FLG*) in the development of CHE.

Methods.—In total, 122 German patients with clearly defined CHE subtypes were screened for the *FLG* variants R501X and 2282del4 by polymerase chain reaction and restriction enzyme digest analysis. The prevalence of these variants in CHE patients was compared with that in 95 healthy individuals.

Results.—Overall, allele frequency and the number of mutation carriers were similar in both the CHE and control groups. When classified according to clearly defined CHE subtypes, however, the nonfunctional *FLG* variants showed an association with CHE involving an aetiological combination of contact allergy and irritant factors [$P = 0 \cdot 04$; P (exact test) $= 0 \cdot 06$; P (difference in rates) $= 0 \cdot 09$; 95% confidence interval (CI) 0–56·8)], or with excessive daily exposure to water and irritants [$P = 0 \cdot 003$; P (difference in rates) $< 0 \cdot 001$; 95% CI 29·3–67·9].

Conclusion.—Heterozygosity for nonfunctional mutations in the *FLG* gene may contribute to the manifestation and maintenance of a particular CHE subtype that is characterized by the combination of allergic and irritant contact dermatitis.

▶ Chronic hand eczema (CHE) is a persistent inflammatory skin condition that is multifactorial. Filaggrin is a structural protein in the stratum corneum that is responsible for protection against water loss and physical and chemical irritants. Past studies have revealed that gene defects in the filaggrin (FLG) protein has been known to impair the skin barrier and contribute to dermatitis. This is a study of 122 German patients with CHE subtypes screened for *FLG* gene variants (R501X and 2282del4) by polymerase chain reaction compared with 95 healthy individuals. Each patient underwent a survey regarding the history, clinical manifestation of hand eczema, course of disease, atopy or contact allergies, and previous and current dermatological treatment. Each patient was genotyped for the 2 *FLG* variants from whole blood performed blinded. Of the 122 patients, 28 patients were diagnosed with allergic contact dermatitis, 25 with irritant contact dermatitis, and 43 with idiopathic CHE. Clinical morphology revealed that 45 patients displayed hyperkeratotic rhagadiform features, 40 patients with dyshidrotic features, and 37 patients had mixed pattern of clinical features. Sixty-nine patients had a persistent CHE course while 49 patients an intermittent and relapsing CHE course. Eleven heterozygous mutation carriers were found in 122 CHE patients. None of the mutation carriers showed signs of ichthyosis or had a history of atopic dermatitis, although 5 individuals had an atopic predisposition. These findings may be due to small group size of mutation carriers. Compared with patients with CHE without the mutation, statistical significance was reached for individuals with a combination type of allergic and irritant contact dermatitis: 5 of 26 patients with simultaneous contact allergic and irritant CHE had a *FLG* gene mutation (R501X or 2282del4; $P = .04$). In addition, a statistically significant association was found for individuals with excessive daily exposure to water or irritants compared with patients with CHE lacking these mutations (R501X or 2282del4; $P = .003$). No other significant association between the different variables, including contact allergy and morphology was observed. Overall, in this cohort of 122 patients with CHE the *FLG* gene mutations were similar in both the CHE and control groups. Therefore, CHE patients were classified according to clinical features, causative factors, and morphological aspects. Patients were diagnosed with 4 main different forms of CHE: allergic contact dermatitis (23%), irritant contact dermatitis (21%), and a combined manifestation of allergic and irritant contact dermatitis (21%) and idiopathic CHE (35%). *FLG* mutations were seen in all the different CHE subtypes. A statistical significant heterozygous association with the *FLG* mutations R501X or 2282del4 was observed [$P = .04$; P (exact test) $= .06$; P (difference in rates) $= .09$, 95%

CI 0-56.8] for individuals suffering from combined irritants and allergic contact dermatitis. Five of 26 patients with a combined contact allergic and irritant CHE had a *FLG* gene mutation (19%), and 5 of 11 *FLG*-mutation carriers were diagnosed with combined irritant and allergic contact dermatitis. These results proposed a relevance of the *FLG* mutations for development of irritant contact dermatitis and allergic sensitization. In this study, authors suggest that heterozygous *FLG* variants do not seem to confer a risk for inflammatory skin disease in general. However, these findings may be limited because there is genetic variation between ethnic groups and results may differ with larger sample sizes of patients. In conclusion, investigators suggest that *FLG* gene may contribute to a particular CHE subtype with a combination of allergic and irritant contact dermatitis.

G. K. Kim, DO
J. Q. Del Rosso, DO

Early introduction of fish decreases the risk of eczema in infants
Alm B, Åberg N, Erdes L, et al (Univ of Gothenburg, Sweden; Skene Hosp, Sweden; et al)
Arch Dis Child 94:11-15, 2009

Background.—Atopic eczema in infants has increased in western societies. Environmental factors and the introduction of food may affect the risk of eczema.

Aims.—To investigate the prevalence of eczema among infants in western Sweden, describe patterns of food introduction and assess risk factors for eczema at 1 year of age.

Methods.—Data were obtained from a prospective, longitudinal cohort study of infants born in western Sweden in 2003; 8176 families were randomly selected and, 6 months after the infant's birth, were invited to participate and received questionnaires. A second questionnaire was sent out when the infants were 12 months old. Both questionnaires were completed and medical birth register data were obtained for 4921 infants (60.2% of the selected population).

Results.—At 1 year of age, 20.9% of the infants had previous or current eczema. Median age at onset was 4 months. In multivariate analysis, familial occurrence of eczema, especially in siblings (OR 1.87; 95% confidence interval (CI) 1.50 to 2.33) or the mother (OR 1.54; 95% CI 1.30 to 1.84), remained an independent risk factor. Introducing fish before 9 months of age (OR 0.76; 95% CI 0.62 to 0.94) and having a bird in the home (OR 0.35; 95% CI 0.17 to 0.75) were beneficial.

Conclusions.—One in five infants suffer from eczema during the first year of life. Familial eczema increased the risk, while early fish introduction and bird keeping decreased it. Breast feeding and time of milk and egg introduction did not affect the risk.

▶ Atopic eczema is a common skin condition with genetic and environmental influences contributing to its existence. Certain types of food and the time period of food introduction may influence the onset of eczematous dermatitis in atopic individuals. Dairy products, omega-3 fatty acids, and a diet containing lactobacilli have been suggested to have a protective factor against the development of atopy. This is a prospective longitudinal cohort study of infants born in western Sweden with 8176 families randomly selected to answer questionnaires after 6 and 12 months of birth and with 4921 infants having completed the study. Patients were asked questions concerning family, environment, perinatal history, tobacco, breastfeeding, food introduction, and prevalence of diseases in the first year of life. The study concluded that 1 in 5 infants had eczema at a mean onset of 4 months with a strong association with a family history of eczema. They also observed benefits of introducing fish before 9 months of age, while short duration of breastfeeding, keeping furry pets, or age at which eggs or milk were introduced did not affect the risk of developing eczema. In the multivariable analysis, significant risk factors were maternal eczema, a sibling with eczema, a bird in the home, introduction of fish before 9 months of age, and allergy to cow milk. Because data was analyzed using questionnaires alone there was some uncertainty about the exact prevalence of eczema since an official diagnosis by a trained physician was not conducted by this study. The strongest risk factor for eczema was a family history of eczema, maternal eczema in particular, which was also consistent with past studies. Although this study does emphasize the benefits of early introduction of omega-3 fatty acids in fish, there was no correlation found with a certain type of fish or any other products that contained omega-3 fatty acids. In addition, the authors could not find that breastfeeding was a protective factor for eczema, which is a conclusion that was made without knowing how much breast milk was given to these infants and for how long. Because this was a study based on questionnaires, it would have also been beneficial to see if these children had professionally diagnosed eczema. It would have also been of interest to follow these children for a longer duration of time to evaluate if early dietary introduction of fish continued to have a protective effect or if these children developed eczema later on in life.

G. K. Kim, DO
J. Q. Del Rosso, DO

Cornulin, a marker of late epidermal differentiation, is down-regulated in eczema

Liedén A, Ekelund E, Kuo I-C, et al (Karolinska Institutet, Stockholm, Sweden; Natl Univ of Singapore; et al)
Allergy 64:304-311, 2009

Background.—Eczema is a common chronic inflammatory skin disorder which shows strong genetic predisposition. To identify new potential molecular determinants of the disease pathogenesis, we performed a gene expression study in an eczema mouse model. This analysis identified a marked down regulation of the cornulin gene (*CRNN*), a member of the epidermal differentiation complex, in the eczema-like skin. We then investigated *CRNN* as an eczema candidate gene and studied its polymorphism and the expression in the skin of eczema patients.

Methods.—An eczema-like phenotype was induced in mice by allergen (Der p2) patching. Gene expression analysis was performed with the subtractive suppression hybridization method and validated by real time PCR and the transmission disequilibrium test was used to test for genetic associations in 406 multiplex eczema families.

Results.—Der p 2 patched mice developed a localized eczema and a Th 2 skewed systemic response. Real time PCR analysis confirmed a down regulation of *CRNN* mRNA in eczema-like skin in the mouse model and in human eczema. The *CRNN* polymorphism rs941934 was significantly associated with atopic eczema in the genetic analysis ($P = 0.006$), though only as part of an extended haplotype including a known associated variant (2282del4) in the filaggrin gene.

Conclusions.—*CRNN* mRNA expression is decreased in eczematous skin. Further studies are needed to verify whether the associated cornulin polymorphism contribute to the genetic susceptibility in eczema.

▶ Cornulin, like filaggrin, is a product of the so-called fused gene family located on human chromosome 1. These proteins are similar in structure, are expressed during epidermal differentiation, and appear to be involved in maintenance of normal epidermal barrier function. Several recent studies have convincingly demonstrated a highly significant association between loss-of-function mutations of the filaggrin gene and susceptibility to atopic eczema. In this elegant study, Liedén et al showed that skin cornulin expression was dramatically reduced in their previously described and well-characterized murine model of atopic eczema. Further studies revealed a similar significant down-regulation of cornulin mRNA in the lesional skin of patients with eczema, compared with nonlesional skin from the same patients, healthy donor skin, and both lesional and nonlesional skin from patients with psoriasis.

Next, the investigators examined the allelic distribution of 6 single-nucleotide polymorphisms (SNP) within the cornulin gene locus in subjects with eczema. The individuals studied were siblings belonging to a large number of informative families. Their eczema was designated atopic or nonatopic based on IgE levels. Genotyping of these patients revealed a highly significant association between the rare (minor) allele of one cornulin SNP in subjects with atopic eczema, whereas no association was found in patients with nonatopic eczema. However, further analysis revealed an association with atopic eczema only in those subjects with both the risk allele of cornulin and the deletion mutation of filaggrin associated with eczema, which was most likely due to linkage disequilibrium between the two. Further studies of the role of cornulin in eczema are clearly warranted.

G. M. P. Galbraith, MD

What causes flares of eczema in children?
Langan SM, Silcocks P, Williams HC (Univ of Nottingham, UK)
Br J Dermatol 161:640-646, 2009

Background.—Although eczema affects 2–20% of children worldwide, there is little direct evidence on the role of environmental factors in disease flares.

Objectives.—We sought to identify which environmental factors might worsen eczema.

Methods.—Sixty children aged 0–15 years with eczema were studied intensively for up to 9 months. Daily electronic diaries and portable data loggers were used to record indoor exposures, and external meteorological data were obtained from a local monitoring centre. The primary outcome was a daily 'bother' score. Autoregressive moving average models were used to study the impact of exposures on eczema severity for individuals. Random effects modelling pooled estimated regression coefficients across participants.

Results.—Increased severity was associated with nylon clothing [pooled regression coefficient $0 \cdot 23$, 95% confidence interval (CI) $0 \cdot 03$–$0 \cdot 43$], dust $(0 \cdot 53, 0 \cdot 23$–$0 \cdot 83)$, unfamiliar pets $(0 \cdot 22, 0 \cdot 10$–$0 \cdot 34)$, sweating $(0 \cdot 24, 0 \cdot 09$–$0 \cdot 39)$ and shampoo $(0 \cdot 07, 0 \cdot 01$–$0 \cdot 14)$. The latter was enhanced in cold weather $(0 \cdot 30, 0 \cdot 04$–$0 \cdot 57)$. Body-site specificity was observed for nylon clothing, (trunk $P = 0 \cdot 02$, limbs $P = 0 \cdot 03$), wool clothing (trunk $P = 0 \cdot 03$, but not limbs $P = 0 \cdot 62$) and unfamiliar pets (hands $P < 0 \cdot 001$). A combination of any three of seven likely variables was associated with disease worsening (pooled regression coefficient $0 \cdot 41$, 95% CI $0 \cdot 20$–$0 \cdot 63$).

Conclusions.—This exploratory study suggests that nylon clothing, dust, unfamiliar pets, sweating and shampoos may play a direct role in worsening eczema in children with eczema. Combinations of exposures acting in concert may also be important. Such knowledge may be useful to families with eczema and could lead to better strategies for preventing flares.

▶ Eczema can cause significant morbidity to many children with many exacerbating factors. This is a study of 60 children between the age of 0 to 15 with a history of eczema followed for 9 months that electronically recorded external factors that caused them to have flares of eczema. Patients were required to put their flares in a daily diary and changes to medications, including a "step up" move to a higher potency corticosteroid, was also noted. The authors found that increased disease severity correlated with direct contact to nylon, dust exposure, unfamiliar pets, sweating, and shampoo exposure. Eczema flares were worse with shampoo exposure and cold water; in addition, worsening of hand eczema was associated with pets. In this study, nylon and wool clothing were associated with worsening eczema that was site specific to the trunk. Association with worsening of eczema and washing a child's hair during bath time was also seen in correlation with low temperatures. Swimming in chlorinated water was also seen with disease worsening and a need to step up to a higher potency topical corticosteroid treatment. This study was interesting in that it introduced a novel electronic diary to track precipitating factors for eczema patients, and findings also suggested that there may be multiple culprits that induce eczema flares.

G. K. Kim, DO

J. Q. Del Rosso, DO

Filaggrin haploinsufficiency is highly penetrant and is associated with increased severity of eczema: further delineation of the skin phenotype in a prospective epidemiological study of 792 school children
Brown SJ, Relton CL, Liao H, et al (Royal Victoria Infirmary, UK; Newcastle Univ, UK; Univ of Dundee, UK)
Br J Dermatol 161:884-889, 2009

Background.—Null mutations within the filaggrin gene (*FLG*) cause ichthyosis vulgaris and are associated with atopic eczema. However, the dermatological features of filaggrin haploinsufficiency have not been clearly defined.

Objectives.—This study investigated the genotype–phenotype association between detailed skin phenotype and *FLG* genotype data in a population-based cohort of children.

Methods.—Children (n = 792) aged 7–9 years were examined by a dermatologist. Features of ichthyosis vulgaris, atopic eczema and xerosis were recorded and eczema severity graded using the Three Item Severity score. Each child was genotyped for the six most prevalent FLG null mutations (R501X, 2282del4, R2447X, S3247X, 3702delG, 3673delC). Fisher's exact test was used to compare genotype frequencies in phenotype groups; logistic regression analysis was used to estimate odds ratios and penetrance of the *FLG* null genotype and a permutation test performed to investigate eczema severity in different genotype groups.

Results.—Ten children in this cohort had ichthyosis vulgaris, of whom five had mild–moderate eczema. The penetrance of *FLG* null mutations with respect to flexural eczema was $55\cdot6\%$ in individuals with two mutations, $16\cdot3\%$ in individuals with one mutation and $14\cdot2\%$ in wild-type individuals. Summating skin features known to be associated with FLG null mutations (ichthyosis, keratosis pilaris, palmar hyperlinearity and flexural eczema) showed a penetrance of 100% in children with two FLG mutations, 87·8% in children with one FLG mutation and 46·5% in wild-type individuals ($P < 0·0001$, Fisher exact test). FLG null mutations were associated with more severe eczema ($P = 0·0042$) but the mean difference was only 1–2 points in severity score. Three distinct patterns of palmar hyperlinearity were observed and these are reported for the first time.

Conclusions.—Filaggrin haploinsufficiency appears to be highly penetrant when all relevant skin features are included in the analysis. FLG null mutations are associated with more severe eczema, but the effect size is small in a population setting.

▶ Filaggrin is a protein expressed by keratinocytes that contributes to moisture retention in the stratum corneum principally through production of natural moisturizing factor (NMF). Loss of function (null) mutations within the gene encoding filaggrin gene (*FLG*) causes ichthyosis vulgaris and is associated with atopic eczema. This is a study investigating the genotype-phenotype relationship with the *FLG* gene in a population-based cohort study of 792 children aged 7 to 9 years of age. Each child was genotyped for the 6 most prevalent *FLG* null mutations. Odds ratios and penetrance of the *FLG* null genotype and permutation tests were performed to investigate eczema severity in different genotype groups. Features of ichthyosis vulgaris, atopic eczema, and xerosis were recorded and severity grading was done according to the Three Item Severity score. Ichthyosis, keratosis pilaris, palmar hyperlinearity, and flexural eczema may be associated with *FLG* null mutations suggesting a highly penetrant haploinsufficiency: 100% of individuals with 2 *FLG* null mutations and 87.8% of individuals with one *FLG* null mutations showed one or more of these skin features compared with 46.5% of wild-type individuals, which was a statistical difference ($P < .0001$). *FLG* null heterozygotes exhibited a milder skin phenotype than the *FLG* null homozygotes. The findings suggest that 85% to 100% of individuals carrying one or more *FLG* null mutations may demonstrate a sign of filaggrin haploinsufficiency, although they are often asymptomatic. Incomplete penetrance (<100%) implies that other factors, both genetic and environmental, may contribute to filaggrin haploinsufficiency in eczema where the penetrance is much lower than in ichthyosis/keratosis pilaris, palmar hyperlinearity, and eczema group. Keratosis pilaris and palmar hyperlinearity are each independently associated with *FLG* null mutations in this cohort. Limitations in this study include variation in genotypes between populations of people and within ethnic groups, which was not mentioned. Findings may be inconsistent due to this variation. This study also did not have age matched controls, which would have been useful in evaluating the nature of the *FLG* null mutation. In conclusion, authors suggest that *FLG* mutations are associated with more severe eczema in this population of patients and introduced a novel observation of 3 distinct patterns of palmar hyperlinearity.

J. Q. Del Rosso, DO
G. K. Kim, DO

Filaggrin mutations in the onset of eczema, sensitization, asthma, hay fever and the interaction with cat exposure

Schuttelaar MLA, Kerkhof M, Jonkman MF, et al (Univ of Groningen, the Netherlands; et al)
Allergy 64:1758-1765, 2009

Background.—Filaggrin gene (*FLG*) mutations contribute to the development of eczema and asthma, but their contribution to sensitization and hay fever remains unclear.

Methods.—FLG mutations R501X, 2282del4 and R2447X were genotyped in the Prevention and Incidence of Asthma and Mite Allergy birth cohort ($n = 934$) to evaluate longitudinally, for up to 8 years, their association with eczema, sensitization, asthma, hay fever and their interaction with cat exposure.

Results.—The combined *FLG* mutations were significantly associated with eczema at all ages when occurring in the first year of life (OR = 2.0; 95% CI: 1.4–2.8). Combined *FLG* mutations were associated with both atopic and nonatopic eczema, as well as asthma (OR = 3.7; 95% CI: 1.8–7.5). When the *FLG* 2282del4 mutation was analysed separately, it was significantly associated with the development of eczema during the first year, having eczema up to 8 years and sensitization at the age of 8 years, which was enhanced by early-life cat exposure (ORs being 8.2; 95% CI: 2.6–25.9, 6.0; 95% CI: 3.2–11.3 and 5.4; 95% CI: 1.2–23.6 respectively). FLG 2282del4 was significantly associated with hay fever from the age 5 years onwards (OR = 3.9; 95% CI: 1.5–10.5).

Conclusions.—*FLG* mutations are associated both with atopic and nonatopic eczema starting in the first year of life. *FLG* mutations combined with eczema in the first year of life are associated with a later development of asthma and hay fever, a clear example of the atopic march. We confirm that cat exposure enhances the effect of a *FLG* mutation on the development of eczema and sensitization.

▶ Filaggrin (*FLG*) is a protein that contributes to maintaining the integrity and function of the stratum corneum. Hence, *FLG* is an important component of epidermal barrier function. Abnormalities of *FLG* can serve as important factors in the pathogenesis of eczema. Past studies have suggested that *FLG* mutations contribute to the development of eczema, asthma, and hay fever. Two prevalent loss-of-functions of *FLG* variants (R501X and 2282del4) have been known to have strong predisposing factors for eczema and concomitant asthma. This is a study of 934 patients evaluated longitudinally for up to 8 years with the

FLG mutations (R501X, 2282del4, and R2447X) genotyped in the Prevention and Incidence of Asthma and Mite Allergy birth cohort in association with eczema, sensitization, asthma, hay fever, and their interaction with cat exposure evaluated. In this study, children from atopic mothers were more frequently heterozygous for the 2282del4 mutation than children from nonatopic mothers (6.9% vs 2.5%; $P < .01$). The carrier frequency of the combined genotype was significantly higher in children with eczema than those without eczema at the age of 4 years (20.9% vs 7.5% [$P = .000004$]). The combined genotype was significantly associated with the incidence of eczema in the first year of life only ($P < .001$). The difference between the first year and subsequent years was significant ($P = .007$). The overall association of 2282del4 with the presence of eczema was significantly stronger in children with a cat at home ($P = .024$). *FLG* mutations were associated with both atopic and nonatopic eczema, as well as asthma (OR = 0.7; CI: 1.8-7.5). Overall, the combined genotype was significantly associated with asthma at the age of 0 to 8 years ($P = .003$). Results revealed that *FLG* gene mutations are associated with eczema at the age of 0 to 8 years when occurring in the first year of life. However, the higher risk of asthma and hay fever in children with *FLG* variants can be explained by the high risk of early eczema. *FLG* gene mutations were seen in both atopic and nonatopic eczema in the first year of life and was also associated with a later development of asthma/hay fever. This longitudinal analysis demonstrated that the association between 2282del4 and eczema was stronger in children with a cat at home. However, the mechanism by which cat exposure drives the development of eczema in *FLG* mutation carriers is still unclear. The authors propose that this study may indicate that *FLG* carriers should avoid exposure to cats to reduce the risk of developing eczema and sensitization. In conclusion, a disturbed barrier function due to *FLG* gene mutations may enable allergens to penetrate into the skin more easily and contribute to the development of sensitization, asthma, and seasonal rhinitis (hay fever).

J. Q. Del Rosso, DO

G. K. Kim, DO

The allergic sensitization in infants with atopic eczema from different countries
de Benedictis FM, on behalf of the EPAAC Study Group (Salesi Children's Hosp, Ancona, Italy; et al)
Allergy 64:295-303, 2009

Background.—No study has compared allergic sensitization patterns in infants with atopic eczema from different countries. The aim of this study was to investigate the patterns of allergic sensitization in a cohort of infants with atopic eczema participating in a multicentre, international study.

Methods.—Two thousand one hundred and eighty-four infants (mean age 17.6 months) with atopic eczema from allergic families were screened in 94 centres in 12 countries to participate in a randomized trial for the early prevention of asthma. Clinical history, Severity Scoring of Atopic Dermatitis Index, measurements for total serum IgE and specific IgE antibodies to eight food and inhalant allergens were entered into a database before randomization to treatment. A history of type of feeding in the first weeks of life and exposure to animals was recorded.

Results.—A total of 52.9% of the infants had raised total IgE, and 55.5% were sensitized to at least one allergen. There was a wide difference in the total IgE values and in the sensitization rates to foods and aeroallergens among infants from different countries. The highest prevalence rates of allergen-sensitized infants were found in Australia (83%), the UK (79%) and Italy (76%). Infants from Belgium and Poland consistently had the lowest sensitization rates. In each country, a characteristic pattern of sensitization was found for aeroallergens (house dust mite > cat > grass pollen > *Alternaria*), but not for food allergens.

Conclusions.—In infants with atopic eczema, there is a wide variation in the pattern of allergic sensitization between countries, and data from one country are not necessarily generalizable to other countries.

▶ The authors of this study successfully investigated the pattern of allergic sensitization in infants with atopic eczema from different countries and compared the sensitization patterns in this study population with sensitization patterns evaluated in the ETAC study completed 10 years earlier. This study also provided an opportunity to examine the possible relationship between exposure to environmental factors and allergic sensitization. However, while the authors have presented thorough data on the prevalence of allergen sensitization in different countries, the reviewers have a lack of analysis on why certain countries may have exhibited greater sensitization patterns than others. Perhaps this topic requires further investigation.

The limitations of this study include the substantial differences in the number of screened infants between the different countries and the lack of uniform approach in screening methodology in the different countries. Additionally, the patient population selected for this study had high genetic risk of atopy, and therefore the data from this study may not be applicable to low-risk individuals.

J. Levin, DO
J. Q. Del Rosso, DO

Medium-dose ultraviolet (UV) A1 vs. narrowband UVB phototherapy in atopic eczema: a randomized crossover study

Gambichler T, Othlinghaus N, Tomi NS, et al (Ruhr-Univ of Bochum, Germany)
Br J Dermatol 160:652-658, 2009

Background.—Ultraviolet (UV) A1 and narrowband (NB)-UVB have been reported to be effective treatments for atopic eczema (AE).

Objectives.—We aimed to compare the efficacy of medium-dose UVA1 and NB-UVB mono-phototherapy in patients with AE.

Methods.—A randomized double-blind controlled crossover trial (ClinicalTrials.gov Identifier: NCT00419406) was conducted in which patients with AE received a 6-week course of both medium-dose UVA1 and NB-UVB. Clinical efficacy was assessed using the Six Area, Six Sign, Atopic Dermatitis (SASSAD) score and a visual analogue scale for pruritus. Assessment of health-related quality of life was performed using the Skindex-29. Total immunoglobulin E (IgE) and eosinophilic cationic protein (ECP) were evaluated at baseline and after each phototherapy course.

Results.—Twenty-eight patients who completed both UVA1 and NB-UVB phototherapy courses on an intention-to-treat basis were analysed according to the crossover design. Both interventions were associated with significant clinical improvement but there was no significant difference between treatments with respect to the mean ± SD relative reduction (RR) of the clinical scores (SASSAD, $43 \cdot 7 \pm 31 \cdot 4\%$ vs. $39 \cdot 4 \pm 24 \cdot 1\%$, $P = 0 \cdot 5$; pruritus score, $16 \pm 61 \cdot 8\%$ vs. $25 \cdot 2 \pm 30 \cdot 5\%$, $P = 0 \cdot 5$, respectively). There was no significant difference in the mean ± SD RR of the Skindex-29 after UVA1 and NB-UVB phototherapy ($12 \cdot 7 \pm 18 \cdot 8\%$ vs. $16 \cdot 5 \pm 17 \cdot 6\%$, $P = 0 \cdot 1$). Changes in the total IgE and ECP levels following UVA1 and NB-UVB did not differ significantly ($P = 0 \cdot 3$ and $P = 0 \cdot 9$, respectively).

Conclusions.—A 6-week course of NB-UVB and UVA1 phototherapy of AE resulted in significant clinical improvement. With regard to efficacy and tolerability, both phototherapeutic modalities may be considered comparably good.

▶ There are many treatments for atopic eczema (AE) with a variety of topical and systemic therapy, including phototherapy. This is a randomized double-blind controlled crossover study comparing the efficacy of medium dose UVA1 versus narrow band UVB (narrowband ultraviolet B [NB-UVB]) mono-phototherapy for 6 weeks in patients with atopic eczema. There was a 2-week washout period for patients who were on other therapies such as topical agents. Those that were pregnant, had a history of skin cancer or dysplastic nevi, were photosensitive or with Fitzpatrick skin type I, or had a history of autoimmune disease were excluded. AE was assessed using a Six Area Six Sign Atopic Dermatitis (SASSAD) score including erythema, lichenification, excoriation, dryness, cracking, and exudation. Only subjects having a score over 20 were included in the study, with the most severe being 180.

They also incorporated a health-related quality of life analysis and serological measurement of total immunoglobulin E (IgE) and eosinophilic cationic protein (ECP) levels in the serum, collected at baseline and at the end of the study. Both treatments of UVA1 and NB-UVB phototherapy were well tolerated by the patients. Mild erythema was observed in 1 patient's treatment with UVA1 and 3 patients who received NB-UVB. No significant reduction in serological markers of IgE or ECP levels was found at the end of the study. It was concluded that UVA1 and NB-UVB might be comparably effective in AE. A strength of this study included not allowing patients to use any other forms of treatment along with phototherapy, which is commonly observed in other studies. Although this study found phototherapy to be effective in AE, there is some long-term risk such as photocarcinogenesis, which was not explored in this trial. Although UVA1 and NB-UVB were both found to be effective in the treatment of AE, it is difficult for some patients to have access to phototherapy as these modalities may not be available in all dermatology offices.

G. K. Kim, DO
J. Q. Del Rosso, DO

Increased stratum corneum serine protease activity in acute eczematous atopic skin
Voegeli R, Rawlings AV, Breternitz M, et al (DSM Nutritional Products Ltd, Basel, Switzerland; AVR Consulting Ltd, Cheshire, UK; Friedrich Schiller Univ, Jena, Germany)
Br J Dermatol 161:70-77, 2009

Background.—Atopic dermatitis (AD) is a chronic inflammatory disease associated with changes in stratum corneum (SC) structure and function. The breakdown of epidermal barrier function in AD is associated with changes in corneocyte size and maturation, desquamation, lipid profiles, and some protease activities.

Objectives.—The purpose of this study was: (i) to examine physiological changes in lesional (L) skin of acute eczematous AD, compared with non-lesional (NL) AD skin and healthy (H) skin, using sequential tewametry and SC protein analysis to estimate SC thickness; and (ii) to assess which serine proteases might be involved in pathogenesis.

Methods.—Six subjects with H skin, six AD patients with NL skin and six AD patients with mild to moderate eczema (L skin) were enrolled. Skin was assessed using several noninvasive techniques but SC thickness was estimated using tewametry and SC protein content of D-Squame strippings. SC integrity was determined by sequential tape stripping (D-Squame) and infrared densitometry. Kallikreins, plasmin, urokinase and leucocyte elastase protease activities together with a novel SC tryptase-like enzyme activity were quantified.

Results.—Transepidermal water loss (TEWL) levels after D-Squame stripping were elevated in L compared with NL and H skin at all sampling points $(P < 0·05)$. Conversely, the amount of SC removed by sequential tape stripping was decreased in L skin, indicating increased intracorneocyte cohesion $(P < 0·05)$. By correlating 1/TEWL values and SC removed as an estimate of SC thickness, a significantly thinner SC was observed in L compared with NL and H skin $(P < 0·05)$. Elevated extractable serine protease activity was measured in AD skin in the order: SC tryptase-like enzyme $(45×)$, plasmin $(30×)$, urokinase $(7·1×)$, trypsin-like kallikreins $(5·8×)$ and chymotrypsin-like kallikreins $(3·9×)$. Leucocyte elastase activity was not detected in H and NL skin but was observed in AD SC samples (L skin). All enzymes were elevated in the deeper layers of L SC compared with NL and H SC samples. All consistently elevated SC protease activities were significantly correlated with the bioinstrumental data.

Conclusions.—We report increased serine protease activities in acute eczematous AD, especially in deeper layers of the SC, including SC tryptase-like enzyme, plasmin, urokinase and leucocyte elastase activities. These elevations in protease activities were associated with impaired barrier function, irritation, and reduced skin capacitance. Increased SC cohesion was apparent despite elevated TEWL during tape stripping, which would indicate reduced SC thickness in acute eczematous lesions of AD. Indeed, this was observed using an estimate of SC thickness.

▶ Voegeli et al previously reported that activity of certain proteases in healthy human stratum corneum correlated positively with increasing transepidermal water loss and negatively with skin hydration.[1] In this study, they extended their investigation to include subjects with atopic dermatitis. Although the number of subjects studied was small, the results were dramatically (and significantly) different in lesional atopic dermatitis skin when compared with normal skin and non-lesional patient skin. The major findings were that lesional skin showed increases in both water loss and protease activities, particularly tryptase-like and plasmin, and conversely, decreases in hydration and thickness of the stratum corneum. This study differed from their previous investigation in that baseline and sequential measurements were taken after subjecting the skin to 5, 10, and 15 applications of tape stripping, which removes the surface layers of the stratum corneum and results in local perturbation of barrier function. The data thus obtained clearly showed the highest levels of enzyme activities in the last strippings taken from lesional skin, ie, from the deeper layers of the stratum corneum.

The role of serine proteases in the pathogenesis of atopic dermatitis remains to be clarified, as does the cause of their increased activity in this disease. The authors suggest that a deficiency of protease inhibitor(s) could account for this in part, as it appears to in Netherton syndrome; this condition is associated with mutations of the serine protease inhibitors of the Kazal type 5 (*SPINK5*) gene, a member of the gene family of serine protease inhibitors of the Kazal type. Interestingly, atopic dermatitis is one manifestation of Netherton disease. However, studies of possible associations between atopic dermatitis and *SPINKS5* gene polymorphisms have yielded conflicting results.[2] Nevertheless, these authors propose that serine protease inhibitors could be of therapeutic benefit in patients with atopic dermatitis.

G. M. P. Galbraith, MD

References

1. Voegeli R, Rawlings AV, Doppler S, Schreier T. Increased basal transepidermal water loss leads to elevation of some but not all stratum corneum serine proteases. *Int J Cosmetic Science.* 2008;30:435-442.
2. Hubiche T, Ged C, Benard A, et al. Analysis of SPINK-5, KLK 7, and FLG genotypes in a French atopic dermatitis cohort. *Acta Derm Venereol.* 2007;87: 499-505.

IL-17 in atopic eczema: Linking allergen-specific adaptive and microbial-triggered innate immune response
Eyerich K, Pennino D, Scarponi C, et al (IDI-IRCCS, Rome; et al)
J Allergy Clin Immunol 123:59-66, 2009

Background.—Patients with atopic eczema (AE) regularly experience colonization with *Staphylococcus aureus* that is directly correlated with the severity of eczema. Recent studies show that an impaired IL-17 immune response results in diseases associated with chronic skin infections.

Objective.—We sought to elucidate the effect of IL-17 on antimicrobial immune responses in AE skin.

Methods.—T cells infiltrating atopy patch test (APT) reactions were characterized for IL-17 secretion to varying stimuli. IL-17–dependent induction of the antimicrobial peptide human β-defensin 2 (HBD-2) in keratinocytes was investigated.

Results.—Approximately 10% of APT-infiltrating T cells secreted IL-17 after phorbol 12-myristate 13-acetate (PMA)/ionomycin stimulation. Among these, 33% belonged to the newly characterized subtype T_H2/IL-17. Despite the capacity to secrete IL-17, specific T-cell clones released only low amounts of IL-17 on cognate allergen stimulation, whereas IL-4, IFN-γ, or both were efficiently induced. IL-17 secretion was not enhanced by IL-23, IL-1β, or IL-6 but was enhanced by the *S aureus*–derived superantigen staphylococcal enterotoxin B. Both healthy and AE keratinocytes upregulated HBD-2 in response to IL-17, but coexpressed IL-4/IL-13 partially inhibited this effect. *In vivo*, additional application of staphylococcal enterotoxin B induced IL-17 in APT reactions, whereas IL-4, IFN-γ, and IL-10 were marginally regulated. Induced IL-17 upregulated HBD-2 in human keratinocytes *in vivo*.

Conclusion.—IL-17–capable T cells, in particular T_H2/IL-17 cells, infiltrate acute AE reactions. Although IL-17 secretion by specific T cells is tightly regulated, it can be triggered by bacteria-derived superantigens. The ineffective IL-17–dependent upregulation of HBD-2 in patients with

TABLE 1.—Functional Characterization of APT-Derived IL-171$^+$ T-Cell Clones

	Proliferation		Cytokine Profile (after PMA/Ionomycin Stimulation)							
Clone	SI to Der p 1	SI to SEB	IFN-γ	IL-4	IL-10	IL-13	IL-17	IL-22	TNF-α	Subtype
3	75	45	496	4,285	13,484	13,738	12,494	2,931	7,779	T$_H$2/IL-17
27	1	20	0	3	1,578	947	13,788	2,595	1,596	T$_H$17
60	25	30	5,385	2,922	10,623	13,074	11,000	126	5,348	T$_H$0/IL-17
91	20	15	0	3,252	16,260	18,317	3,519	7,000	4,620	T$_H$2/IL-17
96	40	45	9,946	3,477	16,159	14,302	2,394	3,568	3,840	T$_H$0/IL-17
141	40	1	0	4,710	1,149	20,472	5,500	219	861	T$_H$2/IL-17

Cytokine levels are measured by means of ELISA after PMA/ionomycin stimulation.
SI, Stimulation index to Der p 1 and SEB.

AE is due to a partial inhibition by the type 2 microenvironment, which could partially explain why patients with AE do not clear *S aureus*.

▶ As anticipated, this year has yielded a healthy crop of studies of the role(s) of Th17 lymphocytes in the pathogenesis of various dermatological diseases. In the excellent study described here, the investigators not only obtained strong evidence of a molecular basis for the pathogenic link between *Staphylococcus aureus* colonization and atopic eczema, but also identified subtypes of Th17 cells that have differing activities.

T cells were obtained from allergen-specific patch test lesions induced in patients with atopic eczema and examined for cytokine production. Not surprisingly, most infiltrating T cells were found to express interleukin (IL)-4, whereas only approximately 10% were able to produce IL-17, and most, but not all, of these also expressed IL-22. IL-17 + T-cell clones were derived from these cells; cytokine profiles of the cells revealed several subsets (Table 1). Of particular interest is the Th2/IL-17 subset, which produces IL-4, 10, and 13 (Th2) and IL-17 and 22 (Th17), and accounted for approximately one third of IL-17 producing cells. Induction of IL-17 expression in these cells could not be achieved by challenge with specific allergen, but could be triggered by exposure to staphylococcal superantigen.

IL-17 is a potent stimulus for the production of antimicrobial defensins, and their deficient production in atopic eczema has been suggested to account for the almost invariable colonization of the skin with *S aureus* in this disease. In this study, the authors demonstrated that IL-17-induced defensin induction by keratinocytes could be substantially inhibited by IL-4. Furthermore, while Th17 clones derived from patients with atopic eczema efficiently induced defensin production, cells of the Th2/IL17 subset were comparatively inefficient in this activity. These results highlight the complexity of the interactions between T cell subsets, defensins, and staphylococci in the microenvironment of the skin in atopic eczema.

G. M. P. Galbraith, MD

The treatment of facial atopic dermatitis in children who are intolerant of, or dependent on, topical corticosteroids: a randomized, controlled clinical trial

Hoeger PH, Lee K-H, Jautova J, et al (Catholic Children's Hosp, Wilhelmstift, Hamburg, Germany; Yonsei Univ College of Medicine, Seoul, Korea; Fakultna Nemocnica L. Pasteura, Kosice, Slovakia; et al)
Br J Dermatol 160:415-422, 2009

Background.—Atopic dermatitis (AD) is most prevalent in areas of reduced skin barrier reserve, like face and neck, especially in children. Treatment with topical corticosteroids (TCS) is limited due to heightened risk of treatment-associated side-effects, thus necessitating alternative AD therapies.

Objectives.—The primary study objective was to determine the efficacy of pimecrolimus cream 1% in children with mild-moderate facial AD dependent on/intolerant of TCS. Secondary objectives included effects on overall Eczema Area and Severity Index (EASI), head/neck EASI, pruritus severity and time to clearance of facial AD.

Methods.—A multicentre, double-blind (DB) study of ≤ 6 weeks, followed by a 6-week, open-label (OL) phase was conducted. Two hundred patients (aged 2–11 years) were randomized 1:1 to pimecrolimus cream 1% (n = 99) or vehicle (n = 101) twice daily until clearance of facial AD or for a maximum of 6 weeks (DB phase). Sixteen patients receiving vehicle were allowed to switch to the OL phase at day 22.

Results.—Significantly more pimecrolimus-treated vs. vehicle-treated patients were cleared/almost cleared of facial AD (Investigators' Global Assessment 0/1): 74·5% vs. 51·0%, $P < 0.001$ (day 43) [57·1% vs. 36·0%, $P = 0.004$ (day 22)]. Median time to clearance was 22·0 vs. 43·0 days (pimecrolimus vs. vehicle, respectively). Statistically significant differences for pimecrolimus vs. vehicle were also seen on head/neck EASI, overall EASI, and head/neck pruritus scores. Adverse events were mainly mild–moderate, occurring with similar frequency in both treatment groups.

Conclusions.—In children with facial dermatitis intolerant of/dependent on TCS, pimecrolimus cream 1% effectively controls eczema and pruritus and is well tolerated.

▶ This trial covers the younger age group (2-11 years) providing the evidence for the efficacy of 1% pimecrolimus in mild to moderate facial atopic dermatitis that had already been published for the older teenager and adult age groups in 2007 . Although the trial design was identical, the younger children showed a better and faster clearance of facial atopic dermatitis than older children and adults, a finding consistent with previous studies showing greater efficacy in atopic dermatitis of the head and neck. Interestingly, children in the vehicle group had a better clearance than the older children and adults in the treatment group. The study also showed a decrease in pruritus and a good short-term safety profile; however, what remains elusive, but needed, is the study for the youngest age group (< 2 years old).

S. Hill, MD

S. Fallon Friedlander, MD

Itch characteristics in atopic dermatitis: results of a web-based questionnaire
Dawn A, Papoiu ADP, Chan YH, et al (Wake Forest Univ School of Medicine, Winston-Salem, NC; et al)
Br J Dermatol 160:642-644, 2009

Background.—Itch significantly impairs the quality of life of patients with atopic dermatitis. However, only a few previous studies have examined the specific characteristics of itch in atopic dermatitis.

Objective.—To examine the frequency, intensity and perceived characteristics of pruritus among individuals with atopic dermatitis.

Methods.—Questionnaire reliability and validity were established in pilot testing. Survey participants completed the comprehensive, web-based 'Characteristics of itch' questionnaire. Participants provided anonymous demographic information and answered questions regarding itch intensity, frequency, timing, duration, location, associated symptoms and itch descriptors.

Results.—A total of 304 individuals with atopic dermatitis completed the web-based questionnaire. Itch occurred at least once daily in 91% of the individuals surveyed. Of the 32 itch descriptors rated by survey participants, 31 demonstrated a statistically significant positive correlation with the participants' ratings of itch intensity ($P < 0.001$). More than half the survey participants reported pain (59%) and heat sensation (53%) associated with itch.

Conclusion.—The questionnaire was found to be a useful tool in characterization of itch. Pain appears to be an important component of atopic dermatitis. The strong correlation between itch descriptors and itch intensity suggests that such descriptors serve as strong indicators of the symptomatology in atopic dermatitis.

▶ Although it may seem obvious that itching is the hallmark of atopic dermatitis (AD), this article provides some insights into the subjective and emotional motivations behind the drive to scratch. This is the first time I have heard the phrase "pleasure for scratching," which for many patients with eczematous disorders can be significant when no other remedies are available. Another interesting observation in this survey of patient answers to a questionnaire was the demographics of those involved, which should remind the reader that AD affects the middle class married male as much as it does a less fortunate patient without access to proper hygiene or moisturizing routines.

The real question then points to compliance of nonprescription strategies for prevention such as bathing, moisturizing, and avoidance of triggers in the management of AD that may further reduce the drive to scratch and therefore deprive patients of that pleasure. This article should suggest to the dermatologists that itching in the condition known as "the itch that rashes" should be managed more aggressively.

N. Bhatia, MD

First experience with enteric-coated mycophenolate sodium (Myfortic®) in severe recalcitrant adult atopic dermatitis: an open label study
van Velsen SGA, Haeck IM, Bruijnzeel-Koomen CAFM, et al (Univ Med Centre Utrecht, The Netherlands)
Br J Dermatol 160:687-691, 2009

Background.—Severe atopic dermatitis (AD) is often treated successfully with oral immunosuppressive drugs such as ciclosporin (CsA) or oral corticosteroids. However, some patients develop adverse effects or are unresponsive to these first-choice oral immunosuppressive drugs.

Objectives.—To evaluate whether enteric-coated mycophenolate sodium (EC-MPS) is an effective treatment in patients with severe, recalcitrant AD.

Methods.—Ten patients with severe, recalcitrant AD were treated with EC-MPS 720 mg twice daily for 6 months. All patients had to discontinue other oral immunosuppressive drugs due to adverse effects ($n = 8$) or nonresponsiveness ($n = 2$). Disease activity was monitored using the Severity Scoring of Atopic Dermatitis (modified SCORAD) index and the Leicester Sign Score (LSS). Additionally, the level of serum thymus and activation-regulated cytokine (TARC) was measured. During treatment, safety laboratory examination was performed. Total serum immunoglobulin E (IgE) was followed during treatment. Use of topical corticosteroids was recorded before and during treatment.

Results.—Compared with baseline, the mean scores for disease activity significantly decreased during treatment with EC-MPS [modified SCORAD ($P = 0·04$), LSS severity ($P = 0·01$), LSS extent ($P = 0·01$)]. In addition, serum TARC levels and total serum IgE levels significantly decreased after treatment compared with before ($P = 0·03$; $P = 0·05$). Disease activity decreased after approximately 2 months of treatment and stabilized during the 6-month treatment period. No differences in the amount of topical corticosteroids used in the 6 months prior to treatment compared with the 6-month treatment period were found ($P = 0·4$). None of the patients discontinued use of EC-MPS and only mild adverse effects were seen.

Conclusions.—In this study EC-MPS at a dose of 720 mg twice daily for 6 months has proven to be an effective and well-tolerated treatment for patients with severe, recalcitrant AD.

▶ Atopic dermatitis (AD) is a common chronic skin condition that is characterized by recurrent, pruritic, erythematous skin lesions with a profound effect on the quality of life. There is also a subset of patients who are unresponsive to traditional treatment. This is a study of 10 patients with severe, recalcitrant AD treated with enteric-coated mycophenolate sodium (EC-MPS) for 6 months. It has been shown that mycophenolate mofetil (MMF) is effective in the treatment of severe AD and is safer than cyclosporine because of the relative lack of nephrotoxic side effects, as seen with the latter agent. Unfortunately, MMF is known to have gastrointestinal (GI) side effects such as diarrhea and abdominal pain, which has been known to occur in 45.5% of renal transplant patients. Therefore, EC-MPS was designed to reduce the gastrointestinal side effects of MMF. The patients included in this study were not responsive to potent topical corticosteroids and/or UV phototherapy, and all patients had failed on immunosuppressive drugs due to nonresponsiveness or side effects. Complete blood cell count, lymphocyte subsets, total bilirubin, alkaline phosphatase, aminotransferase (ASAT and ALAT), electrolytes, creatinine, urea, and cholesterol panel were evaluated in the subjects. Patients were also asked if they had any subjective adverse effects at each visit. All patients reported a gradual improvement over 4 to 8 weeks of treatment with a 40% improvement in disease activity, and improvements continued to stabilize over the 6-month period. Adverse reactions observed were diarrhea, mild nausea, flatulence, mild headache, and tiredness, and 1 patient reported concentration problems. Patients also continued with the same topical corticosteroids; however, the authors did not attribute improvements to topical corticosteroids because there were no changes in potencies or regimens used. A limitation was that the study size was small. However, based on this study, it was concluded that the incidence of GI side effects was much lower with EC-MPS, and no laboratory abnormalities were observed during the 6-month course. They also found that a small but significant decrease in total serum IgE and a significant decrease in serum thymus and activation-regulated cytokine (TARC), which was used as a marker for disease activity, decreased over time. The potential for long-term susceptibility to opportunistic infection and malignancies, such as lymphoma, was not addressed.

G. K. Kim, DO
J. Q. Del Rosso, DO

Three Years of Italian Experience of an Educational Program for Parents of Young Children Affected by Atopic Dermatitis: Improving Knowledge Produces Lower Anxiety Levels in Parents of Children with Atopic Dermatitis

Ricci G, Bendandi B, Aiazzi R, et al (Univ of Bologna, Italy)
Pediatr Dermatol 26:1-5, 2009

The chronic course of atopic dermatitis is a problem for children and their families: it can be extremely disabling, and may cause psychologic problems for both child and family. As atopic dermatitis affects 10% of the pediatric population, pediatricians and dermatologists spend much time on the treatment of this disease, which requires a multidisciplinary approach. To improve the quality of life of children and families affected by atopic dermatitis we have offered an educational program to the parents of young children affected by the disease. The program consists of six meetings at weekly intervals involving a pediatric allergist, a dermatologist, and a psychologist. Our experience has been positive. This type of program may help to improve the quality of life of families with children affected by atopic dermatitis. Lower levels of anxiety were observed among parents at the end of the program. We believe that educational programs of this type, in association with conventional treatment, can be useful in the long term management of the disease. They may be considered to improve the quality of life of the family and children and to create more interaction and compliance between physicians, parents, and children.

▶ Atopic dermatitis is a chronic skin condition affecting 10% to 15% of the pediatric population under 5 years of age. While medical treatment is an obvious component, Ricci et al provide a persuasive consideration for physicians in treating atopic dermatitis, namely, to improve the quality of life of the patients and families through education of the condition. Positive improvements were reported, especially to anxiety levels, and suggest that patient and family education is a valuable element in treatment. While notable, the applicability of the study has its limitations, especially for smaller practitioners and sole practitioners with restricted resources and time. The educational program consisted of six 90-minute sessions involving a dermatologist, pediatric allergist, and psychologist in addition to the parents and patients, as well as multiple questionnaires. Also, while there was an improvement noted in quality of life for both parents and patients, the study was limited to children aged 5 months to 5 years (mean age of 18 months) over 6 treatments. Questionnaires relating to the infants quality of life were necessarily answered by the parents. Given the chronic nature of this condition, an interesting follow-up study as to whether there is a long-term benefit to such an educational program as perceived by the patient may be insightful. Additionally, a study including older children would allow the patient to independently evaluate the importance of such a program. Participation may also be a variable element. Most mothers (of the 30 participating families) were able to attend every session, but not all fathers, secondary to work obligations. The success of such a program may change depending on demographics such as single-family households or families of both working parents. Thus, this additional modality may be more of a hopeful consideration than practical. The program also is more time intensive than what may be practical in ambulatory practice. Overall, however, the article serves as an important reminder of the importance of both patient and family education, especially when treating pediatric dermatologic conditions.

B. D. Michaels, DO

J. Q. Del Rosso, DO

Cobalt-containing alloys and their ability to release cobalt and cause dermatitis
Julander A, Hindsén M, Skare L, et al (Stockholm Centre for Public Health, Sweden; Univ Hosp, Sweden)
Contact Dermatitis 60:165-170, 2009

Background.—Cobalt, nickel, and chromium are important skin sensitizers. However, knowledge about cobalt exposure and causes of cobalt sensitization is limited.

Objectives.—To study release of cobalt, nickel, and chromium from some cobalt-containing hard metal alloys and to test reactivity to the materials in cobalt-sensitized patients.

Methods.—Discs suitable for patch testing were made of some hard metal alloys. Cobalt, nickel, and chromium release from the materials was determined by immersion in artificial sweat (2 min, 1 hr, 1 day, and 1 week). Patch test reactivity to the discs and to serial dilutions of cobalt and nickel was assessed in previously patch-tested dermatitis patients (19 cobalt positive and 18 cobalt-negative controls).

Results.—All discs released cobalt, nickel, and chromium. Some discs released large amounts of cobalt (highest concentration: 290 μg/cm^2/ week). Seven discs elicited three or more positive test reactions.

Conclusions.—The concentration of released cobalt was high enough to elicit allergic contact dermatitis in cobalt-sensitized patients. As the materials in the discs are used in wear parts of hard metal tools, individuals with contact allergy to cobalt may develop hand eczema when handling such materials.

▶ This study is an important reminder of the much needed vigilance required for patients with positive patch tests to metals, particularly cobalt, as well as nickel and chromium. While the concentration of a particular element in a metal allow may influence the release of the allergenic material, there are numerous factors that may facilitate the bioavailability of these haptens on the skin, such as sweat. These issues pose particular challenges to clinicians, because the assessment of allergens in any metal object is very difficult. While the dimethylglyoxime test allows patients to readily analyze metal articles for the presence of nickel, there are few practical approaches for the cobalt or chromium allergic patient to make a similar appraisal. For patients with hand dermatitis, this could further complicate the prognosis as some of these metal allergens, particularly chromium, are associated with poorer outcomes.[1]

D. E. Cohen, MD, MPH

Reference

1. Hald M, Agner T, Blands J, Ravn H, Johansen JD. Allergens associated with severe symptoms of hand eczema and a poor prognosis. *Contact Dermatitis.* 2009;61: 101-108.

Ichthyosis vulgaris: novel *FLG* mutations in the German population and high presence of CD1a+ cells in the epidermis of the atopic subgroup
Oji V, Seller N, Sandilands A, et al (Univ of Münster, Germany; Univ of Dundee, UK; et al)
Br J Dermatol 160:771-781, 2009

Background.—Ichthyosis vulgaris (IV) is a genetic disorder with a prevalence of 1 : 250–1000 caused by filaggrin (*FLG*) mutations, which also predispose to atopic diseases.

Objectives.—To study the genotype/phenotype relationship in IV and to analyse whether the suggested skin barrier defect is associated with differences of epidermal dendritic cells.

Patients/Methods.—We evaluated a cohort of 26 German patients with IV, established an IV severity score and analysed epidermal ultrastructure, histology, filaggrin and CD1a antigens. Mutations were screened by restriction enzyme analysis. Particular sequencing techniques allowed the complete *FLG* analysis to reveal novel mutations.

Results.—The combined null allele frequency of R501X and 2282del4 was 67·3%. Patients also showed the mutations S3247X and R2447X as well as five novel *FLG* mutations: 424del17 and 621del4 (profilaggrin S100 domain), 2974delGA (repeat 2), R3766X (repeat 10_1) and E4265X (repeat 10_2). Their combined allele frequency in controls was < 0·7%. No mutation was found in one IV patient, all in all ~27% were heterozygous, and the majority (~69%) showed two null alleles. The IV severity score and ultrastructure showed a significant correlation with genotypes. Interestingly, CD1a cell counts showed a significant difference between nonatopic and atopic IV patients both with eczema and without eczema.

Conclusions.—We confirm that the mutations R501X and 2282del4 represent the most frequent genetic cause in German IV patients. The novel mutations are probably population and family specific. The observed differences of CD1a cells support the hypothesis that there is a barrier defect that predisposes to atopic manifestations, possibly independent of atopic eczema.

▶ Ichthyosis vulgaris (IV) is a disorder that has been associated with atopic disease in the past. Patients with IV may have mild orthohyperkeratosis of the epidermis and reduced or absent stratum granulosum (SG). Also, the hallmark of IV is represented by abnormally low numbers of often crumbly keratohyaline (KH) granules. This is a cohort study of 26 IV German patients with analysis of disease severity, epidermal ultrastructure, histology, filaggrin, and CD1a antigens. Authors were interested in evaluating the expression of CD1a+ cells in skin biopsies of patients with IV with and without atopic disease compared with normal skin. All patients were questioned about a history of eczema, allergic rhinoconjunctivitis, and asthma. Patients also had IV severity score based on clinical presentation. The combined risk allele frequency of R501X and 2282del4 was 67.3% giving a highly significant difference compared with healthy controls ($P < 5 \times 10^{-5}$). This study revealed that *FLG* null alleles R501X and 2282del4 have a high combined risk allele frequency (67.3%) in German IV patients. The combined allele frequency in 376 healthy German controls was 4.6% with 2282del4 being more common than R501X. The complete *FLG* sequencing analysis revealed 5 novel *FLG* mutations with a low frequency in the control population. *FLG* analysis confirmed a genotype with 2 null alleles in 18 patients (69.2%), one mutation in 7 patients (26.9%), and 1 female patient did not show any mutation (3.9%). The IV severity score ranging from 5 to 12 showed a mean value of 7.3 in all patients with IV. Those patients having one *FLG* mutation had a mean score of 5.1 in contrast to patients with 2 mutations, who showed a mean score of 7.8 ($P = .0053$). The frequency of atopic disorders in patients in IV with one *FLG* mutation was 71.4%, and the atopy frequency in the double null allele carriers was 66.7%. Atopic disorders in general were present in two thirds of the cohort in this study. Allergic rhinitis or high IgE level was present in 42%, but only 6 of these patients with IV reported a history of eczema. This suggests that allergic sensitization in *FLG* deficiency may develop apart from eczema, which reveals that *FLG* mutation confer a substantial risk for allergic rhinitis independent of eczema. Limitations to this study were the small study size and low ethnic diversity, which could have affected the data. Another limitation is a single institute site. The correlation of filaggrin antigen and histological stratum corneum (SC) with the risk of allele frequency was not consistent. However, the ultrastructure assessed by electron microscopy revealed a correlation of genotype and keratohyaline granules morphology. This revealed that there may be other genes involved in the pathogenesis of IV implying genetic heterogeneity between different populations. Although these results are seen in this group of individuals, results may vary with other ethnic groups due to genetic variability. Also, atopic patients with a history of eczema showed a significantly increased rate of CD1a+ cells compared with nonatopic IV skin. Authors confirmed that R501X and 2282del4 were the most frequent genetic mutations seen in German

IV patients. They also noted that differences in CD1a cell may confirm a barrier defect that predisposes patients to atopic manifestations independent of atopic eczema.

G. K. Kim, DO
J. Q. Del Rosso, DO

Allergic contact dermatitis to the hair dye 6-methoxy-2-methylamino-3-aminopyridine HCl (INCI HC Blue no. 7) without cross-sensitivity to PPD
Søsted H, Nielsen NH, Menné T (Univ of Copenhagen, Hellerup; Dermatology Clinic, Bagsværd)
Contact Dermatitis 60:236-237, 2009

---

p-Phenylenediamine (PPD) is used as a screening agent for hair dye contact allergy in the European baseline series. Evaluations based on the exposure from consecutively patch-tested patients generally confirm that PPD is an acceptable screening agent for hair dye allergy.

6-Methoxy-2-methylamino-3-aminopyridine HCl (INCI name HC Blue no. 7; CAS 83732-72-3) is used as a precursor in oxidative hair dye products. In 2003, an opinion from the EU Commission's Scientific Committee on Cosmetic and Non-Food Products (SCCNFP) indicated that the substance is normally used by the consumer at a maximum final concentration of 1% when mixed with hydrogen peroxide. The opinion of the SCCNFP was that 'The information (at that time) submitted (to the committee) is insufficient to allow an adequate risk assessment to be carried out. Accordingly, the SCCNFP considers that it is not possible to assess the safe use of the substance'. As of 2008, there is no upper limit for the use of the substance regulated in the EU Cosmetics Directive.

According to the cosmetics industry, the amount of HC Blue no. 7 used in hair dye products is more than 2000 kg per year. The local lymph node assay shows that the substance has sensitizing properties with an EC3 value 5.6% (E. Hoting, Schwarzkopf & Henkel GmbH, Hamburg, personal communication). The compound can be classified as a strong sensitizer.

The following case concerns the first reported case of contact allergy to HC Blue no. 7 in a consumer.

▶ p-Phenylenediamine (PPD) is a common allergen. Most allergic contact dermatitis (ACD) to hair dyes is caused by PPD or its chemical relatives. This report discusses an unrelated chemical as a cause of hair dye allergy. It is important to keep in mind when thinking about a potential case of hair-dye allergy, that other ingredients in the hair dyeing product, especially preservatives, fragrances, and other dyes, in addition to PPD, may cause the allergic dermatitis.

J. F. Fowler, Jr, MD

Three Times Weekly Tacrolimus Ointment Reduces Relapse in Stabilized Atopic Dermatitis: A New Paradigm for Use

Paller AS, Eichenfield LF, Kirsner RS, et al (Northwestern Univ Feinberg Med School/Children's Memorial Hosp, Chicago, IL; Rady Children's Hosp-San Diego/Univ of California, San Diego; Univ of Miami Miller School of Medicine, Miami, FL; et al)

Pediatrics 122:e1210-e1218, 2008

Objective.—Long-term, safe and effective therapeutic options for managing the chronic relapsing nature of atopic dermatitis are essential for improving patient quality of life. To minimize the risks of continued topical corticosteroid usage and potentially reduce the incidence of flares, we tested the efficacy and safety of a rotational paradigm of initial brief application of topical corticosteroid followed by long-term intermittent application of non-steroidal tacrolimus ointment to previously inflamed sites of dermatitis.

Methods.—In this 2-phase study, patients who were 2 to 15 years of age and had moderate to severe atopic dermatitis were randomly assigned to 4 days of twice-daily double-blind therapy with either alclometasone ointment 0.05% or tacrolimus ointment 0.03% (Phase I acute), followed by up to 16 weeks of twice-daily open-label tacrolimus ointment 0.03% (Phase I short-term). Patients whose disease stabilized underwent new randomization to double-blind tacrolimus ointment 0.03% or vehicle applied once daily, 3 times per week to clinically normal-appearing skin for up to 40 weeks (Phase II). Corticosteroid use was prohibited.

Results.—Of 206 randomly assigned patients, 152 completed Phase I; 105 of 152 were randomly assigned into Phase II (68 tacrolimus ointment and 37 vehicle). There were no differences in adverse events between alclometasone and tacrolimus (Phase I) or between tacrolimus and vehicle (Phase II). In the acute period, alclometasone-treated patients showed greater improvement in atopic dermatitis signs and symptoms; thereafter, when all patients applied tacrolimus ointment (short-term), there were no differences. In Phase II, tacrolimus-treated patients had significantly more disease-free days compared with vehicle, significantly longer time to first relapse, and significantly fewer disease relapse days.

Conclusions.—For patients with stabilized moderate to severe atopic dermatitis, long-term intermittent application of tacrolimus ointment to normal-appearing but previously affected skin was significantly more effective than vehicle at maintaining disease stabilization, with a safety profile similar to vehicle.

▶ Atopic dermatitis is a common and distressing inflammatory skin disease in children. It is characterized by exacerbations and remissions of dry and eczematous, pruritic skin. In treating children with atopic dermatitis, a delicate balance between efficacy and safety must be maintained. Although a number of therapeutic regimens are available depending on the severity of the disease, the mainstay of treatment thus far has been intermittent use of topical corticosteroids along with emollients. This article describes a new paradigm for topical corticosteroid and nonsteroidal therapy, the latter with topical tacrolimus ointment. Specifically, authors state that patients with moderate to severe atopic dermatitis showed greater improvement when using alclometasone for acute exacerbations followed by a 3 times weekly maintenance application of tacrolimus ointment 0.03% to previously affected skin. In other words, following stabilization of initial flare with corticosteroid use, patients apply tacrolimus once daily, 3 times a week to recurrently affected but normal appearing skin. The safety profile was reported to be similar to vehicle. Overall, this was a valuable study with adequate number of randomly assigned patients ($N = 206$) and with a follow-up period up to 40 weeks.

S. Bellew, DO

J. Q. Del Rosso, DO

Prevalence and risk factors for allergic contact dermatitis to topical treatment in atopic dermatitis: a study in 641 children

Mailhol C, Lauwers-Cances V, Rancé F, et al (Paul Sabatier Univ, Toulouse, France; Dept of Epidemiology and Methodology in Clinical Res, Toulouse, France; Toulouse Univ, Paediatric Hosp, Toulouse, France)
Allergy 64:801-806, 2009

Background.—There is little information regarding the risk of sensitization associated with topical atopic dermatitis (AD) treatment.

Objectives.—To assess the frequency of sensitization to topical treatment of AD in children and to determine risk factors associated with skin sensitization.

Methods.—Six hundred and forty-one children with AD were systematically patch tested with seven agents of common topical treatment: chlorhexidine, hexamidine, budesonide, tixocortol pivalate, bufexamac, sodium fusidate and with the current emollient used by the child. The following variables were recorded: age, sex, age at onset of AD, associated asthma, severity of AD, and history of previous exposure to topical agents used in the treatment of AD. Skin prick tests to inhalant and food allergens were used to explore the IgE-mediated sensitization.

Results.—Forty-one positive patch tests were found in 40 patients (6.2%). Allergens were emollients (47.5%), chlorhexidine (42.5%), hexamidine (7.5%), tixocortol pivalate and bufexamac (2.5% each). Risk factors associated with sensitization to AD treatment were AD severity [OR: 3.3; 95% confidence interval (CI):1.5–7.1 for moderate to severe AD], AD onset before the age of 6 months (OR: 2.7; 95% CI: 1.2–6.1), and IgE-mediated sensitization (OR: 2.5; 95% CI: 1.1–5.9).

Conclusions.—Topical treatment of AD is associated with cutaneous sensitization. Antiseptics and emollients represent the most frequent sensitizers and may be included in the standard series in AD children when contact dermatitis is suspected. Risk factors associated with sensitization to AD topical treatments are AD severity, early AD onset and IgE-mediated sensitization.

▶ The pathophysiology of atopic dermatitis (AD) and allergic contact dermatitis (ACD) are quite different. Over the years many studies have looked at the proportion of atopic patients in population groups who have ACD. Some studies have looked at prevalence of ACD in atopic persons.

This article purports to assess atopics for ACD to topical treatments. And it does that, but only in a very narrow and limited manner. The authors have chosen only 7 potential allergens. They have totally ignored the many allergens in topical vehicles, including preservatives and fragrances. They have not even looked for allergy to many active ingredients, such as several corticosteroids, topical antibiotics, etc. The results, as far as they go, show a low amount of sensitization to all tested allergens, although chlorhexidine did show enough allergy to be of interest.

Most authorities think that atopics are somewhat less likely to become sensitized (because of their innate immunologic makeup), but this may be counterbalanced by the fact that they tend to use many more topical agents than nonatopics. This higher level of exposure to potential allergens increases the likelihood of ACD, even in persons who may be inherently less sensitizable.

Unfortunately, this article does not add much to our knowledge on this topic, except for the few ingredients that they looked at. The article would have more impact if more potential allergens were included in the evaluation.

J. F. Fowler, Jr, MD

Regulatory T cells in atopic dermatitis: epidermal dendritic cell clusters may contribute to their local expansion

Szegedi A, Baráth S, Nagy G, et al (Univ of Debrecen, Med and Health Science Centre, Hungary; et al)
Br J Dermatol 160:984-993, 2009

Background.—Regulatory T cells (Tregs) have an essential role in tolerance and immune regulation. However, few and controversial data have been published to date on the role and number of these cells in atopic dermatitis (AD).

Objectives.—To investigate the number of CD4+CD25+FOXP3+ Tregs and interleukin 10-producing T regulatory type 1 (Tr1) cells in patients with AD.

Methods.—Peripheral blood and skin biopsy samples from atopy patch test (APT)-positive patients with acute- and chronic-phase AD were investigated. Immunohistochemistry was applied to identify CD4+CD25+FOXP3+ Tregs in the skin, while flow cytometry was used to detect CD4+CD25highFOXP3+ Tregs and Tr1 cells in the peripheral blood.

Results.—In the peripheral blood samples of patients with AD significantly elevated numbers of Tr1 cells were found. Although neither the absolute number nor the percentage of CD4+CD25highFOXP3+ Tregs showed significant alteration in the peripheral blood of patients, increased numbers of FOXP3+ Tregs were detected in skin biopsy specimens. All of the APT-positive skin samples showed epidermal dendritic cell aggregates, morphologically consistent with so-called Langerhans cell microgranulomas, which also contained intermingled FOXP3+ Tregs.

Conclusions.—Tr1 cell numbers were elevated in the peripheral blood and increased numbers of CD4+CD25highFOXP3+ Tregs were detected in the skin of patients with AD. The epidermal dendritic cell clusters in APT-positive lesional skin showed a close connection to the FOXP3+ Tregs.

▶ The role of regulatory T-cells (Tregs) is explored in this article as well as a comprehensive review on the expression of important markers such as forkhead transcription factor (FOXP3), which is a signature marker of regulatory T-helper cells, compared with other T-helper cell lines identified by CD4 and CD25 staining. The shift of T-helper cells to the Th2 profile is observed in atopic states. What is interesting in the article is also comparison with findings in psoriasis and chronic atopic dermatitis (AD), where the cellular balance favors lymphocytes of the Th1 profile. Populations of regulator T-cells displaying the FOXP3 antigen were high in the epidermis but not found in the peripheral blood in AD, compared with Tregs that stained positive for interleukin (IL)-10, secreted in high levels in Th2 immune diseases.

The reader should have a basic understanding of these balances when approaching the findings presented, but the conclusions presented by the author are important for demonstrating how the immune system attempts to balance cellular inflammation. The activation of the regulatory cells and, more importantly, the dendritic cells that promote their activity, by contact antigens discussed (eg, dust mites) may suggest new targets for therapeutics in lesional skin as well as systemic therapies given the changes in the peripheral blood.

N. Bhatia, MD

Contact hypersensitivity and allergic contact dermatitis among school children and teenagers with eczema
Czarnobilska E, Obtulowicz K, Dyga W, et al (Jagiellonian Univ Med College, Krakow, Poland)
Contact Dermatitis 60:264-269, 2009

Background.—Patch testing is an essential procedure in the investigation of eczema in children.

Objectives.—To analyse the frequency of contact hypersensitivity and allergic contact dermatitis among Polish children with eczema.

Patients/Methods.—During an allergy screening programme involving 9320 children aged 7 and 16 years, 12.6% reported symptoms of chronic/recurrent eczema. From this group, a representative sample of 229 eczema children underwent patch testing: 96 children aged 7 years and 133 teenagers aged 16 years. Patch testing was with 10 allergens: methylchloroisothiazolinone/methylisothiazolinone (MCI/MI), nickel sulfate, mercury ammonium chloride, thimerosal, cobalt chloride, potassium dichromate, lanolin, fragrance mix I, *Myroxylon pereirae* (balsam of Peru), and colophonium.

Results.—49.4% tested children were found patch test (PT) positive. 43.8% of 7 year olds with eczema were PT positive, with sensitization to nickel sulfate (30.2%), thimerosal (10.4%), cobalt chloride (8.3%), fragrance mix I (7.3%), MCI/MI (6.3%), potassium dichromate (6.3%), *M. pereirae* (3.1%), mercury ammonium chloride (2.3%), and colophonium (1.0%). 52.6% teenagers were PT positive, with sensitization to nickel sulfate (23.3%), thimerosal (27.8%), cobalt chloride (10.5%), potassium dichromate (6.0%), mercury ammonium chloride (2.3%), *M. pereirae* (1.5%), and MCI/MI (0.8%). The final diagnosis of allergic contact dermatitis was confirmed in 36% of 7 year olds and 26% of 16 year olds.

Conclusions.—Every second child with eczema is PT positive, whereas every third child is finally diagnosed with allergic contact dermatitis.

▶ Allergic contact dermatitis and contact hypersensitivity were thought to be more prevalent in the adult population. New data from the previous 5 years, including this study, prove that allergic contact dermatitis is equally prevalent in the pediatric population. Results from a previous study done by the North American Contact Dermatitis Group[1] and other studies, demonstrated that children with atopic dermatitis are equally prevalent to develop allergic contact dermatitis compared with nonatopics. The prevalence found in this study for contact sensitization among patients with atopic dermatitis is slightly lower than those found in different North American pediatric contact dermatitis series, where about 50% of their patients had atopic dermatitis. The levels of sensitization or contact hypersensitivity among atopic patients from this study were not higher than the general population of children tested to date. Patch test relevance was lower than reported in other studies, probably suggesting that children with atopic dermatitis could be at increased risk for contact hypersensitivity and not for allergic contact dermatitis, when compared with nonatopic children. This study does not compare the rate between atopic and nonatopic children, which makes it difficult to assess any significant differences between the 2 groups. The rates of positive reactions to the 10 different allergens tested are similar to those previously reported. No clear definition of the diagnosis of eczema was given, which puts in question the true diagnosis. Allergic contact dermatitis should be part of the differential diagnosis of children with eczema that do not improve with standard therapies or have a history consistent with contact dermatitis; in these cases patch testing should be recommended.

C. Matiz, MD

S. Fallon Friedlander, MD

Reference

1. Zug KA, McGinley-Smith D, Warshaw EM, et al. Contact allergy in children referred for patch testing: North American Contact Dermatitis Group data, 2001-2004. *Arch Dermatol.* 2008;144:1329-1336.

Effects of skin care with shower therapy on children with atopic dermatitis in elementary schools

Mochizuki H, Muramatsu R, Tadaki H, et al (Gunma Univ, Maebashi, Gunma, Japan)
Pediatr Dermatol 26:223-225, 2009

For elementary school children with atopic dermatitis, a skin care program using shower therapy was performed during the school lunch break for 6 weeks from June to July in 2004 and 2005. All 53 participants showed an improvement in their atopic dermatitis during the 6-week periods studied. Skin care with daily showering at an elementary school was thus found to be effective for the treatment of atopic dermatitis.

▶ This article suggests a helpful adjuvant treatment option for children with atopic dermatitis (AD) that can be implemented during school hours. However, the improvement in AD may be from additional application of emollients rather than the showering itself. Participation in such a study may have also resulted in overall increased compliance with other treatments occurring at home. This case series had no control population with which to compare the study group, and because there was no blinding of school nurses, an observer bias may have occurred in evaluation of improvement in skin conditions.

Overall, this study showed a practical method of adding a skin care regimen to an elementary school. This appears to have had a positive effect on patients and families with AD, both in regards to skin improvement and adherence to a skin care regimen.

S. Guide, MD
S. Fallon Friedlander, MD

The Relationship Between Sensory Hypersensitivity and Sleep Quality of Children with Atopic Dermatitis

Shani-Adir A, Rozenman D, Kessel A, et al (Haemek Med Ctr, Afula, Israel; Bnai-Zion Med Ctr, Haifa, Israel; et al)
Pediatr Dermatol 26:143-149, 2009

This study aims to investigate the impact of sensory hypersensitivity in children with atopic dermatitis (AD) and to evaluate a possible relationship between sensory hypersensitivity, sleep quality and disease severity in AD. Fifty-seven AD patients and 37 healthy children, aged 3–10 years, participated in this study. Disease severity was assessed using the Severity Scoring of Atopic Dermatitis (SCORAD) Score. The sensory profile was assessed using the Short Sensory Profile (SSP) and sleep characteristics were evaluated using the Children's Sleep Habits Questionnaire (CSHQ). The AD group demonstrated significantly worse sleep quality compared with the controls in the following CSHQ subscales: sleep duration; parasomnias; sleep disordered breathing and daytime sleepiness. Sensory hypersensitivity was correlated with lower sleeping quality. Severity Scoring of Atopic Dermatitis Scores was positively correlated with sleep anxiety and with parasomnias. Sensory hypersensitivity and disturbed sleep patterns were common in the children with AD that participated in this study. A possible common underlying mechanism of hyperarousability may account for both phenomena. Evaluation of AD children should also refer to their sensory processing abilities and sleep habits to create optimal intervention programs that will be better focused on the child and family needs.

▶ Atopic dermatitis can have a lasting negative impact on the quality of life for children affected with this disorder. It is the chronic nature of the disease as well as the unavailability of curative treatment that most frustrates patients and their families. Children are often left with extreme sensations of pruritus and pain, which interrupts sleep and limits activities of daily living. Moreover, previous studies indicate that children with atopic dermatitis often have developmental impairments that may be secondary to impaired sleep patterns.[1] This study further examines the relationship between sensory hypersensitivity and the quality of sleep in atopic patients. In fact, it is suggested that a common mechanism of hyperarousability is shared in both sensory hypersensitivity and sleep disturbance in children with atopic dermatitis. Data for this study were performed using parent-reported answers to questionnaires on their child's sleeping pattern and their responses to sensory stimuli. It should be kept in mind that parents may under or overreport their child's behavior. An important point for clinicians is to have a multidisciplinary approach in treating atopic dermatitis patients. In conjunction with treating symptom severity, also address sensory hypersensitivity by avoiding extremes in temperature, friction of tight clothing, and decreasing light and sound stimuli.

S. Bellew, DO

J. Q. Del Rosso, DO

Reference

1. Krishna MT, Mavroleon G, Hogate ST. *Essentials of Allergy.* London: Martin Dunitz Ltd; 2001.

Neonatal colonization with *Staphylococcus aureus* is not associated with development of atopic dermatitis

Skov L, Halkjaer LB, Agner T, et al (Copenhagen Univ Hosp Gentofte, Denmark; et al)
Br J Dermatol 160:1286-1291, 2009

Background.—*Staphylococcus aureus* in atopic skin has been associated with exacerbation of eczema.

Objectives.—To investigate a possible association between neonatal colonization with *S. aureus* and the risk of atopic dermatitis (AD) during the first 3 years of life.

Materials and Methods.—The study participants were 356 children born of mothers with asthma from the Copenhagen Prospective Study on Asthma in Childhood. Swabs from the vestibulum nasi and the perineum were cultured at 1 month and 1 year, from acute eczema, and from parents (vestibulum nasi and pharynx). AD development and severity were monitored prospectively.

Results.—Of the neonates, 5·3% had positive swabs for *S. aureus* cultured from the vestibulum nasi (51·3%) and/or the perineum (11·3%). Forty-two per cent developed AD, but without association between colonization with *S. aureus* at 1 month of age and risk of developing AD at 3 years of age. There was a 70% concordance for *S. aureus* carriage between neonates and parents. At 1 year of age 11·3% children had swabs positive for *S. aureus*. Fourteen per cent of children tested at the 1-year visit developed AD after the visit but before 3 years of age, but again, there was no association between colonization with *S. aureus* and the risk of AD. In children seen at acute visits the severity of AD measured by scoring of atopic dermatitis (SCORAD) was significantly higher in children with a positive culture for *S. aureus* in lesions.

Conclusions.—Colonization with *S. aureus* at 1 month of age is not associated with an increased risk of developing AD during the first 3 years of life.

▶ Previous studies have demonstrated that colonization with *Staphylococcus aureus* is increased in patients with atopic dermatitis (AD) and is often associated with an acute exacerbation of eczema or increased severity of eczema according to the severity scoring of atopic dermatitis index (SCORAD). The primary aim of this prospective longitudinal cohort was to determine if colonization with *S aureus* in neonates increases the risk of developing AD in the first 3 years of life. The results of this study did not show a correlation between the colonization of skin with *S aureus* in neonates with the development of AD during the first 3 years of life. However, in agreement with previous studies they did find a concordance for *S aureus* carriage between parents and neonates, in acute exacerbation AD skin lesions, and in severe eczematous neonates.

This study design would have been stronger if in addition to testing children of mothers with atopy the authors also included data from children born to mothers without atopy as a control group. Comparing the 2 sets of data might shed additional light to the role of *S aureus* colonization in neonates and the development of AD.

Infantile eczema commonly arises between 2 months to 2 years of age. According to this study, its development may not be correlated or predicted by the colonization of neonate with *S aureus*. However, because an association has been demonstrated between the colonization of *S aureus* and AD, it would be interesting to have followed these same children for longer than 3 years to possibly find a correlation between *S aureus* colonization and the development of childhood or adolescent/adult eczema. Perhaps the colonization of *S aureus* is a better predictor of the development of eczema later in life.

While this study's focus was not the clinical management of eczema, it should be noted that in agreement with previous studies, there was a correlation between the presence of *S aureus* in acute eczema exacerbation and many severe cases of eczema. Perhaps further investigation into the value of the empirically treating *S aureus* in acute eczema exacerbations and severe eczema cases (by SCORAD) even without signs of infection are needed.

J. Levin, DO

J. Q. Del Rosso, DO

Fluocinolone Acetonide 0.01% in Peanut Oil: Safety and Efficacy Data in the Treatment of Childhood Atopic Dermatitis in Infants as Young as 3 Months of Age

Dohil MA, Alvarez-Connelly E, Eichenfield LF (Univ of California, San Diego; Univ of Miami, FL)
Pediatr Dermatol 26:262-268, 2009

Fluocinolone acetonide 0.01% in a blend of refined peanut and mineral oils has been established as effective and safe treatment for atopic dermatitis in patients 2 years and older, including those with peanut sensitivity, for several years. We sought to study the safety of fluocinolone acetonide 0.01% oil and its potential for adrenal axis suppression in infants as young as 3 months of age. A controlled, open-label study was performed in children aged 3 months to 2 years with moderate to severe atopic dermatitis at two academic pediatric dermatology centers. Patients received topical fluocinolone acetonide 0.01% oil twice daily to affected areas involving a minimum of 20% body surface ratio for 4 weeks. Cortisol stimulation testing was performed at baseline and at the end of the treatment phase. Patients were monitored for medication use and adverse events. Efficacy was assessed using the Investigator Global Severity and Response scales. Thirty-two patients with moderate to severe atopic dermatitis were recruited into the study and 30 were evaluated with the Physician's Global Improvement Assessment tool. The mean body surface ratio treated for all age groups was 48%. Eighty-three percent of patients had marked or better improvement scores by week 2 and 96% by week 4, with 40%

completely cleared. No adrenal suppression occurred in the 24 patients that met inclusion criteria for hypothalamus-pituitary axis (HPA) axis analysis. No relevant adverse events occurred. Results of this study support the safety and efficacy of fluocinolone acetonide 0.01% in refined peanut oil vehicle, for infants as young as 3 months of age with atopic dermatitis. No evidence of adrenal suppression or adverse local effects was demonstrated after 4 weeks of twice daily treatment.

▶ Atopic dermatitis (AD) affects many children and can profoundly affect quality of life. This is an open-label study involving 32 pediatric patients aged 3 months to 2 years with moderate to severe AD involving at least 20% of total body surface area. Patients applied fluocinolone acetonide 0.01% in peanut oil twice daily for 4 weeks to areas affected by AD. Patients were also evaluated by global severity and response and watched for local adverse events, with none experiencing any relevant adverse events, such as atrophy or telangiectasia. Evaluation of the hypothalamic pituitary axis (HPA) with the analysis of cortisol levels demonstrated no cases of suppression. Although topical corticosteroids have remained the primary treatment for AD, consideration of potential adverse side effects is important clinically. This study was designed to address these safety concerns specifically using fluocinolone acetonide 0.01% in peanut oil in children, including very young infants. The efficacy, tolerability, and safety of this agent in AD showed excellent clinical response and very favorable safety in childhood AD.

G. K. Kim, DO
J. Q. Del Rosso, DO

Filaggrin mutations that confer risk of atopic dermatitis confer greater risk for eczema herpeticum

Gao P-S, Rafaels NM, Hand T, et al (Johns Hopkins Univ School of Medicine, Baltimore, MD; et al)
J Allergy Clin Immunol 124:507-513, 2009

Background.—Loss-of-function null mutations R501X and 2282del4 in the skin barrier gene, filaggrin (*FLG*), represent the most replicated genetic risk factors for atopic dermatitis (AD). Associations have not been reported in African ancestry populations. Atopic dermatitis eczema herpeticum (ADEH) is a rare but serious complication of AD resulting from disseminated cutaneous herpes simplex virus infections.

Objective.—We aimed to determine whether *FLG* polymorphisms contribute to ADEH susceptibility.

Methods.—Two common loss-of-function mutations plus 9 *FLG* single nucleotide polymorphisms were genotyped in 278 European American patients with AD, of whom 112 had ADEH, and 157 nonatopic controls. Replication was performed on 339 African American subjects.

Results.—Significant associations were observed for both the R501X and 2282del4 mutations and AD among European American subjects ($P = 1.46 \times 10^{-5}$, 3.87×10^{-5}, respectively), but the frequency of the R501X mutation was 3 times higher (25% vs 9%) for ADEH than for AD without eczema herpeticum (EH) (odds ratio [OR], 3.4; 1.7-6.8; $P = .0002$). Associations with ADEH were stronger with the combined null mutations (OR, 10.1; 4.7-22.1; $P = 1.99 \times 10^{-11}$). Associations with the R501X mutation were replicated in the African American population; the null mutation was absent among healthy African American subjects, but present among patients with AD (3.2%; $P = .035$) and common among patients with ADEH (9.4%; $P = .0049$). However, the 2282del4 mutation was absent among African American patients with ADEH and rare (<1%) among healthy individuals.

Conclusion.—The R501X mutation in the gene encoding filaggrin, one of the strongest genetic predictors of AD, confers an even greater risk for ADEH in both European and African ancestry populations, suggesting a role for defective skin barrier in this devastating condition.

▶ Eczema herpeticum (EH) is a recognized presentation of herpes simplex virus (HSV) infection occurring in patients with of atopic dermatitis (AD). EH is a disseminated infection associated with significant morbidity. Two common mutations in the gene encoding filaggrin (*FLG*) are R501X and 2282del4, which have been associated with the risk of AD and related traits. However, little is known regarding the relevance of *FLG* mutations in populations of African descent because most studies have been performed in populations of European or Asian descent. Previous reports suggest that African-American individuals with *FLG* mutations may be less common. This is a study of 278 European American patients with AD, with 112 having ADEH, and 157 nonatopic controls genotyped for 2 common loss-of-function mutations of *FLG* plus 9 *FLG* single nucleotide polymorphisms. Replication was performed on 339 African-American subjects compared with 177 healthy African-American controls. Authors sought to evaluate if *FLG* polymorphisms contributed to ADEH susceptibility. There was an associated with AD and R501X and 2282del4 mutations in European American subjects. The frequency of R501X mutation was 3 times higher for ADEH than for AD without EH. The 501X mutation was completely absent among 152 healthy African-American subjects, but 6 patients with AD among 188 successfully genotyped individuals (3.2%) were heterozygotes for the mutation. The R501X mutation was significantly associated with AD among African-American subjects ($P = .0351$), as observed in the European Americans. Despite the small number of patients with ADEH ($N = 32$), 9.4% of this group carried the mutation and the minor allele frequency was considerably higher (4.7%), resulting in a stronger association for EH ($P = .0049$) as observed in the European American subjects. There was not an observed association between the deletion mutation (2282del4) and AD or ADEH among African-American subjects. This is likely due to very low frequency of 2282del4 mutation among African-American healthy controls (<1%) and patients with AD (3.2%). This study of *FLG* polymorphisms in

2 independent and ethnically diverse populations of patients with AD demonstrated that the functional R501X mutation confers an added risk of ADEH. Furthermore, they observed a significant association between the 2282del4 mutation and AD and ADEH among European American patients, but this association was completely absent among the African-American patients with EH. Importantly, the combined R501X and 2282del4 mutations further enhanced the association for AD ($P = 1.21 \times 10^{-8}$) and ADEH ($P = 1.99 \times 10^{-11}$) among European American patients suggesting the combination of these 2 mutations may contribute to an increased risk of AD and EH. The results of this study highlight the importance of skin barrier function in antiviral response. The association between EH and *FLG* gene mutations may direct in aiding viral penetration and have functional consequences relevant to infectivity.

G. K. Kim, DO

J. Q. Del Rosso, DO

IL-23 and T$_H$17-mediated inflammation in human allergic contact dermatitis

Larsen JM, Bonefeld CM, Poulsen SS, et al (Univ of Copenhagen, Denmark; et al)

J Allergy Clin Immunol 123:486-492, 2009

Background.—IL-17–producing T$_H$ (T$_H$17) cells are key mediators of chronic inflammation in mice. Recent studies have implicated T$_H$17-mediated inflammation in the pathogenesis of human autoimmune diseases; however, the involvement of T$_H$17 cells in allergic disorders remains largely elusive.

Objective.—To investigate T$_H$17-mediated inflammation in human beings with allergic contact dermatitis; in particular, the innate response of keratinocytes to contact allergen, the induction of allergen-specific T$_H$17 cells, and the presence of T$_H$17-related effector cells in inflamed skin.

Methods.—Human keratinocytes were stimulated with nickel *in vitro* followed by measurements of IL-23 and IL-12 production by quantitative PCR and ELISA. Allergen-specific memory T cells from the blood of individuals with nickel allergy and healthy controls were identified and characterized by using a short-term *ex vivo* assay. Nickel patch test lesions and normal skin were analyzed for the expression of T$_H$17-related cells and molecules by using immunohistochemistry.

Results.—Keratinocytes were found to produce IL-23, but no detectable IL-12, in a response to nickel stimulation. Memory T cells isolated from peripheral blood of individuals with nickel allergy, but not healthy controls, contained T$_H$17 and T$_H$1 cells proliferating in response to nickel-pulsed DCs. Inflamed skin of nickel-challenged allergic individuals contained infiltrating neutrophils and cells expressing IL-17, IL-22, CCR6, and IL-22R.

Conclusion.—Our results demonstrate the involvement of T_H17-mediated immunopathology in human allergic contact dermatitis, including both innate and adaptive immune responses to contact allergens.

▶ Allergic contact dermatitis is in fact a contact hypersensitivity reaction to haptens, which historically has been considered to represent a T_H1 lymphocyte mediated response. Previous studies in mouse models have strongly implicated an additional role for T_H17 cells in this event. In this study, Larsen et al investigated T_H17 activity in human contact sensitivity to nickel. They first elected to investigate the ability of dermal keratinocytes to express interleukin (IL)-23 in response to exposure to nickel: IL-23 is a potent inducer of T_H17 cell proliferation and production of IL-17 and IL-22, which characterize this cell type. Primary keratinocyte cultures obtained from healthy donors responded to nickel challenge with IL-23 production, and additional studies showed that recombinant IL-23 induced proliferation of both T_H1 and T_H17 cells in human memory T-cell cultures derived from healthy individuals. Of particular interest was the further finding that exposure of memory T cells to nickel presented by autologous dendritic cells resulted in proliferation of IL-17$^+$ cells (T_H17) and interferon-γ^+ cells (T_H1) in patients with nickel sensitivity but not healthy controls. Finally, immunofluorescence revealed the presence of IL-17 and IL-22 positive cells in lesional skin of nickel sensitive patients; the presence of interferon-γ^+ cells was not investigated.

G. M. P. Galbraith, MD

Different effects of pimecrolimus and betamethasone on the skin barrier in patients with atopic dermatitis
Jensen J-M, Pfeiffer S, Witt M, et al (Univ of Kiel, Germany; Microscopy Services, Flintbek; et al)
J Allergy Clin Immunol 123:1124-1133, 2009

Background.—Genetic defects leading to skin barrier dysfunction were recognized as risk factors for atopic dermatitis (AD). It is essential that drugs applied to patients with AD restore the impaired epidermal barrier to prevent sensitization by environmental allergens.

Objectives.—We investigated the effect of 2 common treatments, a calcineurin inhibitor and a corticosteroid, on the skin barrier.

Methods.—In a randomized study 15 patients with AD were treated on one upper limb with pimecrolimus and on the other with betamethasone twice daily for 3 weeks.

Results.—Stratum corneum hydration and transepidermal water loss, a marker of the inside-outside barrier, improved in both groups. Dye penetration, a marker of the outside-inside barrier, was also reduced in both drugs. Electron microscopic evaluation of barrier structure displayed prevalently ordered stratum corneum lipid layers and regular lamellar body extrusion in pimecrolimus-treated skin but inconsistent extracellular lipid bilayers and only partially filled lamellar bodies after betamethasone treatment. Both drugs normalized epidermal differentiation and reduced epidermal hyperproliferation. Betamethasone was superior in reducing clinical symptoms and epidermal proliferation; however, it led to epidermal thinning.

Conclusion.—The present study demonstrates that both betamethasone and pimecrolimus improve clinical and biophysical parameters and epidermal differentiation. Because pimecrolimus improved the epidermal barrier and did not cause atrophy, it might be more suitable for long-term treatment of AD.

▶ The understanding of atopic dermatitis has changed over the past decade. What was once an allergic disease has become a collection of defects in immunity, the innate immune system, and the barrier function of the skin. This new science has turned out to support some time honored practices like minimizing bathing and maximizing moisturization, and has put others in a critical light (such as soaking baths to hydrate the skin). This article studies the effect of 2 types of therapy on skin's barrier function. A mid potency topical corticosteroid was compared with pimecrolimus, and effects on disease and skin barrier function were measured. The corticosteroid worked a bit better but caused more issues related to epidermal barrier integrity. The authors logically suggest that the pimecrolimus would be a more sensible long-term maintenance drug than the corticosteroid. Do I believe it? Yes. Will pharmacy plans care that it is a better way to manage eczema and now allow coverage? I doubt it. The practical take-home message from this article may be that corticosteroid minimization, especially with prolonged therapy, is helpful to the epidermal barrier, even if third party payers refuse to cover the better drug.

G. Webster, MD, PhD

Effect of sequential applications of topical tacrolimus and topical corticosteroids in the treatment of pediatric atopic dermatitis: An open-label pilot study

Kubota Y, Yoneda K, Nakai K, et al (Kagawa Univ, Japan; et al)
J Am Acad Dermatol 60:212-217, 2009

Background.—The efficacy of combination therapy with topical corticosteroids and tacrolimus in the treatment of atopic dermatitis remains to be established.

Objective.—Our aim was to determine whether a regimen of sequential application of topical corticosteroids and topical tacrolimus is effective in the treatment of pediatric atopic dermatitis. A second goal was to assess the impact of this treatment regimen on quality of life (QOL) and the response shift on QOL changes.

Methods.—The study regimen consisted of 3 phases. In the induction phase, patients were treated for a 2-week period with application of

0.03% tacrolimus ointment in the morning and application of a strong- or weak-potency corticosteroid ointment in the evening. In the transitional phase, they were treated for an additional 2 weeks with 0.03% tacrolimus ointment twice daily on weekdays and concurrent application of tacrolimus and a topical corticosteroid ointment on weekend days. In the maintenance phase, the corticosteroid ointment was discontinued and 0.03% tacrolimus ointment was applied twice daily for an additional 2 weeks. Daily application of tacrolimus ointment was then discontinued and replaced by an emollient with application of 0.03% tacrolimus ointment only when necessary for an additional 6 weeks. The Eczema Area and Severity Index score, Investigators' Global Assessment, severity of pruritus and sleep disturbance scores, and QOL evaluation were measured. After 12 weeks, the patients completed a retrospective version of the pretreatment QOL evaluation for analysis of response shift bias.

Results.—Eczema Area and Severity Index scores decreased by the sixth week, and continued improvement was observed during an additional 6-week period. Both the pruritus and sleep disturbance scores decreased throughout the study. Of patients, 90% showed marked clinical improvement at week 6 and 96% at week 12. On the Children's Dermatology Life Quality Index and the Infant's Dermatology QOL Index survey, mean QOL scores improved after completion of therapy at week 12. The mean difference between the pretest and the retrospective pretest scores indicated the presence of a response shift bias.

Limitations.—This was an uncontrolled, open-label study. Conclusions are limited by the small sample size.

Conclusions.—A fixed sequential regimen of application of tacrolimus ointment with tapering of topical corticosteroids may limit the long-term use and adverse effects of topical corticosteroids, while maintaining clinical control of pediatric atopic dermatitis and improving the QOL. The finding of a response shift bias suggests that parents/guardians underestimate the seriousness of skin disease and its impact on QOL.

▶ This article illustrates the effectiveness of adding a topical immunomodulator to achieve clearance and maintenance in atopic dermatitis patients. A practical method of adding tacrolimus ointment to a regimen and subsequently tapering patients off steroids is suggested. Their aim is to show that combination therapy may not only be more effective than monotherapy, but it may also better enable steroid-free maintenance therapy. A longer follow-up period and evaluation of relapse rate in this study would have been helpful. The conclusions that can be drawn from this study are extremely limited by the absence of a control group and alternate methods of therapy for comparison of treatment efficacy as well as disease relapse. Stratification of treatment and/or response based on body surface involvement might also have been helpful in developing an algorithm for treatment and maintenance of patients with persistent and intermittent disease.

A particularly interesting component of this study is the response shift noted in the quality of life evaluation. It has been suggested that patients with chronic diseases become tolerant of their disease states and adjust their expectations accordingly. Through retrospective evaluation of quality of life, it was shown that this response shift and improvement is even greater than patients themselves realize prior to treatment initiation.

S. Guide, MD

S. Fallon Friedlander, MD

Patient-Oriented SCORAD: A Self-Assessment Score in Atopic Dermatitis. A Preliminary Feasibility Study
Vourc'h-Jourdain M, Barbarot S, Taieb A, et al (Clinique Dermatologique, CHU Hôtel-Dieu, Nantes, France; Service de Dermatologie, CHU Bordeaux, France; et al)
Dermatology 218:246-251, 2009

Background.—The SCORing Atopic Dermatitis (SCORAD) index is used worldwide to assess the severity of atopic eczema. Patient involvement in the treatment process is of major current interest. There are very few validated patient self-assessment tools for atopic dermatitis (AD).

Objective.—To develop a self-assessment score for AD patients, the patient-oriented SCORAD (PO-SCORAD) based on the SCORAD index, and to assess its acceptability in a pilot study.

Methods.—A multicenter working group decided on the initial form of the PO-SCORAD. A prospective, single-center pilot study was then carried out to assess its acceptability and validity. A SCORAD and a PO-SCORAD were applied at baseline and after 18 days; the acceptability of the tool was assessed by questionnaire, its validity by comparing SCORAD and PO-SCORAD on both visits.

Results.—The study involved 15 children and 18 adults. 80% of the respondents found the questions clear and the form easy to fill in; 96% spent less than 10 min on it. A correlation was found between the SCORAD and the PO-SCORAD.

Conclusion.—This study shows that self-assessment is feasible in AD, and that there is a correlation between the physician and the patient scores. This study was the first step in validating the PO-SCORAD.

▶ The SCORing Atopic Dermatitis (SCORAD) index is used to assess the severity of atopic dermatitis (AD). There has been more attention to assess objective clinical signs of AD in patients and using patients in disease assessment. This is a prospective, single-center pilot study that involved 15 children and 18 adults using a patient-oriented SCORAD (PO-SCORAD) to assess its validity in correlation with the physician's SCORAD. The PO-SCORAD falls into 3 parts: an assessment of the extent of disease; parameters related to severity; and an evaluation of subjective symptoms. They also assessed the extent of the disease by shading areas of involvement and a description of the area involved according to the size of their hand. They were also asked questions concerning dryness, inflamed lesions, edema, and lichenification. Lichenification and edema were difficult for patients to assess, but over 82.8% of patients did not think that the testing was difficult overall. This pilot study found that self-assessment in atopic dermatitis was feasible. One aspect that was problematic was that the questionnaires were not distributed with an explanation or an illustration of the severity index for atopic dermatitis. The authors did solve this problem by including a picture of what they considered to be crusting and oozing lesions for the next similarly performed study. The correlations between PO-SCORAD and SCORAD were significant but modest. The authors also pointed out that their sample size was small and that there was a need for larger scale studies to see if PO-SCORAD and SCORAD have a strong correlation. In future studies, it would also be prudent to train patients and physicians on how to score lesions, including use of representative photographs, so that results are more uniform.

G. K. Kim, DO

J. Q. Del Rosso, DO

Lymphoma among patients with atopic dermatitis and/or treated with topical immunosuppressants in the United Kingdom

Arellano FM, Arana A, Wentworth CE, et al (Risk MR, LLC, Bridgewater, NJ; Risk MR Pharmacovigilance Services, SL, Zaragoza, NJ; et al)
J Allergy Clin Immunol 123:1111-1116, 2009

Background.—Atopic dermatitis (AD) has been associated with an increased risk of lymphoma.

Objectives.—To assess the risk of lymphoma associated with AD and use of topical corticosteroids (TCS) or topical calcineurin inhibitors (TCI) in a database allowing medical record validation.

Methods.—We conducted a nested-case control study using the United Kingdom–based The Health Improvement Network (THIN) database. We excluded patients with established risk factors for lymphoma. Cases of lymphoma were identified and classified after review of the medical records and hospital discharge files.

Results.—In the study population of 3,500,194 individuals, we identified 2738 cases of lymphoma (1722 non-Hodgkin lymphoma [NHL], 466 Hodgkin disease, 550 indeterminate cases; overall, 188 had cutaneous involvement) and 10,949 matched controls. AD was associated with an increased lymphoma risk (odds ratio [OR], 1.83; 95% CI, 1.41-2.36). In patients with AD referred to a dermatologist, the OR further increased (OR, 3.72; 95% CI, 1.40-9.87). We did not find any cases of lymphoma in TCI users; however, the number of patients exposed to TCI was insufficient to study any possible association between lymphoma and these drugs. TCS use was associated with an increased lymphoma risk (OR, 1.46; 95% CI, 1.33-1.61). The risk increase was dependent on TCS potency (OR for high-potency TCS, 1.80; 95% CI, 1.54-2.11). The increased risk involved both Hodgkin disease and NHL, especially NHL with skin involvement (OR for high-potency TCS, 26.24; 95% CI, 13.49-51.07).

Conclusion.—Our results show an association between lymphoma—especially skin lymphoma—and use of TCS. The risk increased with duration of exposure and potency of TCS.

▶ In the past, there has been an association between atopic dermatitis (AD) and non-Hodgkin lymphoma (NHL) in adults. This is a nested-case control population study of 3 500 194 with 2738 cases of lymphoma (1722 NHL, 466 Hodgkin disease, 550 indeterminate cases, and 188 with cutaneous involvement) and 10 949 matched controls. The objectives of the study were to evaluate if atopic individuals in the United Kingdom that were treated with topical immunosuppressants such as topical corticosteroids (TCS) or topical calcineurin inhibitors (TCI) had an increased risk of lymphoma. Those that were included had a history of AD and filled at least one prescription of TCS or TCI, with no other associated risk for lymphoma. Compared with nonuse, exposure to TCS was associated with an increased lymphoma risk that was potency-dependent (odds ratio [OR], 1.96: 95% CI, 1.62-2.37 for high potency TCS). The use of TCS was associated with a high risk of NHL with cutaneous involvement. The OR for users of low-potency TCS was 5.35 (95% CI, 3.34-8.57), whereas the risk for high-potency TCS users was 26.24 (95% CI, 13.49-51.07). The OR ranged from 3.85 (95% CI, 2.22-6.66) in users with less than 30 days of exposure to 82.91 (95% CI, 9.29-740) in users with more than 2 years of TCS exposure. Duration of TCS exposure also showed a strong association with the risk of lymphoma with cutaneous involvement. The association became stronger with increasing duration of exposure, whereas the association could not be observed in patients treated with low-potency TCS. Clobetasol was the most frequently prescribed higher potency TCS. Limitations to this study were that authors could not evaluate the cumulative amount of TCS use, and compliance of medication could not be verified. Authors could not evaluate whether the use of lower potency corticosteroids for a longer period of time would also be a risk for lymphoma. This study suggests that there may be a downside to over treatment of a disease with high potency topical corticosteroids. In addition, the use of TCI and the risk of lymphoma are still unknown because the number of patients exposed to TCI was insufficient to evaluate. Future studies will be needed to evaluate other diseases that require topical corticosteroid use to assess if patients with atopic dermatitis have an inherent risk of lymphoma or if higher potency corticosteroids pose a true risk for lymphoma.

G. K. Kim, DO
J. Q. Del Rosso, DO

The Course of Life of Patients with Childhood Atopic Dermatitis
Brenninkmeijer EEA, Legierse CM, Sillevis Smitt JH, et al (Univ of Amsterdam, The Netherlands)
Pediatr Dermatol 26:14-22, 2009

Atopic dermatitis mainly covers the period of infancy to adulthood, an important period in the development of an individual. The impairment of quality of life and the psychological wellbeing of children with atopic dermatitis have been well documented but so far no data exist about the impact of atopic dermatitis in childhood on fulfilling age-specific developmental tasks and achieving developmental milestones during this period, referred to as the course of life. The aims of this study were to: (i) assess the course of life and define the disease-related consequences in young adult patients with childhood atopic dermatitis and (ii) determine whether the severity of atopic dermatitis is predictive for the course of life, the disease-related consequences and quality of life later in life. Adult patients who grew up with atopic dermatitis were asked to complete a medical history questionnaire, the Skindex-29, the "course of life" questionnaire and a subjective disease-specific questionnaire. Patients with severe atopic dermatitis in childhood showed a significant delayed social development in their course of life. The results of the disease-specific questionnaire demonstrated remarkable high percentages of psycho-social consequences and physical discomfort caused by atopic dermatitis in childhood. Patients showed a severely negative impact of atopic dermatitis on their current quality of life. This is the first study that applied the "course of life" questionnaire in atopic dermatitis. More insight in the course of life, disease-specific consequences and quality of life of atopic dermatitis is of high importance, especially in case of severe atopic dermatitis.

▶ This article looks at the quality of life issues that occur with moderate to severe atopic dermatitis (AD). The changes in the quality of life and the course of life are examined. Developmental questions are very useful to examine and understand these common dermatoses that can influence development. This article identifies a decrease in patient well being and perceived quality of life with AD. One area that would have been nice to address within the article would be to compare the course of life with other conditions along with AD. The comparison of the severity of atopic disease with the consequences of this disease and the quality of life are demonstrated. This looks at atopic disease and its effect fulfilling age specific developmental milestones. This study should alert physicians to be prepared to find resources that will enable the family and the patient to deal with this chronic condition. It showed the severity of atopic disease is predictive of later consequences in childhood and a clear difference demonstrated between moderate and severe atopic disease and both the skindex quality of life and the course of life developmental milestones. This article is the first in the concept in the course of life evaluation, which is more comprehensive about social development. It allows us to look at the developmental parameters that are modified with the effect of the disease and the severity of the disease. Children with AD have demonstrated fewer milestones in their social development. It points out the need for an overall approach to the clinical care of these patients and the systematic evaluation of both the physical and the psychosocial consequences of this condition and the control of this disease and improving the quality and course of life parameters.

L. Cleaver, DO

Contact allergies in haemodialysis patients: a prospective study of 75 patients

Gaudy-Marqueste C, Jouhet C, Castelain M, et al (Höpital Sainte Marguerite, Marseille, France)

Allergy 64:222-228, 2009

Background.—Haemodialysis exposes patients to many potentially sensitizing allergens.

Objectives.—The primary objective of this study was to evaluate the prevalence of delayed hypersensitivity in a population of haemodialysis patients. Secondary objectives were to identify the possible risk factors for contact sensitization and to propose a series of skin tests adapted to haemodialysis patients.

Methods.—A prospective monocentric study was carried out in a nonselected population of haemodialysis patients. For each patient, medical history of atopy and allergic contact dermatitis, ongoing treatments (including topical ones), presence of eczema at the site of vascular access for haemodialysis were recorded. Allergological investigation included delayed hypersensitivity tests (European Environmental and Contact Dermatitis Research Group battery, tests GERDA, additional list and a battery of antiseptics and other dialysis-specific allergens) and latex skin prick test.

Results.—Seventy-five patients (41 men, 34 women, mean age of 65 years old), with a mean 3.8 years under dialysis, were included. Nineteen patients (25%) had at least one positive skin test and 13 (17%) a positive patch test to at least one allergen relative to dialysis process including eight tests to lidocaine–prilocaine cream and three to povidone–iodine. Tests results seemed clinically relevant since nine patients had localized pruritus at the fistula site and six patients active eczema around it.

Conclusion.—Contact sensitizations are frequent in haemodialysis patients and are linked to vascular access conditioning especially the use of lidocaine–prilocaine cream. Designing a specific test battery could help to diagnose the potential allergens and subsequently to give advice to avoid contact with sensitizing agents.

▶ Hemodialysis patients are a special population of individuals that because of the chronicity of exposure to unusual allergens may present with difficult to diagnose eczematous type lesions or pruritus. Patients who present in the clinic with potential hypersensitivity reactions may need more expansive patch testing to include rare allergens such as anesthetics, antiseptics, and preservatives unique to the recurring hemodialysis experience.

D. E. Cohen, MD, MPH

A correlation found between contact allergy to stent material and restenosis of the coronary arteries
Svedman C, Ekqvist S, Möller H, et al (Malmö Univ Hosp, Sweden; et al)
Contact Dermatitis 60:158-164, 2009

Background.—Metallic implants, stents, are increasingly being used especially in patients with stenosis of the cardiac vessels. Ten to thirty per cent of the patients suffer from restenosis regardless of aetiology. We have shown increased frequency of contact allergy to stent metals in stented patients.

Objectives.—To we evaluate whether contact allergy to stent material is a risk factor for restenosis.

Methods.—Patients with stainless steel stents, with or without gold plating, were epicutaneously tested and answered a questionnaire. The restenosis rate was evaluated.

Results.—We found a correlation between contact allergy to gold, gold stent, and restenosis (OR 2.3, CI 1.0–5.1, $P = 0.04$). The risk for restenosis was threefold increased when the patient was gold allergic and stented with a gold-plated stent. An increased degree of chest pain in gold-allergic patients stented with gold-plated stent was found.

Conclusions.—We found a correlation between contact allergy to gold, gold-stent, and restenosis. It may be of importance to consider contact allergy when developing new materials for stenting.

▶ Svedman et al report on an unusual manifestation of delayed type hypersensitivity to metal allergens. While we typically encounter reports and epidemiologic studies as they relate to eczematous or spongiotic dermatitis following contact with a provocative allergen,[1-2] this article evaluates an entirely different biological response to cell-mediated immunity to classically described contact allergens. What's more, gold allergy has remained a controversial topic in the contact dermatitis arena largely because of disagreements regarding the relevance of positive patch tests to gold, and its association to the dermatitis being evaluated. The study recruited consecutive patients who underwent percutaneous coronary interventions with either unplated stainless steel (nickel) stents or gold electroplated stents. After provocative patch tests, a risk of restenosis was associated with gold allergy and gold stenting. No association was noted with nickel allergy and nickel stents. Other investigators have correlated higher blood levels of gold in stented patients with higher rates of positive patch tests. In aggregate, these findings challenge the dogma that delayed type hypersensitivity reactions to classical contact allergens are confined to eczematous reactions and may have more far reaching consequences that could influence the bioengineering of implantable prostheses of all types.

D. E. Cohen, MD, MPH

References

1. Ekqvist S, Lundh T, Svedman C, et al. Does gold concentration in the blood influence the result of patch testing to gold? *Br J Dermatol.* 2009;160:1016-1021.
2. Ekqvist S, Svedman C, Lundh T, Möller H, Björk J, Bruze M. A correlation found between gold concentration in blood and patch test reactions in patients with coronary stents. *Contact Dermatitis.* 2008;59:137-142.

Tacrolimus ointment 0.1% in the treatment of allergic contact eyelid dermatitis

Katsarou A, Armenaka M, Vosynioti V, et al (Univ of Athens, Greece)

J Eur Acad Dermatol Venereol 23:382-387, 2009

Background.—Tacrolimus inhibits T-lymphocyte activation and dermal Langerhans' cells, without the side-effects of corticosteroids. The safety profile of tacrolimus makes it a promising therapeutic option for dermatitis affecting the delicate periorbital skin.

Objective.—To access the efficacy and tolerability of tacrolimus ointment 0.1% in the treatment of allergic contact eyelid dermatitis.

Patients and Methods.—Twenty adults (16 women, 4 men) with eyelid dermatitis and with at least one positive patch test reaction to relevant contact allergens were treated with topical tacrolimus in a prospective, open-label, non-comparative clinical study. Dermatitis was graded at baseline, at day 30 and day 60, using a 4-point grading system for the following parameters: erythema, oedema, scaling, lichenification, fissuring (investigator assessment) and burning/stinging and pruritus (patient assessment).

Results.—All patients completed the study. Erythema, oedema, scaling and lichenification showed improvement from baseline to 30 days of treatment ($P < 0.001$), but fissuring was not significantly affected. At 60 days, no further improvement of these investigator parameters was observed. Patient parameters improved significantly by day 30 ($P < 0.004$) and there was a trend for further improvement at the end of 60 days (for burning, $P = 0.046$; for pruritus, $P = 0.059$). Ten per cent of patients mentioned burning and itching, at the application site, during the first days of treatment. No other adverse events were observed.

Conclusion.—Topical tacrolimus is a promising alternative in patients with allergic contact eyelid dermatitis. Therapy was effective by 1 month and was well tolerated. These preliminary results merit a larger, controlled, study.

▶ The treatment of eyelid dermatitis can be problematic, as physicians are understandably reluctant to use topical corticosteroids, especially potent ones, around the eyes. Prolonged use of such preparations can cause local atrophy and telangiectasia, increase ocular pressure, and predispose to cataracts. In recent years, topical calcineurin inhibitors have been used as an alternative to topical steroids for various indications, especially atopic dermatitis. In this study, Katsarou et al examined the therapeutic efficacy of topical tacrolimus ointment 0.1%, in patients with allergic contact dermatitis of the eyelids. Patients with atopic dermatitis were excluded. Although the results were promising, the short duration of application (30 days) precludes evaluation of long-term efficacy and adverse events. As the authors acknowledge, this study should be considered preliminary in nature; a larger prospective, placebo-controlled trial comparing conventional therapy versus tacrolimus would be beneficial. Considering the medicolegal climate surrounding these drugs, it is doubtful whether one will be forthcoming.

B. H. Thiers, MD

Contact sensitization to fragrances in the general population: a Koch's approach may reveal the burden of disease
Thyssen JP, Menné T, Linneberg A, et al (Gentofte Univ Hosp, Denmark)
Br J Dermatol 160:729-735, 2009

Background.—Contact sensitization to fragrance mix (FM) I and *Myroxylon pereirae* (MP) is common among European patients with dermatitis. Recently, FM II was included in the European baseline series as an additional marker of fragrance sensitization.

Objectives.—This literature review aims to assess the prevalence of fragrance sensitization in the general population, and to suggest how future population-based studies and questionnaires should be constructed, better to assess the prevalence and burden of fragrance sensitization. This is of relevance as it is often difficult to establish causality in biological systems.

Methods.—A systematic review of the literature was carried out by searching Pubmed-Medline, Biosis and contact dermatitis textbooks.

Results.—Nineteen studies were identified, of which 13 were performed among adults. Sample sizes varied between 82 and 2545 tested subjects, and 11 648 subjects were tested in total. The median prevalence of FM and MP sensitization among adults was 2·3% (women, 1·7%; men, 1·3%) and 1·1% (women, 1·4%; men, 0%), respectively.

Conclusions.—Based on the reliability of patch test data from the general population and exposure data obtained from patients with dermatitis, the prevalence and burden of fragrance sensitization in the general population is significant (Table 1).

▶ The authors, particularly Dr Thyssen, have been seriously reviewing available data looking at contact allergy prevalence in the general population. Most data on prevalence of positive patch tests, such as the data generated by the North American Contact Dermatitis Group, is developed from patch testing patients

TABLE 1.—The Prevalence of Contact Sensitization to Fragrance Mix (FM) I and *Myroxylon pereirae* (MP; Balsam of Peru) among Children and Adults in the General Population

First Author	Year of Publication	Country	Population	n	Age	Female / Male (%)	Allergens Used for Patch Testing	Patch Test Reading Done at Day	Positive Reaction to FM I, Total, % (95% CI)	Positive Reaction to FM I, Females, %	Positive Reaction to FM I, Males, %	Positive Reaction to MP, Total, % (95% CI)	Positive Reaction to MP, Females, %	Positive Reaction to MP, Males, %
Studies performed in children and adolescents														
Weston[24]	1986	U.S.A.	Children	314	6 months–18 years	47·1	Standard series	3	–	–	–	1·5 (0·5–3·7)	–	–
Barros[48]	1991	Portugal	Schoolchildren	562	5–14 years	49·6	Standard series	2	1·8 (0·9–3·2)	1·4	2·1	0·4 (0·04–1·3)	0·7	0
Dotterud[18]	1995	Norway	Schoolchildren	424	7–12 years	–	Epiquick test	2	–	–	–	0	0	0
Bruckner[22]	2000	U.S.A.	Infants	85	6 months–5 years	43·2	TT	4, 5	0	0	0	0	0	0
Mortz[20]	2002	Denmark	Schoolchildren	1146	12–16 years	54·1	TT	3[a]	1·8 (1·1–2·8)	1·6	2·1	0·6 (0·3–1·3)	0·3	1·0
Jöhnke[19]	2004	Denmark	Unselected infants	543	0–18 months	49·4	TT	2, 3, 4	0·6 (0·1–1·6)	0	1·1	–	–	–
Studies performed in adults														
Forsbeck[8]	1968	Sweden	Twins	202	43–82 years	83·1	Standard series[b]	3	–	–	–	1 (0·1–3)	0·7	1·5
Magnusson[23]	1979	Sweden	Patients awaiting hip surgery	274	Mean 65 years	60	Standard series[b]	3	–	–	–	4·7 (2·6–8·0)	7·2	3
Seidenari[49]	1990	Italy	Male cadets	593	18–28 years	–	Standard series	3	0·5 (0·1–0·5)	–	0·5	0	–	0
Nielsen[11]	1992	Denmark	General population	567	15–69 years	49·2	TT	2	1·1 (0·4–2·3)	1·0	1·1	1·1 (0·4–2·3)	1·4	0·7
Mangelsdorf[10]	1996	U.S.A.	Old healthy volunteers	82	68–87 years	57·3	Standard series	2, 3	10 (4·8–18·3)	–	–	9 (3·5–16·8)	–	–
Greig[9]	2000	Australia	Healthy adult voluteers	219	18–82 years	61	Standard series	2, 4/5/6	4·1 (1·9–7·7)	4·5	3·5	2·3 (0·8–5·3)	3	1·2
Nielsen[12]	2001	Denmark	General population	469	15–41 years	58·8	TT	2	2·3 (1·2–4·2)	3·2	1	1·3 (0·4–2·7)	2·2	0
Schäfer[13]	2001	Germany	General population	1141	28–78 years	50·4	Standard series	3	11·4 (9·6–13·4)	–	–	2·4 (1·6–3·4)	–	–
Bryld[6c]	2003	Denmark	Twins	627	20–44 years	62·3	TT	3	1·3 (0·6–2·5)	1·3	1·3	0·2 (0–0·9)	0·3	0

Spiewak[14]	2005	Poland	Randomly selected students	135	18–19 years	54	Standard series[b]	2	–	–	0	0	0
White[15]	2007	Thailand	General population	2545	18–55 years	61·5	Standard series[d]	2	2·7[d]	2·1[d]	–	–	–
Svedman[21]	2007	Sweden	Stented patients	484	42–89 years	21·3	Standard series	3, 7	4·9	5·0	15·3 (12·2–18·8)	22·3	13·4
Dotterud[7]	2007	Norway	General population	1236	18–69 years	55·8	TT	3	1·7	1·8	0·4 (0·1–0·9)	0·6	0·2

Editor's Note: please check the original article for the full reference.
[a]Forty children were not read at day 3, but rather on day 2, 4 or 7. Some were also read by parents who had been previously instructed.
[b]Subsets of allergens from the standard series.
[c]Calculations made on subjects without hand eczema.
[d]Patch test results from testing with isoeugenol, *Evernia prunastri* and MP. CI, confidence interval; TT, True test; –, not given.

who present for diagnostic patch testing because of symptoms of dermatitis. In this self or physician-selected group, we expect to see a higher rate of allergy than in the general population. In fact, fragrance allergy ranks among the top 5 most common findings in these patch-test reports from the United States, with prevalence rates close to 10%.

As expected, fragrance allergy in the general population is less frequent. However, the data presented show that 1 to 3% of the populations examined in these studies is allergic to fragrances. This is a significant number, especially considering the widespread use of fragranced skin-care and household products around the world.

An area not examined in this article, but one of concern to many patients, is intolerance of airborne fragrance exposure, leading to upper respiratory discomfort. This complaint is also common and is probably unrelated to allergic contact dermatitis.

J. F. Fowler, Jr, MD

Delayed reactions to reusable protective gloves
Pontén A, Dubnika I (Malmö Univ Hosp, Sweden)
Contact Dermatitis 60:227-229, 2009

The materials in plastic protective gloves are thought to cause less contact allergy than rubber gloves. Our aim was to estimate the frequency of delayed reactions to different types of reusable protective gloves among dermatitis patients. 2 × 2 cm pieces of polyvinyl chloride (PVC) gloves, nitrile gloves, and natural rubber latex (NRL) gloves were tested as is in consecutive dermatitis patients tested with the baseline series. Among 658 patients, 6 patients reacted to PVC gloves and 6 patients to the NRL gloves. None reacted to both these types of gloves. Five of six patients with reactions to rubber gloves reacted to thiuram mix in the baseline series. Delayed reactions to reusable PVC gloves may be as common as to reusable NRL gloves. In contrast to most reactions to the NRL glove, the reactions to the PVC glove had no obvious association with reactions to any allergen(s) in the baseline series.

▶ Hand dermatitis is a vexing clinical scenario and can be a dilemma with regard to elucidating the causative agent, if in fact, the dermatitis is related to allergic contact dermatitis. Patch testing is the most reliable method of detecting delayed type hypersensitivity to haptens that patients may contact in their activities of routine daily living and work.[1] Allergy to rubber gloves and personal protective equipment is generally detected with standard allergen patch testing. This study reminds us that despite apparently negative patch tests, reactions may occur to items that contain heretofore unknown allergens and therefore are not readily detectable causes of a dermatitis. Patch testing to products as is may be useful, but the clinician should proceed with caution and ensure that products that are applied to the skin in this method are established to be safely used under these circumstances.

D. E. Cohen, MD, MPH

Reference

1. Warshaw EM, Ahmed RL, Belsito DV, et al. North American Contact Dermatitis Group. Contact dermatitis of the hands: cross-sectional analyses of North American Contact Dermatitis Group Data, 1994-2004. *J Am Acad Dermatol.* 2007;57:301-314.

Contact dermatitis in car repair workers

Attwa E, El-Laithy N (Zagazig University, Egypt)
J Eur Acad Dermatol Venereol 23:138-145, 2009

Background.—Occupational contact dermatitis (OCD) is a common skin disorder with a poor prognosis.

Objectives.—The objectives of this study were to (1) estimate the prevalence of CD among car repair workers, (2) study some risk factors associated with CD, and (3) conduct an intervention skin care education program.

Subjects and Methods.—A cross-sectional study was conducted in 87 car repair workers with regular and direct exposure to chemicals at the industrial zone in Zagazig City, Egypt and 76 unexposed assembly book-sellers. All workers were subjected to a questionnaire and clinical examination, and those who were diagnosed clinically as CD were patch tested. Intervention study with a skin care education program was carried out on 47 car repair workers. Re-evaluation of the intervention group after 5 months was done.

Results.—The total prevalence of CD among car repair workers (18.4%) was significantly higher compared with their controls (3.9%), with the highest prevalence among car mechanics (24.1%) and painters (20.7%); 16.1% of them reported recurrent dermatitis in the last 12 months. Nickel accounted for most positive patch test reactions (33.3%). A significant association was noticed between the prevalence of CD and age, smoking, atopic background and duration of work. After the intervention study, a significantly higher knowledge level about CD was reported.

Conclusion.—The most important risk factors for OCD among the car repair workers are atopic background and long duration of work. Skin care education program is an important tool for prevention of CD and control of exposure to substances hazardous to the skin.

▶ This comparative cross-sectional study or car repair workers with regular occupational exposure to chemicals and bookshop salespersons (control group) with no history of chemical exposures evaluated the prevalence and risk factors for occupational contact dermatitis (CD). The higher prevalence of CD in car repair workers (18.4%) as compared with controls (3.9%) is not surprising. The prevalence of atopic dermatitis (AD) in mechanics was slightly higher than in painters (24.1% vs 20.7%), with nickel being the predominant allergen (33.3%). This is significant in that presence of nickel in tools can be evaluated in advance, and other measures can be taken to reduce exposures as recurrent dermatitis was common overall (16.1%). Important risk factors for CD in car repair workers were atopic background and long duration of work. An intervention program inclusive of education on skin care, proper use of protective equipment, and use of gloves, barrier creams, and paper towels was shown to markedly reduce the intensity of signs and symptoms of occupational CD and the number of workers who experienced recurrent CD. This study supports the importance of education on CD prevention in the workplace along with programs, which provide protective materials and equipment.

J. Q. Del Rosso, DO

Contact allergy in chronic leg ulcers: results of a multicentre study carried out in 423 patients and proposal for an updated series of patch tests
Barbaud A, Collet E, Le Coz CJ, et al (Univ Hosp of Nancy, France; Bocage Hosp, Dijon, France; Hospices Civils, Strasbourg, France; et al)
Contact Dermatitis 60:279-287, 2009

Background.—There is a lack of prospective studies investigating contact sensitization in patients with chronic leg ulcers.

Objectives.—To determine the frequency of contact sensitization in patients with chronic leg ulcers using a special series of patch tests and to determine whether the number of sensitizations was correlated with the duration of the chronic leg ulcers.

Patients/Methods.—Multicentre study carried out in patients with chronic leg ulcers; patch tests with the European baseline series and with an additional 34 individual allergens or mixes and 3 commercial products.

Results.—Of the 423 patients (301 women, 122 men, mean age 68.5 years) with chronic leg ulcers, 308 (73%) had at least one positive patch test with 3.65 positive patch tests per patient. The main allergens were *Myroxylon pereirae* (41%), fragrance mix I (26.5%), antiseptics (20%), and corticosteroids (8%). The number of positive tests per patient was not correlated with the cause of ulcer but was increased with the duration of the ulcer with a statistical difference between the group of the <1 year compared with the group >10 years duration.

Conclusions.—From this large prospective multicentre study, polysensitization is frequent in patients with chronic leg ulcers, increasing with the duration of the ulcer. We propose avoidance of topical antiseptics and ointments containing perfumes in patients with chronic leg ulcers and an updated patch test series for investigating these patients.

▶ Chronic leg ulcers are commonly encountered in dermatology practice. This article sheds light on the possibility that agents we use to treat ulcers may be perpetuating the chronic nature of the lower extremity ulcer. The strength of this multicenter prospective study is that it met its objective by illustrating the increased frequency of sensitization to substances in dressings or topical medications used on patients with chronic leg ulcers. In fact, authors were able to show that the number of sensitizations per patient positively correlated with the duration of the ulcer. Polysensitization was an important finding in chronic leg ulcer patients. Although testing was performed in 4 different centers, no statistically significant difference between populations were noted. Authors suggest that all patients with chronic leg ulcers should be patch tested for contact allergens. The apparent limitation to this is that many dermatology practices are not equipped to conduct patch testing on a regular basis. The cost versus benefit of patch testing all patients with chronic leg ulcers may also warrant more detailed study.

S. Bellew, DO

J. Q. Del Rosso, DO

Treatment of *Staphylococcus aureus* Colonization in Atopic Dermatitis Decreases Disease Severity
Huang JT, Abrams M, Tlougan B, et al (Northwestern Univ, Feinberg School of Medicine, Chicago, IL;)
Pediatrics 123:e808-e814, 2009

Objectives.—The goals were to determine the prevalence of community-acquired methicillin-resistant *Staphylococcus aureus* colonization in patients with atopic dermatitis and to determine whether suppression of *S aureus* growth with sodium hypochlorite (bleach) baths and intranasal mupirocin treatment improves eczema severity.

Methods.—A randomized, investigator-blinded, placebo-controlled study was conducted with 31 patients, 6 months to 17 years of age, with moderate to severe atopic dermatitis and clinical signs of secondary bacterial infections. All patients received orally administered cephalexin for 14 days and were assigned randomly to receive intranasal mupirocin ointment treatment and sodium hypochlorite (bleach) baths (treatment arm) or intranasal petrolatum ointment treatment and plain water baths (placebo arm) for 3 months. The primary outcome measure was the Eczema Area and Severity Index score.

Results.—The prevalence of community-acquired methicillin-resistant *S aureus* in our study (7.4% of our *S aureus*–positive skin cultures and 4% of our *S aureus*–positive nasal cultures) was much lower than that in the general population with cultures at Children's Memorial Hospital

(75%–85%). Patients in the group that received both the dilute bleach baths and intranasal mupirocin treatment showed significantly greater mean reductions from baseline in Eczema Area and Severity Index scores, compared with the placebo group, at the 1-month and 3-month visits. The mean Eczema Area and Severity Index scores for the head and neck did not decrease for patients in the treatment group, whereas scores for other body sites (submerged in the dilute bleach baths) decreased at 1 and 3 months, in comparison with placebo-treated patients.

Conclusions.—Chronic use of dilute bleach baths with intermittent intranasal application of mupirocin ointment decreased the clinical severity of atopic dermatitis in patients with clinical signs of secondary bacterial infections. Patients with atopic dermatitis do not seem to have increased susceptibility to infection or colonization with resistant strains of *S aureus*.

▶ The objective of this study was to examine if the combination of dilute sodium hypochlorite (bleach baths) and intranasal mupirocin ointment treatment in patients with atopic dermatitis (AD) would decrease the disease severity and infection rates. Although a small study size, the conclusions drawn are valid that chronic use of dilute bleach baths and intermittent intranasal mupirocin application does have positive correlation with clinical improvement of AD with clinical signs of secondary bacterial infections. Patients in the nonplacebo group used 0.5 cup of 6% bleach to full bathtub of water for 5 to 10 minutes twice weekly. Mupirocin ointment was applied twice a day for 5 consecutive days each month by the patients and their household members. Patients in the placebo group used petrolatum ointment and plain water baths. No patient withdrew from the study due to adverse events. Patients in the treatment group showed significantly greater mean reducations from baseline in Eczema Area and Severity Index (EASI) scores, compared with the placebo group at each visit. Of interest, the mean EASI score for the head and neck (sites that were not submerged in bleach baths) did not decrease for patients in the treatment group. Patients and their parents should be educated on dilute bleach baths as adjunctive therapy for atopic dermatitis. It is effective and also inexpensive with minimal adverse effects.

S. B. Momin, DO

J. Q. Del Rosso, DO

Corticosteroids' Effect on the Height of Atopic Dermatitis Patients: A Controlled Questionnaire Study
Thomas MW, Panter AT, Morrell DS (UNC-CH School of Medicine; Univ of North Carolina-Chapel Hill)
Pediatr Dermatol 26:524-528, 2009

To investigate if children treated with topical corticosteroids have a significantly shorter height than the height of children not treated with corticosteroids and to see if corticosteroids affect the ability for treated children to meet growth potential defined as midparental height. Parents of patients attending the UNC's Dermatology clinic completed the survey. The patient's height and siblings' heights were measured by staff. Parents' heights were self reported as were the child's diagnosis of atopic dermatitis, and duration of use of corticosteroids. The patient's height was standardized using CDC charts. Additionally, the midparental height was calculated and standardized. The difference between present and predicted standardized heights was calculated; 151 surveys yielded data on 83 girls and 63 boys (ages 2–21 yrs). The standing height and the difference in standing height and midparental scores were not significantly different among: (i) children with and without atopic dermatitis; and (ii) children treated and not treated with corticosteroids. The overall height of children examined in this survey who were treated with topical corticosteroids appears to be unaffected.

▶ The goal of this study was to examine the relationship between treatment of atopic dermatitis (AD) with topical corticosteroids and the patient height. No statistical significant differences were observed between patients who were or who were not diagnosed with AD in either the standardized height or midparental height. The midparental height equation was used to determine whether topical corticosteroids were reducing height when compared with a child's genetic potential. Midparental height was also used because the children were from the same regional area and to minimize factors such as body mass index, socioeconomic factors, and general health by assuming that parents and children shared many of these factors. There were no significant differences in mean standing heights or predicted heights for patients treated with corticosteroids versus those who were not treated, irrespective of whether or not they had AD. Standing height was not significantly associated with potency levels of the topical corticosteroids. It was possible to examine the relationship between height and topical corticosteroids to see if a higher potency topical corticosteroid affects the mean height by breaking the patients into groups by potency. Mean standing height did not significantly differ between patients with AD and their siblings without AD and did not differ between patients who used topical corticosteroids compared with their untreated siblings. A limitation as stated in the article was that the study did not look at growth velocity; therefore, it is not possible to conclude whether the topical corticosteroid had any effect on rate of growth. Another limitation stated in the article was that the study included children over the age of 16, an age where some children have reached physical maturity. Therefore, it is impossible to conclude whether topical corticosteroid have an effect on prepubertal children who may later experience catch up growth during puberty.

S. B. Momin, DO
J. Q. Del Rosso, DO

Thiuram patch test positivity 1980–2006: incidence is now falling

Bhargava K, White IR, White JML (St John's Inst of Dermatology, London, UK)
Contact Dermatitis 60:222-223, 2009

Thiurams are accelerators commonly used in the manufacture of natural rubber latex (NRL) products, including medical NRL gloves. The thiuram mix (tetramethylthiuram disulfide, tetraethylthiuram disulfide, tetramethylthiuram monosulfide, and dipentamethylenethiuram disulfide, each at 0.25%) is used as a marker of rubber accelerator contact allergy. Although carbamates are frequently used accelerators, for some years, the carba mix has not been included in the baseline series of contact allergens. From the 1980s, there has been an increasing use of NRL gloves because of 'Universal Precautions', resulting in an increased incidence of contact allergy to thiurams.

Healthcare workers account for a significant proportion of those with hand dermatitis and thiuram sensitization. For the period 1989–1995, our group demonstrated a significant increase in the incidence of thiuram positivity in healthcare workers but no increase in other individuals using NRL gloves (e.g. housewives). We suggested that gloves with higher levels of accelerator residues, due to insufficient technical processing, were being introduced to meet the rapidly increasing demand in healthcare settings. We have now looked at our more recent data to determine whether higher quality gloves (reduced accelerator residues) and/or the widespread availability of non-NRL gloves have altered trends in thiuram positivity.

▶ Thiurams are a family of chemicals used in the manufacture of a variety of rubber products, including rubber gloves. They are found in both latex and nitrile gloves. This report follows the prevalence of patch test reactions to thiuram in a general patch test population and in health care workers. In both groups, the prevalence of allergy to thiuram rose from the late 1980s through the 1990s, then fell over the last few years. The authors speculate that this may be explained by increased use of vinyl gloves and higher quality processing of rubber gloves, especially in health care settings.

The weakness of this report is that it is from only one center, albeit the preeminent patch testing center in the United Kingdom.

J. F. Fowler, Jr, MD

Are we biased when reading a doubtful patch test reaction to a 'clear-cut' allergen such as the thiuram mix?
Uter W, Frosch PJ, Becker D, et al (Univ of Erlangen-Nürnberg; Univ of Witten and Klinikum Dortmund gGmbh; Univ Hospital of Mainz; et al)
Contact Dermatitis 60:234-235, 2009

The authoritative chapter on how to perform a patch test by Wahlberg and Lindberg states that 'Reading of patch tests is based on morphological criteria only. Reading of a patch test ... is a question of strictly following objective criteria'. The reading of a patch test is the first of three successive steps: (i) reading, (ii) interpretation as allergic versus nonallergic (irritant or unclear), and (iii) the evaluation of clinical relevance in those patch test reactions deemed allergic. However, the comparison of ratings of a 'Patch test quiz' before and after unblinding the nature of the substance seems to indicate that knowledge of what is being tested may compromise the strict application of objective criteria mandatory in the first step.

▶ Interpretation of patch tests is inherently somewhat subjective. A "borderline, doubtful, or questionable" test should show nonpalpable erythema, whereas a positive test (1 + or more) should have some papules or infiltration. However, experienced patch-testers know that certain allergens such as carbamate mix and cobalt often give an "irritant" reaction of mild erythema. Contrast that with most other allergens that almost never give irritant reactions.

This study looks at behavior of patch test readers when they know the identity of an allergen, as opposed to reading a patch test (on photographs) without such knowledge. A significant number of readers rated the patch test as questionable when they did not know that the allergen was a "nonirritant" but changed the rating to 1 + once they learned the allergen's identity.

Frankly, I do not find this surprising. Interpretation of patch tests requires both the art and science of dermatology. The thoughtful dermatologist will use all available information to decide when to call a positive patch test. There are 2 major weaknesses of this article. First, the reactions were graded from photographs—and no matter how good they are, photos do not substitute for live patient assessment. Second, nondermatologists were included in the panel.

In conclusion, while an interesting observation, this report is not surprising and should probably not change patch test reader's behavior.

J. F. Fowler, Jr, MD

Do 'cinnamon-sensitive' patients react to cinnamate UV filters?

Pentinga SE, Kuik DJ, Bruynzeel DP, et al (VU Univ Med Ctr, Amsterdam, The Netherlands)
Contact Dermatitis 60:210-213, 2009

Background.—Use of sunscreens has increased dramatically worldwide, and some sunscreen chemicals may be allergens. Ultraviolet (UV) filters are added to various cosmetic products. Cinnamate UV filters are structurally related to cinnamon-related fragrances.

Objective.—The purpose of this study was to determine if 'cinnamon-sensitive' patients show positive photopatch tests to cinnamate UV filters and, therefore, should avoid these UV filters.

Method.—We photopatch tested cinnamon-sensitive patients ($n = 18$) with cinnamon, cinnamon-related fragrances, *Myroxylon pereirae*, and two cinnamate UV filters.

Results.—No positive photopatch test to cinnamate UV filters was found (95% confidence interval 0–13%).

Discussion.—The risk of developing unwanted allergic contact dermatitis because of cinnamate UV filters in cinnamon-sensitive patients seems to be low, but our study population was small. Therefore, we recommend cinnamon-sensitive patients to perform a use test, for example the repeated open application test, before using cosmetic products containing cinnamate UV filters. In addition, physicians and patients should be aware that many sunscreens contain (cinnamon-related) fragrances and could, therefore, elicit allergic contact dermatitis in cinnamon-sensitive patients, independently from other potential sensitizing components of the sunscreen (Table 1).

▶ Fragrances are among the most common causes of allergic contact dermatitis. Cinnamon-related fragrance components are likewise among the most common fragrance allergens. Cinnamate derivatives are common sunscreen agents. We have always wondered if these ultraviolet (UV) filters would cross-react with fragrance allergens. This study evaluated 18 patients with cinnamon-related allergy with photopatch tests to cinnamate UV filters.

None of the patients reacted to the photopatch tests.

This suggests that we do not have to worry about allergy to cinnamate sunscreen filters in our many fragrance-allergic patients. However, we must remember that other fragrance agents in sunscreen products may well cause allergic contact dermatitis in these patients. The major limitation in this report is the relatively small number of patients.

J. F. Fowler, Jr, MD

TABLE 1.—Results of Patch Test and Photopatch Tests in 18 Patients

Category	Substances[a]	Maximum Patch Test Scores[b]					Total Positive Patch Tests	Percentage Positive Patch Tests (%)	Total Positive Photopatch Tests	Percentage Positive Photopatch Tests (%)	Upper Limit Percentage, Positive Photopatch Test, 95% CI[c]
		−	?+	+	++	+++					
Cinnamon	Cinnamon (30%)	11	1	2	3	1	6	33	1	6	
Cinnamon-related fragrances	Amyl cinnamal (2%)	16	0	1	1	0	2	11	0	0	
	Benzyl cinnamate (5%)	17	1	0	0	0	1	6	0	0	
	Cinnamal (2%)	14	0	0	2	2	4	22	0	0	
	Cinnamyl alcohol (2%)	12	1	1	3	1	5	28	2	11	
	Coumarin (5%)	17	0	0	0	1	1	6	1	6	
	Eugenol (2%)	14	1	1	0	2	3	17	1	6	
	Hexyl cinnamal (10%)	16	1	0	1	0	1	6	0	0	
Fragrance marker	Isoeugenol (2%)	13	2	0	2	1	3	17	1	6	
	Myroxylon pereirae (25%)	9	1	2	3	3	8	44	1	6	
Cinnamate UV filters	Ethylhexyl methoxycinnamate (10%)	18	0	0	0	0	0	0	0	0	13.1
	Isoamyl-p-methoxycinnamate (10%)	18	0	0	0	0	0	0	0	0	13.1

CI, confidence interval; UV, ultraviolet.
[a]Vehicle: petrolatum.
[b]−, negative; ?+, doubtful (or follicular); +, weak positive; ++, strong positive; +++, extreme positive.
[c]Only computed for cinnamate UV filters.

Delayed hypersensitivity to corticosteroids in a series of 315 patients: clinical data and patch test results

Baeck M, Chemelle J-A, Terreux R, et al (Université Catholique de Louvain, Brussels, Belgium; Univ of Lyon, France; et al)
Contact Dermatitis 61:163-175, 2009

Background.—Corticosteroids may cause immediate or delayed hypersensitivity. In 1989, based on structural and clinical characteristics, we put forward a classification of corticosteroids into four cross-reacting groups, namely group A, B, C, and D, the latter later subdivided into two subgroups, i.e. D1 and D2. The constituents on the D-ring of the corticosteroid-molecule are considered to have a central role for binding to skin proteins and for cross-reactions patterns; however, halogenation of the molecules is also interfering.

Objective.—To study the clinical data and analyse simultaneous positive reactions obtained in a large group of corticosteroid-allergic patients.

Methods.—Patch tests were performed with the baseline series, to which hydrocortisone butyrate and prednisolone caproate were added, as well as with the corticosteroids to which the patients had been exposed. Three hundred and forty subjects with a presumed or proven corticosteroid allergy were further investigated with an extended series containing 72 molecules.

Results.—Out of 11 596 patients investigated, 315 subjects reacted positively to at least 1 corticosteroid-molecule, with most of them presenting with multiple positive reactions.

Conclusion.—A prevalence of corticosteroid allergy of 2.7% was found. Despite validity of the ABCD (sub)classification in many cases, possible adjustments may have to be considered.

▶ Corticosteroids have been known to produce allergic and delayed hypersensitivity reactions. It is also difficult to determine which specific corticosteroids a patient has been exposed to in the past. Based on structural and clinical characteristics, corticosteroids have been classified into cross-reacting groups, A, B, C, D1, and D2. This is a study of 11 596 patients patch tested to hydrocortisone butyrate, prednisolone caproate, and other corticosteroids to which the patient has been exposed from 1990-2008. Sixty-six corticosteroids, including those from the baseline series, and 2 sex hormones (progesterone and testosterone) were tested. Ethanol was the vehicle used to test all corticosteroid molecules and petrolatum for tixocortol pivalate and budesonide. Ethanol and ethanol/dimethyl sulfoxide (DMSO) were also used as controls. In this study, 11 596 patients were studied using patch testing with 315 subjects reacting positively to at least one corticosteroid molecule, and 267 patients (85%) reacted to more than one corticosteroid. Among the 315 positive reacting patients, 74 were men (24%), and 241 (76%) were women. The most frequent occupations of the corticosteroid allergic patients were: housewife (18%), office work (17%), retired (7%), housekeeping (6%), education (5%), student (5%), and health care (4%). Atopic history was found in 108/315 patients (34%) (atopic eczema

23%, asthma 11%, and rhinoconjunctivitis 19%) and familial atopy in 119/315 patients (38%). Personal atopy history and contact allergy were found to be significant (*P* < .01). The skin was the most frequent sensitization route in 235 of 315 patients. Twenty-two patients (7%) were probably sensitized by inhalation corticosteroids, 15 were taking care of patients who used corticosteroids on a regular basis. Nineteen (6%) patients became sensitized by ophthalmic preparations. Affected areas were hand (25%), legs (21%), face (20%), feet (17%), and generalized (14%). Patch test results revealed that 191 (61%) reacted to budesonide, 135 (43%) to tixocortol pivalate, 96 (31%) to hydrocortisone 17-butyrate, and 70 (22%) to prednisolone caproate. Notably, 266 of 315 patients (84%) also reacted to other allergens; the most frequent being fragrance mix (29%), nickel (23%), *Myroxylon Pereira* (19%), and lanolin (17%). The investigators found that 3 times more women than men had corticosteroid allergy, which differed significantly from the total population of patients tested. They also observed that there was a significant difference in the prevalence of personal atopic background and that this was a risk factor for corticosteroid allergy. Results revealed that there is cross reactivity between corticosteroids. One limitation to this study was that weak irritant reactions to DMSO/ethanol could not be completely ruled out. Most patients were sensitized by the cutaneous route, which is consistent with past studies. The prevalence of corticosteroid allergy was found to be 2.7% in this study and suggest that the ABCD classification may need some modification.

G. K. Kim, DO

J. Q. Del Rosso, DO

Association between positive patch tests to epoxy resin and fragrance mix I ingredients
Andersen KE, Christensen LP, Vølund A, et al (Univ of Southern Denmark; Skovholmvej Charlottenlund, Denmark)
Contact Dermatitis 60:155-157, 2009

Background.—Both epoxy resin (diglycidyl ether of bisphenol A) and fragrance mix I are included in the European baseline series of contact allergens. A significant association between positive reactions to epoxy resin and fragrance mix has been reported by others.

Objective.—To investigate and possibly reproduce this association with the use of TRUE® test data and supplementary tests with fragrance mix ingredients from the Department of Dermatology, Odense University Hospital.

Materials and Methods.—Six thousand one hundred and fifteen consecutive eczema patients tested from 1995 to 2007 were included, and test results from all patients tested with fragrance mix ingredients were analysed.

Results.—One hundred and forty-five (2.4%) were positive to epoxy resin and 282 (4.6%) were positive to fragrance mix I. Nineteen were positive to both giving an odds ratio of 3.3, which is significant

(95% CI 2.0–5.4). Analysis of association to individual fragrance mix ingredients showed a significant association to α-amyl cinnamal and isoeugenol.

Conclusions.—The significant association between positive reactions to epoxy resin and fragrance mix I was reproduced. However, the clinical implications are not clarified, and even though the association may be coincidental, the fact that it can be reproduced with a different patch test system and in a different population speaks against a random result. Further studies may help to interpret the association.

▶ This study was designed to further explore the reported association of positive patch tests to fragrances and epoxy resin. Other reports came from centers using allergens in petrolatum, while this article reported on testing with *true* test panels. The sample size was quite large (over 6000 patients). As in previous reports, there was a correlation between patch test reactions to each of these allergens (odds ratio 3.3).

While this article confirms that there is a statistical correlation between these 2 very different allergens, it does not help us understand why this should occur. There are some chemical similarities in an aromatic ring structure between several of the fragrance mix components and epoxy resin. Because there do not seem to be any clinical reasons for these 2 allergens to react in the same patients, these chemical similarities may explain the findings.

J. F. Fowler, Jr, MD

Patch Tests in Children with Suspected Allergic Contact Dermatitis: A Prospective Study and Review of the Literature
de Waard-van der Spek FB, Oranje AP (Erasmus MC-Sophia Children's Hosp, Rotterdam, The Netherlands)
Dermatology 218:119-125, 2009

Aims.—The results of patch testing in children visiting our out-patient clinic with suspected allergic contact dermatitis (ACD) were prospectively investigated and compared with those reported in the literature. A review of the literature on patch testing and ACD in children is provided.

Methods.—Children were patch tested using the TRUE® test, supplemented with tixocortol-17-pivalate, budesonide and 3 commonly used emollients. Supplementary patch tests were undertaken on indication.

Results.—Seventy-nine children (31 boys and 48 girls) were patch tested. Of the patients tested, 40 (51%) had 1 or more positive allergic patch test reactions. Twenty-two (55%) of these 40 children suffered from atopic dermatitis, 9 (23%) from hand or foot dermatitis, and 9 (23%) from other skin ailments. Nickel was the most common contact allergen, but many other common and less common allergens were noted to give positive patch tests in patients.

Conclusion.—Sensitization to contact allergens may begin in infancy and continue to be more common in toddlers and young children. In recalcitrant atopic dermatitis, especially at the age of 5 years and over, patch tests are indicated. Good information on preventing the development of ACD in children is useful for caregivers.

▶ Allergic contact dermatitis (ACD) is a common disease in children that can occur at any age in childhood, including in infancy. This is a prospective study of results obtained from patch testing of 79 children who had suspected ACD as compared with results found in literature. There were 40 patients (51%) who patch tested positive for one or more allergens, with 55% exhibiting atopic dermatitis. All patients with suspected ACD by history, or by localization, or with uncontrolled or deteriorating atopic dermatitis, were patch tested using recognized criteria. Subjects included for patch testing were refractory atopic dermatitis in 47 patients, localized hand and/or foot eczema without atopy in 18 patients, and other clinical presentations in 14 patients (localized eczema on the lower leg, perioral dermatitis, pruritus, suspected contact allergic reaction to several topical drugs). Nickel was found to be the most common contact allergen in children younger than 18 years of age. In atopic and non-atopic children with foot eczema, they studied allergies to components in the patient's own shoes in addition to various known allergens and found that 6 patients were allergic to their own shoes and that 3 patients were atopic. This study supports the notion that ACD is common in children with both atopic and non-atopic dermatitis. They also found that ACD is common in atopic children, because they are exposed to more sensitizers due to a damaged epidermal barrier and the use of several topical medications and skin care products. This study also confirmed that ACD increases with age similar to that reported in other studies suggesting that children with atopic dermatitis are exposed to more sensitizers over time. They also explored the possibility of early sensitization at as young as 6 years of age related to skin piercing, dental braces, and exposure to hospital metal rails. The authors suggest that patch testing should be considered in any child with eczematous or nonspecific dermatitis that is difficult to control. It was also suggested that children should be tested strictly based on the indication used in a standardized protocol and that a negative patch test result does not exclude contact dermatitis. Although patch testing may be limited as to what potential allergens can be tested, it is a good indication to help a child with future avoidance. It was also pointed out that resistant foot dermatitis can be an indication of allergies to chemicals or material from the shoes.

This is important as an eczematous foot eruption may erroneously be treated as tinea pedis empirically, especially by non-dermatologists who are not aware that dermatophyte infections other than tinea capitis are rare in children. A limitation of this study was that the authors did not describe what they considered to be a true positive patch test result, as patch testing results do vary in intensity. Some reactions may look strongly positive with the presence of blisters, whereas others may look equivocal with minimal erythema. There was also no discussion of possible false positives and any measures to exclude such results from the study.

G. K. Kim, DO
J. Q. Del Rosso, DO

Differential effects of skin nerves on allergic skin inflammation

Vieira dos Santos R, Metz M, Lima HC, et al (Charité-Universitätsmedizin Berlin, Charitéplatz, Germany)
Allergy 64:496-502, 2009

In this study, we report – for the first time – a quantitative assessment of all four features of allergic skin inflammation (i.e. rubor, calor, tumor, and pruritus) in allergen- and histamine-induced skin responses in the absence and presence of fully functional sensory skin nerves, and we show that sensory skin nerves differentially modulate allergic inflammatory reactions in human skin.

▶ Neuroimmune interactions in the manifestations of atopic skin reactions have been the subject of increasing interest in recent years. It is generally accepted that activation of primary afferent nerves by diverse local insults or reflexes can result in the release of bioactive neuropeptides such as substance P from sensory nerve endings. These peptides can modulate the functions of a variety of cells such as mast cells (degranulation) and vascular smooth muscle cells (vasodilation). In fact the flare or erythema of the wheal-and-flare reaction observed in a positive skin test for allergy is thought to be due in large part to the production of neuropeptides stimulated by axonal reflex. Several previous studies have revealed that the flare reaction can be largely inhibited by surgical sensory denervation, neuropeptide antagonists, or the administration of local anesthetics. This publication by Vieira dos Santos et al similarly reports that skin test erythema in atopic human volunteers was significantly reduced, but not abrogated, by the application of lidocaine/prilocaine cream, whereas the effect on the wheal or pruritus associated with the skin test response was not affected. Some inhibition of skin temperature elevation was also found and stated to be statistically significant: the methodology used for statistical analysis was not given.

G. M. P. Galbraith, MD

Toll-like receptor 2 is important for the T_H1 response to cutaneous sensitization

Jin H, Kumar L, Mathias C, et al (Harvard Med School, Boston; et al)
J Allergy Clin Immunol 123:875-882, 2009

Background.—Atopic dermatitis and allergic contact dermatitis are skin disorders triggered by epicutaneous sensitization with protein antigens and contact sensitization with haptens, respectively. Skin is colonized with bacteria, which are a source of Toll-like receptor (TLR) 2 ligands.

Objective.—We sought to examine the role of TLR2 in murine models of atopic dermatitis and allergic contact dermatitis.

Methods.—TLR2$^{-/-}$ mice and wild-type littermates were epicutaneously sensitized with ovalbumin (OVA) or contact sensitized with oxazolone (OX). Skin histology was assessed by means of hematoxylin and eosin staining and immunohistochemistry. Ear swelling was measured with a micrometer. Cytokine mRNA expression was examined by means of quantitative RT-PCR. Antibody levels and splenocyte secretion of cytokines in response to OVA stimulation were measured by means of ELISA. Dendritic cells were examined for their ability to polarize T-cell receptor/ OVA transgenic naive T cells to T_H1 and T_H2.

Results.—In response to OVA sensitization, TLR2$^{-/-}$ mice experienced skin infiltration with eosinophils and CD4$^+$ cells, as well as upregulation of T_H2 cytokine mRNAs that was comparable with that seen in wild-type littermates. In contrast, epidermal thickening, IFN-γ expression in the skin, IFN-γ production by splenocytes, and IgG2a anti-OVA antibody levels were impaired in TLR2$^{-/-}$ mice. After OX ear challenge, contact sensitized TLR2$^{-/-}$ mice exhibited defective ear swelling with impaired cellular infiltration, decreased epidermal thickening and local IFN-γ expression, and impaired OX-specific IgG2a responses. Dendritic cells from TLR2$^{-/-}$ mice induced significantly lower production of IFN-γ but normal IL-4 and IL-13 production in naive T cells.

Conclusions.—These results indicate that TLR2 promotes the IFN-γ response to cutaneously introduced antigens.

▶ This is a careful and thorough investigation of the role of toll-like receptor 2 (TLR2) in the pathogenesis of atopic and contact dermatitis. TLR2 recognizes a wide variety of microbial-associated ligands, and is expressed by numerous cell types, both immune and nonimmune, including dendritic cells and keratinocytes. In general, TLR2 activation tends to result in polarization of T lymphocytes toward T_H1 responses through the production of interferon-gamma. Although acute atopic dermatitis is primarily a T_H2 event, a predominantly T_H1 response is observed in contact dermatitis. Several previous studies provided evidence of inhibition of allergic responses by TLR2 activation. Jin et al investigated the hypothesis that TLR2 activation promotes a T_H1 response to antigens and haptens introduced cutaneously, using a TLR2 knockout murine model. The results clearly showed that while the knockout mice were able to mount a normal T_H2 response to ovalbumin, their T_H1 response was significantly compromised. This was particularly evident in the marked reduction of IFN-γ production in these mice when compared with wild-type animals, which also occurred in mice challenged with the hapten oxazolone. Thus, TLR2 signaling appears to play a role in T_H1 responses in the skin, at least in mice.

An interesting additional finding in these studies was the upregulation of TLR2 itself in the skin of mice subjected to antigen/hapten challenge. The application of oxazolone to the skin resulted in a 7-fold increase of TLR2 mRNA expression, while tape stripping of the skin before exposure to ovalbumin caused a 3-fold increase. The authors compare this scenario with scratching (which, as we have all been told, will only make things worse).

G. M. P. Galbraith, MD

The prevalence and morbidity of sensitization to fragrance mix I in the general population

Thyssen JP, Linneberg A, Menné T, et al (Univ of Copenhagen, Denmark; Glostrup Univ Hosp, Denmark; et al)
Br J Dermatol 161:95-101, 2009

Background.—The prevalence of sensitization to fragrance mix (FM) I and *Myroxylon* pereirae (MP, balsam of Peru) has decreased in recent years among Danish women with dermatitis.

Objectives.—This study investigated whether the decrease could be confirmed among women in the general population. Furthermore, it addressed the morbidity of FM I sensitization.

Methods.—In 1990, 1998 and 2006, 4299 individuals aged 18–69 years (18–41 years only in 1998) completed a premailed questionnaire and were patch tested to FM I and MP. Data were analysed by logistic regression analyses and associations were expressed as odds ratios (ORs) with 95% confidence intervals (CIs).

Results.—The prevalence of FM I and MP sensitization followed an inverted V-pattern among women aged 18–41 years (i.e. an increase from 1990 to 1998, followed by a decrease from 1998 to 2006). Logistic regression analyses showed that 'medical consultation due to cosmetic dermatitis' (OR 3·37, 95% CI 1·83–6·20) and 'cosmetic dermatitis within the past 12 months' (OR 3·53, CI 2·02–6·17) were significantly associated with sensitization to FM I.

Conclusions.—In line with trends observed in Danish patients with dermatitis, our results supported a recent decrease in the prevalence of FM I and MP sensitization in Denmark. The study also showed that fragrance sensitization was associated with self-reported cosmetic dermatitis and use of health care related to cosmetic dermatitis.

▶ *Myroxylon pereirae* (MP) and fragrance mix I (FM I containing cinnamal, cinnamyl alcohol, geraniol, isoeugenol, eugenol, hydroxycitronellal, evernia prunastri, and alpha-amyl cinnamal) are important diagnostic markers in contact sensitization. This is a study during the years of 1990, 1998, and 2006 with 4299 individuals aged 18 to 69 years who completed a questionnaire and were patch tested to FM I and MP. The sensitization to FM I and MP were stratified by sex and age. This study showed that the prevalence of sensitization to FM I and MP decreased among women aged 18 to 41 between the years 1998-2006. They also found that the prevalence of cosmetic dermatitis was higher in the youngest age group (18-41 years), and higher among women compared with men. Products most frequently reported by both men and women included deodorants (26.1%), scented lotions (11.5%), perfumes (9.2%), and body wash and shampoo (9.1%). Analysis also showed that cosmetic dermatitis was associated with sensitization to FM I, female sex, atopic dermatitis, and age. The prevalence of cosmetic dermatitis was higher among women than men, which may be explained by a more frequent use of cosmetic products, and there was an increase in dermatitis from deodorants, scented lotions, perfumery, and make-up products more often for women than for men. These self-reported dermatitis reactions are certainly related to irritant and allergic reactions, which was emphasized by the observation that atopic dermatitis was associated with self-reported dermatitis in the regression analyses. The prevalence of self-reported cosmetic dermatitis did not decrease together with the prevalence of FM I and MP sensitization between 1998 and 2006. This can be due to other ingredients being used in fragrances. It could also be due to overall use of cosmetic products increasing in Denmark during the past 20 years with an increasing number of irritants and allergic reactions to preservatives. There may also be an increased awareness of skin problems in the population today as compared with 20 years ago. This study showed that FM I sensitization was strongly associated with the occurrence of self-reported cosmetic dermatitis. This study confirmed the decrease of FM I and MP sensitization observed among women with dermatitis in Denmark.

G. K. Kim, DO
J. Q. Del Rosso, DO

Topical Peroxisome Proliferator Activated Receptor Activators Accelerate Postnatal Stratum Corneum Acidification

Fluhr JW, Man M-Q, Hachem J-P, et al (Veterans Affairs Med Ctr, San Francisco, CA; et al)
J Invest Dermatol 129:365-374, 2009

Previous studies have shown that pH declines from between 6 and 7 at birth to adult levels (pH 5.0–5.5) over 5–6 days in neonatal rat stratum corneum (SC). As a result, at birth, neonatal epidermis displays decreased permeability barrier homeostasis and SC integrity, improving days 5–6. We determined here whether peroxisome proliferator-activated receptor (PPAR) activators accelerate postnatal SC acidification. Topical treatment with two different PPARα activators, clofibrate and WY14643, accelerated the postnatal decline in SC surface pH, whereas treatment with PPARγ activators did not and a PPARβ/δ activator had only a modest effect. Treatment with clofibrate significantly accelerated normalization of barrier function. The morphological basis for the improvement in barrier function in PPARα-treated animals includes accelerated secretion of lamellar bodies and enhanced, postsecretory processing of secreted lamellar body contents into mature lamellar membranes. Activity of β-glucocerebrosidase increased after PPARα-activator treatment. PPARα activator also improved SC integrity, which correlated with an increase in corneodesmosome density and increased desmoglein-1 content, with a decline in serine protease activity. Topical treatment of newborn animals with a PPARα activator increased secretory phospholipase A2 activity, which likely accounts for accelerated SC acidification. Thus, PPARα activators accelerate neonatal SC acidification, in parallel with improved permeability homeostasis and SC integrity/cohesion. Hence, PPARα activators might be useful to prevent or treat certain common neonatal dermatoses.

▶ This is an interesting article from a group of investigators that has published widely in the field of peroxisome proliferator-activated receptors (PPARs) and liver X receptors (LXRs) and their roles in epidermal physiology. PPARs and LXRs are related lipid-activated nuclear receptors that act as transcription factors, and have been shown to be involved in regulation of both metabolic and inflammatory pathways. Activation of LXR and PPAR isoforms α and β/δ has been previously reported to regulate keratinocyte differentiation and enhance the formation and homeostasis of the epidermal barrier in neonatal rodents. Receptor activation has also been shown to be involved in the formation of the lipid matrix of the stratum corneum (SC) by the stimulation of lamellar body secretion and epidermal lipid synthesis. The authors postulated that these activities would be associated with enhanced acidification of the SC, which has also been shown to result in improved barrier function and integrity. In a previous report, Fluhr et al described the accelerated acidification of the SC, and improved permeability barrier recovery and SC function after disruption in neonatal rats treated with topical LXR activators.[1] In addition, the acidification was blocked by inhibition of secretory phospholipase A2 (PLA2) activity. This article describes very similar results with the application of PPAR activators. Interestingly, activators of the α and β/δ isoforms, but not the γ isoform of PPAR produced these effects.

It is generally accepted that the relatively acidic environment of the SC favors the colonization of normal flora and discourages the growth of pathogenic organisms. These studies of the role of nuclear receptors in the development of this environment hold therapeutic implications. It is noteworthy that PPAR agonists have been shown to be efficacious in animal models of irritant contact dermatitis and in human atopic eczema.[2]

G. M. P. Galbraith, MD

References

1. Fluhr JW, Crumrine D, Mao-Qiang M, Moskowitz DG, Elias PM, Feingold KR. Topical liver X receptor activators accelerate postnatal acidification of stratum corneum and improve function in the neonate. *J Invest Dermatol*. 2005;125: 1206-1214.
2. Schmuth M, Jiang YJ, Dubrac S, Elias PM, Feingold KR. Peroxisome proliferator-activated receptors and liver X receptors in epidermal biology. *J Lipid Res*. 2008; 49:499-509.

Topical Treatments with Pimecrolimus, Tacrolimus and Medium- to High-Potency Corticosteroids, and Risk of Lymphoma
Schneeweiss S, Doherty M, Zhu S, et al (Harvard School of Public Health, Boston, MA; i3 Drug Safety, Waltham, MA; et al)
Dermatology 219:7-21, 2009

Background/Aims.—A potential risk of lymphoma associated with the use of topical calcineurin inhibitors is debated. We assessed the risk of lymphoma among patients treated with topical pimecrolimus, tacrolimus or corticosteroids.

Methods.—We conducted a cohort study using health insurance claims data. Cohorts of initiators of topical pimecrolimus, tacrolimus and corticosteroids, along with cohorts of persons with untreated dermatitis and randomly sampled enrollees were identified from January 2002 to June 2006. Lymphomas were identified using insurance claims and adjudicated by medical records review. We adjusted for confounders by propensity score matching.

Results.—Among 92,585 pimecrolimus initiators contributing 121,289 person-years of follow-up, we identified 26 lymphomas yielding an incidence of 21/100,000 person-years. This incidence of lymphoma was similar to that among tacrolimus users (rate ratio, RR = 1.16; 95% confidence interval, CI = 0.74–1.82) as well as corticosteroid users (RR = 1.15; 95% CI = 0.49–2.72). All three topical treatments were associated with an increased risk of lymphoma compared with the general population ($RR_{Pim} = 2.89$; $RR_{Tac} = 2.82$; $RR_{Cort} = 2.10$) suggesting increased detection of preexisting lymphomas.

Conclusion.—This study did not find an increased risk of lymphoma among initiators of topical pimecrolimus relative to other topical agents during an average follow-up of 1.3 years. Longer-term studies may be needed.

▶ Tacrolimus ointment was approved for use in atopic dermatitis by the Food and Drug Administration (FDA) in December 2000, and pimecrolimus cream was approved for use in mild to moderate atopic dermatitis by the same agency in December 2001. Possessing anti-inflammatory properties similar to topical corticosteroids, but lacking the side effects of thinning of the skin and striae formation, use of these agents, especially by nondermatologists was exceptional.

Use of pimecrolimus cream rose 10-fold over a period of 3 years, with pediatricians writing about a third of all prescriptions. The rate of pimecrolimus prescribing among pediatricians rose 62% between June 2002 to May 2003 and June 2003 to May 2004.[1]

On January 2006, the FDA issued a public health advisory and mandated labeling changes to inform prescribers and patients of a potential malignancy risk, including skin cancer and lymphoma, from use of these topical agents. Of concern was animal data where lymphomas developed after oral administration, case reports of cancer in a small number of patients, and an observed incidence of increased cancers (including lymphoma) among those taking the drugs to prevent rejection of solid-organ transplants.

Admittedly, systemic absorption when tacrolimus ointment or pimecrolimus cream is applied to the skin is small, but measurable. Data seeking to quantify any possible risk of lymphoma in users of topical formulations are scarce. In this article, funded by Novartis, the maker of topical pimecrolimus cream (Elidel), the authors sought to use a large amount of health insurance claim data to assess the incidence of lymphoma among uses of pimecrolimus cream, tacrolimus ointment, and topical steroids. It is interesting that while no increased risk of lymphoma was identified for the immune response modifiers relative to topical steroids, an increased risk of lymphoma when compared with the general population was identified. The authors attribute this observation to either unobserved factors, a possible increased risk of lymphoma in the setting of atopic dermatitis, or cutaneous forms of lymphoma that were misclassified as dermatitis in the first place. However, the chief limitation of this study, in my mind, is the relatively brief follow-up period of just 1.3 years. Clearly, long-term studies will be necessary to fully investigate the safety of topical formulations of these agents.

W. A. High, MD, JD, MEng

Reference

1. Gorman RL. FDA advises using 2 atopic dermatitis drugs only as labeled. *AAP News*. 2005;26:32.

Dermal Dendritic Cells, and Not Langerhans Cells, Play an Essential Role in Inducing an Immune Response
Fukunaga A, Khaskhely NM, Sreevidya CS, et al (Univ of Texas, Houston)
J Immunol 180:3057-3064, 2008

Langerhans cells (LCs) serve as epidermal sentinels of the adaptive immune system. Conventional wisdom suggests that LCs encounter Ag in the skin and then migrate to the draining lymph nodes, where the Ag is presented to T cells, thus initiating an immune response. Platelet-activating factor (PAF) is a phospholipid mediator with potent biological effects. During inflammation, PAF mediates recruitment of leukocytes to inflammatory sites. We herein tested a hypothesis that PAF induces LC migration. Applying 2,4-dinitro-1-fluorobenzene (DNFB) to wild-type mice activated LC migration. In contrast, applying DNFB to PAF receptor-deficient mice or mice injected with PAF receptor antagonists failed to induce LC migration. Moreover, after FITC application the appearance of hapten-laden LCs (FITC$^+$, CD11c$^+$, Langerin$^+$) in the lymph nodes of PAF receptor-deficient mice was significantly depressed compared with that found in wild-type mice. LC chimerism indicates that the PAF receptor on keratinocytes but not LCs is responsible for LC migration. Contrary to the diminution of LC migration in PAF receptor-deficient mice, we did not observe any difference in the migration of hapten-laden dermal dendritic cells (FITC$^+$, CD11c$^+$, Langerin$^-$) into the lymph nodes of PAF receptor-deficient mice. Additionally, the contact hypersensitivity response generated in wild-type or PAF receptor-deficient mice was identical. Finally, dermal dendritic cells, but not LCs isolated from the draining lymph nodes after hapten application, activated T cell proliferation. These findings suggest that LC migration may not be responsible for the generation of contact hypersensitivity and that dermal dendritic cells may play a more important role.

▶ The opening line of this article says a lot: dendritic cells are professional antigen presenting cells, whereas Langerhans cells (LCs) are immature... These concepts, as well as the identification of platelet-activating factor (PAF) as an important stress-induced mediator in WBC recruitment, especially in terms of expression on keratinocytes to induce migration, and the fact that dermal dendritic cells did not need any influence from PAF or other mediator to stimulate immune responses, undo some of the conventional suppositions from immunology where it was presumed that the LCs (marked by langerin/ CD207) were in fact the main player in creating hypersensitivity responses.

Dermal dendritic cells are hypothesized to be labelled as negative for epidermal growth factor-negative and CD8-α and are CD11c and hapten-positive but CD205 intermediate. The tests performed on mice that either expressed PAF or not were their critical end points but in reality based on the activation of the immune responses in UVB and PUVA that were tested here, these markers could have significant impacts on future psoriasis therapies, or explain why topical steroids that stabilize LCs may not provide sufficient suppression of an immune response, whereas systemic therapies that affect the dermal dendritic cells might have more impact. Finally, the progression of squamous cell carcinoma (SCC) from early photodamaged skin may be delayed if the ultraviolet-induced suppression of LCs, as demonstrated here, may be reinstituted with the reactivation of dermal dendritic cells, perhaps by inducing PAF or some other mediator's activity, to survey for tumor antigen in earlier stages.

N. Bhatia, MD

Children's clothing fasteners as a potential source of exposure to releasable nickel ions

Heim KE, McKean BA (Nickel Inst, Toronto, Ontario, Canada)
Contact Dermatitis 60:100-105, 2009

Background.—Cutaneous nickel allergy in the very young is not well documented or characterized. A significant number of individuals are nickel sensitized by their mid-teenage years. Recent studies suggest that children may become sensitized to nickel at an early age.

Objectives.—The purpose of this study was to investigate nickel release from children's clothing fasteners as one potential route of exposure of pre-school age children to nickel ions.

Patients/Methods.—Fasteners from new and used children's clothing purchased in the USA were tested using the dimethylglyoxime (DMG) and EN1811 tests for nickel ion release.

Results.—Of 173 fasteners tested, 10 (6%) tested positive using the DMG test for nickel release. EN 1811 standardized nickel release testing of these 10 items demonstrated that 70% (4% of all fasteners tested) released nickel in excess of the European Nickel Directive release limit (0.5 µg/cm^2/week). Ten randomly selected DMG-negative fasteners were also EN 1811 tested, of which 30% of fasteners exceeded the European Nickel Directive release limit. Therefore, not less than 6% of the fasteners tested released excessive nickel.

Conclusion.—This study concluded that clothing fasteners purchased in the USA could be a source of early childhood exposure to releasable nickel.

▶ Nickel is a ubiquitous allergen with significant rates of positive patch tests (sensitization) in young children cited throughout the international data. However, sources of nickel exposure among infants and children remain debatable. The authors sought to determine whether clothing fasteners represent a potential source of releasable nickel ions capable of causing childhood sensitization reactions. They found that out of 173 metal fasteners from new and used children's clothing purchased in the United States, a minimum of 6% released amounts of nickel that exceeded the European Union's (EU) Nickel Directive limit of 0.5 µg/cm^2/week. Since young children outgrow their clothing rapidly and are thus potentially exposed to multiple nickel-releasing fasteners, metal clothing fasteners can be a significant source of childhood nickel sensitization. Avoidance of such fasteners can help reduce early exposure to nickel, thereby theoretically preventing sensitization to an allergen that is otherwise difficult to avoid.

Although this study makes an interesting point, the clinical relevance of the data remains unclear. One issue lies in the fact that the EU Nickel Directive limit, which was derived from adults, is used as the standard to which the rate of nickel release from the fasteners is compared, even though it is unknown whether the EU's limit is equally relevant to young children as it is to adults. Additionally, there is no specific discussion on the threshold of elicitation, the level of nickel exposure at which sensitized patients will actually develop a clinical dermatitis. Without this knowledge, the only conclusion that can be drawn is that clothing fasteners are a potential source of nickel exposure in young children that may lead to sensitization, but the risk of developing a clinically relevant cutaneous reaction from this exposure is undetermined. Further studies (a prospective longitudinal study or clinical cases) would be necessary to prove that clothing fasteners are capable of eliciting cutaneous nickel allergy.

J. Hsu
S. Fallon Friedlander, MD

2   Psoriasis and Other Papulosquamous Disorders

Rates of new-onset psoriasis in patients with rheumatoid arthritis receiving anti-tumour necrosis factor α therapy: results from the British Society for Rheumatology Biologics Register
Harrison MJ, the British Society for Rheumatology Biologics Register Control Centre Consortium, on behalf of the BSRBR (The Univ of Manchester, United Kingdom; et al)
Ann Rheum Dis 68:209-215, 2009

Background.—Anti-tumour necrosis factor (TNF)α treatments improve outcome in severe rheumatoid arthritis (RA) and are efficacious in psoriasis and psoriatic arthritis. However recent case reports describe psoriasis occurring as an adverse event in patients with RA receiving anti-TNFα therapy.

Objectives.—We aimed to determine whether the incidence rate of psoriasis was higher in patients with RA treated with anti-TNFα therapy compared to those treated with traditional disease-modifying antirheumatic drugs (DMARDs). We also compared the incidence rates of psoriasis between the three anti-TNFα drugs licensed for RA.

Methods.—We studied 9826 anti-TNF-treated and 2880 DMARD-treated patients with severe RA from The British Society for Rheumatology Biologics Register (BSRBR). All patients reported with new onset psoriasis as an adverse event were included in the analysis. Incidence rates of psoriasis were calculated as events/1000 person years and compared using incidence rate ratios (IRR).

Results.—In all, 25 incident cases of psoriasis in patients receiving anti-TNFα therapy and none in the comparison cohort were reported between January 2001 and July 2007. The absence of any cases in the comparison cohort precluded a direct comparison; however the crude incidence rate of psoriasis in those treated with anti-TNFα therapy was elevated at 1.04 (95% CI 0.67 to 1.54) per 1000 person years compared to the rate of 0 (upper 97.5% CI 0.71) per 1000 person years in the patients treated with DMARDs. Patients treated with adalimumab had a significantly higher rate of incident psoriasis compared to patients treated with etanercept (IRR 4.6, 95% CI 1.7 to 12.1) and infliximab (IRR 3.5, 95% CI 1.3 to 9.3).

Conclusions.—Results from this study suggest that the incidence of psoriasis is increased in patients treated with anti-TNFα therapy. Our findings also suggest that the incidence may be higher in patients treated with adalimumab.

▶ The British Society for Rheumatology Biologics Register is a mandatory registry for rheumatoid arthritis patients treated with biologics in the United Kingdom. It constitutes one of the largest prospective observational cohorts of patients treated with tumor necrosis factor-α (TNF-α) blockers. The results of this study are therefore important and quite revealing. It should not come as a surprise that there are many cases of TNF-α blocker-induced psoriasis, as there have been many case reports of patients treated with TNF-α for rheumatoid arthritis who have gone on to develop psoriasis. The information presented here is clinically important because dermatologists have to recognize this syndrome that clearly exists.

It is tempting to speculate that the entity called TNF-α-induced psoriasis simply represents previously existing psoriasis in patients with rheumatoid or psoriatic arthritis whose skin disease has gone undiagnosed. The significant numbers of cases that have been reported, the distinctive distribution of lesions, and the exacerbation by TNF-α blockers, which generally treat psoriasis support the existence of TNF-α blocker-induced psoriasis. Palmoplantar psoriasis has been a recurring phenotype in published case reports of TNF-α-induced psoriasis, and is reported in several of the patients in this cohort.

The strength of this study lies in the numbers of patients followed. The only weakness is understandable and that is the attempt to explain why this condition occurs. The authors make it clear that their explanations are speculative. This is important reading for every dermatologist.

M. Lebwohl, MD

Ustekinumab, a human interleukin 12/23 monoclonal antibody, for psoriatic arthritis: randomised, double-blind, placebo-controlled, crossover trial
Gottlieb A, Menter A, Mendelsohn A, et al (Tufts Med Ctr, Boston, MA; Baylor Univ Med Ctr, Dallas, TX; LLC, Malvern, PA; et al)
Lancet 373:633-640, 2009

Background.—Since some patients with psoriatic arthritis do not respond to typical drug treatments, alternatives are needed. Findings suggest that interleukins 12 and 23 might affect clinical symptoms and pathological joint changes of psoriatic arthritis. Ustekinumab is a human monoclonal antibody that inhibits receptor-binding of these cytokines. We aimed to assess the efficacy and safety of ustekinumab for psoriatic arthritis in this phase II study.

Methods.—We undertook a double-blind, randomised, placebo-controlled, crossover study at 24 sites in North America and Europe. Patients with active psoriatic arthritis were randomly allocated via interactive voice response system to either ustekinumab (90 mg or 63 mg) every week for 4 weeks (weeks 0–3) followed by placebo at weeks 12 and 16 (n = 76; Group 1) or placebo (weeks 0–3) and ustekinumab (63 mg) at weeks 12 and 16 (n = 70; Group 2). The first 12 weeks of the study were placebo-controlled. Masking was maintained to week 16 infusion, and patients were followed up to week 36. The primary endpoint was ACR20 response at week 12. Analysis was by intention to treat. This trial is registered with ClinicalTrials.gov, number NCT00267956.

Findings.—At week 12, 32 (42%) patients in Group 1 and ten (14%) in Group 2 achieved the primary endpoint (difference 28% [95% CI 14·0–41·6]; p = 0·0002). Of 124 (85%) participants with psoriasis affecting 3% or more body surface area, 33 of 63 (52%) in Group 1 and three of 55 (5%) in Group 2 had a 75% or greater improvement in psoriasis area and severity index score at week 12 (47% [33·2–60·6]; p < 0·0001). During the placebo-controlled period (weeks 0–12), adverse events arose in 46 (61%) patients in Group 1 and 44 (63%) in Group 2; serious adverse events were recorded in three (4%) Group 2 patients (none in Group 1).

Interpretation.—Ustekinumab significantly reduced signs and symptoms of psoriatic arthritis and diminished skin lesions compared with placebo, and the drug was well tolerated. Larger and longer term studies are needed to further characterise ustekinumab efficacy and safety for treatment of psoriatic arthritis.

▶ Among the biologic therapies, inhibitors of tumor necrosis factor (TNF) are well established as effective for both psoriasis and psoriatic arthritis (PsA). As therapies with novel mechanisms of action are introduced for psoriasis, it is of scientific and clinical value to determine their efficacy for PsA. Ustekinumab is a human immunoglobulin monoclonal antibody that binds with high affinity to the shared P40 subunit of human interleukins 12 and 23, inhibiting their binding to the interleukin 12Rβ1 receptor on the surface of T cells, NK cells, and antigen-presenting cells and preventing subsequent receptor signaling and activation of the receptor-bearing cell. This therapy has been shown to be safe and effective for the treatment of psoriasis. The authors of this phase II study assessed the safety and efficacy of ustekinumab in patients with active PsA. They found that ustekinumab significantly reduced signs and symptoms of PsA and diminished skin lesions compared with placebo, and the drug was well tolerated. The authors noted that their data suggest that interleukin 12/23 P40 cytokines could have an important role in the pathogenesis of PsA and other arthritides. A larger phase III study will be necessary to validate these findings. However, the data from this study indicate that ustekinumab may be a reasonable choice in those with psoriasis and PsA, especially if they have failed anti-TNF therapy.

J. Weinberg, MD

Epidemiology and clinical pattern of psoriatic arthritis in Germany: a prospective interdisciplinary epidemiological study of 1511 patients with plaque-type psoriasis

Reich K, Krüger K, Mössner R, et al (Dermatologikum Hamburg, Germany; Rheumatological Practice, Munich, Germany; Georg-August-Univ, Göttingen, Germany, et al)
Br J Dermatol 160:1040-1047, 2009

Background.—Because psoriatic arthritis (PsA) usually develops years after the first manifestation of skin symptoms, in many cases the initial diagnosis of PsA depends on the dermatologist.

Objectives.—To investigate the prevalence and clinical pattern of PsA in a daily practice population of patients with psoriasis.

Methods.—Patients were enrolled in an observational prospective cross-sectional cohort study at 48 community and academic centres. Demographic and medical parameters were recorded, including severity of skin symptoms (Psoriasis Area and Severity Index, PASI), previous and current treatments, concomitant diseases, and the impact of psoriasis on productivity and health-related quality of life (Dermatology Life Quality Index, DLQI). Patients with joint symptoms were referred to a rheumatologist for diagnosis and to record the activity and pattern of arthritis.

Results.—Among 1511 patients 20·6% had PsA; in 85% of the cases PsA was newly diagnosed. Of these patients more than 95% had active arthritis and 53·0% had five or more joints affected. Polyarthritis (58·7%) was the most common manifestation pattern, followed by oligoarthritis (31·6%) and arthritis mutilans (4·9%). Distal interphalangeal involvement was present in 41·0% and dactylitis in 23·7% of the patients. Compared with patients without arthritis, patients with PsA had more severe skin symptoms (mean PASI 14·3 vs. 11·5), a lower quality of life (mean DLQI 11·6 vs. 7·7) and greater impairment of productivity parameters.

Conclusions.—The findings are consistent with a high prevalence of undiagnosed cases of active PsA among patients with psoriasis seen by dermatologists. As many of these patients also have significant skin symptoms, treatment strategies are required that are equally effective in the control of skin and joint symptoms of psoriasis.

▶ This study investigated the prevalence and clinical pattern of psoriatic arthritis (PsA) among patients attending a dermatologist for plaque-type psoriasis and found a prevalence of PsA of 20.6%. The authors noted that the actual prevalence might be higher as 144 patients with suspected joint involvement did not consult a rheumatologist and therefore the diagnosis of PsA could not be confirmed. This data is within the accepted range for the incidence of PsA, although the incidence varies in different studies in different populations. Differences in the reported incidences may be explained by geographical and ethnic differences, different characteristics of the investigated patients with psoriasis, and differences in the applied diagnostic criteria of PsA. A key finding of the study is a high prevalence of undiagnosed cases of active PsA among patients with psoriasis seen by dermatologists. This should reemphasize the need for close patient follow-up and patient education in those who have psoriasis and therefore may be at risk for the development of PsA. Referral to a rheumatologist in those patients with joint or significant joint stiffness ("morning gel") may be a consideration.

J. Weinberg, MD

Time Trends in Epidemiology and Characteristics of Psoriatic Arthritis Over 3 Decades: A Population-based Study
Wilson FC, Icen M, Crowson CS, et al (College of Medicine, Rochester, MN)
J Rheumatol 36:361-367, 2009

Objective.—To determine time trends in incidence, prevalence, and clinical characteristics of psoriatic arthritis (PsA) over a 30-year period.

Methods.—We identified a population-based incidence cohort of subjects aged 18 years or over who fulfilled ClASsification of Psoriatic ARthritis (CASPAR) criteria for PsA between January 1, 1970, and December 31, 1999, in Olmsted County, Minnesota, USA. PsA incidence date was defined as the diagnosis date of those who fulfilled CASPAR criteria. Age- and sex-specific incidence rates were estimated and age- and sex-adjusted to the 2000 US White population.

Results.—The PsA incidence cohort comprised 147 adult subjects with a mean age of 42.7 years, and 61% were men. The overall age- and sex-adjusted annual incidence of PsA per 100,000 was 7.2 [95% confidence interval (CI) 6.0, 8.4] with a higher incidence in men (9.1, 95% CI 7.1, 11.0) than women (5.4, 95% CI 4.0, 6.9). The age- and sex-adjusted incidence of PsA per 100,000 increased from 3.6 (95% CI 2.0, 5.2) between 1970 and 1979 to 9.8 (95% CI 7.7, 11.9) between 1990 and 2000 (p for trend < 0.001). The point prevalence per 100,000 was 158 (95% CI 132, 185) in 2000, with a higher prevalence in men (193, 95% CI 150, 237) than women (127, 95% CI 94, 160). At incidence, most PsA subjects had oligoarticular involvement (49%) with enthesopathy (29%).

Conclusion.—The incidence of PsA has been rising over 30 years in men and women. Reasons for the increase are unknown, but may be related to a true change in incidence or greater physician awareness of the diagnosis.

▶ Criteria for ClASsification of Psoriatic ARthritis (CASPAR) were recently published[1] and represent a simplified tool for this inflammatory joint disease that is associated with psoriasis. In the presence of inflammatory joint, spine, or entheseal disease, psoriatic arthritis is diagnosed when 3 points are present. Two points are given for current psoriasis or history of psoriasis in the patient or in a first- or second-degree relative. One point is given for onycholysis, pitting or hyperkeratosis of the nail bed; another point for a negative rheumatoid factor; another point for active or past dactylitis, which presents as swelling of an entire digit; and X-ray evidence of juxta-articular new bone formation, which is assigned one point. The sensitivity and specificity of the CASPAR criteria have been shown to be high, not only in established psoriatic arthritis, but also in early psoriatic arthritis. This is the first article to apply CASPAR criteria to a large geographically defined patient database over a 30-year period.

It is interesting that the incidence of psoriatic arthritis increased from 3.6 per 100 000 between 1970 and 1979 to 9.8 per 100 000 in the decade from 1990-2000. At incidence, 49% of patients had oligoarticular disease and 29% enthesopathy.

If the incidence of psoriatic arthritis were truly increasing at this rapid rate, the results reported in this article would be extremely important. Annual incidence estimates for psoriatic arthritis vary substantially. As the authors point out, estimates range from 3 to 23 per 100 000 with higher estimates in recent years. For the first time, we have a class of drugs, the tumor necrosis factor-α (TNF-α) inhibitors, which has been shown to prevent the radiographic progression of joint disease in psoriatic arthritis. Four TNF blockers have been approved to treat psoriatic arthritis: adalimumab, etanercept, golimumab, and infliximab. With the approval of each drug, there has been heightened awareness of psoriatic arthritis, with substantial marketing efforts by the pharmaceutical companies making those drugs. Undoubtedly, those marketing efforts have contributed to the rising awareness of psoriatic arthritis, but the study results reported in this article predated the approval of any of those drugs for psoriatic arthritis by several years.

M. Lebwohl, MD

Reference

1. Taylor W, Gladman D, Helliwell P, Marchesoni A, Mease P, Mielants H; CASPAR Study Group. Classification criteria for psoriatic arthritis: development of new criteria from a large international study. *Arthritis Rheum.* 2006;54:2665-2673.

Outcomes of methotrexate therapy for psoriasis and relationship to genetic polymorphisms
Warren RB, Smith RL, Campalani E, et al (The Univ of Manchester, UK; St Thomas' Hosp, London, UK)
Br J Dermatol 160:438-441, 2009

Background.—The use of methotrexate is limited by interindividual variability in response. Previous studies in patients with either rheumatoid arthritis or psoriasis suggest that genetic variation across the methotrexate metabolic pathway might enable prediction of both efficacy and toxicity of the drug.

Objectives.—To assess if single nucleotide polymorphisms (SNPs) across four genes that are relevant to methotrexate metabolism [folypolyglutamate synthase (*FPGS*), gamma-glutamyl hydrolase (*GGH*), methylenetetrahydrofolate reductase (*MTHFR*) and 5-aminoimidazole-4-carboxamide ribonucleotide transformylase (*ATIC*)] are related to treatment outcomes in patients with psoriasis.

Methods.—DNA was collected from 374 patients with psoriasis who had been treated with methotrexate. Data were available on individual outcomes to therapy, namely efficacy and toxicity. Haplotype-tagging SNPs ($r^2 > 0.8$) for the four genes with a minor allele frequency of > 5% were selected from the HAPMAP phase II data. Genotyping was undertaken using the MassARRAY spectrometric method (Sequenom®).

Results.—There were no significant associations detected between clinical outcomes in patients with psoriasis treated with methotrexate and SNPs in the four genes investigated.

Conclusions.—Genetic variation in four key genes relevant to the intracellular metabolism of methotrexate does not appear to predict response to methotrexate therapy in patients with psoriasis.

▶ Single nucleotide polymorphisms (SNPs) can cause variations in response to drugs, vaccines, and predisposition to certain diseases. Methotrexate is a commonly used drug in rheumatology and dermatology with past studies showing mixed results with SNPs interfering with efficacy and toxicity. This was a retrospective cohort study of 375 patients with psoriasis on methotrexate and investigating 47 haplotype-tagging and 3 functional SNPs in 4 genes involved in methotrexate intracellular metabolism; folypolyglutamate synthase (FPGS); gamma-glutamyl hydrolase (GGH); methylenetetrahydrofolate reductase (MTHFR); and 5-aminoimidazole-4-carboxamide ribonucleotide transfomylase (ATIC). Patients were stratified as either (i) responders those who had clinical improvement using the Psoriasis Area and Severity Index (PASI) > 75% reduction in PASI from the start of methotrexate therapy versus (ii) nonresponders—those who had < 50% improvement in PASI while on therapy. Methotrexate toxicity is measured by monitoring liver enzymes (liver function tests [LFTs]) for hepatoxicity, and gastrointestinal (GI) toxicity is measured by subjective reports from patients including nausea, vomiting, or diarrhea. The study group consists of 94% Caucasian and 6% Chinese/Asian. Findings are consistent with no statistical significance of SNPs for the enzymes FPGS, GGH, MTHFR, and ATIC in terms of efficacy and toxicity to methotrexate. There was also no significant statistical difference in terms of efficacy or toxicity for those who took folic acid supplementation and for those who did not. There were many limitations to this study including subjective GI reports from patients about side effects being harder to quantify without knowing for sure if methotrexate was the culprit. It was also unknown whether these patients were on other medications at the time or had experienced GI symptoms from other possible illnesses. It was also unknown whether or not these patients had a history of previous liver disease and if there were any criteria used to exclude such individuals, because it is well known that those with hepatic fibrosis could also have normal LFTs. Abnormal LFTs can be a measure of liver insult from multiple potential sources; a more accurate measurement would be a liver biopsy. Although the authors acknowledge that variations in SNPs could potentially affect the metabolism of methotrexate, there were no efforts to check if SNP variations increased or decrease methotrexate levels by actually checking blood levels of methotrexate. In addition, there are other dangerous side effects of methotrexate, such as leukopenia, anemia, and thrombocytopenia, which were not evaluated in relation to methotrexate therapy in this article. Although the authors claim that variations in SNP didn't have an effect on LFTs and GI symptoms, it is of importance to note that other significant side effects could have potentially occurred without documentation by the authors. Methotrexate toxicity can also take months to years to develop in some individuals. In this study there was a diverse range of end points used, which was also problematic because the cumulative dosage of methotrexate in these patients was unknown. Another limitation is the lack of diversity in this study group, with 95% of the study subjects being Caucasian. SNPs are known to vary between different patient populations and ethnicities, and a more diverse group of individuals could have yielded different results.

G. K. Kim, DO

J. Q. Del Rosso, DO

The Role of Online Support Communities: Benefits of Expanded Social Networks to Patients With Psoriasis
Idriss SZ, Kvedar JC, Watson AJ (Ctr for Connected Health, Boston)
Arch Dermatol 145:46-51, 2009

Objective.—To determine the demographics, usage patterns, attitudes, and experiences of online support site users.

Design.—Online survey.

Patients.—A total of 260 subjects recruited from 5 online psoriasis support groups.

Main Outcome Measures.—An exploratory analysis was performed to determine demographic and disease characteristics of online support site users. Perceived benefits were also documented.

Results.—The mean (SD) age of respondents was 40.1 (11.5) years (range, 18-75 years), most (75.7%) were white, female (60.4%), and college educated (84.3%). Key factors associated with use of online support sites included availability of resources (95.3%), convenience (94.0%), access to good advice (91.0%), and the lack of embarrassment when dealing with personal issues (90.8%). The most common activities were posting messages (65.0%) and searching for information (63.1%). Nearly half of all respondents perceived improvements in their quality of life (49.5%) and psoriasis severity (41.0%) since joining the site. Intensity of participation in online support activities was associated with improved quality of life ($P = .002$), but not with improvements in psoriasis severity.

Conclusions.—Our data demonstrate that psoriasis virtual communities offer users both a valuable educational resource and a source of psychological and social support. Such benefits could be further enhanced by physician engagement within these communities.

▶ This study provides a hypothesis generated, exploratory cross-sectional analysis to determine the demographics and disease characteristics of online support users and the perceived benefits of such networks. It was found that psoriasis online virtual communities offer both a valuable educational resource and a source of psychological and social support. The study examined 5 online sites.

This article, although a study, serves to alert physicians to the use of online virtual communities as a component of overall psoriasis management. Thus, the strength of the article is in its ability to effectively advocate for an additional tool in the treatment of the psychosocial aspects of psoriasis, an area that may often be overlooked in ambulatory care. However, given that over 0.6% to 4.8% of the world population is affected by psoriasis, the study size of 260 patients is relatively small to determine if the online virtual communities are indeed a valuable resource of support, and ultimately representative of the global attitudes of patients with psoriasis. Additionally, of the 5 Web sites reviewed, the study was only able to estimate a response rate from 2 Web sites, which garnered a 25.7% and 13.8% response rate for each site. Further, of the responding patients, most were white, college-educated females. This further adds to the question as to the true efficacy of the site in providing appropriate support for many other patient types inflicted with psoriasis. In concluding that the sites provide a valuable educational tool, the determination may be limited to those who are facile with computers, and also those who have access to use of a computer. Of the Web sites reviewed, none were formally moderated by a health care provider or coach, and admittedly the study was not able to address the issue of whether participating in the online groups actually had an objectively measurable effect on psoriasis itself or quality of life.

Nonetheless, the article provides an awareness of an underused modality in the treatment of the psychological and social aspects of psoriasis with some potential benefits demonstrated. Given the popularity of the Internet and the advocacy of articles such as this, the potential benefits to others may grow in the future, and improvements in Web sites are also likely to develop.

B. D. Michaels, DO

J. Q. Del Rosso, DO

Long-term maintenance treatment of moderate-to-severe plaque psoriasis with infliximab in combination with methotrexate or azathioprine in a retrospective cohort
Dalaker M, Bonesrønning JH (Trondheim Univ Hosp, Norway)
J Eur Acad Dermatol Venereol 23:277-282, 2009

Background.—Effective, fast-acting and safe therapies are needed for long-term maintenance treatment of psoriasis. In October 2005, infliximab was approved for the treatment of moderate-to-severe plaque psoriasis, but long-term data are limited.

Objective.—To evaluate the effectiveness of infliximab, used in combination with methotrexate or azathioprine, in maintaining clinical benefit in patients with moderate-to-severe psoriasis.

Methods.—The medical charts of 23 patients treated with infliximab from August 2001 to February 2007 were retrospectively reviewed. Most patients received either infliximab 3 mg/kg (17 of 23) or 5 mg/kg (1 of 23) in combination with methotrexate, while 5 of 23 patients received infliximab 5 mg/kg in combination with azathioprine. Psoriasis Area Severity Index (PASI) score and adverse events were recorded at every infliximab infusion visit at the hospital.

Results.—Patient data were available for a minimum of 4 weeks and up to 5 years and 5 months. At week 14, 91.3% achieved PASI 50, 69.6% achieved PASI 75, and 39.1% achieved PASI 90. Only two patients discontinued therapy due to loss of response: one after 15 months and one after 3 years. All other patients displayed a good clinical response (≥ PASI 50) and were still receiving this regimen at last observation. Combination regimens of infliximab with methotrexate or azathioprine were well tolerated, and only one patient discontinued therapy because of an adverse event (lung embolism) after two infusions with infliximab.

Conclusions.—Long-term (> 1 year) maintenance therapy of infliximab combined with methotrexate or azathioprine is effective and well tolerated for moderate-to-severe plaque-type psoriasis.

▶ Tumor necrosis factor-α (TNF-α) is believed to play an important role in the pathogenesis of psoriasis. Infliximab is a TNF-α antagonist, which has been shown to be highly effective for the treatment of psoriasis. This is a retrospective cohort study reviewing the medical charts of 23 patients treated with infliximab from 2001 to 2007 for moderate-to-severe plaque psoriasis in combination with methotrexate or azathioprine. Infliximab was used in combination with other drugs to use the lowest effective dose of infliximab and reduce toxicity. A 3-week washout period was allowed for all patients to receive another biological agent. Those who did not tolerate methotrexate were given azathioprine. Activity of erythrocyte enzyme thiopurine methyltransferase was assessed before azathioprine treatment to avoid increased risk for bone marrow suppression. The Psoriasis Area and Severity Index (PASI) score was evaluated by a dermatologist at each visit, and patients were followed up for a minimum of 4 weeks and a maximum of 5 years and 5 months during the chart review. After 1 year of therapy, 12 of 15 patients (80%) achieved PASI 50. No adverse events were observed that were directly related to treatment, including hepatotoxicity and bone marrow suppression. This study showed that methotrexate or azathioprine in combination with other biological agents may have additive benefit for treatment of psoriasis, similar to results seen with rheumatoid arthritis.

G. K. Kim, DO

J. Q. Del Rosso, DO

Trends in incidence of adult-onset psoriasis over three decades: A population-based study
Icen M, Crowson CS, McEvoy MT, et al (College of Medicine, Rochester, MN; et al)
J Am Acad Dermatol 60:394-401, 2009

Background.—Incidence studies of psoriasis are rare, mainly due to lack of established epidemiological criteria and the variable disease course. The objective of this study is to determine time trends in incidence and survival of psoriasis patients over three decades.

Methods.—We identified a population-based incidence cohort of 1633 subjects aged ≥18 years first diagnosed with psoriasis between January 1, 1970 and January 1, 2000. The complete medical records for each potential psoriasis subject were reviewed and diagnosis was validated by either a confirmatory diagnosis in the medical record by a dermatologist or medical record review by a dermatologist. Age- and sex-specific incidence rates were calculated and were age- and sex-adjusted to the 2000 US white population.

Results.—The overall age- and sex-adjusted annual incidence of psoriasis was 78.9 per 100,000 (95% confidence interval [CI]: 75.0-82.9). When psoriasis diagnosis was restricted to dermatologist-confirmed subjects, the incidence was 62.3 per 100,000 (95% CI: 58.8-65.8). Incidence of psoriasis increased significantly over time from 50.8 in the period 1970-1974 to reach 100.5 per 100,000 in the 1995-1999 time period ($P = .001$). Although the overall incidence was higher in males than in females ($P = .003$), incidence in females was highest in the sixth decade of life (90.7 per 100,000). Survival was similar to that found in the general population ($P = .36$).

Limitations.—The study population was mostly white and limited to adult psoriasis patients.

Conclusion.—The annual incidence of psoriasis almost doubled between the 1970s and 2000. The reasons for this increase in incidence are currently unknown, but could include a variety of factors, including a true change in incidence or changes in the diagnosing patterns over time.

► In this population-based study, the authors describe trends in the incidence of psoriasis over time and report, for the first time, that the incidence of psoriasis increased significantly over the 3 decades between 1970 and 2000. They note that the reasons for this increase in incidence are unknown, but could include a number of factors, including a true change in incidence or changes in the diagnosing patterns in this population. The authors speculate that some of the reasons for increased diagnosis might include the following: psoriasis patients seek care later in the course of disease; improved access to medical care; and increased awareness of the disease state. Their findings also indicate that the age-and sex-specific incidence of psoriasis is in general higher in males than in females, except for the sixth decade of life, suggesting the potential role of sex hormones in the etiology of psoriasis. This is an intriguing study, although it is limited for many of the reasons listed. It would be interesting to see if this trend continues to occur, and also if similar studies in different communities in the United States and abroad show similar findings. It is also interesting that survival was similar to the general populations, in contrast to other published data.[1]

J. Weinberg, MD

Reference

1. Gelfand JM, Troxel AB, Lewis JD, et al. The risk of mortality in patients with psoriasis: results from a population-based study. *Arch Dermatol.* 2007;143: 1493-1499.

Three-year registry data on biological treatment for psoriasis: the influence of patient characteristics on treatment outcome

Driessen RJB, Boezeman JB, van de Kerkhof PCM, et al (Radboud Univ Nijmegen Med Centre, the Netherlands)
Br J Dermatol 160, 670-675, 2009

Background.—The course of biological treatment in clinical practice may be highly different from treatment schedules in clinical trials. Treatment modifications and patient characteristics may influence treatment safety and efficacy. So far, long-term results from the use of biological treatment in clinical practice are lacking.

Objectives.—To report short- and long-term efficacy and safety data on biologics, especially etanercept, used in daily clinical practice. Special attention has been paid to patient characteristics that may have influenced the response to therapy.

Methods.—Prospectively collected registry data of all patients with psoriasis treated with biologics in the Radboud University Nijmegen Medical Centre outpatient clinic were used for analysis. Patient and treatment characteristics were surveyed. Efficacy and safety of etanercept for up to 3 years were analysed. Moreover, the influence of patient characteristics on etanercept treatment response was studied.

Results.—The analysed cohort, consisting of 118 patients, went through 142 treatment episodes in total. Patients treated with biologics had an extensive medical history. Optimization of biological treatment was established in various ways, including treatment switches and introduction of concomitant therapies. Short-term etanercept efficacy analysis showed a mean Psoriasis Area and Severity Index (PASI) improvement at week 24 of 59·7%. No significant influence of gender, age, baseline PASI, body mass index, number of previous systemic therapies or duration of psoriasis was found on week 24 efficacy results, although trends were discernible. The efficacy of etanercept remained stable for up to 156 weeks. Long-term daily practice treatment with etanercept was only occasionally accompanied by major safety concerns.

Conclusions.—The current study demonstrates that etanercept is able to improve psoriasis symptoms for a considerable time, and that serious side-effects are infrequent. The influence of patient characteristics on treatment response is limited.

▶ The evaluated cohort, consisting of 118 patients, went through 142 treatment episodes in total. While of value, this study is limited by the fact that the overwhelming number of patients followed were treated with etanercept. Inclusion of an increased number of patients on other therapies would have been interesting. Therefore, efficacy analyses in this study focused on etanercept. The authors noted that efficacy results may be overestimated, as only patients with available long-term efficacy data were included for analysis. After the first 24 weeks of therapy, the effect remained stable during the next 132 weeks of treatment, which leads to the conclusion that etanercept has the potential to improve psoriasis symptoms for a considerable time. This is an interesting study. However, in clinical practice, a number of patients treated long-term with etanercept do demonstrate loss of efficacy, with some degree of breakthrough. The long-term safety is consistent with the established safety profile of this drug.

J. Weinberg, MD

Evaluation of the clinical and immunohistological efficacy of the 585-nm pulsed dye laser in the treatment of psoriasis
Noborio R, Kurokawa M, Kobayashi K, et al (Nagoya City Univ Graduate School of Med Sciences, Japan)
J Eur Acad Dermatol Venereol 23:420-424, 2009

Background.—The 585-nm pulsed dye laser (PDL) therapy is useful for the patients with psoriasis. PDL treatment is based on selective photothermolysis of the dermal vasculature.

Objective.—The objectives of this study were to evaluate the clinical and immunohistological effects of PDL on psoriasis and to examine the association between psoriatic dermal vasculature and the clinical effects.

Methods.—Eleven patients with recalcitrant psoriasis were treated with 585-nm PDL. Biopsy specimens obtained before and after treatment were stained with CD31. All microvessels to the depth of 400 μm from the rete ridge were counted and the internal diameters were measured.

Results.—The mean percent reduction of plaque severity score was 42. The mean microvessel count decreased significantly from 63 to 35.6 ($P < 0.001$). There was a strong positive correlation between the plaque severity score and microvessel number ($P < 0.001$) and a strong negative correlation between the microvessel count of an untreated area and degree of the change in the microvessel count after treatment ($P = 0.005$).

Conclusions.—The findings of this study suggest that PDL treatment improves psoriasis. Moreover, PDL treatment decreased the number of

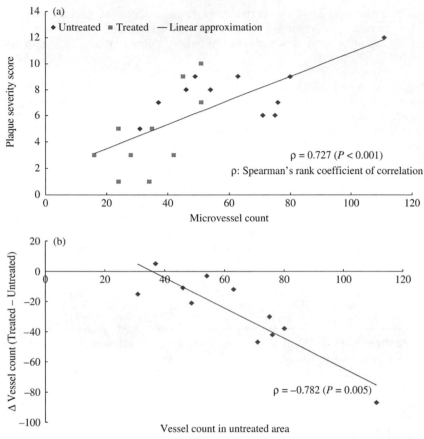

FIGURE 3.—(a) Correlation between plaque severity score and microvessel count ($\rho = 0.727$, $P < 0.001$). ρ: Spearman's rank coefficient of correlation. (b) Correlation between the change in the microvessel count and microvessel count in the untreated area ($\rho = -0.782$. $P = 0.005$). (Courtesy of Noborio R, Kurokawa M, Kobayashi K, et al. Evaluation of the clinical and immunohistological efficacy of the 585-nm pulsed dye laser in the treatment of psoriasis. *J Eur Acad Dermatol Venereol.* 2009;23:420-424.)

dermal papillary microvessels. Dermal papillary microvessels are important pathogenetic targets of psoriasis, and PDL therapy, which selectively targets superficial vessels, is therefore a valid therapeutic approach (Fig 3).

▶ Device treatment of psoriasis is an emerging discipline and is an important part of our therapeutic armamentarium. This provocative study demonstrates that the pulsed dye laser (PDL) diminishes the vascular supply of psoriatic plaques in a predictable way. This effect is at least partially responsible for the efficacy demonstrated by this device. Unfortunately, my experience with this device is variable and not as dependable as our narrow-band ultraviolet B (UVB) or excimer laser treatment of psoriatic plaques. However, when PDL does work, the effects seem to be much more sustained. We still have a lot to learn about the use of PDL in this disease.

E. A. Tanghetti, MD

Immunological effects of stress in psoriasis
Schmid-Ott G, Jaeger B, Boehm T, et al (Hannover Med School, Germany; et al)
Br J Dermatol 160:782-785, 2009

Background.—Psychological stress causes phenotypic changes in circulating lymphocytes and is regarded as an important trigger of the Th1-polarized inflammatory skin disease psoriasis.

Objective.—To study the effects of psychological stress on immunological parameters, i.e. membrane molecules relevant to the pathophysiology of psoriasis, especially cutaneous lymphocyte-associated antigens (CLA) involved in T and natural killer (NK) cells homing in on the skin.

Methods.—The severity of psoriasis was assessed in patients using the Psoriasis Area and Severity Index. Patients with psoriasis ($n = 15$) and healthy volunteers ($n = 15$) were exposed to brief psychological stress in the laboratory. *In vitro* analyses were conducted 1 h before, immediately following and 1 h after stress exposure. Peripheral T- and NK-cell subsets including CD8+ T lymphocytes, CLA+ lymphocytes and lymphocyte function-associated antigen type 1 (LFA-1)+ lymphocytes were analysed by flow cytometry.

Results.—We found a significant stress-induced increase of CD3+ T lymphocytes in patients with psoriasis only. Analyses of T-cell subsets revealed that this increase was observable for cytotoxic CD8+ T lymphocytes and CLA+ CD3+ lymphocytes. The total number of circulating NK cells (CD16+, CD56+) increased immediately after stress in both groups whereas only patients with psoriasis showed a significant increase in CLA+ NK cells.

Conclusions.—A higher stress-induced increase of CLA+ T and CLA+ NK cells in the circulation of patients with psoriasis might point to an increased ability of T and NK cells in the presence of psoriasis to home in on the skin during mental stress. Further studies are needed to verify these relationships in more detail and to investigate the time point at which these cells accumulate within lesional skin, and whether or not psychotherapy improves the quality of life of patients with psoriasis and influences stress-dependent parameters.

▶ The aim of this study was to determine the effects of psychological stress on immunological membrane markers that may have relevant pathophysiology to psoriasis.

Fifteen patients with stable chronic plaque psoriasis and without psoriatic arthritis were matched according to sex, social status, educational background, and age to 15 healthy control subjects. Each group was exposed to standardized methods of mental stress and analysis of T-cell, and natural killer (NK)-cell subsets was conducted by flow cytometry 1 hour before, during the stress, and 1 hour after the stress exposure. Analysis demonstrated an increase in CD3+ T cells (including cutaneous lymphocyte-associated antigens [CLA]+ T cells) and CLA+ NK cells in psoriasis patients only. The authors believe that it may be a higher stress-induced release of CLA+ T and CLA+ NK cells in the circulation of patients with psoriasis that may increase the ability of T cells and NK cells to hone in on the skin during mental stress. Other studies investigating the effects on stress in atopic dermatitis and Th2-associated diseases have also found an increase in CLA+ lymphocytes.

The authors speculate whether the stressed induced increase in CLA+ lymphocytes is a result of increased interleukin (IL)-2 or IL-12 and the rapid activation of α-1,3-fucosyltransferase-VII or if these cells are redistributed upon stress leading to higher levels in circulation.

While this study was conducted on a small number of subjects, the experiment was well designed and the preliminary findings may have significant clinical application. Further investigation is recommended to confirm these results on a larger patient population and also may help determine whether or not psychotherapy can influences stress dependent parameters in psoriasis patients.

J. Levin, DO

J. Q. Del Rosso, DO

Evaluation of the Efficacy of Acitretin Therapy for Nail Psoriasis

Tosti A, Ricotti C, Romanelli P, et al (Univ of Bologna, Italy; Univ of Miami, FL; et al)
Arch Dermatol 145:269-271, 2009

Objective.—To evaluate the therapeutic efficacy of ac-itretin in patients with isolated nail psoriasis.

Design.—Open study involving 36 patients with moderate to severe nail psoriasis treated with acitretin.

Setting.—University-based outpatient dermatology clinic specializing in nail diseases.

Patients.—A total of 27 men and 9 women (mean age, 41 years) with nail psoriasis.

Intervention.—Therapy consisted of acitretin, 0.2 to 0.3 mg/kg/d, for 6 months.

Main Outcome Measures.—Clinical evaluation, and Nail Psoriasis Severity Index (NAPSI) and modified NAPSI scores before therapy, every 2 months during therapy, and 6 months after treatment.

Results.—The mean percentage of reduction of the NAPSI score after treatment was 41%; the mean percentage of reduction of the modified NAPSI score of the target nail was 50%. Clinical evaluation at 6 months showed complete or almost complete clearing of the nail lesions in

9 patients (25%), moderate improvement in 9 (25%), mild improvement in 12 (33%), and no improvement in 6 (11%).

Conclusion.—Results from low-dose acitretin therapy show NAPSI score reductions comparable with those studies evaluating biologic drugs for nail psoriasis and suggest that low-dose systemic acitretin should be considered in the treatment of nail psoriasis.

▶ Although nail psoriasis is common, the results of treatment of nail psoriasis are often disappointing. Unfortunately, there is little information addressing the efficacy of systemic therapies in patients with diffuse and severe nail involvement in the absence of skin disease. This study demonstrated a 46% reduction in the Nail Psoriasis Severity Index (NAPSI) score after 20 weeks of low-dose acitretin therapy. This result is comparable with the other systemic therapies for nail psoriasis. Other studies indicate that adalimumab and infliximab can produce more than a 50% reduction of the NAPSI score after 20 weeks of treatment.

The results of this study are promising although only a small group of patients was evaluated. Systemic therapy for the treatment of psoriasis limited to nails only warrants a thorough risk versus benefit assessment; however, nail involvement can be symptomatically problematic and/or psychosocially devastating to some patients. Oral acitretin, like any oral retinoid therapy, can have severe side effects and likely should be reserved for severe cases of nail psoriasis and/or after other safer modalities have been tried.

In addition to major side effects, oral retinoid therapy can be associated with many unpleasant "nuisance side effects," although these are less common with low-dose acitretin therapy. It would be interesting to evaluate the patient relevant benefit of oral retinoid use for nail psoriasis therapy versus the side effect profile.

J. Levin, DO

J. Q. Del Rosso, DO

Psoriasis and risk of incident myocardial infarction, stroke or transient ischaemic attack: an inception cohort study with a nested case-control analysis
Brauchli YB, Jick SS, Miret M, et al (Univ Hosp Basel, Switzerland; Boston Univ School of Medicine, Lexington, MA; Merck Serono International SA, Geneva, Switzerland)
Br J Dermatol 160:1048-1056, 2009

Background.—Systemic inflammation may increase the risk for cardiovascular diseases in patients with psoriasis, but data on this risk in patients with early psoriasis are scarce.

Objectives.—To assess and compare the risk of developing incident myocardial infarction (MI), stroke or transient ischaemic attack (TIA) between an inception cohort of patients with psoriasis and a psoriasis-free population.

Methods.—We conducted an inception cohort study with a nested case–control analysis within the U.K.-based General Practice Research Database. The study population encompassed 36702 patients with a first-time recorded diagnosis of psoriasis 1994–2005, matched 1 : 1 to psoriasis-free patients. We assessed crude incidence rates (IRs) and applied conditional logistic regression to obtain odds ratios (ORs) with 95% confidence intervals (CIs).

Results.—Overall, the IRs of MI (n = 449), stroke (n = 535) and TIA (n = 402) were similar among patients with or without psoriasis. However, the adjusted OR of developing MI for patients with psoriasis aged < 60 years was 1·66 (95% CI 1·03–2·66) compared with patients without psoriasis, while the OR for patients aged ≥ 60 years was 0·99 (95% CI 0·77–1·26). The adjusted ORs of developing MI for patients of all ages with ≤ 2 or > 2 prescriptions/year for oral psoriasis treatment were 2·48 (95% CI 0·69–8·91) and 1·39 (95% CI 0·43–4·53), with a similar finding for stroke and TIA.

Conclusions.—The risk of developing a cardiovascular outcome was not materially elevated for patients with early psoriasis overall. In subanalyses, however, there was a suggestion of an increased (but low absolute) MI risk for patients with psoriasis aged < 60 years, mainly with severe disease.

▶ Psoriasis is characterized as an inflammatory disease with the activation of cytokines, tumor necrosis factor-α, and acute phase C-reactive proteins. It has been theorized that there is an increased incidence of atherosclerosis and transient ischemic attack (TIA) in psoriasis patients due to elevated inflammatory processes driven by proinflammatory cytokines. This is a nested case-controlled analysis within the United Kingdom population database to quantify the risk of and incident of myocardial infarction (MI), stroke, or TIA diagnosis in patients after a first-time recorded psoriasis diagnosis compared with a matched population without psoriasis. Patients that were excluded were those with a previous history of ischemic heart disease, cerebrovascular disease, cancer, or HIV before psoriasis diagnosis. Then, these individuals were followed until they developed a first-time diagnosis of MI, stroke, or TIA, or until their medical record ended. Results revealed that patients with psoriasis were more likely to be current smokers and overweight compared with controls. Past studies have shown that there is an increased risk for cardiovascular events in patients with severe hospitalized forms of psoriasis, which was also found in this study. They also concluded that there was no evidence for an overall increased risk of MI, stoke, or TIA associated with psoriasis. Although they mentioned that there was a slight elevated risk associated with severe psoriasis, the definition of severe psoriasis was defined by the use of oral agents or ultraviolet (UV) treatment, but no clinical scale to measure psoriatic lesions and severity was mentioned. This is problematic because it is unknown whether psoriasis in these patients was well controlled and what the actual extent of severity was. There were also findings to suggest that MI risk was elevated in patients under 60 years of age independent of other cardiovascular risk factors. The risk was not related to duration of psoriasis but tended to be higher for patients with less intense oral treatment (<2 prescription/year) possibly due to disease-modifying antirheumatic drugs (DMARDs), reducing disease activity in the skin and having systemic anti-inflammatory effects thereby reducing cardiovascular morbidity and mortality. Some limitations of this study were that there was no measurement of cardiovascular status of control and psoriasis patients before and after the study was conducted. Therefore, previous atherosclerotic lesions could not be predicted. In addition, it is unknown whether or not psoriasis patients could have had previous unrecognized psoriatic lesions before this study. The study also had a short follow-up period of 4 to 6 years, which was another limitation since chronic systemic inflammatory disease may take years before its effects can be seen in the heart or other organs. Also, just because a patient didn't have a stroke or an MI at the end of the study does not mean that they have no risk at all to have one of these events occur in the future.

G. K. Kim, DO

J. Q. Del Rosso, DO

Plaque thickness and morphology in psoriasis vulgaris associated with therapeutic response
Rakkhit T, Panko JM, Christensen TE, et al (Univ of Utah School of Medicine, Salt Lake City; et al)
Br J Dermatol 160:1083-1089, 2009

Background.—The Utah Psoriasis Initiative (UPI) is an expanding database that is being used to identify and characterize phenotypic variants of psoriasis and explore genotype–phenotype relationships. We recently reported distinct morphological variants of psoriasis that are characterized by thickness of lesions (induration) in the untreated state.

Objectives.—To explore the clinical relevance of these morphological variants.

Methods.—For these analyses, we used the phenotypic data from 282 additional subjects gathered at enrolment into the UPI and compared their phenotype with that of the original 500 patients reported previously. The analysis was further expanded via a longitudinal follow-up of 286 subjects from the original 500 case cohort.

Results.—Firstly, the initial findings were confirmed. Expansion of the cohort used for the original observation by about 50% and reanalysis showed that there was no alteration in the proportions of patients expressing thin- and thick-plaque disease phenotypes. Secondly, analysis of the larger cohort showed that this morphological phenotype had clinical relevance: those patients with thin-plaque disease were more likely to report a complete therapeutic response to topical corticosteroids and phototherapy. In contrast, plaque thickness did not appear to be a factor in response to systemic agents.

Conclusions.—Using a patient's baseline plaque morphology to choose a primary treatment modality may result in earlier disease improvement and reduce the cost of therapy.

▶ The authors sought to evaluate plaque thickness and morphology, and their association with therapeutic responses to different modalities. Analysis of the larger cohort in this study demonstrated that morphological phenotype had clinical relevance: those patients with thin-plaque disease were more likely to report a complete therapeutic response to topical corticosteroids and phototherapy. In contrast, plaque thickness did not appear to be a factor in response to systemic agents. The authors speculated that systemic therapy eradicates lesions of psoriasis in a fashion that is independent of the pathological events that determine thickness. They further postulate that these findings are likely to modulate therapeutic considerations in the selection of treatment regimens and need to be considered when interpreting data from clinical trials where phenotypic differences have generally not been a consideration.

However, it is unclear if this study will significantly alter our approach to psoriasis patients. Further follow-up of this cohort and additional studies will help to confirm these findings.

J. Weinberg, MD

Efficacy and Safety of Combination Acitretin and Pioglitazone Therapy in Patients With Moderate to Severe Chronic Plaque-Type Psoriasis: A Randomized, Double-blind, Placebo-Controlled Clinical Trial
Mittal R, Malhotra S, Pandhi P, et al (Postgraduate Inst of Med Education and Res, Chandigarh, India)
Arch Dermatol 145:387-393, 2009

Objective.—To evaluate the efficacy and safety of combination therapy with acitretin and pioglitazone hydrochloride in patients with moderate to severe chronic plaque-type psoriasis.

Design.—Randomized, double-blind, placebo-controlled clinical trial.

Setting.—A tertiary care referral hospital.

Patients.—The study included patients of either sex (age range, 18-65 years) with moderate to severe chronic plaque-type psoriasis. Patients were excluded if they were of child-bearing potential or if they had impaired liver or renal function, hyperlipidemia, diabetes mellitus, coronary artery disease, or a body mass index greater than 30 (calculated as weight in kilograms divided by height in meters squared). Of the 62 patients screened, 41 were randomly assigned to 2 groups: 22 to an acitretin (25 mg) plus placebo group and 19 to an acitretin (25 mg) plus pioglitazone hydrochloride (15 mg) group.

Main Outcome Measure.—Change in Psoriasis Area and Severity Index score between the 2 groups from baseline to 12 weeks.

Results.—After 12 weeks of therapy, the percentage of reduction in the Psoriasis Area and Severity Index score was 64.2% in the acitretin plus pioglitazone group and 51.7% in the acitretin plus placebo group. The majority of the adverse events were mild to moderate except for 1 possibly unrelated episode of acute myocardial infarction in a 49-year-old woman in the acitretin plus placebo group.

Conclusions.—Pioglitazone has a potential beneficial antipsoriatic effect and may provide a convenient, efficacious, and relatively safe option to combine with acitretin, although further studies are needed.

Trial Registration.—clinicaltrials.gov Identifier: NCT00395941.

▶ Thiazolidinediones (TZDs) have potential beneficial therapeutic effects in psoriasis. Pioglitazone hydrochloride is a TZD that is used as insulin sensitizer in patients with type 2 diabetes mellitus. TZDs have been shown to inhibit proliferation and to induce differentiation in various in vitro and murine models of psoriasis.[1,2] A number of recent clinical studies, including 3 open-label studies and 1 randomized, double-blind, placebo-controlled, prospective study, have demonstrated evidence of some therapeutic benefit of TZDs in psoriasis.[1,3-5]

This study provides important insights into the beneficial effect of pioglitazone in combination with acitretin for therapy of moderate to severe chronic plaque-type psoriasis. The authors note that pioglitazone may offer a convenient, efficacious, and relatively safer alternative for combining with acitretin than currently available immunosuppressive agents, although this theory needs to be proved by further studies. In addition, the long-term safety of pioglitazone therapy in patients with chronic plaque-type psoriasis needs to be established. The growing body of literature on this novel therapy for psoriasis points toward an increasing role in clinical practice once more data is available.

J. Weinberg, MD

References

1. Ellis CN, Varani J, Fisher GJ, et al. Troglitazone improves psoriasis and normalizes models of proliferative skin disease: ligands for peroxisome proliferators-activated receptor-gamma inhibit keratinocytes proliferation. *Arch Dermatol.* 2000;136:609-616.
2. Demerjian M, Man MQ, Choi EH, et al. Topical treatment with thiazolidinediones, activators of peroxisome proliferator-activated receptor-gamma, normalizes epidermal homeostasis in a murine hyperproliferative disease model. *Exp Dermatol.* 2006;15:154-160.
3. Pershadsingh HA, Sproul JA, Benjamin E, Finnegan J, Amin NM. Treatment of psoriasis with troglitazone therapy. *Arch Dermatol.* 1998;134:1304-1305.
4. Robertshaw H, Friedmann PS. Pioglitazone: a promising therapy for psoriasis. *Br J Dermatol.* 2005;152:189-191.
5. Shafiq N, Malhotra S, Pandhi P, Gupta M, Kumar B, Sandhu K. Pilot trial: pioglitazone versus placebo in patients with plaque psoriasis (the P6). *Int J Dermatol.* 2005;44:328-333.

Palmoplantar psoriasis: A phenotypical and clinical review with introduction of a new quality-of-life assessment tool
Farley E, Masrour S, McKey J, et al (Baylor Univ Med Ctr, Dallas, TX)
J Am Acad Dermatol 60:1024-1031, 2009

Background.—Palmoplantar psoriasis is associated with significant quality-of-life issues. Its epidemiology and phenotypical expression remain ill defined.

Objective.—We reviewed the literature and our clinical experience and developed a new quality-of-life assessment tool.

Methods.—We conducted a retrospective review of 150 patients with palmoplantar psoriasis.

Results.—In all, 78 (52%) patients displayed predominantly hyperkeratotic palmoplantar lesions, 24 (16%) pustular, 18 (12%) combination, and 30 (20%) had an indeterminate phenotype. In 27 (18%) patients, lesions were confined to the palms and soles. A new quality-of-life index was constructed to characterize disease severity. In all, 27 (18%) had mild, 72 (48%) moderate, and 51 (34%) severe disease involvement. Palmoplantar disease severity appeared independent from the degree of body surface area involvement.

Limitations.—This was a retrospective review. The quality-of-life index remains to be statistically verified in prospective clinical studies.

Conclusion.—Defining morphologic subtypes together with the use of a specific quality-of-life assessment tool in patients with palmoplantar psoriasis will improve our understanding and treatment of this recalcitrant form of psoriasis.

▶ Although isolated palmoplantar psoriasis (PPP) affects less than 5% of the body surface area (BSA), it can significantly affect a patient's quality of life due to its recalcitrant nature. There is data lacking on PPP and the impact on a patient's quality of life. This is a retrospective review of 150 patients with significant PPP in a psoriasis clinic in Dallas using a new assessment tool, the Palmar-Plantar Quality-of-Life Index, to help quantify the quality of life in individuals. Significant disease was defined as moderate-to-severe psoriasis, having at least 50% of a single palmoplantar surface involved. The 2 main objectives for this study were to examine the subtypes of palmoplantar psoriasis: hyperkeratotic, purely pustular, or mixed variants. In addition, the extent to which other parts of the body were involved and disease severity were also noted. A single clinician did the examination for uniformity purposes. The thick, scaly, hyperkeratotic variety was the dominant phenotype present in 78 (52%) patients. Twenty-four (16%) patients had purely pustular variant, and 18 (12%) patients had a mixed phenotype that was composed of both hyperkeratotic plaques and pustules, whereas 30 (20%) patients were considered indeterminate. A total of 27 (18%) out of 150 patients had only hand and foot involvement. The remaining 123 (82%) had involvement elsewhere, with 50 (33%) patients having less than 10% BSA involvement. The quality of life index, 51 (34%) of the patients were severely affected by their disease. In all,

72 (48%) were moderately affected, with only 27 (18%) showing mild impact. A total of 142 (95%) of palmoplantar patients had at some stage required systemic therapy for their psoriasis. This study illustrated that patients with palmoplantar psoriasis may have devastating disease especially if their dominant hand is significantly affected or if the soles of their feet have multiple painful fissures, making ambulation difficult. With this is mind, the authors sought to create a quality of life index especially for this group of patients. Limitations included a single institute site with no age matched comparison group. In the future, there needs to be larger prospective trials conducted to fully assess the quality of life in these patients. This will allow for evidence-based recommendations concerning treatments for PPP and validation for aggressive therapy.

G. K. Kim, DO

J. Q. Del Rosso, DO

A retrospective analysis of treatment responses of palmoplantar psoriasis in 114 patients

Adişen E, Tekin O, Gülekon A, et al (Gazi Univ, Ankara, Turkey)

J Eur Acad Dermatol Venereol 23:814-819, 2009

Background.—Treatment options remain unsatisfactory for patients with palmoplantar psoriasis (PP) and palmoplantar pustular psoriasis (PPP).

Aim.—To evaluate the therapeutic responses of PP and PPP patients that were treated in our psoriasis polyclinic between 2003 and 2007.

Methods.—This retrospective study comprised PP ($n = 62$) and PPP ($n = 52$) patients. Treatments were individualized according to patient compliance and associating systemic diseases. The effect of systemic treatments was grouped as follows: 'no improvement': patients unresponsive for the present treatment; 'partial improvement': < 50% decrease in severity or affected area; 'moderate improvement': 50–75% decrease in severity or affected area, and 'marked improvement': > 75% decrease of the disease compared to baseline.

Results.—In the PP group, 17 of 62 patients showed marked improvement to topical agents, while the remaining patients required systemic agents including oral retinoids ($n = 24$), local psoralen plus ultraviolet A (PUVA; $n = 12$), methotrexate ($n = 9$) and cyclosporine ($n = 2$). Marked improvement was achieved in 53%, 45%, 47% and 100%, respectively. In these patients, two ($n = 10$), three ($n = 5$), or four ($n = 5$) systemic agents were used alternately.

In the PPP group, 18 of 52 patients achieved marked improvement by topical agents. Patients that required systemic agents were treated with colchicum ($n = 19$), local PUVA ($n = 8$), methotrexate ($n = 4$), oral retinoids ($n = 3$) and cyclosporine ($n = 2$). These treatments achieved a marked improvement in 60%, 33%, 57%, 83%, and 50% of the patients, respectively. In the course of the disease, 18 patients required two and 3 patients required three systemic agents alternately.

Conclusions.—Although the success rates appeared to be high, the high number of patients who required multiple systemic agents emphasized the fact that localized forms of psoriasis were resistant to therapy.

▶ Palmoplantar psoriasis and palmoplantar pustular psoriasis are notoriously difficult to treat. The latter observation is confirmed in this retrospective study of 114 patients treated between 2003 and 2007 in a psoriasis clinic in Ankara, Turkey. Only 27% of patients in the palmoplantar psoriasis group and 35% of patients in the palmoplantar pustular psoriasis group showed marked improvement to topical agents compared with 53% and 83% of patients treated with oral retinoids, 47% and 57% treated with methotrexate, and 50% and 100% treated with cyclosporine for palmoplantar psoriasis and palmoplantar pustular psoriasis respectively. Marked improvement to topical or oral PUVA ranged from 0% to 53%. The one conclusion that can be derived from this article is that the treatment of palm and sole psoriasis remains difficult, but there are many therapeutic options available. Sixty percent of patients treated with palmoplantar pustular psoriasis achieved marked improvement with oral colchicine.

While the information presented here is clinically relevant and mirrors the experiences of others treating psoriasis of the palms and soles, there are a number of serious flaws to the study. There was not a consistent approach to the management of these patients so that the results can't be generalized to every patient who presents with psoriasis of the palms and soles. Patients with severe disease, for example, might be treated more aggressively with drugs like methotrexate, accounting for the lower response rate with that drug. In typical practices, female patients of childbearing potential are not treated with oral retinoids. Other variations in presentation might explain the different response rates reported here. Furthermore, several treatments available in other parts of the world were not considered here. For example, the excimer laser is not mentioned, nor were biologic therapies used. Also, many of the patients required 2 or 3 systemic agents so it may not be entirely clear which agent ultimately resulted in improvement of psoriasis.

M. Lebwohl, MD

Association of Psoriasis With Coronary Artery, Cerebrovascular, and Peripheral Vascular Diseases and Mortality
Prodanovich S, Kirsner RS, Kravetz JD, et al (Univ of Miami Miller School of Medicine, FL; Yale Univ School of Medicine, New Haven, CT)
Arch Dermatol 145:700-703, 2009

Objective.—To examine the cardiovascular risk factors in patients with psoriasis and the association between psoriasis and coronary artery, cerebrovascular, and peripheral vascular diseases.

Design.—Observational study.

Setting.—Large Department of Veterans Affairs hospital.

Patients.—The study included 3236 patients with psoriasis and 2500 patients without psoriasis (controls).

Main Outcome Measures.—Using *International Classification of Diseases, Ninth Revision, Clinical Modification,* codes, we compared the prevalence of traditional cardiovascular risk factors and other vascular diseases as well as mortality between patients with psoriasis and controls.

Results.—Similar to previous studies, we found a higher prevalence of diabetes mellitus, hypertension, dyslipidemia, and smoking in patients with psoriasis. After controlling for these variables, we found a higher prevalence not only of ischemic heart disease (odds ratio [OR], 1.78; 95% confidence interval [CI], 1.51-2.11) but also of cerebrovascular (OR, 1.70; 95% CI, 1.33-2.17) and peripheral vascular (OR, 1.98; 95% CI, 1.32-2.82) diseases in patients with psoriasis compared with controls. Psoriasis was also found to be an independent risk factor for mortality (OR, 1.86; 95% CI, 1.56-2.21).

Conclusions.—Psoriasis is associated with atherosclerosis. This association applies to coronary artery, cerebrovascular, and peripheral vascular diseases and results in increased mortality.

▶ This is an excellent study reinforcing the association of psoriasis with coronary artery disease and also establishing a correlation with psoriasis to peripheral artery disease and cerebrovascular disease. The large size of this study gives validity to the conclusions drawn which is that patients with psoriasis have higher prevalence of not only ischemic heart disease but also of peripheral arterial and cerebrovascular diseases. Psoriasis was determined to be an independent risk factor for mortality. Despite some limitations to the study, the information is still valid. One limitation of the study is that approximately 96% of psoriatic patients were men. Men in general are at higher risk for coronary artery, peripheral, and cerebrovascular diseases than compared with women. This is an excellent article not only for dermatologists but also for primary care physicians to be aware that patients with psoriasis appear to need more vigilant screening for atherosclerotic disease.

S. B. Momin, DO

J. Q. Del Rosso, DO

Efficacy and safety of calcipotriol plus betamethasone dipropionate scalp formulation compared with calcipotriol scalp solution in the treatment of scalp psoriasis: a randomized controlled trial

Kragballe K, Hoffmann V, Ortonne JP, et al (Aarhus Univ Hosp, Denmark; Clinical Operations, LEO Pharma A/S, Ballerup, Denmark; Hôpital L'Archet, France; et al)

Br J Dermatol 161:159-166, 2009

Background.—Current topical therapies for scalp psoriasis are difficult or unpleasant to apply, resulting in decreased adherence and efficacy.

Objectives.—To compare the efficacy and safety of once-daily treatment with a combination of calcipotriol $50\,\mu g\,g^{-1}$ plus betamethasone $0\cdot5\,mg\,g^{-1}$ (as dipropionate) (Xamiol®; LEO Pharma A/S, Ballerup, Denmark) and twice-daily calcipotriol $50\,\mu g\,mL^{-1}$ scalp solution in patients with scalp psoriasis.

Methods.—This 8-week, multicentre, randomized, investigator-blind, parallel-group study compared two-compound calcipotriol/betamethasone scalp formulation with calcipotriol scalp solution in patients with moderately severe scalp psoriasis. Primary efficacy outcome was the proportion of patients who achieved 'clear' or 'minimal' disease severity according to investigator's global assessment of disease severity at week 8. Secondary efficacy outcomes and adverse events were also evaluated. Relapse and rebound were assessed in an 8-week, post-treatment observation phase.

Results.—In total, 207 patients received the two-compound scalp formulation and 105 patients received calcipotriol scalp solution. The proportion of patients with 'clear' or 'minimal' disease at week 8 was significantly greater in the two-compound scalp formulation group $(68\cdot6\%)$ than in the calcipotriol scalp solution group $(31\cdot4\%;$ $P < 0\cdot001)$. Improvement was more rapid with the two-compound scalp formulation than with calcipotriol scalp solution. Further evidence of the superiority of the two-compound scalp formulation over the scalp solution was demonstrated through greater improvements in clinical signs and fewer adverse events.

Conclusions.—A once-daily combination of calcipotriol plus betamethasone dipropionate was significantly more effective and better tolerated than twice-daily calcipotriol scalp solution in the treatment of scalp psoriasis.

▶ Psoriasis is a debilitating disease of the skin that can greatly affect the quality of life of affected individuals. Due to its chronic nature and potential for frequent exacerbations, physicians and patients are continuously seeking better, more efficacious treatment alternatives. Traditionally, psoriasis involving the scalp has been treated with either topical corticosteroids, salicylic acid shampoos, tar shampoos, or a vitamin D derivative. Each treatment option has its inherent pros and cons. Topical corticosteroids have a quicker onset of action with patients often noting resolution of symptoms (ie, pruritus) in the first few weeks. However, the side effects associated with long-term continuous corticosteroid use forces us to look toward steroid sparing alternatives. To that end, vitamin D derivatives, including calcipotriol have been investigated. The efficacy of vitamin D derivatives is well documented; however, patients sometimes complained of burning or irritation with application of calcipotriene when used as monotherapy. Thus, this study evaluated the combination therapy of both treatments mentioned above.

The results of the current multicenter randomized study echoed previous reports of combination treatment yielding significantly greater improvement of signs and symptoms than calcipotriol alone. In fact, the combination scalp solution of betamethasone dipropionate with calcipotriol had fewer reported adverse side effects with the benefit of once daily application compared with twice daily use of calcipotriol.

S. Bellew, DO

J. Q. Del Rosso, DO

The prevalence of previously diagnosed and undiagnosed psoriasis in US adults: Results from NHANES 2003-2004
Kurd SK, Gelfand JM (Univ of Pennsylvania School of Medicine, Philadelphia)
J Am Acad Dermatol 60:218-224, 2009

Background.—Psoriasis is a predictor of morbidity. It is important to determine the extent to which psoriasis remains undiagnosed.

Objective.—To determine the prevalence of psoriasis.

Methods.—We conducted a cross-sectional study using the National Health and Nutrition Examination Survey 2003-2004.

Results.—The prevalence of diagnosed psoriasis was 3.15% (95% confidence interval [CI], 2.18-4.53), corresponding to 5 million adults. Approximately 17% of these patients have moderate to severe psoriasis based on body surface area report and 25% rate psoriasis a large problem in everyday life. The prevalence of undiagnosed active psoriasis by conservative estimate was 0.4% (95% CI, 0.19-0.82), corresponding to approximately 600,000 US adults, and 2.28% (95% CI, 1.47-3.50) by a broader definition, corresponding to 3.6 million US adults. Undiagnosed patients had a trend toward being more likely to be male, nonwhite, less educated, and unmarried compared with patients who had received a diagnosis.

Limitations.—The method for determining the presence of psoriasis had limited ability to detect mild disease and only fair interrater agreement.

Conclusion.—More than 5 million adults have been diagnosed with psoriasis. A large number have undiagnosed psoriasis and there are important disparities which may be associated with not receiving medical attention.

▶ Estimates of the prevalence of psoriasis have varied tremendously, with higher estimates occurring at northern latitudes, and lower estimates closer to the equator. In recent years, a telephone survey estimated that the prevalence of psoriasis in adults in the United States was 2.2%, and a mail survey estimated the prevalence of psoriasis at 2.6%. Because many patients may be unaware of their diagnosis, surveys are often inaccurate. This study relies on a United States database called the National Health and Nutrition Examination Survey (NHANES) from 2003-2004. Survey participants, aged 20 years to 59 years, complete an interviewer-administered questionnaire. The diagnosis of psoriasis is determined both by patient interview and by examination of photographs by 2 dermatologists.

Using this methodology, the prevalence of diagnosed psoriasis was 3.5% and undiagnosed active psoriasis was estimated to be 0.4% to 2.28%. Using these numbers, up to 8.6 million United States adults could be affected.

This reported study is based on data that includes both interviews and examination, and is therefore probably more accurate than mail and telephone surveys, and may be the most accurate data available to date in the United States. The main drawback of any study that relies on databases is that it will never be as accurate as direct examination of large numbers of patients with the specific purpose of identifying whether or not they have psoriasis. A strong feature of this study, however, is that it identifies undiagnosed active psoriasis in a substantial proportion of patients. Moreover, the authors of the study clearly recognized that these numbers do not include inactive psoriasis. Until sensitive and specific markers emerge for the multifactorial and genetic disorder that we call psoriasis, we won't know the true prevalence.

M. Lebwohl, MD

Increasing use of more potent treatments for psoriasis

Strowd LC, Yentzer BA, Fleischer AB Jr, et al (Wake Forest Univ School of Medicine, Winston-Salem, NC)
J Am Acad Dermatol 60:478-481, 2009

Background.—Psoriasis therapy has evolved during the past 25 years as newer and more effective medications become available. Furthermore, various combination regimens and approaches have been advocated.

Objective.—We sought to describe patterns of psoriasis treatment from 1986 to 2005.

Methods.—Visits to dermatologists for treatment of psoriasis were identified using National Ambulatory Medical Care Survey data, a representative survey of visits to physician offices in the United States. We focused on medications listed at these visits during the 1986-to-2005 interval to determine how treatment for psoriasis has changed.

Results.—There were an estimated 23.9 million visits for psoriasis during the 20-year study period. As a category, the most common medications used for psoriasis were topical steroids. Dermatologists are prescribing more potent topical steroids compared with nondermatologists. The use of these potent drugs has increased from 1986 to 2005.

There has been growing use of systemic treatments, with biologic therapies introduced in the 2001-to-2005 time period.

Limitations.—National Ambulatory Medical Care Survey data represent national trends in psoriasis treatment and cannot be used to evaluate smaller subpopulations of patients with psoriasis. These data are used to speculate why certain trends in treatment are seen.

Conclusion.—The primary treatment for psoriasis in the late 1980s and early 1990s was mid-potency corticosteroids. Since then, the primary therapies for psoriasis have evolved to include class I ultrapotent topical corticosteroids, vitamin-D analogs, and systemic medications such as methotrexate and biologic agents. These changes in psoriasis management are consistent with patient desire for better disease control.

▶ While the article is significant in the number of patients and study period involved, the conclusions of this article are not surprising. The article concludes that dermatologists are prescribing greater potency topical corticosteroids (vs nondermatologists) as well as oral systemic therapies, vitamin-D analogs, and biologic treatments compared with the late 1980s and early 1990s.

The article, however, further suggests the change in treatment is due in part to the patient's desire for better disease control and a discrepancy between the physician and patient impression of the impact of psoriasis on their quality of life. While this may have merit, a few observations have to be made. First, this certainly cannot be extrapolated to all dermatologists. Secondly, it inherently assumes there was a lack of understanding on the part of dermatologist 20 years ago about the impact of psoriasis on a patient's quality of life, based simply on the change in prescribed medications. Also not entirely considered is the dermatologists' perspective for greater control as additional medications became available or simply the possibility that better data and education were available regarding the treatments that are more effective in controlling psoriasis. Moreover, as noted by the author, biologic agents were not available for comparison in previous years, thus it is not possible to conclude that such agents would have been prescribed in a lesser or greater quantity had they been available.

The article also notes that dermatologists prescribe more potent topical corticosteroids now than nondermatologists, but no data was provided in the article to support this conclusion. Furthermore, the study included all patients with whom psoriasis was listed as 1 of 3 possible diagnoses. It is certainly possible for numerous patients with other diagnoses besides psoriasis to have been included in this study.

Ultimately, the objective of the article to describe patterns of psoriasis treatment from 1986-2005 has been met, although questions regarding its conclusions may be a consideration for further studies.

B. D. Michaels, DO
J. Q. Del Rosso, DO

Lichen planus and dyslipidaemia: a case-control study

Dreiher J, Shapiro J, Cohen AD (Clalit Health Services, Tel Aviv, Israel; Soraski Med Ctr, Tel Aviv, Israel; et al)
Br J Dermatol 161:626-629, 2009

Background.—Previous reports have demonstrated an association between psoriasis and dyslipidaemia.

Objectives.—As lichen planus (LP) is also a chronic inflammatory disorder, we investigated the association between LP and dyslipidaemia in Israel.

Methods.—A case–control study was performed utilizing the database of Clalit Health Services, a large healthcare provider organization in Israel. Patients aged 20–79 years who were diagnosed as having LP were compared with a sample of enrollees without LP regarding the prevalence of dyslipidaemia. Data on other health-related lifestyle factors and comorbidities were collected.

Results.—The study included 1477 patients with LP and 2856 controls without LP. The prevalence of dyslipidaemia was significantly higher in patients with LP (42·5% vs. 37·8%, P = 0·003; odds ratio, OR 1·21, 95% confidence interval, [CI]: 1·06–1·38). A multivariate logistic regression model demonstrated that LP was significantly associated with dyslipidaemia even after controlling for confounders, including age, sex, smoking, hypothyroidism, diabetes, hypertension, socioeconomic status and obesity (multivariate OR 1·34, 95% CI: 1·14–1·57, P < 0·001).

Conclusions.—In the present study, LP was found to be associated with dyslipidaemia.

▶ In this epidemiological study, the authors detail an association between a diagnosis of lichen planus (LP), as rendered by a dermatologist, and dyslipidemia. Diagnosis codes were used for the study; no measure of the lipid levels or lipid profiles were discussed. The control population, twice as large as the population of patients with lichen planus, was selected at random from the same institutional archives and matched for age and sex. The study found an increased prevalence of dyslipidemia among those with lichen planus (LP). These same authors reported similar findings among psoriatics,[1] and it was speculated that this might be the result of a chronic inflammatory state. Hypothyroidism was also found associated with LP, and certainly this fits not only with dyslipidemia, as the authors claim, but also, more generally, with the postulated autoimmune nature of LP. Limitations of the study include complete dependence upon the validity of diagnosis codes. Furthermore, while the authors note controls were screened for lipid abnormalities presumably to satisfy a national programme for quality indicators, the potential for selection bias exists. Additional study will determine the proper weight to place upon this finding, particularly with regard to cardiovascular risk assessment in patients diagnosed with LP.

W. A. High, MD, JD, MEng

Reference

1. Dreiher J, Weitzman D, Davidovici B, Shapiro J, Cohen AD. Psoriasis and dyslipidemia: a population-based study. *Acta Derm Venereol.* 2008;88:561-565.

Treatment of Refractory Oral Erosive Lichen Planus with Topical Rapamycin: 7 Cases
Soria A, Agbo-Godeau S, Taïeb A, et al (Service de Dermatologie-Allergologie, Hôpital Tenon, et; Service de Stomatologie, Hôpital Pitié-Salpétrière, Paris, et; Service de Dermatologie, Hôpital Saint-André, Bordeaux, France)
Dermatology 218:22-25, 2009

Background.—Chronic erosive oral lichen planus (CEOLP) is a painful disease. Topical steroids constitute the mainstay of treatment. Given the reports of a slightly greater risk of squamous-cell carcinoma, rapamycin may be a good candidate for recalcitrant CEOLP, as it has both immunosuppressive and antitumour properties.

Objectives.—To investigate the therapeutic effect and evaluate the blood absorption of topical rapamycin in patients with CEOLP.

Patients and Methods.—We carried out an open prospective study: 7 women with CEOLP applied topical rapamycin (1 mg/ml) on oral erosive lesions twice a day for 3 months. Four patients also had erosive vulvar lesions and applied the same solution on both mucosae. We monitored blood sirolimus levels 15 days after the initiation of treatment. Complete remission was defined by the disappearance of oral erosions and partial remission when the surface of oral erosions was 50% less than the surface of the initial erosion.

Results.—At 3 months, 4 women had complete remission and 2 women had partial remission. One patient stopped treatment due to local discomfort. Only 1 woman had blood sirolimus levels that were detectable.

Conclusion.—Topical rapamycin may be effective in some cases of refractory CEOLP, with negligible absorption into blood and minimal side effects.

▶ The objective of this article was to look at the effectiveness of topical rapamycin in patients with recalcitrant chronic erosive oral lichen planus (CEOLP). The study size was small with 7 patients. All 7 patients chosen were treated unsuccessfully in the past with topical corticosteroids, and 5 out of 7 patients had received at least one course of oral corticosteroids. Rapamycin was effective in 6 patients with 4 having complete remission. Patients with CEOLP are at risk for development of oral squamous cell carcinoma (SCC), and rapamycin is proposed as an alternative therapy as it has antitumor effects. However, no evidence was presented to support that rapamycin-treated patients may have a reduction in the risk of oral SCC development.

The limitation of this study was the small size, but nonetheless the study provides a potentially effective alternative therapy in recalcitrant patients.

S. Bhambri, DO

J. Q. Del Rosso, DO

Lichen Planopilaris: Retrospective Study and Stepwise Therapeutic Approach

Spencer LA, Hawryluk EB, English JC III (Univ of Pittsburgh, PA)
Arch Dermatol 145:333-334, 2009

Lichen planopilaris (LPP) is a primary lymphocytic scarring alopecia that causes inflammation, erythema, pruritus, dysesthesia, and alopecia that can be treatment resistant. After approval from the institutional review board, we performed a retrospective case analysis of alopecia due to LPP to assess possible therapeutic effectiveness.

▶ Lichen planopilaris (LPP) is a scarring alopecia that also causes inflammation, erythema, pruritus, and dysesthesia. This article reports a retrospective case analysis of alopecia due to LPP to assess possible therapeutic effectiveness, defined as absence of reported symptoms, such as pruritus, burning, and dysesthesia; lack of disease progression; reduction in erythema and follicular hyperkeratosis; and the ability to discontinue therapy. This article concludes that an effective therapy for refractory disease remains undetermined, but does support doxycycline and hydroxychloroquine as first-line agents. If no improvement is seen, a switch to mycophenolate mofetil or acitretin therapy may be successful. The limitations of oral acitretin use in females of child-bearing potential must be respected. The results do provide a good therapeutic approach, but the major weakness of this analysis are the small number of cases evaluated. Other limitations are stated in the article such as end points that did not include percentage of scalp hair loss or hair counts.

S. B. Momin, DO

J. Q. Del Rosso, DO

3 Bacterial and Fungal Infections

Staphylococcus lugdunensis, a Common Cause of Skin and Soft Tissue Infections in the Community

Böcher S, Tønning B, Skov RL, et al (Viborg Hosp, Denmark; Statens Serum Institut, Copenhagen, Denmark)
J Clin Microbiol 47:946-950, 2009

Staphylococcus lugdunensis, a rare cause of severe infections such as native valve endocarditis, often causes superficial skin infections similar to *Staphylococcus aureus* infections. We initiated a study to optimize the identification methods in the routine laboratory, followed by a population-based epidemiologic analysis of patients infected with *S. lugdunensis* in Viborg County, Denmark. Recognition of a characteristic *Eikenella corrodens*-like odor on Columbia sheep blood agar combined with colony pleomorphism and prominent β-hemolysis after 2 days of incubation, confirmed by API-ID-32 Staph, led to an 11-fold increase in the detection of *S. lugdunensis*. By these methods we found 491 *S. lugdunensis* infections in 4 years, corresponding to an incidence of 53 per 100,000 per year, an increase from 5 infections per 100,000 inhabitants in the preceding years. Seventy-five percent of the cases were found in general practice; these were dominated by skin abscesses (36%), wound infections (25%), and paronychias (13%). Fifty-six percent of the infections occurred below the waist, and toes were the most frequently infected site (21%). Only 3% of the patients suffered from severe invasive infections. The median age was 52 years, and the male/female ratio was 0.69. Our study shows that *S. lugdunensis* is a common cause of skin and soft-tissue infections (SSTI) and is probably underrated by many laboratories. *S. lugdunensis* should be accepted as a significant pathogen in SSTI and should be looked for in all routine bacteriological examinations, and clinicians should be acquainted with the name and the pathology of the bacterium.

▶ *Staphylococcus lugdunensis* is a coagulase-negative staphylococci (CoNS) bacterium. Infections with *S lugdunensis* tend to run a more severe course, which resemble that of *Staphylococcus aureus* infections rather than that caused by other CoNS. In addition, these organisms are frequently misidentified as *S aureus* because of similar characteristics. In addition, just like *S aureus*,

S lugdunensis can cause acute endocarditis in prosthetic and native valves and is also an important cause of many skin and soft-tissue infections (SSTI).

Over the time period of the study, the incidence of *S lugdunensis* was 53 infections per 100 000 inhabitants per year, in contrast to the value of 5 infections per 100 000 inhabitants per year previously determined. In addition 75% of cases found were in general practice outside of the hospital setting. It is the recommendation of these authors that an *S lugdunensis* infection be treated as seriously as a *S aureus* infection, and appropriate diagnostic methods should be performed routinely on culture and sensitivities.

Although definitive identification of *S lugdunensis* is well described and reliable, this study indicates that one problem is failure to suspect *S lugdunensis* due to its similar clinical appearance to *S aureus*. In addition, *S lugdunensis* is typically susceptible to the same antibiotics that treat *S aureus* such as naficillin, oxicillin, and vancomycin. Although this study does report a 20% resistance to penicillin, 2% methicillin-oxicillin resistance, and a 5% resistance to erythromycin, it is the opinions of the reviewers that it may not be cost-effective to test for *S lugdunensis* with every culture, given its similarity to *S aureus* and it epidemiology.

While the prevalence information and diagnostic method optimizations presented here may be useful in epidemiological studies and situations where identification of the exact pathogen may be necessary, for clinical dermatologists the identification of this pathogen is not entirely necessary as treatment will not be altered. Clearly a cost-benefit analysis needs to be completed before routine cultures and sensitivity includes testing for *S lugdunensis*.

J. Levin, DO

J. Q. Del Rosso, DO

Variability among pediatric infectious diseases specialists in the treatment and prevention of methicillin-resistant *Staphylococcus aureus* skin and soft tissue infections
Creech CB, Beekmann SE, Chen YY, et al (Vanderbilt Univ School of Medicine, Nashville, TN; Univ of Iowa)
Pediatr Infect Dis J 27:270-272, 2008

There are currently no clear consensus recommendations for the treatment and prevention of community-associated methicillin-resistant *Staphylococcus aureus* skin and soft tissue infections in pediatric patients. We surveyed over 100 Pediatric Infectious Diseases consultants and found considerable variability in both the treatment of skin and soft tissue infections and the strategies used for the management of children with recurrent MRSA disease.

▶ This survey of prescribing habits of pediatric infectious disease specialists is of interest to dermatologists, but suffers from serious limitations and raises more questions than it answers. The survey demonstrated a potential practice gap, namely the degree of variability in treatment strategies for primary methicillin-resistant *Staphylococcus aureus* (MRSA) infections and recurrent disease. The data reflect lack of consensus regarding the best treatment, but do not indicate whether this is based on lack of superiority of a given regimen, lack of data, or limitations in the survey tool itself.

Most importantly, only nasal colonization strategies were addressed, although most infections (67%) involved the buttocks or perineum. In these sites, skin carriage is far more relevant than nasal carriage, and treatment of nasal carriage alone has been shown to have little effect on outcomes. The degree to which these issues affected responses cannot be determined. Significant data suggest that treatment of household contacts, teammates, and day-care providers may be more important than addressing the patient's nares, but these were not addressed in the survey tool.

When faced with a recurrent infection with similar sensitivities, 20% of respondents said they would use a different antimicrobial agent, while 31.7% would use the same agent for longer period of time. The most common reasons for failure, of course, would be inadequate drainage, noncompliance, failure to treat an underlying dermatosis, contact with fomites such as towels and soap or direct contact with a carrier. The most compelling reason for a change in the antibiotic would be inducible resistance with clindamycin, but this was not likely to be a major factor in anyone's decision as the vast majority reported that their microbiology labs routinely performed a D-test for inducible clindamycin resistance and that they would have modified therapy based on the test results.

In summary, this report was more thought provoking in regard to how to design a survey tool than for the results reported.

D. M. Elston, MD

Risk Factors for Methicillin-Resistant *Staphylococcal aureus* Skin and Soft Tissue Infections Presenting in Primary Care: A South Texas Ambulatory Research Network (STARNet) Study
Parchman ML, Munoz A (Univ of Texas Health Science Ctr, San Antonio; Munoz Family Medicine Clinic, Austin, TX)
J Am Board Fam Med 22:375-379, 2009

Purpose.—To examine skin and soft tissue infections presenting at 4 primary care clinics and assess if historical risk factors and examination findings were associated with a positive methicillin-resistant *Staphylococcus aureus* (MRSA) culture.

Methods.—During the 10-month observational study (April 2007 through January 2008), physicians in 5 practices across South Texas collected history, physical examination findings, culture results, and antibiotic(s) prescribed for all patients presenting with a skin or soft tissue infection. Analyses were conducted to determine the relationship between historical indicators, location of lesions, and examination findings with a positive MRSA culture.

Results.—Across 4 practices, 164 cases of skin and soft tissue infections were collected during 10 months. Of the 94 with a culture, 63 (67%) were MRSA positive. Patients working in or exposed to a health care setting were more likely to have a culture positive for MRSA, as were those presenting with an abscess. MRSA-positive lesions were also significantly smaller in size.

Conclusions.—Because of the high prevalence of MRSA skin and soft tissue infections among patients presenting to family physicians, presumptive treatment for MRSA may be indicated. However, increasing levels of resistance to current antibiotics is concerning and warrants development of alternative management strategies.

▶ Parchman and Munoz performed a limited observational study to determine whether historical risk factors and examination findings were associated with a positive methicillin-resistant *Staphylococcus aureus* (MRSA) culture. The article found that patients working in or exposed to a health care setting and those patients presenting with an abscess were more likely to have a positive MRSA culture. It was also noted that MRSA positive lesions were smaller in size. With this data, it was suggested that presumptive treatment for MRSA may be indicated. This study should be interpreted with caution for several reasons, including many of which are appropriately noted by the authors themselves. The study interestingly found that those patients who presented with an abscess were 3.4 times more likely to have a MRSA infection versus any other skin lesion and that none of the cultured abscesses were MRSA negative. However, for clarification, the author's note only 4 of the 37 patients who presented without an abscess were cultured. Thus, as not all lesions were cultured, it is difficult to definitively determine and contrast the prevalence of MRSA positivity in other nonabscess lesions. Moreover, a specific and uniform definitional term was not used by all the practitioners participating in the study for either abscess, or skin, or soft-tissue infection. Rather, classification of the lesion was left to the judgment of the individual practitioner. Further, while the authors note that the MRSA positive lesions were smaller, this risk factor arguably needs more specific parameters before being considered as one of the criteria for administering presumptive treatment for MRSA. Other concerns include the limitations of the study by both the size of the study (164 cases) and its geographical restrictions—the study was conducted in 4 primary care clinic settings in South Texas. While these limitations are also emphasized by the authors, a suggestion of a presumptive treatment for MRSA treatment based on the above risk factors itself appears presumptive, especially given the concern regarding increased levels of antibiotic resistance. In the end, however, the study does importantly note the call for development of an alternative management strategy for MRSA in the face of antibiotic resistance.

B. D. Michaels, DO
J. Q. Del Rosso, DO

The Incidence of Methicillin-Resistant *Staphylococcus aureus* **in Community-Acquired Hand Infections**
Wilson PC, Rinker B (Univ of Kentucky College of Medicine, Lexington)
Ann Plast Surg 62:513-516, 2009

Methicillin-resistant *Staphylococcus aureus* (MRSA) has become increasingly prevalent in hand infections. Traditionally, the empiric treatment of hand infections has involved β-lactam antibiotics, which are ineffective against MRSA. Centers for Disease Control recommends empiric coverage of MRSA infections if the local rate of MRSA exceeds 10% to 15%. A retrospective review was performed on all patients admitted for community-acquired soft tissue infections of the hand between 2004 and 2007 at a single institution. The overall incidence of MRSA was 60%. The incidence of MRSA in healthy adults was 64%, healthy pediatric patients was 100%, immunocompromised patients was 45%, and diabetic patients was 20%. The current rates of MRSA would imply that all patients presenting with hand infections should be treated empirically for MRSA. Linezolid is the only oral antibiotic approved by the Food and Drug Administration for treating MRSA, but many studies have reported that trimethoprim-sulfamethoxazole is an effective antibiotic for outpatient treatment of MRSA.

▶ There is little doubt that community-acquired methicillin-resistant *Staphylococcus aureus* (CA-MRSA) infections in the United States are increasing. However, it is important to realize that the prevalence of MRSA infections does vary with respect to the field of medicine practiced. For example, in a study conducted in 2006, using data from emergency departments, a 59% overall prevalence of MRSA was found, while a study in 2008, using data from an outpatient dermatology clinic in Germany, found a 14% overall prevalence of MRSA.[1,2] It was argued that differences in acuity among patients seeking care might explain this discrepancy. Certainly, the recommendation from the Centers for Disease Control (CDC), that empiric coverage of MRSA be commenced for skin and soft tissue infections (SSTI) when the local MRSA rates exceed 10% to 15%, might impact these 2 practice environments differently.[3]

In this study, the authors examined the rate of CA-MRSA in hand infections severe enough to justify admission to a hospital service. This latter fact may introduce a selection bias that must be considered before applying the results directly to dermatology, where hand infections may be, on the whole, somewhat less acute.

Still, the authors found a 60% rate of MRSA infections in 84 patients with hand infections seen over a 4-year period. These MRSA infections were, as most CA-MRSA have been to date, 100% sensitive to trimethoprim/sulfamethoxazole (TMP/SMX) and tetracycline. The authors found also that pediatric patients with hand infections were even more likely to be caused by MRSA than were adult patients with hand infections.

Therefore, while practice environments are different, it may behoove the dermatologist to consider this information when confronted with bacterial infections on the hand, particularly in children, and to consider a management strategy that uses antibiotics known to effectively treat CA-MRSA, including TMP/SMX and the tetracycline family of antibiotics (the latter when the patient is greater than 8-9 years old).

W. A. High, MD, JD, MEng

References

1. Moran GJ, Krishnadasan A, Gorwitz RJ, et al. EMERGEncy ID Net Study Group. Methicillin-resistant S. aureus infections among patients in the emergency department. *N Engl J Med.* 2006;355:666-674.
2. Jappe U, Heuck D, Strommenger B, et al. *Staphylococcus aureus* in dermatology outpatients with special emphasis on community-associated methicillin-resistant strains. *J Invest Dermatol.* 2008;128:2655-2664.
3. Gorwitz RJ, Jernigan DB, Powers JH, et al. *Strategies for Clinical Management of MRSA in the Community: Summary of an Experts Meeting Convened by the CDC.* Atlanta, GA: Centers for Disease Control and Prevention; 2006.

Antimicrobial and Healing Efficacy of Sustained Release Nitric Oxide Nanoparticles Against *Staphylococcus Aureus* Skin Infection
Martinez LR, Han G, Chacko M, et al (Albert Einstein College of Medicine, Bronx, NY)
J Invest Dermatol 129:2463-2469, 2009

Staphylococcus aureus (SA) is a leading cause of both superficial and invasive infections in community and hospital settings, frequently resulting in chronic refractory disease. It is imperative that innovative therapeutics to which the bacteria are unlikely to evolve resistance be developed to curtail associated morbidity and mortality and ultimately improve our capacity to treat these infections. In this study, a previously unreported nitric oxide (NO)-releasing nanoparticle technology is applied to the treatment of methicillin-resistant *SA* (MRSA) wound infections. The results show that the nanoparticles exert antimicrobial activity against MRSA in a murine wound model. Acceleration of infected wound closure in NO-treated groups was clinically shown compared with controls. The histology of wounds revealed that NO nanoparticle treatment decreased suppurative inflammation, minimal bacterial burden, and less collagen degradation, providing potential mechanisms for biological activity. Together, these data suggest that these NO-releasing nanoparticles have the potential to serve as a novel class of topically applied antimicrobials for the treatment of cutaneous infections and wounds.

▶ *Staphylococcus aureus* (SA) is a gram-positive coccus that is responsible for most skin infections both in the emergency room and in the outpatient setting. Topical nitric oxide (NO) has been theorized to be a useful preventative to superficial skin infections, including those caused by methicillin-resistant *SA*

(MRSA). This is a study investigating the application of topically applied NO releasing nanoparticles (NO-np) for the treatment of MRSA wound infections using mouse models. The 2 groups that were evaluated were patients with uninfected skin and patients with skin wounds infected with MRSA. Each group included untreated wounds, treated with np (np without NO precursors), and NO-np treated wounds. Researchers examined the behavior of NO in NO-np and found that it was released immediately after application, and reached a steady-state level after 6 hours lasting until 24 hours. Examiners also determined susceptibility of clinical MRSA and methicillin-sensitive SA (MSSA) strains to NO-np. In addition, it was also found that NO-np treated lesions had increased wound-healing rates (shortened healing time), correlated with a significant decrease in the size of eschars compared with untreated or np groups ($P < .001$) at day 3. MRSA-infected NO-np treated wounds showed significantly a lower microbial count burden than did the untreated wounds ($P < .01$). Additionally, MRSA-infected mice treated with NO-np had a significantly lower microbial count burden than did the untreated or np-treated mice ($P < .01$). Furthermore, NO-np accelerated wound healing by preventing collagen degradation by MRSA in infected tissue upon microscopic examination. Future randomized, double-blinded, placebo-controlled trials in human models should be conducted to fully assess usage of NO-np in the clinical setting. One limitation to this study was that the safety profile of NO-np in humans could not be assessed and the possibility of systemic absorption was not discussed. Investigators suggest that NO may have a role in immunity and aid in wound healing with many implications for the future. This study also revealed the potential of NO-np with the treatment of different types of wounds like burns and decubitus ulcers. Most importantly, this study illustrates NO-np as an antimicrobial agent with activity against resistant bacterial species such as MRSA.

G. K. Kim, DO

J. Q. Del Rosso, DO

Hansen's disease in a general hospital: uncommon presentations and delay in diagnosis
da Costa Nery JA, Schreuder PAM, Castro Teixeira de Mattos P, et al (Univ Gama Filho, Brazil; NLR, Brazil; et al)
J Eur Acad Dermatol Venereol 23:150-156, 2009

Background.—The question was raised as to why 'obvious' signs of leprosy, Hansen's disease (HD), are often missed by medical doctors working in a HD endemic area.

Methods.—This study describes a small sample of patients who were diagnosed with HD during their hospital admission and not before. The discussion is whether the typical early signs and symptoms of HD are just not recognized, or whether unusual presentations confuse the attending physician.

Results.—A total of 23 HD patients were hospitalized during the study period, of which 6 (26%) were only diagnosed with HD during their admission. All were classified as lepromatous leprosy (LL) with a history of signs and symptoms of HD. In nearly all patients, a suspicion of HD might have been raised earlier if a careful history and dermato-neurological examination had been done.

Conclusions.—Multibacillary (MB) HD, especially close to the lepromatous end of the spectrum, may mimic other diseases, and the patient can not be diagnosed without a biopsy or a slit skin smear examination. Clinicians working in a HD endemic area (Rio de Janeiro) do not always include HD in their differential diagnosis, especially when the clinical presentation is unusual. HD should be considered in all patients with skin lesions not responding to treatment, especially when they have neurological deficits, and live or have lived in an HD endemic area. Due to the increase in global travel and immigration, doctors in low endemic areas need to consider HD as a possible diagnosis.

▶ Recently, there has been a high prevalence of Hansen's disease (HD) being misdiagnosed by physicians in certain endemic areas, which has become a major concern. This is a prospective study during the years 2004-2005 in Santa Casa Hospital, Rio de Janeiro, including 23 patients diagnosed with HD both before and after admission to the hospital. The authors wanted to answer why "obvious" signs of HD were missed in an area were HD is endemic. Most of the patients were males within the range of 19 to 72 years. There were 17 patients who had been diagnosed before hospitalization. With a diagnosis of HD, the patients were transferred to the dermatology department for further management. A physical examination, including a dermatological and neurological assessment, was performed, and a slit skin smear and biopsies were taken to diagnose and classify. They also found that early signs and symptoms— including skin lesions and signs of infiltration, numbness, sensory loss, or other neurological deficits—were often not recognized. When a patient did not respond to the initial treatment, HD was still not considered in the differential diagnosis. Conclusions were that special attention should be given to the more uncommon presentations of HD, which are often not recognized in the early stages of the disease. In addition, clinicians tend to pay attention to the more obvious signs of symptoms in his or her own field of expertise without being aware of the systemic involvement of HD. Some unusual presentations may have diffuse and discrete infiltration with loss of body hair but no visible skin nodules. The other clinical manifestations may be rhinitis, alopecia, telangiectasia of face and chest, facial acne or rosacea, and livedoid changes on the lower extremities. Some patients may present with rheumatic symptoms. Another uncommon manifestation is erythema nodosum leprosum (ENL), which is mainly seen in Latin America. The authors also emphasize that it is typical for the evolution of HD involving the upper respiratory tract to start with the involvement of the nose with symptoms of rhinitis. Ulceration of the lower legs can develop before the onset of the more typical lepromatous lesions and heal rapidly when anti-HD treatment is used. In HD, there is also edema of the lower legs, mostly bilateral, which is more evident in the evening. This may proceed by months or even years before the appearance of the more typical HD skin lesions. The authors also discovered that most newly diagnosed patients at the hospital with clear signs and symptoms of HD were ignored by health services. Early signs and symptoms with skin infiltration, numbness, sensory loss, or other neurological deficits must be recognized, and HD should be included in the differential diagnoses, especially in endemic areas.

G. K. Kim, DO

J. Q. Del Rosso, DO

The use of an intermittent terbinafine regimen for the treatment of dermatophyte toenail onychomycosis

Gupta AK, Lynch LE, Kogan N, et al (Sunnybrook Health Sciences Ctr and the Univ of Toronto, Canada; Mediprobe Res Inc, Ontario, Canada)
J Eur Acad Dermatol Venereol 23:256-262, 2009

Objective.—To compare the efficacy and safety of intermittent terbinafine with standard courses of terbinafine and itraconazole for dermatophyte toenail onychomycosis.

Design.—Data from a Canadian study of continuous terbinafine (CTERB) and intermittent itraconazole (III) was compared to an intermittent terbinafine regimen (TOT) using similar protocol to the randomized study.

Interventions.—Terbinafine 250 mg/day for 4 weeks followed by 4 weeks of no terbinafine and then an additional 4 weeks of terbinafine 250 mg/day (TOT); terbinafine 250 mg/day for 12 weeks (CTERB); itraconazole pulse of 200 mg twice daily for 7 days on, 21 days off, three pulses given (III).

Results.—At 72 weeks, mycological cure rates (negative KOH and culture) were 36 of 43 (83.7%), 25 of 32 (78.1%), and 17 of 30 (56.7%), for the TOT, CTERB, and III groups, respectively ($P = 0.01$ for TOT vs. III). Effective cure rates (simultaneous mycological cure and $\leq 10\%$ nail plate involvement) were 34 of 43 (79.1%), 21 of 32 (65.6%), and 11 of 30 (36.7%), respectively ($P < 0.001$ for TOT vs. III; $P = 0.02$ for CTERB vs. III). No significant differences in effective and mycological cure rates were noted between the two terbinafine groups. Adverse events reported were similar to those reported in the respective package inserts. Most adverse events were mild to moderate, transient, and did not require interruption of the drug regimens. No serious adverse events were reported.

Conclusions.—A TOT intermittent terbinafine regimen provided similar efficacy and safety to the gold standard continuous terbinafine regimen and better effective cure rates than pulse itraconazole therapy.

▶ The authors performed an interesting but small study to compare an intermittent terbinafine regimen (250 mg daily for 4 weeks, followed by 4 weeks off, followed by 250 mg daily for a second 4 weeks) with continuous terbinafine treatment (250 mg daily for 12 weeks) and itraconazole pulse therapy (200 mg twice daily for 7 days per month repeated 3 times ["3 pulses"]) for dermatophyte toenail onychomycosis. This article concludes that there is no statistical difference in clinical efficacy and mycological cure rate between continuous and intermittent terbinafine therapy at week 32, 48, or 72. The article under review would have had more valid conclusion if the study size was larger. A larger study not mentioned in the discussion is a randomized, double blind comparison of intermittent versus continuous terbinafine regimens in the treatment of toenail onychomycosis ($N = 2005$). The intermittent regimen was terbinafine 250 mg daily for 3 cycles of 2 weeks of treatment followed by 2 weeks off treatment while continuous therapy was terbinafine 250 mg daily for 12 weeks. This study concluded that intermittent terbinafine regimen was significantly less effective and did not provide any safety advantage.[1] Although terbinafine concentrations remain in the nail for several months after treatment has ceased, does an intermittent course of 2 weeks versus 4 weeks produce a significant clinical difference? The answer is not known and requires further study.

S. B. Momin, DO

J. Q. Del Rosso, DO

Reference

1. Sigurgeirsson B, Elewski BE, Rich PA, et al. Intermittent versus continuous terbinafine in the treatment of toenail onychomycosis: a randomized, double-blind comparison. *J Dermatolog Treat.* 2006;17:38-44.

National epidemiology of cutaneous abscesses: 1996 to 2005
Taira BR, Singer AJ, Thode HC Jr, et al (Stony Brook Univ Med Ctr, NY)
Am J Emerg Med 27:289-292, 2009

Objective.—Little has been reported regarding the national epidemiology of cutaneous abscesses. We examined the National Hospital Ambulatory Medical Care Survey (NHAMCS) national estimates of all emergency department (ED) visits from 1996 to 2005 to determine the trend and the epidemiology of ED abscess visits.
Methods.—Study design: retrospective analysis of NHAMCS databases for 1996 to 2005 available from the National Center for Health Statistics. Subjects: all patients with a first diagnosis of abscess based on the *International Classification of Diseases, Ninth Revision, Clinical Modification,*

diagnosis codes were selected for analysis. Measures: estimated total numbers and percentages of patients by year. Analysis: trends from 1996 through 2005 were examined overall and by demographic factors (eg, age, sex) and abscess characteristics (eg, body region affected). Linear regression was used to evaluate trends.

Results.—Emergency department visits for abscesses more than doubled over the 10-year study period (1.2 million in 1996 to 3.28 million in 2005; trend, $P < .01$). The total number of ED visits increased from 90 million to 115 million over the same period, so that abscess visits are increasing faster than overall visits. Although the frequency of abscesses increased, the demographic and clinical characteristics of ED patients were unchanged over time. About half of ED patients with abscess were male, and about half were between the ages of 19 and 45 years. Annual admissions hovered around 12%. The most common abscess sites coded were the leg, ear, and "unspecified site." About 50% received antibiotics.

Conclusions.—Emergency department visits for abscesses have shown a large increase since 1996; however, demographic and clinical factors are uniform across years.

▶ The focus of this retrospective analysis is whether there was an increase in cutaneous abscesses over a 10-year period (1996-2005). The conclusions were noteworthy—indicating a more than doubling of such abscesses. This finding was, however, based on emergency department (ED) visits, and not necessarily applicable to clinical dermatological practice, although a presumption can be made that such an increase should at least partially correspond to the clinical setting. While there is little doubt that the number of cases have likely increased given the emergence of methicillin-resistant *Staphylococcus aureus* (MRSA) and community-acquired MRSA, there is at least some question as to whether such cases have in fact more than doubled. Namely, the analysis included an ED diagnosis of an abscess based on the entered diagnosis code and not necessarily based on histological confirmation of an abscess or culture results. It was noted, without specific explanation, that there is a potential gradual trend in the way soft-tissue infections are coded. There is simply no way to determine whether the abscess code was also used for other similar cutaneous manifestations, especially without pathological confirmation. This would certainly contribute to the increased number of cutaneous abscesses in the analysis. Furthermore, there is no way to delineate how many of the patients were repeat patients for whom initial treatment was not responsive, particularly given the persistent nature and recurrence of MSRA in carriers. Despite this, the article does elicit further attention to the increasing prevalent nature of this important cutaneous lesion and the need for not only proper recognition, but appropriate diagnosis and treatment.

B. D. Michaels, DO
J. Q. Del Rosso, DO

Trimethoprim-sulfamethoxazole or clindamycin for treatment of community-acquired methicillin-resistant *Staphylococcus aureus* skin and soft tissue infections

Hyun DY, Mason EO, Forbes A, et al (Baylor College of Medicine and Texas Children's Hosp, Houston)
Pediatr Infect Dis J 28:57-59, 2009

The outcome of patients who were treated with oral trimethoprim-sulfamethoxazole or oral clindamycin after hospitalization at Texas Children's Hospital for community-acquired methicillin-resistant *Staphylococcus aureus* skin and soft tissue infections was compared. No significant differences were observed in the percentage of patients who returned to the emergency center or clinics because of worsening or incomplete resolution of the infected site.

▶ Trimethoprim-sulfamethoxazole (TMP-SMZ) and clindamycin are frequently recommended as options for oral therapy for community-acquired methicillin-resistant *Staphylococcus aureus* (CA-MRSA) in skin and soft tissue infections (SSTI) for adults, but its use in the pediatric population has not been reviewed extensively. This is a retrospective chart review of 508 patients admitted to the Texas Children's Hospital for CA-MRSA for SSTI. In the study, all patients received clindamycin intravenously in the hospital upon admission, and 215 patients were given TMP-SMX, and 200 patients were given oral clindamycin as outpatient therapy after discharge. In addition, 94% of patients in the TMP-SMZ group and 86% in the clindamycin group underwent incision and drainage of their abscesses, and the remainder of the patients had spontaneous drainage from their infection sites. Patients with underlying illness predisposing to frequent hospitalization and concurrent infections were excluded. Cultures identified staphylococcal strains from the patient's infection site, but 55% of patients were discharged within 48 hours before antibiotic susceptibility data was available. Patient charts were reviewed for demographic data, clinical presentation, course of hospitalization, any visits to the emergency center or clinics within 30 days of discharge as a result of recurrence, or complications of their SSTI involving the same site. The authors concluded that TMP-SMX and clindamycin may be equivalent as outpatient oral therapies for CA-MRSA SSTI after hospitalization in the pediatric population. Less than 4% of patients from both treatment groups returned to the emergency center for clinics due to incomplete resolution of their infections while on oral antibiotic therapy. Although this is a low recurrence rate, 55% of patients were discharged without knowing whether or not staphylococcal strains were even susceptible. In addition, the low rate of recurrence for both treatment groups could be due to surgical drainage of the infection site, which is a known therapeutic option for most abscesses. It is also controversial whether or not patients need antibiotics after incision and drainage, because most infections will resolve after surgical intervention. In addition, patients were also given intravenous (IV) clindamycin before being discharged, which could be another reason for such low recurrence rates. Another limitation to this study was that those who sought to consult their primary care physicians or other health care professional outside of the hospital system for incomplete resolution or worsening of their infection were not identified through the chart review process. It is also difficult to attribute low infection rates from medication alone because researchers could not monitor compliance of outpatient antibiotic therapy. Additionally, patterns of CA-MRSA susceptibility differ widely among communities across the United States, potentially influencing the variability of outcomes.

G. K. Kim, DO

J. Q. Del Rosso, DO

Antimicrobial Agents for Complicated Skin and Skin-Structure Infections: Justification of Noninferiority Margins in the Absence of Placebo-Controlled Trials
Spellberg B, for the Antimicrobial Availability Task Force of the Infectious Diseases Society of America (Harbor-Univ of California at Los Angeles Med Ctr, Torrance; et al)
Clin Infect Dis 49:383-391, 2009

Background.—The United States Food and Drug Administration requires clinical trial noninferiority margins to preserve a fraction (eg, 50%) of the established comparator drug's efficacy versus placebo. Lack of placebo-controlled trials for many infections complicates noninferiority margin justification for and, hence, regulatory review of new antimicrobial agents. Noninferiority margin clarification is critical to enable new antimicrobial development. In the absence of placebo-controlled trials, we sought to define the magnitude of efficacy of antimicrobial agents and resulting noninferiority margins for studies of complicated skin and skin-structure infection (SSSI).

Methods.—We systematically reviewed literature on complicated SSSI published during 1900–1950 (before widespread penicillin resistance) to define treatment outcomes and confidence intervals (CIs). Antimicrobial efficacy was calculated as the lower limit CI of the cure rate with antimicrobials minus the upper limit CI of the cure rate without antimicrobials.

Results.—We identified 90 articles describing >28,000 patients with complicated SSSI. For cellulitis/erysipelas, cure rates were 66% (95% CI, 64%–68%) without antibiotics and 98% (95% CI, 96%–99%) for penicillin-treated patients, and penicillin reduced mortality by 10%. Cure rates for wound/ulcer infections were 36% (95% CI, 32%–39%) without antibiotics and 83% (95% CI, 81%–85%) for penicillin-treated patients. For major abscesses, cure rates were 76% (95% CI, 71%–80%) without antibiotics and 96% (95% CI, 94%–98%) for penicillin-treated patients; penicillin reduced mortality by 6%.

Conclusion.—Systematic review of historical literature enables rational noninferiority margin justification in the absence of placebo-controlled trials and may facilitate regulatory review of noninferiority trials. Noninferiority margins of 14% for cellulitis/erysipelas, 21% for wound/ulcer infections, and 7% for major abscesses would preserve ≥50% of antibiotic efficacy versus placebo for these complicated SSSI subsets.

▶ There has been a worldwide increase in antimicrobial resistance to topical and systemic antimicrobial agents. Additionally, the concerns have sparked recent controversy over acceptable margins of noninferiority for clinical trials in the development of antibiotics. In this study, the authors sought to define appropriate noninferiority margins for clinical trials of antimicrobial agents in the treatment of skin and skin-structure infections (SSSI). This is a systematic review of peer-reviewed literature on skin infection in the preantibiotic and immediate postantibiotic era (1900-1950). Authors sought to determine the "gold standard" parameters for assessment of an antimicrobial agent relative to no active therapy against SSSI. There were 90 peer-reviewed articles identified describing > 28 000 patients with SSSI. Skin infections were divided into cellulitis, trauma-related infection, and major abscess. Treatment was divided into no active antimicrobial therapy, sulfonamide therapy, and penicillin therapy. The average cure rate for cellulitis/erysipelas was 66% for nonantimicrobial-treated patients, 91% for systemic sulfonamide-treated patients, and 98% for systemic penicillin-treated patients. Penicillin reduced mortality in 10% of patients. Topical or local penicillin-related treatment was less effective than systemic penicillin, resulting in a cure rate of 89% (95% CI, 80%-98%). Heterogeneity was detected in studies reporting cure rates for no antimicrobial therapy or a sulfonamide treatment ($P < .001$ for both). *Staphylococcus aureus* was the most common pathogen isolated, and streptococci was the second most common. The cure rates for wound/ulcer infections were 36%, 73%, or 83% for patients treated with no antimicrobial, a sulfonamide, or penicillin, respectively. Significant heterogeneity in cure rates were detected for all treatment groups ($P < .001$) due to mixture of topical, local versus systemic routes of antimicrobial administration. The preantibiotic era and the immediate postantibiotic era revealed a substantial treatment effect for antimicrobial therapy. Penicillin was more effective than sulfonamides. The authors suggest that due to the low mortality of complicated SSSI treated with antibiotics, it may be reasonable to preserve < 50% of the gold standard comparator's efficacy, resulting in wider noninferiority margins. The clinical benefits would be observed if the agent offered other clinical benefits, such as enhanced antimicrobial activity and safety profile compared with other agents. With the advent of penicillin there has been a 10-fold decrease in mortality rates comparable with those in the modern era, with no notable change during the last 20 years. Limitations of this study include publication bias, retrospective analysis, and large number of single-armed observation studies within the analysis. In addition, noninferiority trials have an inherent weakness compared with superiority trials in that they are not as strongly powered to thoroughly reveal efficacy data or demonstrate assay sensitivity. In conclusion, the authors suggest that noninferiority margins of 14% for cellulitis/erysipelas, 21% for wound/ulcer infections, and 7% for abscesses would preserve > 50% of antibiotic efficacy compared with placebo in SSSI.

G. K. Kim, DO

J. Q. Del Rosso, DO

Epidemiology of Dermatitis and Skin Infections in United States Physicians' Offices, 1993–2005

Pallin DJ, Espinola JA, Leung DY, et al (Brigham and Women's Hosp, Boston MA; Massachusetts General Hosp, Boston, MA; Natl Jewish Med Health, Denver, CO)
Clin Infect Dis 49:901-907, 2009

Background.—Since the discovery of community-associated methicillin-resistant *Staphylococcus aureus* (MRSA), the number of emergency department visits for skin and soft-tissue infection (SSTI) has increased, and one report suggested an increase in the much larger setting of physicians' offices. Dermatitis compromises the cutaneous barrier to microorganisms and may predispose to SSTI. Our objectives were to determine whether office visits for dermatitis or SSTI have become more frequent since the emergence of community-associated MRSA, to describe the age-specific frequency of visits for dermatitis and SSTI, and to determine whether dermatitis is associated with SSTI and whether the association strengthened over time.

Methods.—We analyzed visits for the diagnoses of dermatitis and SSTI by means of codes from the *International Classification of Diseases, Ninth Revision* recorded in the National Ambulatory Medical Care Survey, 1993–2005. We calculated population estimates by year and age group, with 95% confidence intervals (CIs), and examined trends over time. Multivariate logistic regression quantified the association between dermatitis and SSTI and assessed for interaction between dermatitis and year in the prediction of SSTI.

Results.—Dermatitis was diagnosed at 13 million office visits per year (95% CI, 12–14 million office visits per year) over the study period, and SSTI was diagnosed at 6.3 million office visits per year (95% CI, 5.8 million–6.8 million office visits per year). The frequency did not change for either diagnosis over time when expressed as a percentage of all visits (both, $P > .60$). Dermatitis was most common among infants (256 visits per 1,000 population per year; 95% CI, 216–293 visits per 1,000 population per year). The rate of diagnosis of SSTI did not vary importantly by age. Dermatitis was associated with SSTI (odds ratio, 2.54; 95% CI, 1.92–3.35). The association did not strengthen over time.

Conclusions.—The rate of office visits for dermatitis or SSTI did not increase from 1993 through 2005. Dermatitis was associated with SSTI.

This association did not strengthen as community-associated MRSA became prevalent.

▶ Community-associated methicillin-resistant *Staphylococcus aureus* (CA-MRSA) is a common cause of soft-tissue infections (SSTIs) in the United States. Current studies have suggested that there is a rise in SSTIs due to CA-MRSA. This is a study analyzing the association between dermatitis and SSTIs through the International Classification of Diseases, Ninth Revision recorded in the National Ambulatory Medical Care Survey (NAMCS) during 1993-2005. Authors sought to determine whether rates of SSTIs have increased in the physicians' office in certain age-related populations and if those with concurrent dermatitis are at increased risk for SSTIs due to CA-MRSA. Dermatitis was diagnosed at 13 million office visits per year (1.6% of all visits), and SSTIs were diagnosed at 6.3 million office visits per year. Dermatitis was common among infants with no change in the annual rate of dermatitis in the office. SSTIs were diagnosed at 82 million office visits during the study period (0.8% of all visits) with no change in the rate of visits. Atopic dermatitis visits were less common with increasing age ($P < .001$). Patients during this time period made more visits in general but not specifically for SSTI. The frequency of visits for SSTIs varied with age ($P < .001$) and were most common among the elderly. Lack of verification of SSTI with confirmatory microbiological data was a limitation to this study. Most SSTIs were diagnosed on a clinical basis. Authors also did not include the hospital outpatient department sample, which accounted for 6% of all visits in the NAMCS and could have affected the data. SSTI infections before 1993 were not included in this study, which was another limitation. Nevertheless, authors concluded that dermatitis was associated with SSTIs, but the association did not strengthen with the prevalence of CA-MRSA.

G. K. Kim, DO

J. Q. Del Rosso, DO

Terbinafine (250 mg/day): an effective and safe treatment of cutaneous sporotrichosis
Francesconi G, Valle AC, Passos S, et al (Fiocruz, IPEC, Rio de Janeiro, Brazil; Fiocruz, Epidemiology, Rio de Janeiro, Brazil)
J Eur Acad Dermatol Venereol 23:1273-1276, 2009

Background.—There are a few studies on the treatment of sporotrichosis. The standard drug used is itraconazole. However, the use of itraconazole is limited by its interaction with other drugs.

Objective.—To evaluate the effectiveness and safety of 250 mg terbinafine for the treatment of cutaneous sporotrichosis in patients in whom itraconazole use is not possible.

Methods.—We performed a descriptive study of cutaneous sporotrichosis cases treated with 250 mg terbinafine for which itraconazole was contraindicated or resulted in severe or moderate pharmacological inter-actions. Sporotrichosis was diagnosed based on the isolation of *S. schenckii*.

Results.—Fifty patients seen between July 2005 and September 2007 were included. Forty-five (92%) patients reported contact with a sick cat and 47 (94%) presented comorbidities (high blood pressure: 64.0%; diabetes mellitus: 30.0%; dyslipidemia: 16.7%; depression: 10.0%; migraine: 2.1%; Parkinsonís disease: 2.1%; peptic ulcer disease: 2.1%; heart failure: 2.1%, and arrhythmia: 2.1%). All patients used some medication interacting with itraconazole (psycholeptics: 36.0%; antidiabetic agents: 28.0%; hypolipemiant agents: 18.0%; calcium-channel blockers: 16.0%; anticonvulsants: 8.0%; cardiotropic drugs: 6.3%; antacids: 6.3%, and antiparkinsonian agent: 2.1%). Most patients (96%) were cured within a mean period of 14 weeks. The drug was discontinued due to a skin rash in one patient. There were no cases of recurrence of the mycosis within a mean follow-up period of 37 weeks.

Conclusions.—This study suggests that 250 mg/day terbinafine is an effective and well-tolerated alternative to drug therapy of cutaneous sporotrichosis in a population in which itraconazole use is not possible.

▶ The conclusions drawn from this study are that terbinafine is an effective and safe treatment for cutaneous sporotrichosis when use of itraconazole is not possible (ie, possible drug interactions or contraindications), especially because *Sporothrix schenckii* strains have shown excellent in vitro sensitivity to terbinafine. The study's sample size was small, and larger, controlled and randomized trials are necessary to support this conclusion. In 96% of cases, cure was achieved within a mean treatment duration of 14 weeks, with no recurrences noted over a mean follow-up period of 37 weeks. Oral terbinafine therapy was well tolerated.

S. B. Momin, DO

J. Q. Del Rosso, DO

Glucocorticoids Enhance Toll-Like Receptor 2 Expression in Human Keratinocytes Stimulated with *Propionibacterium acnes* or Proinflammatory Cytokines

Shibata M, Katsuyama M, Onodera T, et al (Shiseido Res Ctr, Yokohama, Japan; et al)

J Invest Dermatol 129:375-382, 2009

Toll-like receptors (TLRs) on keratinocytes are important cell surface receptors involved in the innate and acquired immune response to invading microorganisms. In acne vulgaris, TLR2 activation by *Propioni-bacterium acnes* (*P. acnes*) may induce skin inflammation via induction of various proinflammatory molecules that stimulate the invasion of inflam-matory cells. Although corticosteroids themselves exert immunosuppres-sive or anti-inflammatory effects, it is well known clinically that systemic or topical glucocorticoid treatment provokes an acneiform reaction. Nevertheless, the effect of steroids on TLR2 expression in human keratinocytes remains unknown. Here, we found that the addition of glucocorticoids, such as dexamethasone and cortisol, to cultured human keratinocytes increased their TLR2 gene expression. Moreover, these glucocorticoids markedly enhanced TLR2 gene expression, which was further stimulated by *P. acnes*, tumor necrosis factor-α, and IL-1α. Gene expression of mitogen-activated protein kinase (MAPK) phosphatase-1 was also increased by the addition of dexamethasone. By using several inhibitors and activators, we found that TLR2 gene induction by glucocorticoids was mediated by the suppression of p38 MAPK activity following induction of MAPK phosphatase-1. These findings strongly suggest that steroid-induced TLR2 together with *P. acnes* existing as normal resident flora plays an important role in the exacerbation of acne vulgaris as well as in possible induction of corticosteroid-induced acne or in that of rosacea-like dermatitis.

▶ Results of several previous studies have suggested that *Propionibacterium acnes* can activate TLR2 in the skin, triggering an innate inflammatory response, which is manifested clinically as lesions of acne vulgaris. Yet other investigators have shown that glucocorticoids induce TLR2 expression in epithelial cells through pathways involving mitogen-activated protein kinase (MAPK) phosphatase-1, which leads to the inactivation of negative regulators of TLR2 expression. In this study, the investigators use a similar approach to explore the mechanism whereby corticosteroid therapy can trigger or aggravate acneiform skin reactions. The major new findings of this study were that exposure of cultured human keratinocytes to whole, viable *P acnes* resulted in a modest induction of both TLR2 and MAPK phosphate-1 gene expression, as did incubation of the cells with dexamethasone alone. However, cells challenged by bacteria in the presence of dexamethasone resulted in a synergistic, highly significant increase in the expression of both genes. This was abrogated by the addition of a steroid receptor antagonist to the culture. These data hold interesting implications for the interaction between glucocorticoid hormones and innate host defenses against pathogens.

G. M. P. Galbraith, MD

4 Viral Infections (Excluding HIV Infection)

Topical treatment for human papillomavirus-associated genital warts in humans with the novel tellurium immunomodulator AS101: assessment of its safety and efficacy
Friedman M, Bayer I, Letko I, et al (Rambam Med Ctr, Haifa; Tel-Aviv Univ, Israel; Laniado Med Ctr, Netanya, Israel; et al)
Br J Dermatol 160:403-408, 2009

Background.—Various methods are currently used for the treatment of anogenital warts. However, a complete cure is unlikely, and the rate of recurrence is high.

Objectives.—The purpose of this open-label, multicentre trial was to evaluate the safety and clinical efficacy of a new treatment using the immunomodulator ammonium trichloro (dioxoethylene-O,O') tellurate (AS101; Biomas Ltd, Kefar Saba, Israel) 15% w/w cream to clear vulval/perianal condylomata acuminata.

Methods.—Study participants comprised 48 women and 26 men, age range 18–62 years. Of the 48 woman, 44 were diagnosed with vulval condylomata and four with perianal condylomata. All 26 men were diagnosed with perianal condylomata. All the patients in the study received AS101 15% w/w cream twice a day. Maximal treatment duration was 16 weeks. To evaluate the safety and clinical efficacy, patients were examined and lesional areas photographed on a biweekly basis.

Results.—By the end of the treatment, 56 of 74 (76%) patients were considered completely cleared. Complete cure was achieved in 35 of 44 (80%) patients with vulval condylomata and in 21 of 30 (70%) patients with perianal condylomata. No scarring of treated areas was observed. Complete cure was achieved within a time range of 10-109 days. The most frequent side-effects observed were mild-to-moderate itching, soreness, burning and erythema. In post-treatment follow up of up to 6 months, disease recurrence was observed in two patients (4%), at 105 and 144 days following completion of treatment.

Conclusions.—AS101 15% w/w cream is an effective and safe, self-administered therapy used for the treatment of external vulval and perianal warts. The cream is applied topically twice daily for up to 16 weeks. A very low recurrence rate was reported.

▶ This open-label study used a relatively obscure immune modifier to treat external genital warts on nonkeratinized tissue (vulva, perianal skin). Although twice-daily treatment was designed to continue for up to 16 weeks, the median duration of therapy until clearance was actually about 1 month for vulvar and 2 months for perianal lesions. A high clinical cure rate (76%) and low recurrence rate at 3 to 6 months (4%) are both remarkable, as is the good tolerability of this new patient-applied preparation.

Among the shortcomings of the study are the limited follow-up (a year being preferable) and lack of inclusion of male patient with penile external genital warts. The fact that all male patients enrolled exhibited perianal lesions makes one concerned about the possible HIV status of these subjects, a matter not clarified in the article.

Despite these minor problems, this is an interesting publication highlighting a promising new treatment for EGW and, based on the immune mechanism of action (inhibition of IL-10 and upregulation of tumor necrosis factor-α [TNF-α]), possibly other disorders.

T. Rosen, MD

Genital Human Papillomavirus Prevalence and Human Papillomavirus Concordance in Heterosexual Couples Are Positively Associated with Human Immunodeficiency Virus Coinfection
Mbulawa ZZA, Coetzee D, Marais DJ, et al (Univ of Cape Town, South Africa)
J Infect Dis 199:1514-1524, 2009

This study examined the concordance of genital human papillomavirus (HPV) infection in 254 heterosexually active couples and the impact of HIV coinfection. Genital HPV detection was significantly more common among HIV-infected women than among HIV-seronegative women (99 [68%] of 145 women vs. 33 [31%] of 107 women; $P < .001$); similarly, HPV detection was significantly more common among HIV-infected men than among HIV-seronegative men (67 [72%] of 93 and 65 [43%] of 150 men, respectively; $P < .001$). HIV-seronegative male partners of HIV-infected women had a significantly greater prevalence of HPV infection than did HIV-seronegative male partners of HIV-seronegative women (38 [58%] of 65 men vs. 27 [32%] of 85 men; $P = .001$), indicating that HIV coinfection in one partner has a significant impact on the prevalence of HPV genital infection in the other partner. HPV concordance between couples was associated with HIV infection status ($P < .001$, by Pearson's 2 test) and was significantly higher among HIV-infected couples than among HIV-seronegative couples. Typespecific sharing of HPV was associated with HIV concordance status ($P < .024$). HIV-seronegative couples were more likely to share 1 HPV type and were unlikely to share > 1 type, whereas HIV-infected or HIV-discordant couples were more likely to share > 1 HPV type. Women with a high HPV load frequently shared HPV types with their male partners, suggesting that a high HPV load may play a role in HPV transmission between partners. In conclusion, HIV coinfection in one or both sexually active partners increased HPV prevalence and HPV type-specific concordance.

▶ Although the effect of human immunodeficiency virus (HIV) coinfection on the natural course of a given sexually transmitted disease (STD) has been extensively studied, the effect of HIV coinfection on the likelihood of STD transmission to the other partner has not been well documented. This study verified the intuitively obvious: human papillomavirus (HPV) infection is more likely among those who have acquired HIV, all other factors being equal. However, the study also showed that HIV coinfection makes it more likely that an HPV infected individual will pass the HPV to his or her partner, perhaps due to decreased immune response and greater HPV viral load.

Shortcomings of this study include a narrow geographic focus (South Africa), which precludes generalization to worldwide patient populations, and lack of commentary on highly active antiretrovial therapy (HAART) status for any of the HIV coinfected cohort.

T. Rosen, MD

Efficacy of human papillomavirus (HPV)-16/18 AS04-adjuvanted vaccine against cervical infection and precancer caused by oncogenic HPV types (PATRICIA): final analysis of a double-blind, randomised study in young women
Paavonen J, Naud P, Salmerón J, et al (Univ of Helsinki, Finland; Univ Federal of Rio Grande do Sul, Porto Alegre, Brazil; Instituto Mexicano del Seguro Social, Morelos, Mexico; et al)
Lancet 374:301-314, 2009

Background.—The human papillomavirus (HPV)-16/18 AS04-adjuvanted vaccine was immunogenic, generally well tolerated, and effective against HPV-16 or HPV-18 infections, and associated precancerous lesions in an event-triggered interim analysis of the phase III randomised, double-blind, controlled PApilloma TRIal against Cancer In young Adults (PATRICIA). We now assess the vaccine efficacy in the final event-driven analysis.

Methods.—Women (15–25 years) were vaccinated at months 0, 1, and 6. Analyses were done in the according-to-protocol cohort for efficacy (ATP-E; vaccine, n=8093; control, n=8069), total vaccinated cohort (TVC, included all women receiving at least one vaccine dose, regardless of their baseline HPV status; represents the general population, including those who are sexually active; vaccine, n=9319; control, n=9325), and

TVC-naive (no evidence of oncogenic HPV infection at baseline; represents women before sexual debut; vaccine, n=5822; control, n=5819). The primary endpoint was to assess vaccine efficacy against cervical intraepithelial neoplasia 2+ (CIN2+) that was associated with HPV-16 or HPV-18 in women who were seronegative at baseline, and DNA negative at baseline and month 6 for the corresponding type (ATP-E). This trial is registered with ClinicalTrials.gov, number NCT00122681.

Findings.—Mean follow-up was 34·9 months (SD 6·4) after the third dose. Vaccine efficacy against CIN2+ associated with HPV-16/18 was 92·9% (96·1% CI 79·9–98·3) in the primary analysis and 98·1% (88·4–100) in an analysis in which probable causality to HPV type was assigned in lesions infected with multiple oncogenic types (ATP-E cohort). Vaccine efficacy against CIN2+ irrespective of HPV DNA in lesions was 30·4% (16·4–42·1) in the TVC and 70·2% (54·7–80·9) in the TVC-naive. Corresponding values against CIN3+ were 33·4% (9·1–51·5) in the TVC and 87·0% (54·9–97·7) in the TVC-naive. Vaccine efficacy against CIN2+ associated with 12 non-vaccine oncogenic types was 54·0% (34·0–68·4; ATP-E). Individual cross-protection against CIN2+ associated with HPV-31, HPV-33, and HPV-45 was seen in the TVC.

Interpretation.—The HPV-16/18 AS04-adjuvanted vaccine showed high efficacy against CIN2+ associated with HPV-16/18 and non-vaccine oncogenic HPV types and substantial overall effect in cohorts that are relevant to universal mass vaccination and catch-up programmes.

▶ This study evaluates the vaccine that prevents human papillomavirus (HPV) infection subtypes that are most commonly responsible for cervical cancer associated with genital warts. The vaccine is given in 3 injections over 6 months and is currently recommended for girls as young as 11 to 12 years old, as well as females 13 to 26 years old who have not yet been vaccinated. This randomized, double-blinded final analysis of the PApilloma TRIal against Cancer In young Adults (PATRICIA) was performed to assess the vaccine efficacy in this final event-driven analysis. The trial confirmed the efficacy of the HPV-16/18 ASO4-adjuvant vaccine in the prevention of cervical intraepithelial neoplasia grade 2 or more (CIN2+) lesions associated with HPV-16/18 and nonvaccine oncogenic HPV types, including HPV-31, HPV-33, and HPV-45. To note, the 5 types of HPV just mentioned are responsible for causing 82% of cervical cancers. The safety profile of the vaccine was favorable and comparable with the control. Two populations were studied: total vaccinated cohort (TVC) group (women with and without oncogenic HPV infections at baseline) and TVC-naive (women with no evidence of HPV types at baseline). In sum, the HPV vaccine can reduce the cervical cancer incidence and decrease the overall number of colposcopic examinations and cervical excision/ablation procedures.

S. Bellew, DO
J. Q. Del Rosso, DO

Non–Sexually Related Acute Genital Ulcers in 13 Pubertal Girls: A Clinical and Microbiological Study

Farhi D, Wendling J, Molinari E, et al (Université René Descartes–Paris V, Paris, France; Université Pierre et Marie Curie–Paris VI, Paris, France; et al)
Arch Dermatol 145:38-45, 2009

Objective.—To describe the clinical and microbiological features of acute genital ulcers (AGU), which have been reported in virgin adolescents, predominantly in girls.

Design.—Descriptive study. We collected data on the clinical features, sexual history, blood cell count, biochemistry, microbiological workup, and 1-year follow-up.

Setting.—Departments of dermatology of 3 university hospitals in Paris.

Patients.—Thirteen immunocompetent female patients with a first flare of non–sexually transmitted AGU.

Main Outcome Measures.—Clinical and microbiological data, using a standardized form.

Results.—Mean age was 16.6 years (range, 11-19 years). Eleven patients denied previous sexual contact. A fever or flulike symptoms preceded AGU in 10 of the 13 patients (77%), with a mean delay of 3.8 days before the AGU onset (range, 0-10 days). The genital ulcers were bilateral in 10 patients. The final diagnosis was Epstein-Barr virus primary infection in 4 patients (31%) and Behçet disease in 1 patient (8%). No other infectious agents were detected in this series.

Conclusions.—We recommend serologic testing for Epstein-Barr virus with IgM antibodies to viral capsid antigens in non–sexually related AGU in immunocompetent patients. Further microbiological studies are required to identify other causative agents.

► In the past, nonsexually related acute genital ulcers (AGU) were thought to originate from herpes simplex virus (HSV) and aphthosis. However, since the beginning of the 20th century, there is sufficient evidence to suggest other possible etiologies. This is a descriptive study of 13 immunocompetent, self-reported virgin adolescents with seronegativity for HSV and non-sexually transmitted disease (STD) related acute genital ulcers. The authors evaluated the clinical features, systemic signs, virologic work up, final diagnosis, treatment, and response to treatment for AGU. The authors found that 4 of 13 patients (31%) had AGU associated with confirmed Epstein-Barr virus (EBV) infection with clinical characteristics of kissing pattern of the ulcerations present in all 4 of the patients, and with 3 of the 4 having mononucleosis syndrome. This study broadens the differential diagnosis when faced with multiple superficial and nonrelapsing AGU in a population where sexual contact is less likely. Epstein-Barr virus, cytomegalovirus (CMV), Salmonella infection, and toxoplasmosis should also be considered as other causative agents. This study also includes a table of previously reported cases of AGU and allows clinicians to compare and contrast previous reports of AGU with the findings of their study. One aspect that seems to remain problematic is the small sample size and the statement of "reported virgin," which is not clearly defined, with oral sexual history excluded. This information could be useful to the clinician in understanding the pathogenesis of AGU and determining if acute ulcers in the genital region are primary sites of infection, possibly due to physical contact or if EBV migration occurs after a systemic infection, because not all patients who are infected with EBV get AGU. Overall, this study gives an array of potential precipitating factors and the serologic work-up that is needed when investigating nonsexually related AGU.

G. K. Kim, DO
J. Q. Del Rosso, DO

Parental Satisfaction, Efficacy, and Adverse Events in 54 Patients Treated With Cantharidin for Molluscum Contagiosum Infection
Cathcart S, Coloe J, Morrell DS (Univ of North Carolina School of Medicine, Chapel Hill)
Clin Pediatr 48:161-165, 2009

Objective.—To study the efficacy, tolerability, and parental satisfaction of cantharidin in a patient population at a pediatric dermatology referral center.

Methods.—Chart review was completed for 110 patients who presented with molluscum infection and were treated with cantharidin. A total of 54 were available for follow-up by telephone interview regarding adverse effects, parental satisfaction, and overall clearance of the infection.

Results.—Of those who were reachable, 96% improved after treatment with cantharidin. Parental satisfaction was 78%. Patients received an average of 2.2 treatments irrespective of outcome. Overall, 46% of patients experienced adverse events, including pain, pruritus, secondary infection, brisk immune response, and temporary hypopigmentation and 9% experienced an adverse event that they classified as severe.

Conclusions.—The results contribute to the data supporting cantharidin as a safe and effective treatment of molluscum contagiosum. Compared with other treatments, it appears to be equally effective and well-tolerated and should be considered a potential front-line treatment.

▶ Although this article supports the use of cantharidin for molluscum contagiosum (MC) infection that is commonly utilized in practice, it has several weaknesses. In this small retrospective chart review, the patient age ranged from 3 months to 13 years. Parents cannot accurately relay symptoms that the patients experience when they are unable to communicate. There is also recall bias. In this article, cantharidin was not compared with other reported treatments for MC, and parental satisfaction with other therapies used before treatment with cantharidin was not discussed. This article also did not comment on patients' skin color and compare parental satisfaction in darker skinned individuals after treatment. This latter group is more likely to experience persistent dyspigmentation after completion of therapy.

S. Momin, DO
J. Q. Del Rosso, DO

Valacyclovir and topical clobetasol gel for the episodic treatment of herpes labialis: a patient-initiated, double-blind, placebo-controlled pilot trial

Hull C, McKeough M, Sebastian K, et al (Univ of Utah, Salt Lake City)
J Eur Acad Dermatol Venereol 23:263-267, 2009

Background.—Treatment of herpes simplex labialis (HSL) has been associated with modest benefits. This difficulty results from the rapid resolution of the disease accomplished by the immune system, which narrows the window of therapeutic opportunity. The immune response is also responsible for important clinical manifestations, including oedema and pain. The dual role of immune responses (protection, pathology) is well recognized in other infectious diseases. The addition of corticosteroids to antimicrobial agents has been associated with improvement in some of these diseases.

Objective.—We evaluated the combination of oral valacyclovir plus topical clobetasol compared to placebo for recurrent HSL.

Methods.—Eighty-one subjects were screened, randomized, and dispensed medication (valacyclovir 2 g orally twice daily φορ 1 day and clobetasol gel 0.05% twice daily for 3 days). Forty-two patients developed a recurrence and initiated treatment.

Results.—There were more aborted lesions in the valacyclovir–clobetasol arm compared to placebo–placebo (50% vs. 15.8%, $P = 0.04$). Combination therapy reduced the mean maximum lesion size (9.7 vs. 54 mm^2, $P = 0.002$) and the mean healing time of classical lesions (5.8 vs. 9.3 days, $P = 0.002$). We created a composite statistic, area-under-the-curve (AUC) of classical lesion size versus time. There was a reduction in the AUC in the combination arm compared with placebo (23 vs. 193 mm^2, $P < 0.001$). Adverse events were minimal. Secondary and post-treatment recurrences were not increased by combination therapy.

Conclusions.—This pilot study supports the addition of topical corticosteroids to an oral antiviral agent for the treatment of HSL. Larger studies need to confirm the safety and efficacy of this approach.

▶ Unlike genital herpes simplex (HS) infection, orolabial HS infection ("cold sores") has not proven easy to suppress with any of the available acyclovir analogues or immune response modifiers. Thus, a rational approach to this vexing problem is welcome.

In this well executed double-blind, placebo-controlled study, the concomitant use of high-dose valacyclovir and 3 days application of ultrapotent corticosteroid clearly resulted in improvement of clinical parameters of most importance to the patient, most notably maximal lesion size and mean healing time.

The authors readily admit that the optimum regimen is not determined by this study and that it is entirely possible that lower potency topical corticosteroids may suffice. Nonetheless, this convincing investigation offers at least one way in which to lessen the cosmetic and psychosocial burden for those who suffer from orolabial HS infection.

Other minor shortcomings of the study: nearly all patients were Caucasian, and the severity at enrollment was modest (an outbreak about every 3 months). It would be nice to repeat this study in a more ethnically diverse group and with patients who suffer, as many do, near monthly recurrences.

T. Rosen, MD

Changes in the Immune Responses Against Human Herpesvirus-8 in the Disease Course of Posttransplant Kaposi Sarcoma

Barozzi P, Bonini C, Potenza L, et al (Univ of Modena and Reggio Emilia, Modena, Italy; San Raffaele Scientific Inst, Milano, Italy; et al)
Transplantation 86:738-744, 2008

In nine patients with posttransplant Kaposi sarcoma (KS) T-cell responses to human herpesvirus (HHV)-8 latent and lytic antigens, as detected by enzyme-linked-immunospot (Elispot) assay, were absent at disease onset. Virus-specific T-cell responses were detected in six renal recipients at remission after a reduction of calcineurin inhibitors (CIs), and in two HHV-8 seropositive renal recipients without KS. In two liver recipients undergoing switch from CIs to sirolimus (SRL), normalization of the T-cell repertoire and recovery of both HHV-8–specific effector and memory T lymphocytes were associated with complete KS remission. In a renal recipient undergoing SRL conversion, the early recovery of HHV-8–specific effector but not of memory T lymphocytes, was associated only with partial remission. Neither rejection nor changes in graft function were observed after SRL conversion. HHV-8–specific T-cell responses are required to achieve posttransplant KS remission, and may be restored under SRL, while maintaining effective immunosuppression.

▶ The development of Kaposi's sarcoma (KS) is a recognized risk of organ transplantation in patients on immunosuppressive therapy, and is considered to result from reactivation of human herpes virus 8 (HHV-8), now more commonly referred to as Kaposi's sarcoma-associated herpes virus. Several previous studies have shown that reduction of immunosuppressant dose, with or without switching of therapy to the drug sirolimus, can be very efficacious in these patients. Sirolimus, also called rapamycin, is a macrolide drug, which inhibits T- and B-lymphocyte responses to interleukin-2. In this interesting and complex article, Barozzi et al describe their investigations of T-cell responses to HHV-8 and viral load in several groups of subjects.

The first 2 patients were seropositive for HHV-8, but did not develop KS after several years of conventional immunosuppressant therapy. They were found to exhibit specific antiviral T-cell responses and had no detectable circulating virus. Six additional patients who developed KS posttransplant were treated by reduction of conventional immunosuppression with complete remission of the tumors. At the time of diagnosis of KS, antiviral T-cell activity could not be demonstrated in these patients; following remission of disease, they all had such T-cell responses and undetectable viral load. An additional 3 patients with posttransplant KS were treated by switching the immunosuppressant drug regimen to sirolimus. Two of these experienced complete remission with development of antiviral T-cell activity and normalization of the T-cell repertoire. The third patient, who had been previously been treated by reduction of immunosuppression with no effect, had a partial remission upon institution of sirolimus therapy, and also developed T-cell responses to the virus. Lastly, 4 immunocompetent subjects with antibodies to KS (and presumably KS-free) were shown to have specific T-cell responses to KS antigens. These responses were markedly increased compared with those of 10 of the 11 transplant patients described. The results of this study provide important insight into the role of T lymphocytes in the control of posttransplant KS.

G. M. P. Galbraith, MD

5% 5-Fluorouracil Cream for Treatment of Verruca Vulgaris in Children

Gladsjo JA, Alió Sáenz AB, Bergman J, et al (Univ of California, San Diego; Rady Children's Hosp and Health Ctr, San Diego, CA; Univ of British Columbia, Vancouver; et al)
Pediatr Dermatol 26:279-285, 2009

Warts are a common pediatric skin disease. Most treatments show only modest benefit, and some are poorly tolerated because of pain. 5-fluorouracil interferes with deoxyribonucleic acid and ribonucleic acid synthesis, and is used to treat genital warts in adults. Efficacy, safety, and tolerability of topical 5% 5-fluorouracil for treatment of common warts were examined in an open-label pilot study with pediatric patients. Thirty-nine children who have at least two hand warts applied 5% 5-fluorouracil cream (Efudex, Valeant Pharmaceuticals International) once or twice daily, under occlusion for 6 weeks. Assessment of treatment response and side effects was performed at baseline, treatment completion, and 3- and 6-month follow-ups. Hematology measures, liver function tests, and medication blood levels were reassessed at treatment completion. Eighty-eight percent of treated warts improved after 6 weeks of treatment, and 41% of subjects had complete resolution of at least one wart. Treatment response did not differ between once or twice daily applications. Tolerability and patient satisfaction were excellent. No subject had clinically significant blood levels of 5-fluorouracil. At 6 month follow-up, 87% of complete responders had no wart recurrence. Topical 5% 5-fluorouracil is a safe, effective, and well-tolerated treatment for warts in children.

▶ Verruca vulgaris is a common skin condition in children. The efficacy and safety of 5-fluorouracil (5-FU) in children has not been thoroughly investigated. This study included 40 subjects within the range of 4 to 18 years of age with a minimum of 2 verruca vulgaris lesions. At baseline, serum chemistry, complete blood count, and liver function tests were obtained to observe for possible systemic side effects. Half of the patients applied 5-FU once a day and the other half applied it twice a day, under occlusion for 6 weeks. Clinical assessments were made 1, 3, and 6 weeks with posttreatment follow-up performed at 3 and 6 months. The study revealed that 36% of subjects were completely cleared at the 3-month follow-up visit. The frequency of application showed a greater complete resolution of lesions. The most common side effects noted were erythema (33%), hyperpigmentation (26%), and mild erosion (23%), which were all transient. Perception of efficacy was reported as excellent or moderate in 86% of individuals, and 69% were very satisfied with the overall ease and comfort of the treatment. The advantages that 5-FU offers are that it is relatively painless, and parents can administer treatment at home. A major limitation of the study was the absence of a placebo group. This study suggests that 5-FU is a safe, tolerable, and reasonably effective treatment for verruga vulgaris in children.

G. K. Kim, DO
J. Q. Del Rosso, DO

Cantharidin Use Among Pediatric Dermatologists in the Treatment of Molluscum Contagiosum

Coloe J, Morrell DS (Ohio State Univ College of Medicine, Columbus; Univ of North Carolina, Chapel Hill)
Pediatr Dermatol 26:405-408, 2009

Cantharidin is cited often in the dermatology and pediatric literature as a valuable treatment option for molluscum contagiosum (MC). However, there have been no prospective, randomized, vehicle-controlled trials that have been able to quantify cantharidin's efficacy in MC. The purpose of this study was to determine the breadth of usage of cantharidin, most frequently used protocols, and common side effects seen with use of cantharidin. An eighteen question survey was administered to the Society of Pediatric Dermatology. The survey sought to evaluate treatments used in MC and experiences with cantharidin including: protocol, side effects, specific products used, and satisfaction with cantharidin. A total of 300 surveys were distributed via email, 101 surveys were initiated, and 95 (94%) of these were completed. Cantharidin, imiquimod, benign neglect, curettage, cryotherapy, and retinoids were the most common approaches to pediatric MC reported by respondents. Ninety-two percent of respondents reported satisfaction with cantharidin's efficacy, but 79% reported side effects, with discomfort/pain and blistering being the most common. Cantharidin is a common modality in the treatment of MC among pediatric dermatologists. While efficacy data is still lacking, subjective satisfaction with cantharidin is reported. Cantharidin remains a viable treatment option for children with MC.

▶ Molluscum contagiosum (MC) is a self-limiting pediatric viral skin condition that can be unsightly over a period of months to years. Cantharidin is a topical vesicant that produces a small intraepidermal blister that has commonly been used as a treatment option. This is a study of 300 email distributed surveys containing 18 questions addressing different treatments of MC, number of lesions treated, satisfaction of treatment, and side effects seen by pediatric dermatologists. Cantharidin, imiquimod, benign neglect, curettage, cryotherapy, and topical retinoids were the most common approaches to MC lesions. This study revealed that 92% of clinicians were satisfied with the efficacy of cantharidin. Seventy-five percent of respondents reported that they did not occlude the lesions after treating with cantharidin. Fifty percent of respondents had patients return to the clinic every 3 to 4 weeks for reapplication if warranted. Seventy-nine percent of respondents reported that the patients had observed side effects such as rash, subcutaneous nodule in the dermis, fever, and irritability with cantharidin. One patient reported anuria lasting one day after facial application of cantharidin. A limitation to this study was that this was a descriptive survey, and no efficacy data were captured or presented. In addition, no standardized protocol was followed. The amount of cantharidin applied, follow-up visits, and the number of lesions treated varied among physicians. This was also based on subjective reporting, and patient satisfaction was not evaluated with treatment of MC lesions. Also, not every respondent answered all the questions, and recall bias was another limitation to this study. Resolution of lesions could not be directly correlated with application of cantharidin because no controls were provided in this study. In conclusion, this study only revealed that cantharidin was a common treatment modality among pediatric dermatologists with suggestion of subjective satisfaction.

G. K. Kim, DO

J. Q. Del Rosso, DO

Adjuvant Photodynamic Therapy Does Not Prevent Recurrence of Condylomata Acuminata After Carbon Dioxide Laser Ablation—A Phase III, Prospective, Randomized, Bicentric, Double-Blind Study
Szeimies R-M, Schleyer V, Moll I, et al (Regensburg Univ Hosp, Germany; Hamburg Univ Hosp, Germany; et al)
Dermatol Surg 35:757-764, 2009

Background.—Recurrence after therapy for anogenital warts, or condylomata acuminata (CA), is common. Topical photodynamic therapy (PDT) using 5-aminolevulinic acid (ALA) is efficient in the treatment of CA, but one problem with PDT is the limited penetration depth of photosensitizer and light. Pre-PDT vaporization of CA using a carbon dioxide (CO_2) laser may enhance efficacy.

Objectives.—CO_2 laser ablation was followed by ALA-PDT in a phase III prospective randomized bicenter double-blind study to prevent recurrence of CA.

Materials and Methods.—One hundred seventy-five patients with CA received CO_2 laser vaporization plus adjuvant ALA-PDT ($n = 84$) or adjuvant placebo-PDT ($n = 91$). A 20% ALA or placebo ointment was applied to the CA area 4 to 6 hours before CO2 laser vaporization, followed by illumination with red light (600–740 nm, 100 mW/cm^2, 100 J/cm^2).

Results.—Cumulative recurrence rate 12 weeks after treatment was 50.0% in the ALA-PDT group, versus 52.7% in the placebo-PDT group ($p = .72$). No statistically significant difference between groups was detected with regard to recurrence rates up to 12 months after treatment. No major complications were observed.

Conclusion.—Adjuvant ALA-PDT of CA after CO_2 laser ablation was well tolerated, but no significant difference with regard to recurrence rate was observed from CO_2 laser vaporization alone.

▶ This is an excellent example of a thoughtful and well-done study to evaluate the efficacy of 5-aminolevulinic acid (ALA) photodynamic therapy (PDT) after carbon dioxide (CO_2) laser ablation of anal genital warts. Even though adjunctive therapy did not result in an improved outcome, the negative results are worth noting. This study should serve as a model clinical study to investigate combination therapy with a medical device.

E. A. Tanghetti, MD

5 HIV Infection

Antibiotic resistance in *Staphylococcus aureus*-containing cutaneous abscesses of patients with HIV
Krucke GW, Grimes DE, Grimes RM, et al (The Univ of Texas Health Science Ctr, Houston)
Am J Emerg Med 27:344-347, 2009

Purpose.—The aim of this study was to document the resistance patterns found in exudates from cutaneous abscesses of HIV-infected persons.

Basic Procedures.—Patient records were reviewed on 93 culture and sensitivity tests performed on exudates taken from incised and drained abscesses of HIV-infected persons.

Main Findings.—Of the specimens, 84.6% were *Staphylococcus aureus*. Of these, 93.5% were penicillin resistant, 87% oxacillin resistant, 84.4% cephazolin resistant, 84.4% erythromycin resistant, 52.2% ciprofloxacin resistant, and 15.6% tetracycline resistant. Fifty-eight specimens were tested for clindamycin with 29.3% found resistant; 85.7% were methicillin-resistant *S aureus* (MRSA) (defined as resistant to both penicillin G and oxacillin). All specimens were resistant to multiple antibiotics including antimicrobials that might be considered for use in MRSA. No specimens were resistant to trimethoprim-sulfamethoxazole, rifampin, or vancomycin.

Conclusions.—Empiric antimicrobial therapy of HIV-infected persons with cutaneous abscesses must be tailored to the high frequency of antimicrobial drug resistance including MRSA in this population.

▶ The aim of this study was to document the resistance patterns found in exudates from cutaneous abscesses of HIV-infected persons. The investigators retrospectively reviewed the records of 113 consecutive occasions at Houston clinic where HIV patients required incision and drainage of cutaneous abscesses. Of the 113 specimens bacterial growth was seen in 93 cultures, and 77 of these (84.6%) were *Staphylococcus aureus* positive. Of the 77 that were *S aureus*, 69 (74.2%) were methicillin-resistant *S aureus* (MRSA) positive. Although it is expected that community acquired MRSA (CA-MRSA) would be found in HIV-infected patients, its high prevalence was remarkable. Even more interesting and worrisome was the high degree of resistance to antibiotics. All cultures that were *S aureus* positive were resistant to multiple antibiotics, including antimicrobials that might be considered options for use in CA-MRSA. According to the results of this study, the empiric antimicrobial therapy most likely to effectively treat these abscesses in HIV-infected individuals is trimethoprim-sulfamethoxazole alone or in combination with rifampin.

Given the prevalence of MRSA detected in HIV patients in this study and their associated antibiotic resistance, it is recommended by the authors of this study to always ask about patient HIV status or about other risk factors associated with MRSA (such as recent incarceration, hospitalization, residence in a long-term care facility, and military barracks) when seeing a patient with a soft-tissue infection. This information will allow the clinician to use appropriate empiric antimicrobial therapy for patients at risk for CA-MRSA cutaneous infections. This recommendation is in concordance with the American Medical Association, the Infectious Disease Society of America, and the Centers for Diseases Control and Prevention (AMA/CDC/IDSA) guidelines, which state that skin and soft-tissue infections in HIV and high-risk individuals should be treated as if they are CA-MRSA and to use medications that would provide coverage for this type of organism.

This study provides results that are easily applicable to everyday dermatology practice, providing data on the prevalence of *S aureus* and CA-MRSA in abscesses of HIV and high risk associated patients. Antibiotic sensitivity and resistance patterns of these organisms are also discussed. The major limitation of this study is nonrandomized patient selection.

J. Levin, DO

J. Q. Del Rosso, DO

Imiquimod 5% cream for external genital or perianal warts in human immunodeficiency virus-positive patients treated with highly active antiretroviral therapy: an open-label, noncomparative study
Saiag P, Bauhofer A, Bouscarat F, et al (Université Versailles St-Quentin, Boulogne, France; Clinical Res, MEDA Pharma GmbH & Co, Germany; Université Paris, France; et al)
Br J Dermatol 161:904-909, 2009

Background.—Human immunodeficiency virus (HIV)+ patients have an increased risk of anogenital warts. High-risk (HR) human papillomaviruses (HPVs), especially types 16 and 18, are major risk factors for precancerous and cancerous lesions of the anogenital tract, while low-risk (LR) HPVs are associated with benign lesions. Cure of genital warts with ablative techniques, surgical excision, podophyllotoxin or trichloroacetic acid is frequently difficult. Treatment with imiquimod cream showed a total clearance of external genital or perianal warts in about 50% of immunocompetent subjects. However, total clearance was reduced in HIV+ subjects not treated with highly active antiretroviral therapy (HAART).

Objectives.—To assess clinically and by monitoring HPV content the efficacy of 5% topical imiquimod to treat anogenital warts in HIV+ subjects with at least partially restored immune functions.

Methods.—Fifty HIV+ patients successfully treated with HAART (total CD4+ cells ≥ 200 cells mm^{-3} and plasma HIV RNA load $< 10^4$ copies mL^{-1}) with anogenital warts were included. Imiquimod 5% cream was applied on external genital or perianal warts three times weekly for up to 16 weeks. Warts were tested at entry and after treatment for human LR- and HR-HPV DNA.

Results.—Total wart clearance was observed in 16 of 50 (32%) patients at week 16. At enrolment, HPV DNA was present in more than 90% of lesions with a majority of lesions co-infected by HR- and LR-HPV. At study end, the HPV load decreased or became undetectable in 40% of cases studied.

Conclusions.—Imiquimod 5% cream did not show safety concerns and is suitable for use in HIV+ subjects with anogenital warts and successful HAART treatment.

▶ The use of immune response modifiers in transplant patients and HIV-positive patients is a common practice in dermatology, and safety in these populations has been established. However, the reader must remember that although the clearance rates in these studies may not appear striking, the eradication of viral DNA that was once detected in active lesions in 40% of the cases of immunosuppressed population is significant, especially compared with 50% in the immunocompetent population. It is also important to remember that using this class of drugs in a patient that can mount a diminished immune response will involve a reduced success rate and may require more frequent and/or longer applications. The analogy here is like using a laptop computer with only 20% power left: the utilities may still work, but they might be slower. This is supported by the finding that patients not treated with highly active anti-retroviral therapy (HAART) therapy did not experience the same clearance.

N. Bhatia, MD

6 Parasitic Infections, Bites, and Infestations

Demodicosis: A clinicopathological study
Hsu C-K, Hsu MM-L, Lee JY-Y (University Hosp, Tainan, Taiwan; Natl Cheng Kung Univ, Tainan, Taiwan)
J Am Acad Dermatol 60:453-462, 2009

Background.—*Demodex* mites are common commensal organisms of the pilosebaceous unit in human beings and have been implicated in pityriasis folliculorum, rosacea-like demodicosis, and demodicosis gravis.

Objective.—We sought to describe the spectrum of clinicopathological findings and therapeutic responses of demodicosis in Taiwanese patients.

Methods.—We conducted a retrospective study to review clinicopathologic findings and therapeutic responses of 34 cases of diagnosed demodicosis.

Results.—Fifteen cases with positive results of potassium hydroxide examination, standardized skin surface biopsy specimen, and/or skin biopsy specimen, and resolution of skin lesions after anti-*Demodex* treatment were included for final analysis. Nineteen cases were excluded because of insufficient positive data to make a definite diagnosis. There were 4 male and 11 female patients (age 1-64 years, mean age 38.7 years). The disease was recurrent or chronic with a duration ranging from 2 months to 5 years (mean 15.7 months). The skin lesions were acne rosacea-like (n = 8), perioral dermatitis-like (n = 5), granulomatous rosacea-like (n = 1), and pityriasis folliculorum (n = 1). Skin biopsy was performed in 7 patients. Overall, the histopathology was characterized by: (1) dense perivascular and perifollicular lymphohistiocytic infiltrates, often with abundant neutrophils and occasionally with multinucleated histiocytes; (2) excessive *Demodex* mites in follicular infundibula; and (3) infundibular pustules containing mites or mites in perifollicular inflammatory infiltrate. The skin lesions resolved after treatment including systemic metronidazole, topical metronidazole, crotamiton, or gamma benzene hexachloride.

Limitations.—Small sample size and a fraction of patients without long-term follow-up are limitations.

Conclusion.—Demodicosis should be considered in the differential diagnosis of recurrent or recalcitrant rosacea-like, granulomatous rosacea-like, and perioral dermatitis-like eruptions of the face. Potassium hydroxide examination, standardized skin surface biopsy, skin biopsy, or a combination of these are essential to establish the diagnosis.

▶ How many of Koch's postulates are optional? With *Demodex*-associated diseases the time-honored test of causality doesn't work for this hard to quantify member of the normal flora.

The authors present a series of patients with facial eruptions that had large numbers of *Demodex* on histopathology and some measure of response to therapy that could be considered antiparasitic. There was no control group. Some of the drugs used have anti-inflammatory activity as well.

A curiosity with at least some of these cases is their localized distribution. I would (perhaps wrongly) assume that a demodectic eruption would be roughly symmetrical.

Any diagnosis of demodectic skin disease raises more questions for me than it answers. Because *Demodex* is a member of the normal flora, when does its presence become criteria for causality? If one sees it in a basal cell carcinoma, would one say that the mite was at fault? I remain a skeptic.

G. Webster, MD

Dermoscopy of cutaneous leishmaniasis
Llambrich A, Zaballos P, Terrasa F, et al (Hosp de san Pau i Santa Tecla, Tarragona, Spain; Hosp Son Llàtzer, Palma de Mallorca, Spain; et al)
Br J Dermatol 160:756-761, 2009

Background.—Dermoscopy has been proposed as a diagnostic tool in the case of skin infections and parasitosis but no specific dermoscopic criteria have been described for cutaneous leishmaniasis (CL).

Objectives.—To describe the dermoscopic features of CL.

Methods.—Dermoscopic examination (using the DermLite Foto; 3Gen, LLC, Dana Point, CA, U.S.A.) of 26 CL lesions was performed to evaluate specific dermoscopic criteria.

Results.—We observed the following dermoscopic features: generalized erythema (100%), 'yellow tears' (53%), hyperkeratosis (50%), central erosion/ulceration (46%), erosion/ulceration associated with hyperkeratosis (38%) and 'white starburst-like pattern' (38%). Interestingly, at least one vascular structure described in skin neoplasms was observed in all cases: comma-shaped vessels (73%), linear irregular vessels (57%), dotted vessels (53%), polymorphous/atypical vessels (26%), hairpin vessels (19%), arborizing telangiectasia (11%), corkscrew vessels (7%) and glomerular-like vessels (7%). Combination of two or more different types of vascular structures was present in 23 of 26 CL lesions (88%), with a combination of two vascular structures in 13 cases (50%) and three or more in 10 cases (38%).

Conclusions.—Characteristic dermoscopic structures have been identified in CL. Important vascular patterns seen in melanocytic and nonmelanocytic tumours are frequently observed in this infection.

▶ Dermoscopy, also known as dermatoscopy, has found a myriad of uses beyond the study of pigmented lesions. From adnexal tumors to infestations (scabies), a variety of dermoscopic findings have been documented.

In this article, the authors studied leishmaniasis and developed a variety of dermoscopic criteria, including "yellow tears" that of modest use in diagnosing cutaneous leishmaniasis. The new criteria developed, including "yellow tears" and a "white starburst pattern" were present in 53% and 38% of cases, respectively. While leishmaniasis is increasing in certain populations in American health care, such as veterans returning from military duties in Afghanistan and Iraq, dermoscopy might provide important supportive evidence, with comparatively little cost, as the technique is without any real risk to the patient. Still the authors note correctly that features common to cutaneous leishmaniasis are also seen in melanoma, basal cell carcinoma, and squamous cell carcinoma, among others, and, a biopsy is needed for a histopathological final diagnosis. In fact, I would contend that not only is a biopsy needed, but also serious consideration of PCR based testing, now currently offered by the Centers for Disease Control or the Walter Reed Army Institute of Research Leishmania Diagnostic Laboratory.[1,2]

W. A. High, MD, JD, MEng

References

1. Centers for Disease Control. Diagnostic procedures: isolation of Leishmania organisms. http://www.dpd.cdc.gov/dpdx/HTML/DiagnosticProcedures.htm. Accessed November 24, 2009.
2. Walter Reed Army Institute of Research Leishmania Diagnostic Laboratory. Leishmaniasis: information for clinicians. http://www.pdhealth.mil/downloads/cisleishmaniasis.pdf. Accessed November 24, 2009.

Accuracy of Diagnosis of Pediculosis Capitis: Visual Inspection vs Wet Combing
Jahnke C, Bauer E, Hengge UR, et al (Unit of Child and Adolescent Health, Braunschweig, Germany; Charité Univ Medicine, Berlin, Germany; Heinrich-Heine-Univ, Düsseldorf, Germany)
Arch Dermatol 145:309-313, 2009

Objective.—To determine the diagnostic accuracy of visual inspection and wet combing in pediculosis capitis (head lice infestation). Visual inspection of 5 predilection sites (temples, behind the ears, and neck) was performed first, followed by wet combing of hair moistened with conditioner. Presence of mobile stages was defined as active infestation, presence of nits alone as historic infestation.

Design.—Observer-blinded comparison of 2 diagnostic methods.

Setting.—Five primary schools in which head lice infestation was epidemic.

Participants.—A total of 304 students aged 6 to 12 years.

Main Outcome Measures.—Presence of nymph, adults, and nits; sensitivity, predictive value, and accuracy of both methods.

Results.—Visual inspection underestimated the true prevalence of active infestation by a factor of 3.5. The sensitivity of wet combing in diagnosing active infestation was significantly higher than of visual inspection (90.5% vs 28.6%; $P < .001$). The accuracy of the former method was 99.3% and that of the latter method, 95%. In contrast, visual inspection had a higher sensitivity for the diagnosis of historic infestation (86.1% vs 68.4%: $P < .001$).

Conclusions.—Wet combing is a very accurate method to diagnose active head lice infestation. Visual inspection is the method of choice, if one aims to determine the frequency of carriers of eggs or nits.

▶ The diagnosis of pediculosis is usually established by visual inspection, prompted by a history of exposure, scalp pruritus, or posterior cervical lymphadenopathy. False-positive diagnoses are common, and may bar children from school. Common causes of false-positive diagnoses include hair casts, dandruff, and hatched egg cases from a previous infestation. False-negative diagnoses can result in spread of the infestation to other children. This article examined the accuracy of diagnosis by means of visual inspection with that of wet combing. Wet combing has been advocated by some as the gold standard for the diagnosis of pediculosis, but previous data to support this claim have been inconclusive. Wet combing is much less convenient and less likely to be readily accepted by patients and parents. The results of this study suggest that although wet combing is a highly accurate method of identifying infestation with adult lice, visual inspection remains a reasonable means of determining whether patients carry eggs and nits.

Several aspects of the study deserve comment. The 5-zone systematic visual inspection performed in the study seems on the surface to be more thorough than may be performed by many clinicians. Given this systematic inspection, it is somewhat surprising that the sensitivity of visual inspection was only 28.6%. This probably relates to their definition of active infestation. The authors allowed only identification of mobile lice as evidence of active infestation. Had they allowed for identification of ova close to the scalp, the results may have been quite different. Also, this study was performed in a country with little tolerance for louse infestation, and patients had much lower nit loads than in previous studies. Lastly, the hair was parted with the aid of an applicator stick, which allows for much less surface area visualization than inspection with gloved fingers.

Given these limitations, the study has verified the high sensitivity of wet combing, but has not determined the most practical means of inspection for the dermatologist in an office setting, or for school nurses. Based on the results of this study, either method may be acceptable for the office setting, while wet combing should be considered the gold standard for clinical trials.

D. M. Elston, MD

Variable response of crusted scabies to oral ivermectin: report on eight Egyptian patients
Nofal A (Zagazig University, Egypt)
J Eur Acad Dermatol Venereol 23:793-797, 2009

Background.—Several reports have proved the efficacy of oral iver-mectin in the treatment of crusted scabies. However, the response varied greatly between different studies.

Objective.—The aim of this study was to evaluate the response of crusted scabies to oral ivermectin in eight Egyptian patients.

Patients and Methods.—Eight patients with crusted scabies, diagnosed clinically and confirmed microscopically, were involved in this study. Patients received a single oral dose of ivermectin (200µg/kg) and re-examined at 2, 4, 6 and 8 weeks. A second dose of ivermectin was given in case of treatment failure at the end of the second week. A third dose of ivermectin, combined with permethrin 5% and salicylic acid 5% was given at the end of the fourth week for the nonresponders to the second dose.

Results.—Two patients were completely cured after a single dose of iver-mectin, 4 patients required a second dose at a 2-week interval to achieve cure and 2 patients cleared from scabies after the combined therapy. No recurrence was reported at the end of 8 weeks. An inverse relation was observed between the response to ivermectin and the severity of immuno-suppression, crust thickness and mite burden.

Conclusion.—Oral ivermectin is an effective alternative therapy for the treatment of crusted scabies. The response of crusted scabies to oral iver-mectin is variable and combination therapy with topical scabicides and keratolytics seems to be the best choice.

▶ Crusted scabies is a highly contagious variant of scabies due to hyperinfes-tation with *Sarcoptes scabiei*. It results from a failure of the host to experience or relate pruritus due to a blunted immune response or impaired ability to communicate. As a result, proliferation of the mites is unchecked, which can manifest as a psoriasiform and warty dermatosis often in an acral distribution. Lesions are teeming with mites, feces, and scybala due to a prolonged period of proliferation without scratching.

This is a report of 8 patients diagnosed clinically and with microscopic confir-mation with crusted scabies taking ivermectin (200 µg/kg) and re-examined at 2, 4, 6, and 8 weeks. Patients previously on antiscabetic treatment, children weighing less than 15 kg, and pregnant and lactating women were excluded in this study. Close contacts were also given oral ivermectin to minimize risk of reinfestation and patients were informed to launder all infested clothes and bedding at high temperatures. Routine laboratory tests were done before, during, and after therapy to monitor for adverse reactions to ivermectin. Patients considered to be cured were those that had no pruritus, clinical evidence of scabies, or positive skin scrapings. Two patients were completely cured after a single dose of ivermectin. Four patients required a second dose at a 2-week interval, and 2 patients required combination therapy. Two of the patients that were immunocompromised achieved clearance after 3 doses of ivermectin combined with topical scabicides and keratolytics. The variability of the response to treatment corresponded to the variability in immune status. Authors also theorized that crust thickness and extent could interfere with penetration of ivermectin. The management of crusted scabies is challenging. Oral ivermectin is an effective alternative therapy for the treatment of crusted scabies as shown in this study; however, a single dose may not be enough. Crusted scabies is characterized as being therapy resistant with relapses, in which topical remedies alone are often inadequate. As treatment failure is common, the sequential use of several agents may be necessary. This may be attributed to variable immune responses, inadequate application/noncompliance, difficulties in treatment of close contacts, variable penetration of thick crusts, and emergence of resistance. To date, ivermectin is not approved by the FDA for scabies. The optimal dosage, number of doses, interval between repeated doses, and risk of resistance are all questions that are yet to be addressed with future studies.

G. K. Kim, DO

J. Q. Del Rosso, DO

Mucosal leishmaniasis: description of case management approaches and analysis of risk factors for treatment failure in a cohort of 140 patients in Brazil
Amato VS, Tuon FF, Imamura R, et al (Univ of Sao Paulo, Brazil)
J Eur Acad Dermatol Venereol 23:1026-1034, 2009

Background.—Mucosal leishmaniasis is caused mainly by *Leishmania braziliensis* and it occurs months or years after cutaneous lesions. This progressive disease destroys cartilages and osseous structures from face, pharynx and larynx.

Objective and Methods.—The aim of this study was to analyse the significance of clinical and epidemiological findings, diagnosis and treatment with the outcome and recurrence of mucosal leishmaniasis through binary logistic regression model from 140 patients with mucosal leishmaniasis from a Brazilian centre.

Results.—The median age of patients was 57.5 and systemic arterial hypertension was the most prevalent secondary disease found in patients with mucosal leishmaniasis (43%). Diabetes, chronic nephropathy and viral hepatitis, allergy and coagulopathy were found in less than 10% of patients. Human immunodeficiency virus (HIV) infection was found in

7 of 140 patients (5%). Rhinorrhea (47%) and epistaxis (75%) were the most common symptoms. N-methyl-glucamine showed a cure rate of 91% and recurrence of 22%. Pentamidine showed a similar rate of cure (91%) and recurrence (25%). Fifteen patients received itraconazole with a cure rate of 73% and recurrence of 18%. Amphotericin B was the drug used in 30 patients with 82% of response with a recurrence rate of 7%. The binary logistic regression analysis demonstrated that systemic arterial hypertension and HIV infection were associated with failure of the treatment ($P < 0.05$).

Conclusion.—The current first-line mucosal leishmaniasis therapy shows an adequate cure but later recurrence. HIV infection and systemic arterial hypertension should be investigated before start the treatment of mucosal leishmaniasis.

▶ Mucosal leishmaniasis (espundia) is a protozoal disease caused by infection with *Leishmania braziliensis*. I have cared for patients with this disorder in Latin America, and I have witnessed first-hand the devastation it ensues—reaping destruction of the nose and other facial structures; necessitating prolonged, expensive and toxic treatment; sometimes not responding to any treatment in the armamentarium.

In this article, the authors examine a series of 140 patients with espundia all cared for at a single institution in Sao Paulo, Brazil. A variety of diagnostic modalities were used to confirm the diagnosis, but interestingly, polymerase chain reaction (PCR) was not included, although I personally have seen this used by many Latin American centers as a premium diagnostic modality.[1]

The authors note that most patients present with epistaxis and rhinorrhea. This is commensurate with my own anecdotal experience and is certainly not a surprise. The authors also report that N-methyl-glucamine and pentamidine had the highest cure rates, and modest recurrence rates, while amphotericin had a lesser cure rate and the lowest recurrence rate. It is further explained, as amphotericin is known to be a superb agent for treatment of espundia (in fact used for cases that fail other management), that the cure rate in this case was lowered because renal failure, a side-effect of amphotericin, resulted in incomplete treatment. Itraconazole had a lesser cure rate and a higher recurrence rate.

Perhaps the most novel observation made by the authors of this article concerns binary logistical regression, which indicated that treatment failure was associated with either HIV infection or systemic arterial hypertension. Certainly, considering the general immune system dysfunction of HIV, an association with treatment failure is logical and expected. Less clear is why systemic arterial hypertension is associated with treatment failure. The authors speculate that it may be due to antihypertensive agents interfering with inflammatory cascade, but other studies that have found a benefit to coadministration of captopril with N-methyl-glucamine during treatment of cutaneous leishmaniasis seem to undercut this hypothesis. In truth, considering the ubiquitous nature of hypertension, this reader is concerned that some unknown confounder has yet to be identified with regard to this observation.

W. A. High, MD, JD, MEng

Reference

1. Oliveira JG, Novais FO, de Oliveira CI, et al. Polymerase chain reaction (PCR) is highly sensitive for diagnosis of mucosal leishmaniasis. *Acta Trop*. 2005;94:55-59.

7 Disorders of the Pilosebaceous Apparatus

Hair grooming practices and central centrifugal cicatricial alopecia
Gathers RC, Jankowski M, Eide M, et al (Henry Ford Hosp, Detroit, MI)
J Am Acad Dermatol 60:574-578, 2009

Background.—The cause of central centrifugal cicatricial alopecia (CCCA) in African American women remains to be elucidated.

Objective.—This study was designed to determine the hair-grooming practices in African American women with and without CCCA and to evaluate possible etiologic factors.

Methods.—Utilizing a novel survey instrument, the Hair Grooming Assessment Survey, we performed a retrospective comparative survey of the hair-grooming practices of two populations of African American women seen and evaluated at the Department of Dermatology, Henry Ford Hospital in Detroit, MI, between 2000 and 2007. The case group were women with clinical and histologic diagnosis of CCCA, and the control group were those without a history of alopecia.

Results.—All 101 surveys that were returned were analyzed (51 from the case group and 50 from the control group). A strong association was found between the use of both sewn-in hair weaving and cornrow or braided hairstyles with artificial hair extensions and CCCA ($P < .04$, $P < .03$, respectively). Similarly, women with CCCA were more likely to report a history of "damage", typically defined as uncomfortable pulling and tenderness, from both sewn-in and glued-in weaves, and from cornrow or braided hairstyles with artificial hair extensions ($P < .001$, $P < .02$, and $P < .03$, respectively). In contrast to previous anecdotal beliefs, no correlation was found between the use of either hot combing or hair relaxers and the development of CCCA.

Limitations.—Results are limited by patient recall of past hair grooming practices. Also, as hair grooming practices may vary by geographic region, these results may not be generalized to all women of African descent.

Conclusion.—There is a clear difference in both quantitative and qualitative hair grooming practices among African American women with CCCA.

▶ This retrospective study demonstrates women with central centrifugal cicatricial alopecia (CCCA) were more likely to have worn cornrows or braids with artificial hair extensions, sewn-in or glued-in hair weaves, have worn them for more cumulative years and are more likely to report a history of hair damage (tender scalp or uncomfortable pulling). This study also demonstrates that patients with CCCA were more likely to have a sister with hair loss than a mother, grandmother, aunt or cousin with hair loss, possibly secondary to similar hair-grooming behaviors among members in the same household and of the same generation. This article also states that women who wore their hair natural, without any use of chemicals or heat before the age of 20, had an 86% decrease in the risk of developing CCCA.

S. B. Momin, DO
J. Q. Del Rosso, DO

Increased history of childhood and lifetime traumatic events among adults with alopecia areata
Willemsen R, Vanderlinden J, Roseeuw D, et al (Universitair Ziekenhuis Brussel; Univ Psychiatric Ctr KULeuven, Campus Kortenberg; et al)
J Am Acad Dermatol 60:388-393, 2009

Background.—Whether adult alopecia areata (AA) is associated with childhood or total lifetime traumatic events is not known. Previous studies have investigated only the relationship with recent stressful events.

Objective.—We sought to determine whether patients with AA experience more childhood or total lifetime traumatic events, as measured by the Traumatic Experiences Checklist.

Methods.—Using a case-control study, data on 90 patients with AA and 91 control subjects were analyzed.

Results.—Significantly more patients with AA experienced total lifetime and early childhood traumatic events, with an odds ratio of 2.46 (95% confidence interval 1.15-5.28; $P = .017$) and 2.16 (1.15-4.06; $P = .016$), respectively. In patients with AA, the global impact score related to their traumatic experiences was significantly higher than in control subjects ($P < .001$). In addition, patients with AA experienced significantly more emotionally and physically traumatic events.

Limitation.—This case-control study is susceptible to recall bias and to confounding factors associated with stress caused by AA outbreaks or by a traumatic childhood history.

Conclusion.—Our study documents an increased history of childhood trauma in patients with AA compared with control subjects.

▶ The information provided in this article and the conclusions drawn in this case-control study appear to be valid. More patients with alopecia areata (AA) presented with at least one lifetime traumatic event or one early childhood trauma as well. The mean number of emotional and physical traumatic events were significantly higher in patients with AA but were not significant for sexual traumatic events when compared with the control group. As stated by the authors of the article, there are a few limitations of this study including recall and response bias, stress, and anxiety of the chronic disease itself, and that the influence of childhood traumatic events among individuals can vary. Sexual traumatic events can be physical and emotional as well, but the Traumatic Experiences Checklist (TEC) questionnaire clearly itemizes the presence/absence of all traumatic events. Strengths of the article include a good sample size and the use of a valid and reliable standardized questionnaire.

S. B. Momin, DO

J. Q. Del Rosso, DO

History of atopy or autoimmunity increases risk of alopecia areata
Barahmani N, National Alopecia Areata Registry (The Univ of Texas M. D. Anderson Cancer Ctr, Houston; et al)
J Am Acad Dermatol 61:581-591, 2009

Background.—The association between a history of atopy or autoimmune diseases and risk of alopecia areata (AA) is not well established.

Objective.—The purpose of this study was to use the National AA Registry database to further investigate the association between history of atopy or autoimmune diseases and risk of AA.

Methods.—A total of 2613 self-registered sporadic cases (n = 2055) and controls (n = 558) were included in this analysis.

Results.—Possessing a history of any atopic (odds ratio = 2.00; 95% confidence interval 1.50-2.54) or autoimmune (odds ratio = 1.73; 95% confidence interval 1.10-2.72) disease was associated with an increased risk of AA. There was no trend for possessing a history of more than one atopic or autoimmune disease and increasing risk of AA.

Limitations.—Recall, reporting, and recruiting bias are potential sources of limitations in this analysis.

Conclusion.—This analysis revealed that a history of atopy and autoimmune disease was associated with an increased risk of AA and that the results were consistent for both the severe subtype of AA (ie, alopecia totalis and alopecia universalis) and the localized subtype (ie, AA persistent).

▶ Although it is not as common to screen for atopy as thyroid diseases, autoimmune diseases, or hematological diseases, it is important to consider the atopic diathesis as an immune trigger for variants of alopecia areata. These are: (1) the physiological similarities in immune profiles (chronic stage T helper 1 [Th1] profile and IgE autoimmunity against keratinocytes, similar to end-stage atopic dermatitis); (2) correlation to more severe states such as alopecia totalis; and (3) the immunological similarities to autoimmunity based on pathogenesis and response to immunosuppressive therapies.

By contrast, there is no indication for changing management strategies for objective screening except for taking the complete history. However, the information presented might suggest that given the high prevalence of patients considered atopic there should be heightened surveillance and a lower threshold to administer systemic therapies to counteract the immune mechanisms at work.

N. Bhatia, MD

Efficacy of fixed low-dose isotretinoin (20 mg, alternate days) with topical clindamycin gel in moderately severe acne vulgaris
Sardana K, Garg VK, Sehgal VN, et al (Maulana Azad Med College and Lok Nayak Hosp Delhi; Sehgal Nursing Home, Delhi)
J Eur Acad Dermatol Venereol 23:556-560, 2009

Background.—In view of the potentially serious side-effects of standard isotretinoin (0.5–1.0 mg/kg per day) therapy for acne, we studied the safety and efficacy of low-fixed dose isotretinoin plus topical 1%clindamycin gel in the treatment of moderate grade of acne.

Methods.—In this prospective, non-comparative study, 320 adult patients, with moderately severe acne were enrolled and treated with fixed-dose isotretinoin at 20 mg every alternate day (approximately 0.15 mg/kg/day to 0.28 mg/kg/day) for 6 months along with topical clindamycin gel. All female patients were assessed for polycystic ovarian disease. Patients were followed up for 6 months.

Results.—A total of 305 patients completed the study. Overall, patients received a mean of 38.4 mg/kg cumulative dose of isotretinoin, and very good results were observed in 208 (68.20%), while good response was seen in 59 (19.34%) of patients. Failure of the treatment occurred in 38 (12.46%), while relapses occurred in 50 (16.39%) of patients. Relapses were commoner in females, and 37 of 43 (86.04%) patients had polycystic ovarian disease. Though mild chelitis (91%) and xerosis (43%) were common, laboratory abnormalities in the form of elevated hepatic enzymes (5%) and elevated serum lipids (6%) were rare.

Conclusion.—Six months of treatment with fixed-dose, alternate-day isotretinoin (20 mg) plus topical 1%clindamycin gel was found to be effective in the treatment of moderate acne in adult patients, with a low incidence of side-effects.

▶ Sardana et al performed a prospective study of 320 patients and determined that low-dose isotretinoin (20 mg every other day) combined with topical clindamycin was effective in the treatment of moderately severe acne in adult patients with a low incidence of side effects. The study is suggested as the first study to compare this combination of medications for acne vulgaris, although the effectiveness of low-dose isotretinoin monotherapy has been studied and its use with a topical retinoid. While the study showed efficacious results, there are several questions that remain and may be useful to address in further studies:

(1) There were 320 patients that began the study, and 305 of those patients completed the study. In the 15 patients that dropped out or could not be followed, there is no indication as to whether this was secondary to treatment ineffectiveness. Additionally, in the 305 patients that did complete the study, 38 were treatment failures (and required either additional treatment time or an increase in dosage), and 50 patients relapsed (most of which had polycystic ovarian disease).

(2) This was a prospective noncomparative study, and although it summarized a review of other studies showing the efficacy of isotretinoin monotherapy in low dose usage as well as another study using the low-dose oral retinoid in combination with a topical retinoid, a comparison of head-to-head studies comparing isotretinoin versus other topical medications would provide additional evaluation of efficacy.

(3) There is no sure way to gather whether the efficacy of the treatment was due to the combination of the low-dose isotretinoin/topical clindamycin, or whether the outcome could be attributed to simply just the low-dose isotretinoin. A head-to-head study using patients applying low-dose isotretinoin monotherapy versus the combination therapy would again provide additional merit. To the article's credit, there is a summary of studies listing the efficacy of low-dose isotretinoin monotherapy. The purpose of listing the additional studies is to compare the efficacy of low-dose isotretinoin/topical clindamycin versus results reported with oral isotretinoin monotherapy. In Sardana's study the average dose of isotretinoin was 0.15 to 0.28 mg/kg/day with an efficacy rate of 87.64 %. In a study by Amichai et al, subjects used 0.3 to 0.4 mg/kg/day of low-dose isotretinoin monotherapy, resulting in a higher efficacy rate of 92.6% to 94.8%.[1] The question remains as to whether this somewhat small difference in dosage is enough to warrant applying an additional medication such as topical clindamycin. Further, there is no indication in Sardana's study to determine whether the side effect profile was any better or worse than in the Amichai study, warranting the addition of topical clindamycin. Lastly, it is not accurate to compare results from different studies, due to differences in study design and patient populations.

Overall, however, this study provides some data for adding an additional modality in the treatment of acne vulgaris that has not otherwise been examined.

B. D. Michaels, DO

J. Q. Del Rosso, DO

Reference

1. Amichai B, Shemer A, Grunwald MH. Low-dose isotretinoin in the treatment of acne vulgaris. *J Am Acad Dermatol.* 2006;54:644-646.

An exploratory study of adherence to topical benzoyl peroxide in patients with acne vulgaris

Yentzer BA, Alikhan A, Teuschler H, et al (Wake Forest Univ School of Medicine, Winston-Salem, NC)

J Am Acad Dermatol 60:879-880, 2009

This study provides objective documentation of teenagers' poor adherence to topical acne treatment. While the study population was small, it was well powered to detect the large decline in adherence that occurs in just 6 weeks. Improvement in acne probably does not explain the decreasing use of medication, because benzoyl peroxide is not expected to clear acne that quickly. While the role of disease improvement could be assessed if disease severity measures had been included over the course of treatment, doing so could have affected the subjects' adherence behavior. A strength of this study is that subjects were not informed they were in a clinical trial in order to determine the adherence of typical patients as opposed to clinical trial subjects; because of this, a high dropout rate was anticipated. If patients lost to follow-up are less adherent than those who do follow up or if adherence continues to decrease over time, these data may actually overestimate how often typical acne patients' apply medication. Development and testing of new ways to improve acne patients' adherence are acutely needed.

▶ Some of the best things come in small packages. This gem of an article is praiseworthy not only for its content, but also for its pithy presentation. We need more short and to-the-point articles like this one.

The discordance between phase 3 study results and real-world results is an ongoing problem. We are all aware of medications that pass Food and Drug Administration (FDA) scrutiny but are worthless in everyday practice. I'm sure you have your own list. FDA has added investigators' global assessments in an attempt to introduce a real-world grading to the approval process and that has been helpful, but still study results often are better than those in my office.

Compliance is certainly part of the problem. Drugs must be used if they are to work, and this article shows that teens are noncompliant with acne therapy and that compliance falls with time. How can this be improved? Perhaps a between-visits phone call from a nurse would help, or maybe just emphasizing to patients that acne medications must be used for many months and that noncompliance promotes the disease. In my office, I spend more time in an acne visit talking about the medicines and how to use them than anything else.

G. Webster, MD

Differences in Acne Treatment Prescribing Patterns of Pediatricians and Dermatologists: An Analysis of Nationally Representative Data
Yentzer BA, Irby CE, Fleischer AB Jr, et al (Wake Forest Univ School of Medicine, Winston-Salem, NC)
Pediatr Dermatol 25:635-639, 2008

Background.—Acne vulgaris is a very common disease process that is seen frequently by both pediatricians and dermatologists. However, treatment may be different depending on specialty.

Objectives.—To compare pediatricians' and dermatologists' patterns of treatment for acne vulgaris.

Methods.—National Ambulatory Medical Care Survey data on office visits to pediatricians and dermatologists for acne vulgaris were analyzed from 1996 to 2005.

Results.—During this 10-year time period, dermatologists managed an estimated 18.1 million acne visits and pediatricians managed an estimated 4.6 million acne visits. Dermatologists prescribed topical retinoids considerably more frequently than did pediatricians (46.1% of acne visits for dermatologists vs 12.1% for pediatricians).

Conclusions.—There is an opportunity for pediatricians to play a greater role in the management of patients with acne. A shift toward greater use of topical retinoids by pediatricians would be more in line with the practice of dermatologists and with current acne treatment consensus guidelines.

▶ The purpose of this study was to assess how acne in adolescents is managed by dermatologists and pediatricians in the United States. National Ambulatory Medical Care Survey data on office visits to pediatricians and dermatologists for acne vulgaris were analyzed from 1996-2005. The data indicate that pediatricians see the majority of acne patients before age 12, while most cases of acne in patients between 12 and 18 years of age are seen by dermatologists. These data point out the disparity in the use of topical retinoids between pediatricians and dermatologists and suggest that increased use of topical retinoids by pediatricians may lead to improved patient outcomes and perhaps a decreased need for referral to a dermatologist. The methods used are sound, keeping in mind the limitations of a retrospective review of estimates of patient visits, which cannot provide insights into the reasons behind the discrepancy in practice patterns. It is possible that patterns have changed since 2005. The article provides reasonable estimates for the numbers of acne visits and their distribution between dermatologists and pediatricians. The conclusions that pediatricians can incorporate topical retinoids into the care of acne patients is reasonable and supported by multiple studies and widespread clinical experience.

D. Thiboutot, MD

Efficacy of an oral contraceptive containing EE 0.03 mg and CMA 2 mg (Belara®) in moderate acne resolution: a randomized, double-blind, placebo-controlled Phase III trial
Plewig G, Cunliffe WJ, Binder N, et al (Ludwig-Maximilians-Universität, München, Germany; Leeds General Infirmary, UK; Grünenthal GmbH, Aachen, Germany)
Contraception 80:25-33, 2009

Background.—The study was conducted to assess the effects of the monophasic combined oral contraceptive containing ethinyl estradiol (EE) 0.03 mg and chlormadinone acetate (CMA) 2 mg (EE/CMA) on papulopustular acne of the face, décolleté (low neck) and back; on moderate comedonal acne of the face; and on seborrhea, alopecia and hirsutism.

Study Design.—Three hundred seventy-seven women were randomized (2:1) to receive EE/CMA ($n = 251$) or placebo ($n = 126$) for six medication cycles. Due to the placebo-controlled, double-blind design of the trial, condoms were supplied for contraception. The primary efficacy end point was defined as a reduction of at least 50% in the number of papules and/or pustules of the face from admission to Medication Cycle 6.

Results.—In total, 64.1% (161/251) of subjects treated with EE/CMA responded compared with 43.7% (55/126) of those taking placebo (p=.0001). The median reduction in papules/pustules on the face at Cycle 6 compared with admission was 63.6% (EE/CMA) compared with 45.3% (placebo group). For comedonal lesions of the face, the reduction in lesion numbers was 54.8% (EE/CMA) compared with 32.4% (placebo). Moderate papulopustular acne of the décolleté decreased by 92.9% (EE/CMA) vs. 50% (placebo group) and of the back by 86.0% and 58.3%, respectively. For these skin conditions, the p values for the relative difference between groups vs. baseline were <.05 at Cycles 3 and 6, in favor of EE/CMA. As part of a self-assessment rating, at least 70.5% (EE/CMA) vs. 41.3% (placebo) reported an at least satisfactory improvement of their moderate acne. Even 39.8% of women taking EE/CMA reported an "excellent improvement" or "complete resolution" of moderate acne compared with 12.7% taking placebo.

Conclusion.—In addition to its contraceptive efficacy described elsewhere, EE/CMA is an effective treatment for moderate papulopustular acne and other androgen-related skin disorders.

▶ Combination oral contraceptives are effective in the treatment of acne in female patients. This phase III study is the first to examine the effects of a monophasic oral contraceptive containing ethinyl estradiol (EE) (0.03 mg) and chlormadinone acetate (CMA) (2 mg) EE/CMA on acne and seborrhea compared with placebo in large numbers of women. CMA is an antiandrogen with structural similarity to cyproterone acetate, each of which is available in Europe and other areas, but not in the United States. The data demonstrate superiority of EE/CMA over placebo in terms of reduction of inflammatory lesions and noninflammatory lesions with a significantly greater proportion of subjects in the EE/CMA arm achieving at least a 50% reduction in lesions. Improvements in seborrhea were also noted, but the numbers of women with hirsutism were small with some women demonstrating marked improvement. Overall, this agent is currently used in Europe for acne treatment, and these data support its superiority to placebo.

D. Thiboutot, MD

Efficacy of a combined oral contraceptive containing 0.030 mg ethinylestradiol/2 mg dienogest for the treatment of papulopustular acne in comparison with placebo and 0.035 mg ethinylestradiol/2 mg cyproterone acetate

Palombo-Kinne E, Schellschmidt I, Schumacher U, et al (Jenapharm GmbH & Co, Germany; Bayer Schering Pharma AG, Berlin, Germany)
Contraception 79:282-289, 2009

Background.—Acne is a multifactorial disease characterized by androgenic stimulation of sebaceous glands. Therefore, combined oral contraceptives (COCs) containing anti-androgenic progestogens are suitable candidates for acne treatment. This study aimed to show that a COC containing the anti-androgen dienogest (DNG) is superior to placebo and not inferior to a COC containing the potent anti-androgen cyproterone acetate (CPA) in improving mild to moderate acne.

Study Design.—Healthy women between 16 and 45 years old with mild to moderate facial acne were randomly assigned to receive ethinylestradiol (EE)/DNG ($n = 525$), EE/CPA ($n = 537$) or placebo ($n = 264$) for six cycles in a multinational, multicenter, three-arm, double-blind and randomized trial. The primary efficacy variables were the percentages of change (from baseline to cycle 6) in inflammatory and total lesion count and the percentage of patients with acne improvement according to the Investigator Global Assessment.

Results.—All primary analyses proved that EE/DNG was superior to placebo and non-inferior to EE/CPA ($p < .05$). For *inflammatory* lesions, the reduction ($\pm SD$) rates were $-65.6 \pm 29.9\%$ for EE/DNG, $-64.6 \pm 31.2\%$ for EE/CPA and $-49.4 \pm 41.0\%$ for placebo. For *total* lesions, the reduction rates were $-54.7 \pm 26.3\%$ for EE/DNG, $-53.6 \pm 27.5\%$ for EE/CPA and $-39.4 \pm 33.6\%$ for placebo. The percentages of patients with improvement of facial acne were 91.9% for EE/DNG, 90.2% for EE/CPA and 76.2% for placebo.

Conclusion.—EE/DNG was superior to placebo, in spite of the prominent placebo effects, and as effective as EE/CPA in the treatment of mild to moderate acne, thus proving a valid option for the treatment of acne in women seeking oral contraception.

▶ Oral contraceptives (OCs) are a mainstay in the hormonal treatment of acne in women. This study compares the efficacy of a combination OC (COC) containing the progestogen dienogest with placebo and to a gold standard in acne treatment, an OC containing the antiandrogen cyproterone acetate (CPA). The 6-month study was conducted in large numbers of women and was statistically powered to detect superiority to placebo and noninferiority to the combined OC containing CPA. Patients had mild to moderate acne and had on average 20 ± 10 inflammatory acne lesions. An unusually high placebo effect was noted in terms of inflammatory lesion count reduction (about 50%), perhaps related to the relatively small numbers of inflammatory lesions at baseline. Despite this, the ethinylestradiol (EE)/anti-androgen dienogest (DNG) COC was statistically superior to placebo and noninferior to EE/CPA. Although sebum production appeared to decrease in all groups, there were no statistical differences between active treatments and placebo, most likely due to smaller sample size and the known variability of sebum assessments. Safety profiles were similar. One case of ischemic stroke was noted in the EE/DNG arm. OCs and hormonal replacement therapies containing dienogest or products containing CPA are available in Europe and Australia.

D. Thiboutot, MD

Periocular dermatitis: a report of 401 patients
Temesvári E, Pónyai G, Németh I, et al (Semmelweis Univ, Budapest, Hungary)
J Eur Acad Dermatol Venereol 23:124-128, 2009

Background.—Periocular contact dermatitis may appear as contact conjunctivitis, contact allergic and/or irritative eyelid and periorbital dermatitis, or a combination of these symptoms. The clinical symptoms may be induced by several environmental and therapeutic contact allergens.

Objectives.—The aim of the present study was to map the eliciting contact allergens in 401 patients with periocular dermatitis (PD) by patch testing with environmental and ophthalmic contact allergens.

Methods.—Following the methodics of international requirements, 401 patients were tested with contact allergens of the standard environmental series, 133 of 401 patients with the *Brial* ophthalmic basic and supplementary series as well.

Results.—Contact hypersensitivity was detected in 34.4% of the patients. Highest prevalence was seen in cases of PD without other symptoms (51.18%), in patients of PD associated with ophthalmic complaints (OC; 30.4%), and PD associated with atopic dermatitis (AD; 27.9%). In the subgroup of PD associated with seborrhoea (S) and rosacea (R), contact hypersensitivity was confirmed in 17.6%. Most frequent sensitisers were nickel sulphate (in 8.9% of the tested 401 patients), fragrance mix I (4.5%), balsam of Peru (4.0%), paraphenylendiamine (PPD) (3.7%), and thiomersal (3.5%). By testing ophthalmic allergens, contact hypersensitivity was observed in nine patients (6.7% of the tested 133 patients). The most common confirmed ophthalmic allergens were cocamidopropyl betaine, idoxuridine, phenylephrine hydrochloride, Na chromoglycinate, and papaine.

Limitations.—Patients with symptoms of PD were tested from 1996 to 2006.

Conclusions.—The occurence of contact hypersensitivity in PD patients was in present study 34.4%. A relatively high occurence was seen in cases of PD without other symptoms, in PD + OC and in PD + AD patients. The predominance of environmental contact allergens was remarkable: most frequent sensitizers were nickel sulphate, fragrance mix I, balsam of Peru, thiomersal, and PPD. The prevalence of contact hypersensitivity to ophthalmic allergens did not exceed 1.5%.

▶ Periocular contact dermatitis can easily simulate other skin conditions, leading to misdiagnosis. Periocular contact dermatitis can also occur with other concomitant skin diseases and can present as conjunctivitis, irritant eyelid dermatitis, and periorbital dermatitis caused by a variety of environmental allergens such as cosmetics, pigments, metals, and additives in creams. Elimination of the allergen can be challenging because many ophthalmic preparations, cosmetics, and cream formulations contain several ingredients. This is a study of 401 patients with periocular dermatitis (PD), who underwent patch testing with environmental and ophthalmic contact allergens. Contact hypersensitivity was confirmed in 34.4% of patients, with the highest frequency being those that had PD and atopic dermatitis (AD). Environmental allergens and ophthalmic contact allergens in patients with PD and ocular conjunctivitis were also identified. A high percentage (51.18%) of contact hypersensitivity was seen in cases of PD without other symptoms, which is interesting considering that one would expect to observe some reaction in other parts of the face or body in some cases, such as the hands, with handling the allergen. In this study, nickel sulphate, fragrance mix, balsam of Peru, paraphenylendiamine (PPD), and thiomersal were the most frequent sensitizers, which has also been noted in previous studies. This study helps the clinician with diagnosing PD by identifying other associated symptoms like ocular conjunctivitis, atopic dermatitis, and progressive systemic sclerosis. In addition, this study gives a thorough list of possible allergens responsible for PD, encouraging testing geared toward common environmental allergens and emphasizes the importance in uncovering other predisposing factors (ie, atopy, psoriasis, seborrhea, rosacea) that can occur with this disease.

G. K. Kim, DO
J. Q. Del Rosso, DO

Lymph Nodes in Hidradenitis Suppurativa

Wortsman X, Revuz J, Jemec GBE (Hosp del Profesor and Clínica Servet, Santiago de Chile; Henri Mondor Hosp, Paris, France; Univ of Copenhagen, Denmark)
Dermatology 219:22-24, 2009

Background.—Hidradenitis suppurativa (HS) is an inflammatory disease, and yet palpable lymph nodes are rarely found. This may be due to lack of lymph node swelling or to the inability to palpate lymph node regions due to overlying disease. Ultrasound was used to identify and measure regional lymph nodes in HS patients.

Methods.—High-resolution ultrasound scanning was carried out with compact linear 15–7 MHz and linear 12–5 MHz probes in both axillae and inguinal regions following informed consent.

Results.—A total of 198 lymph nodes were identified in 6 HS patients in Hurley stage II and 4 in stage III, and 101 from regional control scans in healthy controls. All the lymph nodes in both HS patients and controls showed a normal oval shape, with a hypoechoic rim and a hyperechoic center, and all were located in the deep subcutaneous tissue. The overall mean lymph node number per region was not significantly different. The overall mean lymph node diameter was not significantly different, but in patients with Hurley stage III disease it was significantly increased (1.3 ± 0.4 cm, p = 0.03).

Conclusion.—Lymph node involvement only occurs with late-stage HS and may therefore reflect secondary infection rather than primary etiological involvement.

▶ Hidradenitis suppurativa (HS) is an idiopathic disease characterized by inflammation with sinus tract formation in the groin and axillae, with prominent scarring as a common sequelae. Immunological response to bacterial infection has been associated with swelling of locoregional lymph nodes, and palpation of these regions is part of the clinical examination. However, palpable lymph nodes are rare in HS. This is a study of 10 patients with HS and 10 healthy control individuals that underwent high-resolution ultrasound scanning for evaluating lymph node size and diameter. A total of 198 lymph nodes were identified in patients with HS and 101 lymph nodes from controls. Of the patients with HS, 6 patients were rated as Hurley stage II and 4 patients were rated as Hurley stage III. Patients were not treated during the examination, and all were without active disease for at least 2 weeks before the study. All lymph nodes in both patients with HS and controls showed normal oval shape with a hypoechoic rim and hyperechoic center. There was no significant increase in the total number of lymph nodes and mean diameter in patients with HS of Hurley stage II. For advanced HS Hurley stage III, more lymph nodes were found that were not significant compared with controls ($P = .03$). Authors suggest that the increase in the number of lymph nodes might suggest a locoregional activation of the immune system that is not due to bacterial infection. However, examinations of lymph nodes were done while patients were without active disease. Future studies would benefit from comparing patients at base line and active disease with bacterial cultures to see if there is a correlation. This could answer the question of whether patients with advanced HS have a slightly increased number of lymph nodes due to the disease itself or due to an active infectious process. In addition, ultrasounds are nonspecific, in that the type of cells in the lymph nodes cannot be detected, and other underlying processes besides HS could cause hyperproliferation of lymph nodes.

G. K. Kim, DO

J. Q. Del Rosso, DO

Primary hyperhidrosis increases the risk of cutaneous infection: A case-control study of 387 patients

Walling HW (Univ of Iowa)
J Am Acad Dermatol 61:242-246, 2009

Background.—Although primary hyperhidrosis (PHH) has been frequently associated with diminished quality of life, the medical consequences of the condition are less well studied.

Objective.—The objective was to study the clinical presentation of PHH and to determine its relationship to cutaneous infection.

Methods.—A retrospective case-control study of patients encountered between 1993 and 2005 with the *International Classification of Diseases, Ninth Revision* diagnosis code for hyperhidrosis (HH) and meeting criteria for PHH was conducted.

Results.—Of 387 patients with PHH included, 59% were female and 41% were male; mean age was 27.3 years (range 2-72). Sites of HH included soles (50.1%), palms (45.2%), and axillae (43.4%). Distributional patterns of HH were isolated axillary (27.6%), palmoplantar (24.3%), isolated plantar (15%), axillary/palmoplantar (5.7%), isolated palmar (5.7%), and craniofacial (5.2%). Axillary HH was more common in female patients ($P = .004$). The mean age of onset (18.6 ± 12.3 years) indicated a mean duration of untreated symptoms of 8.9 years. Age at onset for palmoplantar HH (11.5 ± 8 years) was significantly younger than for axillary HH (20.0 ± 8.3 years; $P < .0001$), whereas onset of craniofacial HH (25.4 ± 13.7 years) was older ($P < .001$). Exacerbating factors included stress/emotion/anxiety (56.7%) and heat/humidity (22%). The overall risk of any cutaneous infection was significantly ($P < .0001$) increased in HH compared with controls (odds ratio [OR] 3.2; 95% confidence interval [CI] 2.2-4.6). Site-specific risks of fungal infection (OR 5.0; 95% CI 2.6-9.8; $P < .0001$), bacterial infection (OR 2.6; 95% CI 1.2-5.7; $P = .017$), and viral infection (OR 1.9; 95% CI 1.2-3.0; $P = .011$) were all increased. Risks of pitted keratolysis (OR 15.4; 95% CI 2.0-117; $P = .0003$), dermatophytosis (OR 9.8; 95% CI 3.4-27.8; $P < .0001$), and verruca plantaris/vulgaris (OR 2.1; 95% CI

1.3-3.6; $P = .0077$) were particularly increased. Association with atopic/eczematous dermatitis (OR 2.9; 95% CI 1.5-55; $P = .019$) was observed.

Limitations.—Retrospective design and single-institution study are limitations.

Conclusions.—Patients with HH are at high risk of secondary infection. Management of HH may have a secondary benefit of decreasing this risk.

▶ Hyperhidrosis (HH) is a condition characterized by sweating beyond what is needed for thermoregulatory demands and environmental conditions. HH can be primary from overactivity of sympathetic nervous system or secondary to a medical condition. This is a retrospective case-control study of patients encountered between 1993-2005 with 288 females and 159 males with an average age of 27.3 years of age evaluating the clinical presentation of primary hyperhidrosis (PHH) and determining its relationship to cutaneous infection. Sites of HH included soles (50.1%), palms (45.2%), and axillae (43.4%). Axillary HH was more common in female patients ($P = .004$). The age at onset of palmoplantar HH was significantly younger than for axillary HH ($P < .001$). In addition, the overall risk of any cutaneous infection was significantly increased ($P < .0001$), including bacterial, fungal, and viral compared with controls. The risks for infections were highest for pitted keratolysis, verruca vulgaris/plantaris, and dermatophytosis. Controlling hyperhidrosis may have a secondary benefit by decreasing the risk of infection. The sites that were most affected were those with the highest densities of eccrine glands, including palmoplantar, craniofacial, and axillary skin. A limitation to this study was that it was a retrospective study done at a single institution. Also, females in this study sought care for HH more commonly than male patients at about a 3:2 ratio. Although there are mounting data with HH and quality of life issues, there are relatively few data regarding the clinical presentation of PHH and association with other dermatologic diseases. In conclusion, demographic features of PHH in this study were comparable with those of population-based surveys conducted with US residents.

G. K. Kim, DO
J. Q. Del Rosso, DO

Clinical characteristics of a series of 302 French patients with hidradenitis suppurativa, with an analysis of factors associated with disease severity
Canoui-Poitrine F, Revuz JE, Wolkenstein P, et al (Université Paris, Créteil, France, Service de dermatologie, Créteil, France; et al)
J Am Acad Dermatol 61:51-57, 2009

Background.—Factors associated with the severity of hidradenitis suppurativa (HS) are not known.

Objective.—We sought to identify factors associated with the severity of HS.

Methodology.—The severity of disease in a series of 302 consecutive patients with HS was assessed using the Sartorius score.

Results.—Atypical locations were more common in men than in women (47.1% vs 14.8%; $P < .001$). Men also had more severe disease (median Sartorius score: 20.5 vs 16.5; $P = .02$). Increased body mass index ($P < .001$), atypical locations ($P = .002$), a personal history of severe acne ($P = .04$), and absence of a family history of HS ($P = .06$) were associated with an increased Sartorius score. The Sartorius score was highly correlated with the intensity and duration of pain and suppuration (all P values $< .001$).

Limitations.—The referral center base of the study may have biased recruitment.

Conclusion.—Our data showed a significant association between the severity of HS and several clinical and behavioral factors. Prospective studies are needed to confirm the prognostic role of these factors.

▶ Hidradenitis suppurativa (HS) is characterized by relapses and chronicity that has been known to adversely affect the quality of patients' lives. The aim of this study was to describe the clinical characteristics and severity of 302 French patients and to identify clinical differences between genders, prevalence of obesity, associated follicular diseases, and atypical locations. The anatomic zones of HS were recorded and classified as either typical locations (axilla, breast, inguinofemoral, perianal, and perineal) or atypical locations (ears, chest, abdomen, and legs). Disease severity was assessed by using the Sartorius severity score, which correlated with intensity, duration of pain, and suppuration. Atypical lesions (41.7% vs 14.8%), severity of disease (median Sartorius score 20.5 vs 16.5), increased body mass index (BMI), and personal history of acne were more common in men compared with women in this study. Women also had more frontal involvement (groin and breast), whereas the involvement of the back (buttocks and perineal) was seen more exclusively in men. There was also a strong association with BMI and severity of HS with 1 U of BMI associated with an increase in 0.84 U in the mean Sartorius score. Limitations to this study were that the Sartorius score is not formally validated for assessing HS severity, but in this study it was positively associated with the Hurley classification. The study also revealed that there may be benefits to future interventional studies in order to assess the value of weight loss in correlation to severity of HS and recognizes that an exclusively surgical approach may not be justified in every case.

G. K. Kim, DO

J. Q. Del Rosso, DO

8 Photobiology

A Controlled Trial of Objective Measures of Sunscreen and Moisturizing Lotion
Elliott T, Nehl EJ, Glanz K (Emory Univ, Atlanta, GA)
Cancer Epidemiol Biomarkers Prev 18:1399-1402, 2009

Taking an alcohol swab of a person's forearm and analyzing it using a spectrophotometer has been shown to be a reliable method for detecting the presence of sunscreen. The aims of this study were to determine if moisturizing lotions or other non-sunscreen products influence the absorbance readings from skin swabs in a controlled setting, and to establish the cutoff point in determining the presence or absence of sunscreen using a crystal cuvette instead of a plastic one. In a controlled trial of 30 volunteer office workers, absorbance readings from two popular brands of sunscreen with sun-protection factors (SPF) of 30 and 45 were compared with absorbance readings from two different moisturizing lotions, one with an SPF of 15 and another with no stated SPF. Moisturizers with SPF 15 tested positive for sunscreen, with absorbance readings (mean, 3.77; min, 3.30) comparable to sunblock with SPF 30 or 45 (mean, 3.51; min, 2.02). Moisturizers with no stated SPF factor tested negative for the presence of sunscreen, with extremely low absorbance readings (mean, 0.06; max, 0.19) similar to control readings. The skin swabbing technique remains a valid and useful method for detecting the presence of sunscreen and does not result in false positives when moisturizers with no stated SPF are present. Using a conservative cutoff point of 0.30 with a crystal cuvette reduces any chance of false-positive readings and remains robust when sunscreen of SPF 15 or higher is present.

▶ Spectrophotometry has been known to be a reliable method for detecting the presence of sunscreen and ultraviolet absorption (UVA). The aim of this study was to determine whether moisturizing lotions or other nonsunscreen products might influence the absorbance readings and to establish the cutoff point in determining the presence or absence of sunscreen. This was a controlled trial of 30 patients using 2 popular brands of sunscreen with sun protection factor (SPF) of 30 and 45 in comparison with moisturizers with SPF 15 and another with no stated SPF. Reports in the past have suggested that people do not apply enough sunscreen to meet the recommended dose of 2 mg/cm^2. Moisturizers with SPF 15 tested positive for sunscreen comparable with SPF 30 or 45, and moisturizers with no SPF tested negative for the presence of sunscreen similar to controls. The authors found that skin swabbing is a useful method for detection of sunscreen and does not appear to result in false positive results. Limitations include the lack of specific testing for residual sunscreen from previous applications. It is still unclear whether very low SPF or residual sunscreen from previous applications may affect absorbance readings. The technique limitations are inability neither to detect sunscreens containing exclusively inorganic ingredients, nor to measure features related to the quality of sunscreen (eg, UVA coverage and waterproof ability) or adequacy of application. In conclusion, this technique may be useful in evaluating behavioral interventions geared toward increase use of sunscreen in patients.

G. K. Kim, DO

J. Q. Del Rosso, DO

Ultraviolet A within Sunlight Induces Mutations in the Epidermal Basal Layer of Engineered Human Skin
Huang XX, Bernerd F, Halliday GM (The Univ of Sydney, New South Wales, Australia; L'Oreal Life Sciences Res, Clichy, France)
Am J Pathol 174:1534-1543, 2009

The ultraviolet B (UVB) waveband within sunlight is an important carcinogen; however, UVA is also likely to be involved. By ascribing mutations to being either UVB or UVA induced, we have previously shown that human skin cancers contain similar numbers of UVB- and UVA-induced mutations, and, importantly, the UVA mutations were at the base of the epidermis of the tumors. To determine whether these mutations occurred in response to UV, we exposed engineered human skin (EHS) to UVA, UVB, or a mixture that resembled sunlight, and then detected mutations by both denaturing high-performance liquid chromatography and DNA sequencing. EHS resembles human skin, modeling differential waveband penetration to the basal, dividing keratinocytes. We administered only four low doses of UV exposure. Both UVA and UVB induced p53 mutations in irradiated EHS, suggesting that sunlight doses that are achievable during normal daily activities are mutagenic. UVA- but not UVB-induced mutations predominated in the basal epidermis that contains dividing keratinocytes and are thought to give rise to skin tumors. These studies indicate that both UVA and UVB at physiological doses are mutagenic to keratinocytes in EHS.

▶ The carcinogenic potential of ultraviolet A (UVA) irradiation is now well recognized, which has contributed to the waning popularity of cosmetic tanning lamps using UVA. This study used a model of human skin consisting of normal human fibroblasts cultured in a collagen matrix and seeded with keratinocytes. As shown in Fig 2, this model morphologically resembles human skin with readily identifiable cell layers. Exposure of the skin model to UVA, UVB, and solar simulated UV (ssUV) irradiation at doses equivalent

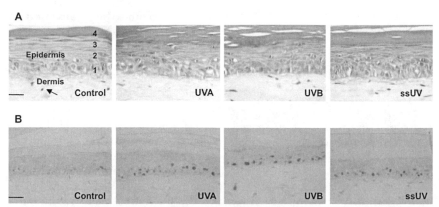

FIGURE 2.—UV radiation does not induce detectable morphological changes in EHS (**A**). Fibroblasts (**arrow**) encased in a type I collagen lattice provides dermal support for the epidermis. EHS collected on day 11, 3 days after the final of four UV exposures, were fixed and H&E-stained. Distinct basal (**1**), spinous (**2**), granular (**3**), and cornified (**4**) layers are recognizable in un-irradiated control, 12.5 J/cm^2 UVA-, 0.1 J/cm^2 UVB-, and 1.4 J/cm^2 ssUV-irradiated EHS. Sections from the same groups of EHS were immunostained for p53 protein (**B**). Anti-CPD immunostaining in adult human skin collected 24 hours after UV irradiation. (Courtesy of Huang XX, Bernerd F, Halliday GM. Ultraviolet A within sunlight induces mutations in the epidermal basal layer of engineered human skin. *Am J Pathol.* 2009;174:1534-1543.)

to those experienced during routine daily activities, all resulted in clearly demonstrable expression of the tumor suppressor p53. It is noteworthy that p53 expression was detected particularly in basal layer cells (Fig 2B), which would be more susceptible to the effects of the longer UVA wavelengths. Furthermore, p53 mutations were detected in 15 of 24 irradiated samples, with similar frequency of occurrence in the UVA, UVB, and ssUV groups. These mutations tended to occur more often in the basal layer of cells in models exposed to UVA, although the numbers were too small to be analyzed for significance. The investigators were also interested in determining whether the different UV wavelengths would promote different types of mutations: the results showed that the most frequently observed mutations in UVA, but not UVB-treated samples involved a A:T > C:G transversion. In addition, approximately 70% of UVA and ssUv-induced mutations were missense, as opposed to only 30% of those induced by UVB. Again, the statistical significance of these findings cannot be determined, but their clinical implications are indisputable.

G. M. P. Galbraith, MD

Photodynamic Therapy With Methyl Aminolevulinate for Prevention of New Skin Lesions in Transplant Recipients: A Randomized Study

Wennberg A-M, Stenquist B, Stockfleth E, et al (Sahlgrenska Univ Hosp, Gothenburg, Sweden; Charité, Univ Hosp Berlin, Germany; et al)
Transplantation 86:423-429, 2008

Background.—Organ transplant recipients on long-term immunosuppressive therapy are at increased risk of non-melanoma skin lesions. Repeated field photodynamic therapy using topical methyl aminolevulinate (MAL) may have potential as a preventive treatment.

Methods.—This open randomized, intrapatient, comparative, multicenter study included 81 transplant recipients with 889 lesions (90% actinic keratoses (AK)]. In each patient, the study treatment was initially administered to one 50 cm area on the face, scalp, neck, trunk, or extremities (n = 476 lesions) twice (1 week apart), with additional single treatments at 3, 9, and 15 months. On each occasion, the area was debrided gently and MAL cream (160 mg/g) applied for 3 hr, before illumination with noncoherent red light (630 nm, 37 J/cm^2). The control, 50 cm^2 area (n = 413 lesions) received lesion-specific treatment (83% cryotherapy) at baseline and 3, 9, and 15 months. Additionally, all visible lesions were given lesion-specific treatment 21 and 27 months in both treatment and control areas.

Results.—At 3 months, MAL photodynamic therapy significantly reduced the occurrence of new lesions (65 vs. 103 lesions in the control area; $P = 0.01$), mainly AK (46% reduction; 43 vs. 80; $P = 0.006$). This effect was not significant at 27 months (253 vs. 312; $P = 0.06$). Hypopigmentation, as assessed by the investigator, was less evident in the treatment than control areas (16% vs. 51% of patients; $P < 0.001$) at 27 months.

Conclusion.—Our results suggest that repeated field photodynamic therapy using topical MAL may prevent new AK in transplant recipients although further studies are needed.

▶ Patients who are on long-term immunosuppressive therapy are at increased risk for developing nonmelanoma skin cancer (NMSC) and precancerous lesions, such as actinic keratosis (AK). Photodynamic therapy using the topical photosensitizer methyl aminolevulinate (MAL-PDT) is reported to be convenient, effective, and a well-tolerated treatment for NMSC. This is an open, randomized, intrapatient multicenter study conducted in 11 outpatient hospital centers in Europe with organ transplant recipients on immunosuppressive therapy for more than 3 years. The aim of this study was to use MAL-PDT as a preventive treatment for new lesions in immunocompromised organ transplant recipients, based on previous clinical evidence. After 3 months there were significantly fewer new lesions in the treatment areas compared with the control areas, with reduction in new AK lesions. Patients who had undergone organ transplantation within 10 years tended to have a better response to MAL-PDT and experienced favorable cosmetic outcomes overall with minimal changes in pigmentation. Adverse events associated with MAL-PDT were erythema, modest pain, and crusting in 75% of patients. Initial effects were seen at 3 months, mainly with a decrease in new AK lesions, particularly in patients who had undergone organ transplantation within 10 years, although this difference was no longer significant at 27 months. In this study, 62% of treated areas remained free from new lesions 12 months later. In contrast, treatment with PDT using blue light and topical aminolevulinic acid showed no preventive effect on the occurrence of new squamous cell carcinoma lesions. Findings suggested that photodynamic therapy is generally very well tolerated by patients that are immunosuppressed. It also offers a more favorable cosmetic outcome and causes less scarring and tissue destruction than cryosurgery (for AK) and surgery (for NMSC), and can be used as a preventative measure for AK lesions.

G. K. Kim, DO

J. Q. Del Rosso, DO

Epidermal Langerhans cells in actinic prurigo: a comparison between lesional and non-lesional skin

Calderón-Amador J, Flores-Langarica A, Silva-Sánchez A, et al (Dept of Cell Biology CINVESTAV-IPN, Mexico city; Dept of Immunology ENCB-IPN, Mexico)
J Eur Acad Dermatol Venereol 23:438-440, 2009

Background.—Actinic Prurigo (AP) is a chronic pruritic dermatosis of unknown cause affecting sun exposed skin in defined ethnic groups with characteristic MHC alleles. However, the cutaneous dendritic cells have not been assessed.

Objective.—To assess in situ the epidermal Langerhans Cell (LC) status in Actinic Prurigo.

Study Design.—Fresh skin samples from three AP patients were used to evaluate in situ the epidermal LC, comparing lesional and non-lesional sites in each subject.

Setting.—AP patients attending the Dermatology Department at the Hospital M. Gea-Gonzalez in Mexico city.

Methods.—Lesional and non-lesional skin samples were taken from each subject to prepare both epidermal sheets and conventional tissue sections. Three markers restricted to LC in epidermis (CD1a, ATPase, MHC-II) were used to quantify the LC per area in epidermal sheets.

Results.—Compared to non-lesional skin from the same subject, a significant reduction in the number of LC per area of epidermis was found in lesional skin; with any of the three markers evaluated.

Conclusion.—The frequency of epidermal LC decreases importantly in lesional skin from AP patients.

▶ The authors describe a small, preliminary study of 3 patients with actinic prurigo. Their finding of decreased numbers of Langerhans cells in lesional epidermis of these patients prompted them to suggest several scenarios, including mobilization and migration of these cells in response to cytokines such as interleukin (IL)-10, or local induction of apoptosis. Further studies are apparently in progress.

G. M. P. Galbraith, MD

Intense Pulsed Light Effects on the Expression of Extracellular Matrix Proteins and Transforming Growth Factor Beta-1 in Skin Dermal Fibroblasts Cultured within Contracted Collagen Lattices

Wong W-R, Shyu W-L, Tsai J-W, et al (Graduate Inst of Clinical Med Sciences; Chang Gung Memorial Hosp, Taipei, Taiwan; et al)
Dermatol Surg 35:816-825, 2009

Background.—Emerging clinical evidence suggests that intense pulsed light (IPL) treatment may exert some beneficial effects on photoaged skin. The molecular mechanisms underlying this IPL effect have not been fully elucidated.

Objective.—To examine the effects of IPL irradiation on normal human dermal fibroblasts grown in contracted collagen lattices.

Methods.—Human skin fibroblasts cultured in contracted collagen lattices were irradiated with IPL with triple pulses of 7 ms with a pulse interval of 70 ms and fluences of 20, 50, and 75 J/cm^2. Twenty-four hours after the irradiation, cell viability, messenger RNA (mRNA), and protein levels of extracellular matrix proteins (e.g., collagen I, collagen III, and fibronectin) and transforming growth factor beta-1 (TGF-b1) were evaluated using dye exclusion, real-time reverse transcriptase polymerase chain reaction, and enzyme-linked immunosorbent assay, respectively.

Results.—A dose-dependent increase in viable cells was demonstrated after the IPL irradiation. There was no significant change in mRNA levels of collagen I and fibronectin. Upregulated expression of collagen III and TGF-β1 in dermal fibroblasts was verified.

Conclusions.—The analytical results presented here provide a potential mechanistic explanation for the mechanism of clinical photorejuvenation effects of IPL that involves the increase of extracellular matrix construction by upregulating the gene expressions of collagen III and TGF-β1.

▶ Intense pulsed light (IPL) therapy uses polychromatic light at wavelengths (greater than 515 nm) that target the dermis with relative sparing of the epidermis. It has been shown to be moderately effective in treatment of several skin conditions, including photodamage and disorders of pigmentation. Despite its popularity, the mechanism underlying its apparent efficacy remains unknown, but it is generally thought to involve a healing response to photothermal injury. Wong et al used an interesting in vitro model to examine the behavior of human dermal fibroblasts in response to an IPL challenge, which approximated what was used clinically. Essentially, this was a continuation of their previously published study of the same model.[1] The major findings in the current investigation were increased expression of collagen III and transforming growth factor beta-1 (TGF-β1) in pooled normal human fibro-blasts exposed to IPL. Although these initial data are interesting and can be placed quite neatly into a molecular model of cellular response to IPL, it may be premature to extrapolate these results, obtained in a system consisting of fibroblasts, collagen and medium, to the in situ complexities of the skin, and the interactions of its many components. It would also be of interest to deter-mine if IPL induced a temperature change in the model, similar to that observed both clinically and in animal studies, because thermal injury is considered to be integral to the therapeutic activity of IPL.

G. M. P. Galbraith, MD

Reference

1. Wong WR, Shyu WL, Tsai JW, Hsu KH, Lee HY, Pang JH. Intense pulsed light modulates the expressions of MMP-2, MMP-14 and TIMP-2 in skin dermal fibro-blasts cultured within contracted collagen lattice. *J Dermatol Sci.* 2008;51:70-73.

9 Collagen Vascular and Related Disorders

Lupus Erythematosus Tumidus: Response to Antimalarial Treatment in 36 Patients With Emphasis on Smoking
Kreuter A, Gaifullina R, Tigges C, et al (Ruhr Univ Bochum, Germany)
Arch Dermatol 145:244-248, 2009

Objective.—To determine the efficacy of antimalarial drug use in patients with lupus erythematosus tumidus.

Design.—Retrospective single-center study.

Setting.—Dermatologic clinic at a university hospital.

Patients.—Thirty-six patients with multifocal lupus erythematosus tumidus.

Intervention.—Treatment with either chloroquine phosphate or hydroxy chloroquine sulfate.

Main Outcome Measures.—Cutaneous Lupus Erythematosus Disease Area and Severity Index score.

Results.—Treatment with antimalarial drugs resulted in a significant reduction in the Cutaneous Lupus Erythematosus Disease Area and Severity Index score, from 4 (range, 2-8) at baseline to 1 (range, 0-6) after 3 months of therapy ($P < .001$). Twenty-two patients (61%) exhibited complete or almost complete clearance of skin lesions, consistent with a clinical score of 0 or 1. No difference in efficacy was noted between the chloroquine-treated group and the hydroxy chloroquine-treated group ($P = .40$). Adverse effects (nausea, dizziness, and headache) occurred only in patients treated with chloroquine. Twenty- eight patients (78%) were smokers, and smokers had a significantly higher mean (SD) clinical score than nonsmokers (5.1 [1.8] vs 3.3 [1.6]; $P = .03$). Moreover, smokers had a significantly lower reduction in clinical score with antimalarial treatment compared with nonsmokers ($r = 0.30$; $P = .03$; 95% confidence interval, -0.05 to 0.57). Eighty-eight percent of nonsmokers (7 of 8 patients) but only 57% of smokers (16 of 28 patients) had a clinical score of 1 or 0 after 3 months of treatment with antimalarial drugs.

Conclusions.—These retrospective study findings demonstrate that antimalarial treatment is highly effective in multifocal lupus erythematosus tumidus. Lower incidence of adverse effects and equal efficacy might favor the use of hydroxychloroquine. Patients who smoke should be encouraged to join smoking cessation programs because they will respond better to antimalarial treatment.

▶ Lupus erythematosus tumidus (LET) is a subset of cutaneous lupus erythematosus (CLE) that presents with annular urticaria-like papules and plaques in sun-exposed areas of the body, with histopathologic characteristics that are distinct. Because of limited information on LET, treatment guidelines are based on CLE with antimalarial drugs recommended as first-line treatment. In the past, there has been evidence suggesting that cigarette smoking interferes with the efficacy of antimalarial drugs in CLE. This is a retrospective study of 36 patients with multifocal LET skin lesions treated with antimalarial drugs, particularly hydroxychloroquine and chloroquine and the effects of smoking on LET patients. Kreuter et al found that hydroxychloroquine and chloroquine were both equally efficacious with LET skin lesions with 83% of patients achieving complete clearance of skin lesions within a treatment period of at least 6 months. Patients reported fewer side effects with hydroxychloroquine when compared with chloroquine. Additional findings suggest that LET nonsmokers compared with smokers have a higher response to antimalarials with lower CLE disease area and severity index scores (CLASI). Limitations of this study included imprecise documentation of patient smoking behavior with some smokers that reduced their smoking to a maximum of 5 cigarettes with clearance of lesions similar to nonsmokers. In future studies, it would be interesting to compare urinary cotinine levels, which is a major metabolite of nicotine, for a more accurate measure of smoking and medication response with antimalarials in LET. This study reiterates the efficacy of antimalarials in LET patients and emphasizes the benefits of smoking cessation for LET patients when using this class of medications.

G. K. Kim, DO

J. Q. Del Rosso, DO

Histopathologic characteristics of neonatal cutaneous lupus erythematosus: description of five cases and literature review
Peñate Y, Guillermo N, Rodríguez J, et al (Hosp Universitario Insular de Gran Canaria, Spain)
J Cutan Pathol 36:660-667, 2009

Background.—Neonatal lupus erythematosus (NLE) is a disease associated with the transplacental transfer of maternal anti-Ro/SSA. The histopathologic characteristics of neonatal lupus have been described as compatible with cutaneous lupus based on isolated cases.

Methods.—We retrospectively review the available literature and compare them with findings obtained in seven biopsies of five cases.

Results.—Erythematous-desquamative lesions and urticaria-like lesions were observed in our series. Two cases showed both types of lesions. Vacuolar alterations at the dermoepidermal interface and adnexal structures were the histopathologic findings on erythematous-desquamative lesions, and a superficial and deep perivascular and periadnexal lymphocytic infiltrate was the major pattern in urticaria-like lesions. One case showed prevalence of eosinophils in the inflammatory infiltrate. Sixty cases have been reported previously. Sixty-five percent presented erythematous-desquamative and 29% urticaria-like lesions. Pathologic findings of erythematous-desquamative lesions were similar to those found in our series, but epidermal vacuolar changes were the predominant histopathologic finding in urticaria-like lesions of cases reported in the literature.

Conclusions.—The majority of cases of NLE show vacuolar alteration at the dermoepidermal interface and adnexal structures. Some cases exhibit a superficial and deep perivascular and periadnexal lymphocytic infiltrate without epidermal alteration, and rare cases may have eosinophils in the infiltrate.

▶ Neonatal lupus erythematosus (NLE) is a disease due to the transplacental transfer of maternal antibodies to the fetus. The consequences of this disease can often be devastating to both the mother and the infant. Adverse sequelae of NLE include atrioventricular block, thrombocytopenia, hepatic dysfunction, pneumonitis, and cutaneous lesions. This is a retrospective review of literature with histological comparison in 5 cases of NLE. Diagnosis was based on identification of autoantibodies in the mother and newborn with clinical and serological correlation. The authors also evaluated for histological features of subacute cutaneous lupus erythematosus (SCLE) and direct immunofluorescence (DIF) testing. Cutaneous morphologic features, biopsies, presence of antinuclear antibodies ([ANA], antiDNA, antiRo, antiLA, antiU1RNP), complement levels, and echocardiogram results were also noted. Physical examination revealed annular erythematous lesions up to 1 cm in diameter, with atrophic centers and scaling borders resolving in 3 months. Skin lesions of NLE were described as similar to those observed in SCLE. There were 2 types of lesions in these patients: erythematous desquamative lesions and urticarial type lesions. In the urticarial-type lesions, biopsies revealed superficial and deep perivascular infiltrate along with interstitial lymphocytic infiltration. Biopsies obtained from erythematous scaling annular lesions revealed epidermal damage with vacuolar alterations of the basement membrane situated at the dermoepidermal junction and at adnexal structures. Other findings such as necrotic keratinocytes and perivascular or periadnexal inflammatory infiltrates were also noted, and dermal mucin deposition was observed with colloidal iron staining. Antibodies were also negative 6 months after examination. Literature review revealed 65% of cases were typically erythematous-desquamative lesions with atrophy followed by the urticarial-type of lesions in 29% of cases. To add, interface changes at the dermoepidermal junction were the most frequently reported histopathologic finding in urticarial-type lesions. Of the 60 reviewed cases in the literature, 41 included immunofluorescence studies. Positive immunofluorescence was found in less than 50% of all reviewed cases, and positive IgM results in the basal layer was observed in 33% of all cases reviewed. In this study, all 5 cases had negative immunofluorescence possibly due to low sensitivity of the antibodies used, short-time duration of dermal IgG deposition, or rapid clearance of antibodies. The reasons for this phenomenon are unknown. Other limitations included a single institution site and the small study and sample size. The researchers concluded that lymphocytes with plasma cells were the main infiltrate in NLE patients rather than lymphohistiocytic. In conclusion, the cases of NLE in this study revealed histological features of classic lupus erythematosus, including vacuolar alteration of the epidermis and adnexal structures with some superficial and deep perivascular and periadnexal lymphocytic infiltrate.

G. K. Kim, DO
J. Q. Del Rosso, DO

Clinical significance of nailfold capillaroscopy in systemic lupus erythematosus: correlation with endothelial cell activation markers and disease activity
Kuryliszyn-Moskal A, Ciolkiewicz M, Klimiuk PA, et al (Med Univ of Bialystok, Poland)
Scand J Rheumatol 38:38-45, 2009

Objective.—To evaluate whether nailfold capillaroscopy (NC) changes are associated with the main serum endothelial cell activation markers and the disease activity of systemic lupus erythematosus (SLE).

Methods.—Serum levels of vascular endothelial growth factor (VEGF), endothelin-1 (ET-1), soluble E-selectin (sE-selectin), and soluble thrombomodulin (sTM) were determined by an enzyme-linked immunosorbent assay (ELISA) in 80 SLE patients and 33 healthy controls.

Results.—Nailfold capillary abnormalities were seen in 74 out of 80 (92.5%) SLE patients. A normal capillaroscopic pattern or mild changes were found in 33 (41.25%) and moderate/severe abnormalities in 47 (58.75%) of all SLE patients. In SLE patients a capillaroscopic score > 1 was more frequently associated with the presence of internal organ involvement $(p < 0.001)$ as well as with immunosuppressive therapy $(p < 0.01)$. Significant differences were found in VEGF $(p < 0.001)$, ET-1 $(p < 0.001)$, sE-selectin $(p < 0.01)$, and sTM $(p < 0.001)$ serum concentrations between SLE patients with a capillaroscopic score >1 and controls. SLE patients with severe/moderate capillaroscopic abnormalities showed significantly higher VEGF serum levels than patients with mild changes $(p < 0.001)$. Moreover, there was a significant positive correlation between the severity of capillaroscopic changes and the Systemic Lupus Erythematosus Disease Activity Index (SLEDAI) $(p < 0.005)$ as well as between capillaroscopic score and VEGF serum levels $(p < 0.001)$.

Conclusions.—Our findings confirm the usefulness of NC as a noninvasive technique for the evaluation of microvascular involvement in SLE patients. A relationship between changes in NC, endothelial cell activation markers and clinical features of SLE suggest an important role for microvascular abnormalities in clinical manifestation of the disease.

▶ The main objectives of this article are to reconfirm the long held concept that changes in nail fold capillaries are a marker for the diagnosis, extent, and severity of the disease process, and particularly to vascular endothelial growth factor levels. The investigators have conclusively achieved their objectives and further applied this new quantitative paradigm so that it can be useful in the clinical setting. The methods are consistent and reproducible and have the potential to predict prognosis, evaluate the stage of the disease, and thereby adjust treatment accordingly. The authors re-emphasize the importance to the practicing clinician of nail fold capillary examination and that it should be performed by them with more regularity, one of the articles strong messages. They did not mention, however, the reliable and relevant ancillary technique of proximal nail fold biopsy in which periodic acid-Schiff (PAS) staining and direct immunofluorescence often clarify a questionable diagnosis.[1,2] This article will hopefully encourage more dermatologists to include nail fold examination as part of their evaluation of possible connective tissue disorders to a degree approached by rheumatologists. Such a simple diagnostic tool is of special value in assessing those patients presenting with Raynaud's phenomenon only as a physical finding.

R. K. Scher, MD

References

1. Minkin W, Rabhan NB. Nail fold capillary microscopy. *J Amer Acad Dermatol.* 1982;7:190-193.
2. Scher RK, Tom DW, Lally EV, et al. PAS positive deposits in nail fold biopsy. *Arch Dermatol.* 1985;121:1406-1409.

Localized scleroderma: A series of 52 patients
Toledano C, Rabhi S, Kettaneh A, et al (France Université Pierre et Marie Curie-Paris)
Eur J Intern Med 20:331-336, 2009

Background.—Localized scleroderma also called morphea is a skin disorder of undetermined cause. The widely recognized Mayo Clinic Classification identifies 5 main morphea types: plaque, generalized, bullous, linear and deep. Whether each of these distinct types has a particular clinical course or is associated with some patient-related features is still unclear.

Methods.—We report here a retrospective series of patients with localized scleroderma with an attempt to identify features related to the type of lesion involved. The medical records of all patients with a diagnosis of localized scleroderma were reviewed by skilled practitioners. Lesions were classified according to the Mayo Clinic Classification. The relationship between each lesion type and various clinical features was tested by nonparametrical methods.

Results.—The sample of 52 patients included 43 females and 9 males. Median age at onset was 30 y (range 1–76). Frequencies of patients according to morphea types were: plaque morphea 41 (78.8%) (including morphea en plaque 30 (57.7%) and atrophoderma of Pasini–Pierini 11 (21.1%)), linear scleroderma 14 (26.9%). Nine patients (17.3%) had both types of localized scleroderma. Median age at onset was lower in patients with linear scleroderma (8 y (range 3–44)) than in others (36 y (range 1–77)) (p = 0.0003). Head involvement was more common in patients with linear scleroderma (37.5%) than in other subtypes (11.1%) (p = 0.05). Atrophoderma of Pasini–Pierini was never located at the head. Systemic symptoms, antinuclear antibodies and the rheumatic factor were not associated with localized scleroderma types or subtypes.

Conclusion.—These results suggest that morphea types, in adults are not associated with distinct patient features except for age at disease onset (lower) and the localization on the head (more frequent), in patients with lesions of the linear type.

▶ Linear scleroderma is rare. The goal of this evaluation was to look at the patients with scleroderma and report the clinical features and identify additional characteristics. The authors reviewed cases over an 11-year period and classified the features, defining 3 major subtypes: plaque, linear, and deep morphea. The trunk (61.5%) and upper limbs (36.5%) were the most common locations observed. Median age of onset was lower in linear and deep morphea than plaque subtype. The article was well written, and the discussion and description was thorough.

S. Bhambri, DO

J. Q. Del Rosso, DO

Effectiveness, side-effects and period of remission after treatment with methotrexate in localized scleroderma and related sclerotic skin diseases: an inception cohort study
Kroft EBM, Creemers MCW, van den Hoogen FHJ, et al (Radboud Univ Med Centre Nijmegen, St Radboud, The Netherlands; Sint Maartens Kliniek Nijmegen, The Netherlands)
Br J Dermatol 160:1075-1082, 2009

Background.—Detailed information is lacking on effectiveness of methotrexate (MTX) in sclerotic skin diseases, side-effects, and duration of remission after discontinuation.

Objectives.—To determine effectiveness, side-effects and period of remission gained by use of MTX in sclerotic skin diseases.

Methods.—All patients with a sclerotic skin disease who were treated with MTX (group A) or MTX with corticosteroids (CS) (group B) between

1995 and 2007 were evaluated. Detailed information was collected on dosage and duration of MTX treatment, concomitant immunosuppressive medication and CS treatment, effectiveness, side-effects, duration of the remission period, and time until restart.

Results.—Fifty-eight patients (A, $n = 47$; B, $n = 11$) were evaluated. Clinical assessment revealed that 38 patients (81%) treated with MTX and 11 patients (100%) treated with MTX + CS showed improvement of sclerotic skin. After one treatment course 51% of the patients treated with MTX and 73% treated with MTX + CS reached remission status with a median follow-up time of 55 and 58 months. Patients showing relapse still responded to a second and even to a third course of MTX. Patients who showed a relapse had received a lower cumulative dose, due to a shorter period of treatment with MTX in the first course. Serious side-effects were seen in six patients (10%).

Conclusions.—MTX was an effective treatment for various sclerotic skin diseases with a long period of remission and relatively low toxicity. Patients showing relapse still responded to a second and third course of MTX.

▶ The objective of this cohort study was to determine the effectiveness, side effects, and period of remission for treatment of sclerotic skin diseases (excluding systemic sclerosis) with methotrexate (MTX). The article does achieve its objectives however, although it is stated as a large cohort study, calling a sample of 47 patients large may be somewhat misleading. Nevertheless, sclerotic skin disorders are relatively uncommon so this report does provide an important addition to the literature. This study effectively selected patients in whom response to treatment would be difficult. Patients included in this study were those who had extensive and/or progressive sclerotic skin diseases, active disease, or sclerotic skin disease that could lead to loss of mobility.

In group A, patients were treated with MTX only, and in group B, patients were treated with a combination of MTX and oral corticosteroids. In the discussion, this article does state that one of the limitations was that patients in these 2 groups were not randomly assigned and the groups were not identical based on disease duration and disease severity. An example of this is that all patients with eosinophilic fasciitis were assigned to group B. The number of patients differed significantly between the 2 groups, which wasn't mentioned as a limitation by the authors. Also, there was no difference in the weekly median dose of MTX between group A and group B, but patients in group B received a significantly higher median cumulative dose of MTX than group A due to longer period of treatment. Therefore, comparing the results for effectiveness and side effects between both groups does not provide a fully accurate representation if one treatment strategy is reported to be superior to the other. Nevertheless, this article does support MTX as an effective treatment for sclerotic skin diseases.

S. B. Momin, DO
J. Q. Del Rosso, DO

Efficacy and safety of pulsed dye laser treatment for cutaneous discoid lupus erythematosus

Erceg A, Bovenschen HJ, van de Kerkhof PCM, et al (Radboud Univ Nijmegen Med Ctr, Netherlands)
J Am Acad Dermatol 60:626-632, 2009

Background.—Treatment of chronic discoid lupus erythematosus (CDLE) with a pulsed dye laser (PDL) has shown promising results, although outcomes in previous studies were not validated and laser parameters were inconsistent.

Objective.—We conducted an open prospective study to assess the efficacy and safety of PDL for the treatment of recalcitrant CDLE, using a validated scoring method and a fixed treatment schedule.

Methods.—Twelve patients with active CDLE lesions were treated with PDL (585 nm, fluence 5.5 J/cm^2, spot size 7 mm) 3 times with an interval of 6 weeks followed by a 6-week follow-up period. Treatment outcomes were evaluated by 3 observers using the validated Cutaneous Lupus Erythematosus Disease Area and Severity Index (CLASI). Cosmetic results and adverse events were recorded.

Results.—A significant decline in "active" CLASI was observed after 6 weeks, after 12 weeks, and at follow-up. Baseline active CLASI was 4.4 ± 0.2 (mean ± SEM), reaching 1.3 ± 0.3 after follow-up ($P < .0001$). Individual scores for erythema and scaling/hypertrophy significantly declined 6 weeks after treatment. The "damage" CLASI (dyspigmentation, scarring, and atrophy) did not show any significant change during or after therapy. The observed clinical improvement was confirmed

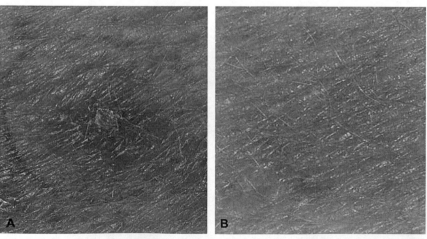

FIGURE 2.—Chronic discoid lupus erythematosus lesion of patient before (A) and after (B) pulsed dye laser treatment, showing slight hyperpigmentation. (Reprinted from Erceg A, Bovenschen HJ, van de Kerkhof PCM, et al. Efficacy and safety of pulsed dye laser treatment for cutaneous discoid lupus erythematosus. *J Am Acad Dermatol.* 2009;60:626-632, with permission from the American Academy of Dermatology.)

by two independent observers by clinical assessment of photographs ($r = 0.87$ and $r = 0.89$; both $P < .05$). The treatment was well tolerated, only minimal pain was reported, and the cosmetic result was fair.

Limitations.—Small sample size and short follow-up duration were limitations.

Conclusion.—PDL treatment is an effective and safe therapy for patients with refractory CDLE (Fig 2).

▶ This study complements previous literature demonstrating the efficacy of the pulsed dye laser (PDL) for treatment of cutaneous discoid lupus erythematosus (CDLE). Not only is this device a safe and effective treatment for refractory CDLE, but also some might consider it the treatment of choice, at least in some patients. When one considers the side effects of chronic topical therapies (ie, corticosteroids) or systemic agents, PDL demonstrates impressive efficacy with few side effects.

E. A. Tanghetti, MD

Incidence of Cutaneous Lupus Erythematosus, 1965-2005: A Population-Based Study

Durosaro O, Davis MDP, Reed KB, et al (Mayo Med School, Rochester, MN; Mayo Clinic, Rochester, MN)
Arch Dermatol 145:249-253, 2009

Objectives.—To assess trends in the cutaneous variants of lupus erythematosus (CLE) and to ascertain the incidence of CLE over the past 4 decades.

Design.—Retrospective population-based study.

Setting.—Community-based epidemiology project.

Patients.—All Olmsted County, Minnesota, residents with any subtype of CLE between January 1965 and December 2005.

Main Outcome Measures.—Incidence of CLE and disease progression to systemic LE (SLE).

Results.—A total of 156 patients with newly diagnosed CLE (100 females and 56 males) were identified between 1965 and 2005. The incidence rate (age and sex adjusted to the 2000 US white population) was 4.30 (95% confidence interval [CI], 3.62-4.98) per 100 000. The age- and sex-adjusted prevalence as of January 1, 2006, was 73.24 (95% CI, 58.29-88.19) per 100 000. Nineteen patients with CLE had disease progression to SLE: cumulative incidence at 20 years, 19%; mean (SD) length to progression, 8.2 (6.3) years. Compared with a previously reported incidence of 2.78 (95% CI, 2.08-3.49) per 100 000 for SLE among Rochester, Minnesota, residents in 1965 through 1992, the incidence of CLE in Rochester was 3.08 (95% CI, 2.32-3.83) per 100 000 in 1965 through 1992.

Conclusions.—The incidence of CLE is comparable to the published incidence of SLE. Our findings double the incidence of the root designation of the disease process known as *LE* (SLE and CLE).

▶ This is a retrospective population-based study that assesses trends in the variants of cutaneous lupus erythematosus (CLE) and the changes in incidence over the past 4 decades. A total of 156 patients were included in the study evaluating age- and sex-adjusted prevalence. This study showed that the incidence of CLE, including subcutaneous lupus erythematosus (SCLE), classic discoid lupus erythematosus (CDLE), bullous lupus erythematosus, and lupus panniculitis, to be 4.30 per 100 000 from 1965 through 2005, with a female predominance and an average onset of 48.5 years of age. The incidence was found to be highest in 1986 through 1995. Data also showed that the incidence of CLE has been stable over the past 40 years. Cutaneous LE had a female predominance during the last 3 decades of this study. Also, 12% of CLE progressed to systemic lupus erythematosus (SLE) with the average time to progression being 8.2 years. One strength of this study was that all forms of lupus erythematosus (LE) were evaluated within a large time span. The limitations of this study were that the Rochester racial profile is not representative of the entire United States because certain ethnicities are underrepresented in that city's population. There is also a higher prevalence of Scandinavian descendents, which cannot be compared with the average city in the United States. There is also a question of latitude with areas that are more sun exposed having higher incidences compared with other geographic locations. Nevertheless, the article elicits an important point, which is that early recognition of CLE is significant in monitoring for transition to the systemic form.

G. K. Kim, DO
J. Q. Del Rosso, DO

Distinct Autoimmune Syndromes in Morphea: A Review of 245 Adult and Pediatric Cases

Leitenberger JJ, Cayce RL, Haley RW, et al (The Univ of Texas Southwestern Med Ctr at Dallas)
Arch Dermatol 145:545-550, 2009

Objective.—To determine the prevalence of extracutaneous manifestations and autoimmunity in adult and pediatric patients with morphea.

Design.—A retrospective review of 245 patients with morphea.

Setting.—University of Texas Southwestern Medical Center–affiliated institutions.

Patients.—Patients with clinical findings consistent with morphea.

Main Outcome Measures.—Prevalence of concomitant autoimmune diseases, prevalence of familial autoimmune disease, prevalence of extracutaneous manifestations, and laboratory evidence of autoimmunity (antinuclear antibody positivity). Secondary outcome measures included demographic features.

Results.—In this group, adults and children were affected nearly equally, and African Americans were affected less frequently than expected. The prevalence of concomitant autoimmunity in the generalized subtype of morphea was statistically significantly greater than that found in all other subtypes combined ($P = .01$). Frequency of a family history of autoimmune disease showed a trend in favor of generalized and mixed subgroups. The linear subtype showed a significant association with neurologic manifestations, while general systemic manifestations were most common in the generalized subtype. Antinuclear antibody positivity was most frequent in mixed and generalized subtypes.

Conclusions.—High prevalences of concomitant and familial autoimmune disease, systemic manifestations, and antinuclear antibody positivity in the generalized and possibly mixed subtypes suggest that these are systemic autoimmune syndromes and not skin-only phenomena. This has implications for the management and treatment of patients with morphea.

▶ This retrospective review of 245 patients with morphea was fraught with certain limitations including the methods of acquisition of medical and family histories, laboratory testing information, recall bias in reporting information by patients and families, the subtype classification being dependent on the treating physician, and the low numbers of patients who were tested for autoantibodies. However, the article did elucidate some important findings. Overall the patients had concomitant rheumatic or other autoimmune disorders 4 times higher than in the general population. The subtype of generalized morphea had significant association with underlying autoimmune disease. Several disorders occurred with greater frequency than expected including psoriasis, systemic lupus erythematosus (SLE), multiple sclerosis, and vitiligo. The generalized and mixed (presence of 2 subtypes of morphea not including generalized subtype) subtypes had the highest frequency of familial autoimmune disease in adults and second highest in children. Rheumatoid arthritis, SLE, and psoriasis were observed with highest frequency in first and second-degree relatives of patients with morphea. Extracutaneous signs including dysphagia, joint pain, and Raynaud's phenomenon are most common in patients with the generalized subtype, while patients with linear disease often have neurologic and ophthalmologic manifestations occurring on the same side as morphea. Pain was reported especially in the generalized subtype. Patients with the generalized and mixed subtypes had the highest frequency of antinuclear antibody (ANA) positivity. The generalized subtype demonstrated a homogeneous ANA pattern, linear and plaque subtype a speckled ANA pattern, and mixed subtype a nucleolar ANA pattern. These are the many important conclusions drawn from this study, strongly supporting that patients with generalized and mixed subtypes of morphea should be aggressively monitored for the presence of systemic manifestations and autoimmune diseases.

S. B. Momin, DO

J. Q. Del Rosso, DO

Complete and Sustained Remission of Juvenile Dermatomyositis Resulting From Aggressive Treatment

Kim S, El-Hallak M, Dedeoglu F, et al (Children's Hosp Boston, MA)
Arthritis Rheum 60:1825-1830, 2009

Objective.—To assess the time needed to achieve sustained, medication-free remission in a cohort of patients with juvenile dermatomyositis (DM) receiving a stepwise, aggressive treatment protocol.

Methods.—Between 1994 and 2004, a cohort of 49 children with juvenile DM who were followed up at a single tertiary care children's hospital using disease activity measures according to a specific protocol received standardized therapy with steroids and methotrexate. If a patient's strength or muscle enzyme levels did not normalize with this initial therapy, additional medications were added in rapid succession to the treatment regimen. The primary outcome measure was time to complete remission. Additional outcome measures were onset of calcinosis, effect of treatment on height, and complications resulting from medications.

Results.—Forty-nine patients were followed up for a mean ± SD of 48 ± 30 months. All but 1 patient received 2 or more medications simultaneously. Transient localized calcifications occurred in 4 patients (8%), and 2 additional patients (4%) had persistent calcinosis. Despite the aggressive therapy, complications associated with treatment were mild and were primarily attributable to steroids. No persistent effect on longitudinal growth was observed. A complete, medication-free remission was achieved in 28 patients; the median time to achievement of complete remission was 38 months (95% confidence interval 32–44 months). None of these patients experienced a disease flare that required resumption of medications during the subsequent period of observation (mean ± SD 36 ± 19.7 months).

Conclusion.—Our findings suggest that aggressive treatment of juvenile DM aimed at achieving rapid, complete control of muscle weakness and inflammation improves outcomes and reduces disease-related complications. In more than one-half of the children whose disease was treated in this manner (28 of 49), a prolonged, medication-free remission was attained within a median of 38 months from the time of diagnosis.

► Juvenile dermatomyositis (JDM) is an inflammatory disease affecting primarily the muscle and skin but can go on to affect other organ systems. Patients with JDM can experience crippling morbidity and limitations with the progression of this disease. Aggressive treatment may help to obtain sustained remission. This is a cohort study of 49 juvenile DM patients between 1994 and 2004 followed up at a single tertiary care children's hospital evaluating an aggressive treatment protocol and assessing the time needed to achieve medication-free remission. Mild disease was treated with high-dose oral prednisone. Those with moderate to severe disease were treated with 3 pulsed doses of intravenous methylprednisolone (MP), methotrexate (MTX), and daily oral prednisone, the latter added until complete response was achieved. Patients were given cyclosporine and intravenous immunoglob-ulin (IVIG) if muscle enzymes did not normalize after 3 months. When muscle enzymes and strength normalized, medications were tapered. Response to treat-ment was rapid, complete, and persistent. A complete, medication free remis-sion was achieved in 28 patients (median time of 39 months) with only 5% of patients relapsing. This study also included both objective and subjective measures making observer bias less likely. The most common adverse side effects included fractures, hypertension, and infections mainly due to systemic corticosteroids. Growth assessment during the disease course revealed a decrease in height percentile during the first year of therapy, and a return to baseline at 48 months. The small sample size of patients was one limitation in this study. Because this was a tertiary center, more severe cases of JDM were seen. In addition, the study also had a short follow-up period with a mean of 36 months. With patients on high dose systemic corticosteroids and immuno-suppressants, patients need to be followed up for a longer period of time. Patients and investigators were not blinded with regard to treatments, which could have also affected the study. Although growth delays normalized, with such visible side effects such as height reduction, parents and patients may not be so willing to comply with therapy. However, researchers found that aggressive treatment aided in the complete control of muscle weakness improving the outcome of JDM.

G. K. Kim, DO

J. Q. Del Rosso, DO

Unmet Patient Needs in Systemic Sclerosis
Rubenzik TT, Derk CT (Thomas Jefferson University, Philadelphia, PA)
J Clin Rheumatol 15:106-110, 2009

Objective.—Assessment of systemic sclerosis patients has not directly addressed functioning from the patient's perspective. With this study, we aim to gain our patient's point of view by using a questionnaire to describe their unmet needs and understanding what demographic parameters influ-ence these.

Methods.—A computer randomization program selected 50 patients, from 242 systemic sclerosis patients actively followed at our rheumatology clinic, to receive a survey about unmet needs. Twenty-five patients responded to the survey. Of 81 questions, 9 provided demographic data, whereas 72 questions addressed physical, daily living, psychologic, spiri-tual, existential, health services, health information, social support, and employment issues. A 4-point scale from no need to high need was used to rate all questions. Significant need was considered any issue for which more than 50% of patients reported a high need. The Fisher exact test was used to compare different demographic variables to unmet patient needs.

Results.—The psychologic/spiritual/existential category had 9 questions reaching significance, the health services category had 5 significant questions, the physical category had 4 significant questions. Patients who had not attended college were more likely to have higher needs than patients who completed a college degree. Unmarried patients reported higher needs in 8 measures as compared with married patients, and patients in rural areas had higher needs in social support needs.

Conclusions.—The greatest prevalence of unmet needs in scleroderma patients were in the psychologic/spiritual/existential domain, such as being unable to do things they used to do, fear that the disease will worsen, anxiety and stress, feeling down or depressed, fears of physical disability, uncertainty about the future, change in appearance, keeping a positive outlook, and feeling in control. Significant differences were observed in unmet needs based on education, marital status, location, knowledge of disease, and age. Understanding each patient's specific unmet needs either through direct questioning or by the use of a questionnaire such as the one used for this study can help clinicians to give better care to each of our patients.

▶ Scleroderma is a heterogenous spectrum of disease ranging from systemic to isolated skin involvement, which can greatly impact a patient's quality of life. This is a study, including 50 randomly selected patients with 25 patients responding to a survey concerning unmet needs regarding daily life with systemic sclerosis. These questionnaires sought to assess the disability index of systemic sclerosis patients. They included psychologic/spiritual/existential category, including anxiety, stress, and fear of worsening disease state. Categories also included physical, daily living, social support, and health services. Patients from rural areas reported higher need in 5 areas of social support possibly due to poor access to social networks. Results found that the greatest prevalence of unmet need was in the psychologic/spiritual/existential domain, which is also a finding seen in unmet needs in systemic lupus erythematosus. This finding reveals the need to address patients' thoughts regarding their disease state in addition to the physical manifestations of scleroderma. This study also found a significant need for guidance on the various phases of the disease, which is an aspect of health information. The authors also found that most patients are lacking psychosocial support and that there were numerous unmet needs in the health services. Patients reported a need for greater and more open discussions with their doctor, having their concerns taken seriously, and knowing when to see their doctor. Results also revealed that patients need help in dealing with their disease state once they are home and away from the clinic. Unmarried patients reported greater unmet needs from physical, psychologic/social/existential, daily living, and social support categories. Although this is a study that is limited by the number of participants, it gives clinicians an opportunity to understand some of the unmet needs in these patients.

G. K. Kim, DO
J. Q. Del Rosso, DO

Risk factors related to the failure of venous leg ulcers to heal with compression treatment

Milic DJ, Zivic SS, Bogdanovic DC, et al (Clinical Ctr Nis, Republic of Serbia; Univ of Nis, Republic of Serbia; et al)
J Vasc Surg 49:1242-1247, 2009

Background.—Compression therapy is the most widely used treatment for venous leg ulcers and it was used in different forms for more than 400 years. Published healing rates of venous ulcers obtained with compression therapy vary widely from 40-95%. According to numerous studies, it has been suggested that the application of external pressure to the calf muscle raises the interstitial pressure resulting in improved venous return and reduction in the venous hypertension. Several risk factors have been identified to be correlated with the failure of venous leg ulcers to heal with compression therapy (longer ulcer duration; large surface area; fibrinous deposition present on >50% of the wound surface and an Ankle Brachial Pressure Index (ABPI) of <0.85.

Methods.—An open prospective single-center study was performed in order to determine possible risk factors associated with the failure of venous ulcers to heal when treated with multi-layer high compression bandaging system for 52 weeks. In the study, 189 patients (101 women, 88 men; mean age 61 years) with venous leg ulcers (ulcer surface > 5 cm^2; duration > 3 months) were included. The study excluded patients with arterial disease (ABPI < 0.8), heart insufficiency with ejection fraction (EF) < 35, pregnancy, cancer disease, rheumatoid arthritis, and diabetes. Based on clinical opinion and available literature, the following were considered as potential risk factors: sex, age, ulceration surface, time since ulcer onset, previous operations, history of deep vein thrombosis, body mass index (BMI), reduction in calf circumference > 3 cm during the first 50 days of treatment, walking distance during the day < 200 meters, calf:ankle circumference ratio < 1.3, fixed ankle joint, history of surgical wound debridement, > 50% of wound covered with fibrin, depth of the wound > 2 cm.

Results.—Within 52 weeks of limb-compression therapy, 24 (12.7%) venous ulcers had failed to heal. A small ulceration surface (<20 cm^2), the duration of the venous ulcer < 12 months, a decrease in calf circumference of more than 3 cm, and emergence of new skin islets on > 10% of wound surface during the first 50 days of treatment were favorable prognostic factors for ulcer healing. A large BMI (>33 kg/m^2), short walking distance during the day (<200 m), a history of wound debridement, and ulcers with deepest presentation (>2 cm) were indicators of slow healing. Calf:ankle circumference ratio < 1.3, fixed ankle joint, and reduced ankle range of motion were the only independent parameters associated with non-healing ($P < .001$).

Conclusion.—The results obtained in this study suggest that non-healing venous ulcers are related to the impairment of the calf muscle pump.

▶ This article provides additional evidence into the most likely risk factors associated with the failure of venous leg ulcers to heal with compression treatment. To this end, the article achieved its objective. The article reviewed 189 patients that completed compression treatment for venous leg ulcers over a 1-year period. Of the numerous factors reviewed, the most significant factors associated with treatment failure were: fixed ankle joint and range of motion of less than 20 degrees as well as calf: ankle circumference <1.3. Not surprisingly, these factors are associated with the impairment of the calf muscle pump. Thus, although compression therapy appears to be an effective treatment modality, the article emphasizes the importance of the calf muscle pump in the etiology of venous leg ulcers and opens the door for future treatment studies in consideration of this important variable. Ultimately, the article provides insightful comparative data and notable considerations in the treatment of venous leg ulcers.

B. D. Michaels, DO
J. Q. Del Rosso, DO

10 Blistering Disorders

Effect of Intravenous Immunoglobulin Therapy on Serum Levels of IgG1 and IgG4 Antidesmoglein 1 and Antidesmoglein 3 Antibodies in Pemphigus Vulgaris
Green MG, Bystryn J-C (New York Univ School of Medicine)
Arch Dermatol 144:1621-1624, 2008

Background.—Intravenous immunoglobulin rapidly decreases serum levels of intercellular antibodies in patients with pemphigus vulgaris. However, little is known about the effects of this therapy on antibodies directed specifically against desmoglein 1 and desmoglein 3 and on the IgG subclasses of these antibodies. This study was conducted to study the effect of intravenous immunoglobulin therapy on serum levels of IgG1 and IgG4 antibodies against desmoglein 1 and desmoglein 3 in patients with pemphigus vulgaris.

Observations.—Within 6 to 16 days after initiating a single cycle of intravenous immunoglobulin therapy in 9 patients, a significant decrease in serum levels of IgG4 and IgG1 antibodies against desmoglein 1 and desmoglein 3 occurred in 60% to 100% of the patients, depending on the antibody subclass and specificity. The median decrease in the antibody levels ranged from 34% to 80%. In addition, most patients (n = 6) showed clinical improvement. The decrease in IgG4 antidesmoglein 3 levels seemed to correlate with improvement in disease activity.

Conclusions.—Intravenous immunoglobulin therapy rapidly lowers serum levels of IgG1 and IgG4 antidesmoglein 1 and desmoglein 3 antibodies. There seems to be a stronger association between the decrease in IgG4 antidesmoglein 3 levels and improvement in clinical activity than with changes in the other antibody levels, which suggests that IgG4 antibodies have a more important role in mediating pemphigus vulgaris.

▶ Administration of intravenous immunoglobulins to patients with pemphigus vulgaris is thought to work by lowering serum levels of pathogenic pemphigus immunoglobulin (IgG) antibodies. Green and Bystryn sought to assess the effect of intravenous IgG on the levels of subclasses of antibodies, specifically IgG antidesmoglein 1 (Dsg1) and IgG antidesmoglein 3 (Dsg3). Their rationale was the assumption that disease activity correlates with both the level and subclass of these antibodies. Both IgG1 and IgG4 antibodies were measured. Patients with disease refractory to prednisone received 1 cycle of intravenous IgG therapy, 400 mg/kg/day, for 5 days. Serum antibody levels were measured at baseline before administration of IgG therapy and 6 to 16 days after initiation of therapy. A rapid decrease in serum levels of both IgG1 and IgG4 anti-Dsg1 and anti-Dsg3 antibodies occurred in most patients. The authors found heterogeneity in the extent of decrease of different IgG subclasses against the same antigen in the same patient, and they inferred that this heterogeneity reflects differences in the way the different subclasses of IgG are affected by intravenous IgG. As IgG4 may represent the subclass of pemphigus autoantibodies that is most pathogenic, selecting IgG preparations with high levels of that subclass might enhance therapeutic efficacy.

B. H. Thiers, MD

Treatment of Juvenile Pemphigus Vulgaris with Intravenous Immunoglobulin Therapy

Asarch A, Razzaque Ahmed A (Tufts Univ School of Medicine, Boston, MA; New England Baptist Hosp, Boston, MA)
Pediatr Dermatol 26:197-202, 2009

We report the clinical response and follow-up on eight patients with juvenile pemphigus vulgaris treated with intravenous immunoglobulin. Six Caucasian females and two Caucasian males ages 15 to 18 (mean 15.5) were treated with intravenous immunoglobulin based on a published protocol. The indications were lack of response and development of serious side-effects to conventional therapy in four, lack of response to dapsone in two, and parental choice in two patients. In seven patients, a prolonged clinical remission was achieved. They received a mean of 28.5 cycles of intravenous immunoglobulin in a mean of 43.4 months and were followed for a mean of 29.8 months after discontinuing treatment. The remaining patient responded, but was lost to follow-up. Mean follow-up was 71.7 months. Six patients experienced mild headache, but no serious side-effects were observed in any patient. Intravenous immunoglobulin is a safe biological agent to use in the treatment of juvenile pemphigus vulgaris. It can be used as monotherapy and has the potential to induce and sustain long-term clinical remissions. In these eight patients, it appears that intravenous immunoglobulin is a safe biological agent without serious, immediate, or long-term side effects. Intravenous immunoglobulin is a valuable agent in the treatment of certain cases of juvenile pemphigus vulgaris.

▶ Pemphigus vulgaris (PV) is a blistering condition that is frequently seen in adults but may be observed in children and adolescent patients. Patients with juvenile PV (JPV) can suffer as a consequence to the disease process and medication side effects. This is a report of 6 Caucasian females and 2 Caucasian males aged 15 to 18 treated with JPV treated with intravenous immunoglobulin (IVIG). All patients had failed conventional treatment and were on other concomitant medication such as prednisone, dapsone, methotrexate, mycophenolate mofetil, and systemic antibiotics before starting IVIG. The indications used for IVIG were lack of response, presence of side effects, and progression of the disease in spite of conventional therapy. IVIG was administered at a dose of 2 g/kg/cycle and patients were observed posttreatment. Researchers also used objective measurements to determine quality of life such as growth retardation, ability to continue normal social life, and performance in school. Clinical response to IVIG was observed at 4.8 to 6.8 months. Once response was achieved, patients were first tapered from other systemic therapies; then IVIG was used as monotherapy and eventually tapered also. Side effects from IVIG were mild, including headaches, nausea, and fatigue. Clinical outcomes were available on only 7 of the 8 patients. Limitations included small sample size and nonrandomized Caucasian patients that were not representative of the population as a whole. In addition, patients did not undergo a wash out period and were on other concomitant medications while on treatment with IVIG. All 7 patients were free of lesions and off systemic therapy, including IVIG and observed for 26 to 36 months in sustained clinical remission. Authors concluded that IVIG was a useful agent in helping treatment resistant JPV patients to achieve remission. However, the high cost of IVIG is not practical for both hospitals and patients. Nevertheless, IVIG's safety profile is also another advantage for patients. This study provides an alternative to JPV patients not responding to conventional therapies with a steroid sparing effect such as growth retardation for younger individuals.

G. K. Kim, DO

J. Q. Del Rosso, DO

Rituximab Exerts a Dual Effect in Pemphigus Vulgaris
Eming R, Nagel A, Wolff-Franke S, et al (Philipps Univ, Marburg, Germany; et al)
J Invest Dermatol 128:2850-2858, 2008

Pemphigus vulgaris (PV) is a severe autoimmune blistering disease affecting the skin and mucous membranes. Autoreactive $CD4^+$ T helper (Th) lymphocytes are crucial for the autoantibody response against the desmosomal adhesion molecules, desmoglein (dsg)-3 and dsg1. Eleven patients with extensive PV were treated with the anti-CD20 antibody, rituximab (375 mg per m^2 body surface area once weekly for 4 weeks). Frequencies of autoreactive $CD4^+$ Th cells in the peripheral blood of the PV patients were determined 0, 1, 3, 6, and 12 months after rituximab treatment. Additionally, the clinical response was evaluated and serum autoantibody titers were quantified by ELISA. Rituximab induced peripheral B-cell depletion for 6–12 months, leading to a dramatic decline of serum autoantibodies and significant clinical improvement in all PV patients. The frequencies of dsg3-specific $CD4^+$ Th1 and Th2 cells decreased significantly for 6 and 12 months, respectively, while the overall count of $CD3^+CD4^+$ T lymphocytes and the frequency of tetanus toxoid-reactive $CD4^+$ Th cells remained unaffected. Our findings indicate that the response to rituximab in PV involves two mechanisms: (1) the depletion of autoreactive B cells and (2) the herein demonstrated, presumably specific downregulation of dsg3-specific CD4⁺ Th cells.

▶ The concept of pemphigus as an autoantibody-mediated disease is well known. Also very much appreciated by both clinicians and researchers is the fact that neither the humoral nor the cell-mediated immune system works in isolation. Numerous mechanisms have been described by which T cells can manipulate and control autoantibody production by B cells, and B cells may have a similar regulatory effect on T cells. It has previously been shown that induction and perpetuation of antibody production in pemphigus may be controlled by dsg1/dsg3-specific autoreactive CD4⁺T cells.[1] Recently published studies have demonstrated the efficacy of rituximab in the treatment of pemphigus vulgaris. The mechanism involved is presumed to involve depletion of autoreactive B cells by the monoclonal anti-CD20 antibody. In this study, Eming et al show that a second mechanism may be important, that is down regulation of dsg3-specific CD4⁺T helper (Th) cells. Similar mechanisms of action may be at play to explain the efficacy of rituximab in other autoimmune diseases, including rheumatoid arthritis, lupus erythematosus, dermatomyositis, and various forms of vasculitis.

B. H. Thiers, MD

Reference

1. Hertl M, Eming R, Vedlman C. T cell control in autoummune bullous skin disorders. *J Clin Invest*. 2006;116:1159-1166.

Diagnosis and Treatment of Stevens-Johnson Syndrome and Toxic Epidermal Necrolysis with Ocular Complications
Sotozono C, Ueta M, Koizumi N, et al (Kyoto Prefectural Univ of Medicine, Japan; et al)
Ophthalmology 116:685-690, 2009

Purpose.—To present a detailed clarification of the symptoms at disease onset of Stevens-Johnson syndrome (SJS) and its more severe variant, toxic epidermal necrolysis (TEN), with ocular complications and to clarify the relationship between topical steroid use and visual prognosis.

Design.—Cross-sectional study.

Participants.—Ninety-four patients with SJS and TEN with ocular complications.

Methods.—A structured interview, examination of the patient medical records, or both addressing clinical manifestations at disease onset were conducted for 94 patients seen at Kyoto Prefectural University of Medicine. Any topical steroid use during the first week at the acute stage also was investigated.

Main Outcome Measures.—The incidence and the details of prodromal symptoms and the mucosal involvements and the relationship between topical steroid use and visual outcomes.

Results.—Common cold-like symptoms (general malaise, fever, sore throat, etc.) preceded skin eruptions in 75 cases, and extremely high fever accompanied disease onset in 86 cases. Acute conjunctivitis and oral and nail involvements were reported in all patients who remembered the details. Acute conjunctivitis occurred before the skin eruptions in 42 patients and simultaneously in 21 patients, whereas only 1 patient reported posteruption conjunctivitis. Visual outcomes were significantly better in the group receiving topical steroids compared with those of the no-treatment group ($P < 0.00001$).

Conclusions.—Acute conjunctivitis occurring before or simultaneously with skin eruptions accompanied by extremely high fever and oral and nail involvement indicate the initiation of SJS or TEN. Topical steroid treatment from disease onset seems to be important for the improvement of visual prognosis.

▶ Although Stevens-Johnson syndrome (SJS) and toxic epidermal necrolysis (TEN) are rare, ocular complications can occur in more than 50% of patients affected by these severe mucocutaneous reactions, resulting in permanent visual impairment or blindness. Unfortunately, there is no universally accepted treatment regimen in patients affected by SJS or TEN. This is a cross-sectional study inclusive of 94 patients with SJS and TEN with ocular complications and a discussion on the clinical manifestation and treatment of SJS and TEN with ocular complications and outcomes affecting vision. In this study, 84/94 (89.4%) of cases were associated with medications, including cold remedies, antibiotics, nonsteroidal anti-inflammatory drugs (NSAIDS), anticonvulsants, and other drugs. They also found that 75 patients experienced common cold-like symptoms preceding the skin eruptions. This study also quantifies prodromal and other symptoms such as genital, oral, and ocular involvement in SJS and TEN. Acute conjunctivitis and oral involvement occurred in all patients and fingernail loss or deformation affected all patients in the acute stage. Other mucous membrane involvement affected the pharynx, respiratory tract, or ear canal. SJS and TEN are often associated with use of medications and can often be mitigated if the inciting agent is identified and discontinued. In addition, there is no standardized ophthalmologic treatment for prevention of ocular complications. The authors in this study concluded that visual outcomes were significantly better in the patients who received treatment with topical corticosteroids during the first week of disease onset compared with those of patients who did not receive topical and/or systemic corticosteroid treatment. They also found that early recognition of the disease helped to decrease the incidence of chronic ocular complications. This article encouraged prompt referral to an ophthalmologist for the prevention of permanent visual loss while using distinctive clinical clues such as the appearance of pseudomembrane formation and corneal or conjunctival epithelial defects as an indicator of ocular involvement. Although ocular improvement with corticosteroid therapy is noted in this study, adverse side effects and resolution of other lesions association with SJS and TEN are not mentioned. While in this study no bacterial cultures were taken, the authors suggest that there may be an association with SJS and TEN and opportunistic bacteria present on the ocular surface, which may be of interest for future research.

G. K. Kim, DO

J. Q. Del Rosso, DO

Successful Treatment of Stevens-Johnson Syndrome with Steroid Pulse Therapy at Disease Onset

Araki Y, Sotozono C, Inatomi T, et al (Kyoto Prefectural Univ of Medicine, Japan)
Am J Ophthalmol 147:1004-1011, 2009

Purpose.—To evaluate the visual prognosis of patients with Stevens-Johnson syndrome (SJS) and its severe variant, toxic epidermal necrolysis (TEN), followed by general and topical high-dose corticosteroids administration from disease onset.

Design.—Prospective, observational case series.

Methods.—Between May 1, 2003 and June 30, 2005, we enrolled 5 patients with SJS or TEN with ocular complications at the acute stage. Intravenous pulse therapy with methylprednisolone (steroid pulse therapy; 500 or 1000 mg/day for 3 to 4 days) was initiated within 4 days from disease onset. Topically, 0.1% betamethasone was applied over 5 times daily for at least 2 weeks. Visual acuity (VA) and slit-lamp microscopic appearance 1 year from disease onset were evaluated.

Results.—At the first examination, corneal or conjunctival epithelial defects and pseudomembranous conjunctivitis were present in all cases. Skin eruptions dramatically improved after steroid pulse therapy. Although ocular inflammation increased for several days, pseudomembranes disappeared and corneal and conjunctival epithelium regenerated within 6 weeks. At the chronic stage, all eyes had clear corneas with the palisades of Vogt (POV), implying the presence of corneal epithelial stem cells. Best-corrected VA was 20/20 or better in all eyes. Five eyes showed superficial punctate keratopathy. No eye had cicatricial changes except for 1 with slight fornix shortening. No significant adverse effects of steroid occurred during all clinical courses.

Conclusions.—Steroid pulse therapy at disease onset is of great therapeutic importance in preventing ocular complications. Topical betamethasone also shows great promise for preventing corneal epithelial stem cell loss in the limbal region and cicatricial changes.

▶ This article deals primarily with amelioration of the ocular manifestations in 4 patients with Stevens-Johnson syndrome (SJS) and one patient with toxic epidermal necrolysis (TEN) using intravenous methylprednisolone initiated within 0 to 4 days of disease onset. The authors noted dramatic improvement of skin function and prevention of serious ocular sequelae. Clearly, the size of this study is a limitation.

While the pendulum of steroid use for treatment of SJS has swung widely over the years, it would appear that for drug-induced disease, when initiated early, high-dose glucocorticosteroids may be beneficial.[1] Overall, this contributor favors administration of glucocorticosteroids to adult patients with SJS caused by drugs, when the disease has been diagnosed promptly (within 24-48 hours), and at sufficiently high dose (> 2 mg/kg daily prednisone or equivalent); but only for a short duration (4-7 days) and with prompt discontinuance at the first sign of infection.[2] The controversy in this area is still too great to support routine use of glucocorticosteroids in TEN. Finally, the article aptly points out that in addition to a dermatologist, an important member of the care team for any person with SJS/TEN is, of course, an ophthalmologist.

W. A. High, MD, JD, MEng

References

1. Tripathi A, Ditto AM, Grammer LC, et al. Corticosteroid therapy in an additional 13 cases of Stevens-Johnson syndrome: a total series of 67 cases. *Allergy Asthma Proc.* 2000;21:101-105.
2. High WA, Nirken MH. Stevens-Johnson syndrome and toxic epidermal necrolysis: management, prognosis, and long-term sequelae. UpToDate Web site. http://www.uptodate.com/online/content/topic.do?topicKey=dermatol/26552#10. Accessed Sep 26, 2009.

Risk Factors for the Development of Ocular Complications of Stevens-Johnson Syndrome and Toxic Epidermal Necrolysis
Gueudry J, Roujeau J-C, Binaghi M, et al (Hôpital Charles Nicolle, Rouen, France; Hôpital Henri Mondor, Créteil, France)
Arch Dermatol 145:157-162, 2009

Objectives.—To describe the acute and late ocular manifestations of toxic epidermal necrosis (TEN), Stevens-Johnson syndrome (SJS), and overlap syndrome and to identify predictors for the development of ocular complications.

Design.—Retrospective cohort study.

Setting.—A single referral unit in a university hospital.

Patients.—The study included 159 patients (mean [SD] age, 49.9 [19.8] years) with TEN and SJS during an 8-year period. Forty-nine patients were contacted at least 15 months after hospital discharge.

Main Outcome Measures.—Records were reviewed for demographics, cause of the condition, and severity of ocular involvement. The patients were contacted to assess late ocular complications.

Results.—A total of 117 patients (74%) had acute ocular involvement, which was mild in 58%, moderate in 8%, and severe in 8%. Patients with TEN had more frequent (odds ratio [OR], 2.7; 95% confidence interval

[CI], 1.06-6.90; $P = .05$) but not more severe (OR, 0.95; 95% CI, 0.20-4.5; $P = .99$) acute ocular involvement. Forty-nine patients were contacted at least 15 months after hospital discharge, and 63% had late ocular complications. Dry eye syndrome was the most common. The mean (SD) Ocular Surface Disease Index score was 32.9 (30.3) (range, 0-97.5). The severity of the acute ocular disease was found to be the only significant risk factor of late complications ($P = .002$), even though 5 patients without acute ocular involvement developed dry eye syndrome.

Conclusions.—Ocular involvement is common in patients with SJS and TEN. Late complications are more frequent in patients with severe initial eye involvement but may also develop in patients without patent initial ocular symptoms.

▶ Why do some patients with Stevens-Johnson syndrome and toxic epidermal necrolysis develop severe ocular complications while others do not? Gueudry et al sought to determine which factors may be predictive of the frequency and severity of ocular complications, including early and late manifestations, and to identify possible ways to predict the development of ocular complications. The methodology used was a retrospective chart review of all patients admitted to their hospital with these conditions between 1994 and 2002. A total of 159 patients were evaluated, with the majority being judged to have mild ocular involvement. The authors could identify no general risk factor, and there was no significant difference in the frequency or severity of long-term ocular complications between patients with Stevens-Johnson syndrome, overlap syndrome, and toxic epidermal necrolysis. Ocular involvement was most often noted during the acute phase of the disease. The most frequent late ocular complication was dry eye syndrome. Clearly, the best strategy to reduce ocular complications of this spectrum of diseases is the hoped for future emergence of better therapies for them. Prospective follow-up is of course necessary for all affected patients.

B. H. Thiers, MD

A randomized double-blind trial of intravenous immunoglobulin for pemphigus

Amagai M, for the Pemphigus Study Group (Keio Univ School of Medicine, Tokyo; et al)
J Am Acad Dermatol 60:595-603, 2009

Background.—Pemphigus is a rare life-threatening intractable autoimmune blistering disease caused by IgG autoantibodies to desmogleins. It has been difficult to conduct a double-blind clinical study for pemphigus partly because, in a placebo group, appropriate treatment often must be provided when the disease flares.

Objective.—A multicenter, randomized, placebo-controlled, double-blind trial was conducted to investigate the therapeutic effect of a single cycle of high-dose intravenous immunoglobulin (400, 200, or 0 mg/kg/d) administered over 5 consecutive days in patients relatively resistant to systemic steroids.

Methods.—We evaluated efficacy with time to escape from the protocol as a novel primary end point, and pemphigus activity score, antidesmoglein enzyme-linked immunosorbent assay scores, and safety as secondary end points.

Results.—We enrolled 61 patients with pemphigus vulgaris or pemphigus foliaceus who did not respond to prednisolone ($\geq$20 mg/d). Time to escape from the protocol was significantly prolonged in the 400-mg group compared with the placebo group ($P < .001$), and a dose-response relationship among the 3 treatment groups was observed ($P < .001$). Disease activity and enzyme-linked immunosorbent assay scores were significantly lower in the 400-mg group than in the other groups ($P < .05$ on day 43, $P < .01$ on day 85). There was no significant difference in the safety end point among the 3 treatment groups.

Limitation.—Prednisolone at 20 mg/d or more may not be high enough to define steroid resistance.

Conclusion.—Intravenous immunoglobulin (400 mg/kg/d for 5 d) in a single cycle is an effective and safe treatment for patients with pemphigus who are relatively resistant to systemic steroids. Time to escape from the protocol is a useful indicator for evaluation in randomized, placebo-controlled, double-blind studies of rare and serious diseases.

▶ Much has been written about the use of intravenous immunoglobulin for a variety of dermatologic indications, including toxic epidermal necrolysis and autoimmune blistering diseases, especially pemphigus vulgaris. Most of the data have been generated from case reports with a low level of evidence or involving a small number of patients receiving multiple treatment cycles. Much needed is a well-controlled, double-blind clinical study to evaluate this innovative therapeutic approach. Amagai et al developed a novel evaluation end point to assess the usefulness of high-dose intravenous immunoglobulin in a single treatment cycle for patients with pemphigus. The study involved 61 patients with pemphigus vulgaris or foliaceus who were unresponsive to high-dose prednisolone. These patients were enrolled in a randomized, multicentric, placebo-controlled, double-blind trial to assess the effect of a single cycle of intravenous immunoglobulin administered over 5 consecutive days. Time to escape from the protocol (TEP) was used as the primary efficacy end point. This was defined as the length of time the patient stayed on the protocol without any additional treatment. Using this parameter, the authors demonstrated that a single cycle of high doses of intravenous immunoglobulin appears to be effective for the treatment of pemphigus in patients who are resistant to systemic steroid therapy.

B. H. Thiers, MD

Clinical and Immunological Follow-Up of Pemphigus Patients on Adjuvant Treatment with Immunoadsorption or Rituximab

Pfütze M, Eming R, Kneisel A, et al (Philipps Univ, Marburg, Germany)
Dermatology 218:237-245, 2009

Background.—Pemphigus vulgaris (PV) is a life-threatening autoimmune blistering skin disease which is associated with pathogenic IgG autoantibodies against desmogleins (Dsg) 1 and 3. Novel therapeutic strategies such as immunoadsorption (IA) or the anti-CD20 antibody rituximab (Rtx) hold promise to be effective in severe or recalcitrant PV.

Patients and Methods.—In the present retrospective study, 6 patients with extensive cutaneous PV were subjected to adjuvant IA treatment while 5 patients with severe mucosal PV received adjuvant Rtx treatment.

Results.—Within 6 months, IA and Rtx induced excellent clinical responses which were associated with a significant reduction of prednisolone doses and a decrease in anti-Dsg-specific IgG. Over a 12-month period, 3 IA-treated patients required additional adjuvant drugs while all of the PV patients on Rtx had no or only minimal residual symptoms.

Conclusion.—The relative therapeutic (long-term) efficacy of IA and Rtx in cutaneous versus mucosal PV needs to be evaluated in a prospective study.

▶ Conventional therapy for severe pemphigus begins with high-dose systemic oral corticosteroids and administration of immunosuppressive steroid-sparing agents such as azathioprine, mycophenolate mofetil, and others. When the latter therapies are not adequate or their side effects are not tolerable, additional therapeutic interventions are necessary. Two of those interventions are described in this study.

Immunoadsorption involves the removal of immunoglobulin G (IgG) autoantibodies. In this study, an adsorber column containing PGAM146 peptide was used with quick and prolonged remissions. IgG antibodies against desmoglein 3 and desmoglein 1, which are the hallmark serologic markers of pemphigus, were reduced by 50% to 70% per immunoadsorption cycle. The second therapy used was rituximab, a chimeric monoclonal antibody against CD-20, which is on the surface of the B lymphocyte.

In this study, the authors measured autoantibody levels and disease activity using the Autoimmune Bullous Skin Disorder Intensity score, a newly introduced tool to assess the severity of pemphigus. The authors did everything they could to accurately assess treatment response because there are no standardized, validated tools to measure the severity of pemphigus vulgaris. This study design is well referenced.

Unfortunately, this study suffers the drawback of every uncommon severe disease. Adjuvant treatments were not standardized so that some patients were on mycophenolate mofetil and others on azathioprine. The study was also not blinded. Nevertheless, the clear clinical response in these difficult-to-treat patients makes this an important contribution to the literature.

M. Lebwohl, MD

Pemphigoid gestationis: early onset and blister formation are associated with adverse pregnancy outcomes

Chi C-C, Wang S-H, Charles-Holmes R, et al (Univ of Oxford, UK; Chang Gung Inst of Technology, Taoyuan, Taiwan; et al)

Br J Dermatol 160:1222-1228, 2009

Background.—It is unclear whether clinical features of pemphigoid gestationis (PG), such as timing of onset and severity, may affect pregnancy outcomes or whether the adverse outcomes in pregnancies complicated by PG are related to or worsened by systemic corticosteroid treatment.

Objectives.—To evaluate the associations of adverse pregnancy outcomes with clinical features, autoantibody titre of PG, and systemic corticosteroid treatment.

Methods.—We conducted a retrospective cohort study recruiting 61 pregnancies complicated by PG from the St John's Institute of Dermatology database which enrolled cases from dermatologists across the U.K., and two tertiary hospitals in the U.K. and Taiwan. Outcome measures included gestational age at delivery, preterm birth, birthweight, low birthweight (LBW, i.e. birthweight < 2500 g), small-for-gestational-age (i.e. birthweight below the 10th percentile for gestational age), fetal loss, congenital malformation, and mode of delivery.

Results.—After controlling for maternal age and comorbidity, decreased gestational age at delivery was significantly associated with presence of blisters ($P = 0·017$) and disease onset in the second trimester ($P = 0·001$). Reduced birthweight was significantly associated with disease onset in the first and second trimesters ($P = 0·030$ and $0·018$, respectively) as was also LBW [adjusted odds ratio (95% confidence interval) $13·71$ ($1·22–154·59$) and $10·76$ ($1·05–110·65$), respectively]. No significant associations of adverse pregnancy outcomes with autoantibody titre or systemic corticosteroid treatment were found.

Conclusions.—Onset of PG in the first or second trimester and presence of blisters may lead to adverse pregnancy outcomes including decreased gestational age at delivery, preterm birth, and LBW children. Such pregnancies should be considered high risk and appropriate obstetric care should be provided. Systemic corticosteroid treatment, in contrast, does not substantially affect pregnancy outcomes, and its use for PG in pregnant women is justified.

▶ Pemphigoid gestationis (PG) is a rare autoimmune dermatosis of pregnancy characterized by intense pruritus and consisting of erythematous urticarial papules, plaques, and blisters on the trunk. Key features in diagnosis are clinical suspicion and perilesional biopsy results. As such, investigation of direct immunofluorescence (DIF) yields a linear band of C3 deposition with or without immunoglobulin G (IgG) along the basement membrane. Results of this retrospective analysis revealed that the presence of blisters and disease onset in the first and second trimesters led to decreased gestational age at delivery and reduced birth weight respectively. These pregnancies should therefore be considered high-risk. In terms of treatment, no significant associations of adverse pregnancy outcomes with systemic corticosteroid were found, nor were there any association with autoantibody titre. Therefore, use of systemic corticosteroids may be warranted in PG patients. As stated by authors, limitations of this study include a relatively small sample size, along with limitations that are inherent to retrospective analysis.

S. Bellew, DO

J. Q. Del Rosso, DO

Risk Factors for Relapse in Patients With Bullous Pemphigoid in Clinical Remission: A Multicenter, Prospective, Cohort Study

Bernard P, Reguiai Z, Tancrède-Bohin E, et al (Hôpital Robert Debré, Reims; Hôpital Saint-Louis, Paris, et al)

Arch Dermatol 145:537-542, 2009

Objective.—To identify prognostic factors for relapse in the first year after cessation of therapy in bullous pemphigoid (BP).

Design.—Prospective, multicenter, cohort study (January 1, 2000, through December 31, 2006).

Setting.—Fifteen French dermatology departments.

Patients.—Patients with BP in remission under low doses of topical or systemic corticosteroids.

Interventions.—Cessation of corticosteroid treatment (day 0) followed by a systematic clinical and immunologic follow-up.

Main Outcome Measures.—The end point was clinical relapse within the first year after cessation of therapy. Associations of clinical, biological, and immunologic (including direct immunofluorescence, serum anti–basement membrane zone autoantibodies, and serum BP180 autoantibodies by enzyme-linked immunosorbent assay [ELISA] on day 0) variables with clinical relapse were assessed by means of univariate and multivariate analyses.

Results.—On day 0, 30 of 114 patients (26.3%) still had a positive result of direct immunofluorescence, 63 of 112 (56.3%) had circulating anti–basement membrane zone autoantibodies, and 34 of 57 (60%) had anti-BP180 antibodies by ELISA. At month 12, 22 patients were dead (n = 11) or lost to follow-up (n = 11), 51 were in remission, and 45 had had relapses (mean interval to relapse, 3.2 months). Factors predictive of relapse within 12 months after cessation of therapy were a positive result of direct immunofluorescence microscopy ($P = .02$), a greater age ($P = .01$), and high-titer ELISA scores ($P = .02$) on day 0. In multivariate analysis, the only factor independently predictive of relapse was a high-titer ELISA score on day 0 (odds ratio, 11.00; 95% confidence interval, 1.29-93.76).

Conclusions.—High-titer anti-BP180 ELISA score and, to a lesser degree, a positive direct immunofluorescence finding are good indicators of further relapse of BP. At least 1 of these tests should be performed before therapy is discontinued.

▶ Bullous pemphigoid (BP) is the most common subepidermal autoimmune bullous disease. The purpose of the study was to look at factors that may put a patient at risk for relapse. Authors looked at data from 15 centers over a period of 6 years. The patient size of 114 was adequate for this type of study. Authors noted that most relapse occurred within 3 months of cessation of therapy with a median interval to relapse of 2.1 months. Studies in the past have failed to identify risk factors for relapse. Authors in this study did notice 2 factors that can put a patient at risk for relapse: positive finding on direct immunofluorescence microscopy and a high titer of BP180 antibodies by enzyme-linked immunosorbent assay (ELISA). These were measured at the time of cessation of therapy. Authors also recommended that at least one of these tests should be measured before the cessation of therapy. The study was well conducted and thorough.

S. Bhambri, DO

J. Q. Del Rosso, DO

Epidermolysis bullosa and the risk of life-threatening cancers: The National EB Registry experience, 1986-2006
Fine J-D, Johnson LB, Weiner M, et al (The Natl Epidermolysis Bullosa Registry, Nashville; et al)
J Am Acad Dermatol 60:203-211, 2009

Background.—Case series have demonstrated that potentially lethal cutaneous squamous cell carcinomas arise in patients with recessive dystrophic epidermolysis bullosa (RDEB), although the magnitude of this risk is undefined.

Methods.—Systematic case finding and data collection were performed throughout the continental United States (1986-2002) by the National EB Registry on 3280 EB patients to determine cumulative and conditional risks for squamous cell carcinoma (SCC), basal cell carcinoma (BCC), and malignant melanoma (MM) within each major EB subtype, as well as the cumulative risk of death from each tumor. Study design was cross-sectional, with a nested randomly sampled longitudinal subcohort (N = 450).

Results.—SCCs arose primarily in RDEB, especially the Hallopeau-Siemens subtype (RDEB-HS), first beginning in adolescence. Less frequently, SCCs occurred in junctional EB (JEB). Cumulative risks rose steeply in RDEB-HS, from 7.5% by age 20 to 67.8%, 80.2%, and 90.1% by ages 35, 45, and 55, respectively. In Herlitz JEB, the risk was 18.2% by age 25. SCC deaths occurred only in RDEB, with cumulative risks in RDEB-HS of 38.7%, 70.0%, and 78.7% by ages 35, 45, and 55, respectively. MM arose in RDEB-HS, with a cumulative risk of

2.5% by age 12. BCCs arose almost exclusively in the most severe EB simplex subtype (Dowling-Meara) (cumulative risk = 43.6% by age 55).

Limitations.—Mutational analyses were performed on only a minority of enrollees in the National EB Registry, preventing evaluation of the possible influence of specific genotypes on the risk of developing or dying from cutaneous SCCs.

Conclusions.—SCC is the most serious complication of EB within adults, especially those with RDEB-HS. By mid-adulthood, nearly all will have had at least one SCC, and nearly 80% will have died of metastatic SCC despite aggressive surgical resection. When compared with SCCs arising within the normal population, the remarkably high risk of occurrence of and then death from SCCs among RDEB patients suggests likely differences in pathogenesis. Additional studies of EB-derived tumors and SCC cell lines may not only provide new insights into the mechanisms of carcinogenesis but also means whereby these particular tumors may be prevented or more effectively treated.

▶ This article makes a significant contribution in bringing to light a major complication of epidermolysis bullosa (EB)—cutaneous life-threatening cancers. The study is comprised of a systematic case finding and data collection of a large sample size of over 3200 patients with EB. This study analyzed all of the patients and delineated the types and subtypes of EB to their associated risk of a particular skin cancer. The data suggested that there is not only an increase in squamous cell carcinoma (SCC) in patients with recessive dystrophic EB (RDEB), and specifically with RDEB-Hallopeau Siemens subtype (RDEB-HS), but also a significant increased risk of mortality secondary to the SCC. The article also found an associated risk of melanoma with RDEB-HS subtype and an increase risk of basal cell carcinoma (BCC) in the EB simplex Dowling-Meara (DM) subtype. With such an intricate analysis, this data underscores the importance of screening patients with EB for skin cancer. The article also made contributions regarding the treatment of choice for SCC in the setting of RDEB and junctional EB. Overall, the article helps focus important attention to a major complication of EB and makes a noteworthy contribution in the literature about this debilitating spectrum of inherited blistering skin diseases.

B. D. Michaels, DO
J. Q. Del Rosso, DO

11 Drug Actions, Reactions, and Interactions

Prevalence of Adrenal Insufficiency Following Systemic Glucocorticoid Therapy in Infants With Hemangiomas
Lomenick JP, Reifschneider KL, Lucky AW, et al (Cincinnati Children's Hosp Med Ctr, OH)
Arch Dermatol 145:262-266, 2009

Objective.—To determine the prevalence of adrenal insufficiency in infants with hemangiomas following treatment with systemic glucocorticoids (GCs).

Design.—Prospective study for 18 months.

Setting.—Hemangioma and vascular malformation center at a tertiary care children's hospital.

Patients.—Sixteen infants with hemangiomas had an adrenal axis evaluation as soon as possible following the completion of GC therapy. Ten healthy control infants were also evaluated for comparison.

Interventions.—Prednisolone at a starting dose of 2 to 3 mg/kg/d for 4 weeks, followed by a tapering period. The mean duration of GC treatment was 7.2 months.

Main Outcome Measure.—Prevalence of adrenal insufficiency in GC-treated subjects as assessed by a combination low-dose/high-dose corticotropin stimulation test.

Results.—Subjects underwent corticotropin testing at a mean of 13 days after the completion of therapy. Only 1 of the 16 GC-treated infants (6%) had adrenal insufficiency. This subject was tested 1 day after GC treatment was stopped, and results from retesting 3 months later were normal. All control subjects had normal adrenal function.

Conclusion.—Infants with hemangiomas are at low risk of adrenal insufficiency following the completion of GC therapy, as used in our hemangioma center.

▶ The study by Lomenick et al suggests that there should be tempered apprehension in using systemic glucocorticoids for infantile hemangiomas when required, noting the findings of a low prevalence of hypothalamic-pituitary-adrenal (HPA) axis suppression after 2 weeks of therapy. An editorial by Sidbury[1] provides a largely reassuring commentary on the effects of systemic glucocorticoids in the treatment of infantile hemangiomas. Sidbury also provides important distinctions in data from other contrasting studies. While the data from Sidbury and the study by Lomenick et al are not definitive on this issue, there is at least some confirming data to partially ease the concern of pediatric referrals to dermatologists for systemic glucocorticoid treatment for infantile hemangiomas when warranted, at least until other larger studies can be performed. Overall, the article is succinct and sheds additional evidence on a contentious issue.

B. D. Michaels, DO
J. Q. Del Rosso, DO

Reference

1. Sidbury R. Hypothalamic-pituitary-adrenal axis suppression in systemic glucocorticoid-treated infantile hemangiomas: putting the risk into context. *Arch Dermatol.* 2009;145:319-320.

Prevalence of Adrenal Insufficiency Following Systemic Glucocorticoid Therapy in Infants With Hemangiomas
Lomenick JP, Reifschneider KL, Lucky AW, et al (Cincinnati Children's Hosp Med Ctr, OH)
Arch Dermatol 145:262-266, 2009

Objective.—To determine the prevalence of adrenal insufficiency in infants with hemangiomas following treatment with systemic glucocorticoids (GCs).

Design.—Prospective study for 18 months.

Setting.—Hemangioma and vascular malformation center at a tertiary care children's hospital.

Patients.—Sixteen infants with hemangiomas had an adrenal axis evaluation as soon as possible following the completion of GC therapy. Ten healthy control infants were also evaluated for comparison.

Interventions.—Prednisolone at a starting dose of 2 to 3 mg/kg/d for 4 weeks, followed by a tapering period. The mean duration of GC treatment was 7.2 months.

Main Outcome Measure.—Prevalence of adrenal insufficiency in GC-treated subjects as assessed by a combination low-dose/high-dose corticotropin stimulation test.

Results.—Subjects underwent corticotropin testing at a mean of 13 days after the completion of therapy. Only 1 of the 16 GC-treated infants (6%) had adrenal insufficiency. This subject was tested 1 day after GC treatment was stopped, and results from retesting 3 months later were normal. All control subjects had normal adrenal function.

Conclusion.—Infants with hemangiomas are at low risk of adrenal insufficiency following the completion of GC therapy, as used in our hemangioma center.

▶ Two previous studies have suggested a relative high frequency of adrenal insufficiency (AI) in infants with hemangiomas following systemic glucocorticoid (GC) therapy. In contrast, the above study found a low prevalence of AI in infants with hemangiomas treated with systemic GC. However, it should be noted that the previous studies both used a morning serum cortisol level to diagnose AI, which is a poor and relatively nonspecific test. This study used a more sensitive and specific combination of tests, the low- and high-dose corticotropin suppression tests, which support the low determined prevalence of AI found in this study. Even further supporting the determined low prevalence is the fact that the one infant who was detected to have AI following GC therapy in this study may have been tested too soon after discontinuing therapy. This infant was tested the day after discontinuing systemic GC therapy. Therefore, depending on when the infant was given his last dose of medication the infant may have had GC still in his system, altering the test.

Although we feel that use of the low- and high-dose corticotrophin suppression tests in this study may provide a more accurate prediction of AI after systemic GS therapy in infants with hemangiomas, there are still several major limitations to this study. The first limitation is the study size of 16 patients, a number too small from which to glean definitive conclusions. Second, the authors failed to standardize when the suppression tests were given. The only requirement for giving the suppression test was that it had to be within 7 days of discontinuing GC therapy. It may also be important to make sure that the suppression test is not given too soon after discontinuing therapy for reasons discussed above. Further experimentation using more standardized methodology and an increased sample size is needed.

J. Levin, DO
J. Q. Del Rosso, DO

Thrombocytopenia associated with the use of anti–tumor necrosis factor–α agents for psoriasis
Brunasso AMG, Massone C (Galliera Hosp, Genoa; Med Univ of Graz, Austria; et al)
J Am Acad Dermatol 60:781-785, 2009

Background.—Thrombocytopenia has been reported to be associated with efalizumab therapy, but has only sporadically been reported with other anti–tumor necrosis factor alfa (TNF-α) agents.

Objective.—To describe the frequency of thrombocytopenia in a cohort of patients who underwent biological therapies for psoriasis.

Methods.—This was a retrospective observational study of 93 patients.

Results.—One hundred eighteen courses of biological therapies were administered to 93 patients. Four of 67 patients who received anti-TNF-α agents developed drug-induced thrombocytopenia during treatment, compared with none of the 51 patients receiving efalizumab therapy. The platelet count recovered after suspension of anti-TNF-α agents in 3 patients and relapsed after re-exposure in two patients. The overall estimated frequency of thrombocytopenia in our cohort was 4.30% (95% confidence interval [CI], 0% to 6.2%).

Limitations.—These findings should be validated in larger studies.

Conclusions.—Drug-induced thrombocytopenia is a potential side effect of anti-TNF-α agents. Immediate monitoring of platelet counts is recommended if autoimmunity is suspected.

▶ This retrospective study brings to light a few important points to remember regarding the safe use of biologic therapies in the treatment of psoriasis. First, along with the recommendations for having tuberculosis skin testing before start of therapy, if there is concern regarding risk of autoimmune reactions, clinicians may obtain a baseline complete blood cell count (CBC) including platelet counts, and also antinuclear antibody testing (ANA) may be considered. Secondly, due to longer follow-up periods of their cohorts, authors were able to highlight that biologic therapy-induced thrombocytopenia can appear much later in onset, up to 32 months. This may explain the higher frequency of thrombocytopenia that was observed in this study compared with previous reports in literature. Although this study showed no incidences of thrombocytopenia in patients on efalizumab therapy, it is important to note that as of June 9, 2009, efalizumab is no longer available in the United States due to increased risk of progressive multifocal leukoencephalopathy (PML).

S. Bellew, DO

J. Q. Del Rosso, DO

Seasonal variation of Stevens-Johnson syndrome and toxic epidermal necrolysis associated with trimethoprim-sulfamethoxazole

Wanat KA, Anadkat MJ, Klekotka PA (Washington Univ School of Medicin, St Louis, MO)
J Am Acad Dermatol 60:589-594, 2009

Background.—Stevens-Johnson syndrome (SJS) and toxic epidermal necrolysis (TEN) are rare and severe cutaneous adverse reactions to medications and infections.

Objective.—We sought to determine whether a seasonal variation to SJS and TEN exists and to define the characteristics in our tertiary referral hospital.

Methods.—A retrospective chart review of 50 patients from 1995 through 2007 was performed and statistically analyzed.

Results.—The most common medication implicated as a cause of SJS/TEN was trimethoprim-sulfamethoxazole (TMX) (26%). A seasonal trend, favoring springtime, was observed for the total number of cases of SJS and TEN ($P = .34$). There was a significant increase in cases due to TMX (53%) occurring in spring compared to other seasons ($P = .002$). These patients were significantly younger (37.8 ± 13.7) than other patients with SJS and TEN (53.7 ± 16.4) ($P = .003$). Their overall mortality (1 death) and average SCORTEN value (1.62 ± 1.6) was also significantly lower ($P = .04$ and 0.03, respectively). Based on outpatient pharmacy records, there was no increase in TMX prescriptions filled during the spring.

Limitations.—The study was limited by reliance on chart data, the use of inpatient records, and number of patients.

Conclusions.—A seasonal variation in SJS and TEN caused by TMX affecting younger patients may exist.

▶ This study was a limited retrospective and observational chart review undertaken to determine an engaging possibility—is there a seasonal variation of Stevens-Johnson syndrome and toxic epidermal necrolysis (TEN) associated with trimethoprim-sulfamethoxazole (TMX). The conclusion of the study is limited and is less than definitive, albeit interesting. The study comprised of 50 patients. Of the 50 patients, 13 patients had TMX implicated as a causative agent. In analyzing the study, 18 cases of SJS/TEN occurred during the spring months of April, May, and June, which itself was not statistically significant versus other months. The study, however, found of the 13 cases caused by TMX, 7 resulted from TMX during the spring months—which was statistically significant. However, as noted, population size is a questionable variable in this study. Namely, while 7 of 13 cases may be statistically significant, it is difficult to conclude a definitive pattern exists based on this limited number of patients. Another consideration is that given the seasonal variations, would this finding be applicable to other geographic locations not only in the United States, but also other countries as well? Finally, the study was also not able to determine the etiology for this trend beyond the correlation of TMX use. Given these limitations, a follow-up study would be intriguing based on a larger patient population to not only determine whether a correlation truly exists between the spring season and TMX causing SJS/TEN, but also to determine the precise etiology.

B. D. Michaels, DO
J. Q. Del Rosso, DO

Cost-Effectiveness of Telavancin versus Vancomycin for Treatment of Complicated Skin and Skin Structure Infections

Laohavaleeson S, Barriere SL, Nicolau DP, et al (Hartford Hosp, CT; Theravance, Inc, South San Francisco, CA)
Pharmacotherapy 28:1471-1482, 2008

Study Objective.—To determine the cost-effectiveness of telavancin versus vancomycin for the treatment of complicated skin and skin structure infections (cSSSIs).

Design.—Pharmacoeconomic analysis conducted from the hospital's perspective using data from the Assessment of Telavancin in Complicated Skin and Skin Structure Infections (ATLAS) phase III clinical trial.

Setting.—One hundred twenty-nine hospitals in the United States and internationally.

Patients.—A total of 1044 clinically evaluable patients who were hospitalized with a cSSSI during the ATLAS trial and who received at least one dose of telavancin or vancomycin in the hospital.

Measurements and Main Results.—Diagnosis-related group–specific hospital bed costs, antibiotic acquisition prices, and cost of vancomycin monitoring were applied to the resource utilization data collected during the ATLAS trial. Infection-related length of stay (LOS_{IR}) and hospitalization costs ($COST_{IR}$) were compared between the telavancin (514 patients) and vancomycin (530 patients) groups. Incremental cost-effectiveness ratios (ICERs) were calculated for the total population and a subset of patients infected with methicillin-resistant *Staphylococcus aureus* (MRSA) by using a 25,000-sample bootstrap analysis. During sensitivity analyses, the daily acquisition price for telavancin was increased from the equivalent to vancomycin ($13.44) to $50, $100, $150, or $200, and the rate of MRSA acquisition was varied between 30% and 75%. The median (interquartile range) LOSIR was 8 days (6–12 days) for both telavancin and vancomycin (p = 0.742), and median (interquartile range) $COST_{IR}$ was $8118 ($6291–11,758) and $8185 ($6474–11,405), respectively (p = 0.560). Similar findings were observed for the MRSA subset. Telavancin cost-effectiveness was greater for the MRSA population versus the total population. During bootstrap analyses of the MRSA population, the ICER for telavancin ranged from dominant (−$9560) to $27,889 as acquisition price was increased.

Conclusions.—Telavancin LOS_{IR} and total $COST_{IR}$ were similar to those of vancomycin for the treatment of cSSSIs. Particularly in those infected with MRSA, telavancin may be more cost-effective than vancomycin over the range of acquisition prices tested.

▶ Dermatologists generally treat uncomplicated skin and skin structure infections, including impetigo, folliculitis, furunculosis, superficial cellulitis, acute paronychia, simple abscesses, ecthyma, and blistering distal dactylitis. The Food and Drug Administration (FDA) defines complicated skin and skin-structure infections as those that affect the deep soft tissue and those that require surgical intervention beyond simple drainage. They also include patients who have significant underlying disease states that complicate their response to treatment, but this definition does not include most infections in diabetic patients, superficial skin, and skin structure infections in patients with HIV infection, or superficial skin and skin structure infections in immunocompromised patients.

Telavancin, unlike vancomycin, is rapidly bacteriocidal by means of cell wall synthesis and disruption of the bacterial membrane. A phase II trial showed noninferiority compared with vancomycin. This study is a pharmacoeconomic analysis of data generated during a separate clinical trial. The cost of the medication was assumed to be anywhere in a range up to $200 per day. There was no difference in length of stay between the treatments, but this relates largely to the methods of the study, as subjects were only included if they were anticipated to require 7 days of treatment. As the greatest cost savings are typically realized through reductions in length of stay, this is a serious limitation.

Cost-effectiveness was found to be greater as the methicillin resistant *Staphylococcus aureus* (MRSA) population increased, but even this conclusion must be challenged, as most of the MRSA strains isolated produced Panton-Valentine leukocidin, suggesting that they were community-acquired strains, and some could have been treated with less expensive oral antibiotics such as trimethoprim-sulfamethoxazole, tetracycline, or clindamycin. At the very least, patients could have had an earlier discharge because of earlier transition to an oral medication. Vancomycin achieves poor intracellular penetration, and has proved inferior to linezolid in several clinical trials. Linezolid is available orally and was not included in the analysis.

Given all of these limitations, data still suggest that in some situations, telavancin may be a cost-effective choice. One way to approach the data is to assume that at a price of $200 per day for telavancin, 24 hospitalized patients would have to be treated at an additional cost of $27 889 to prevent a single vancomycin failure. Fortunately, most outpatient MRSA infections can still be treated with drainage and oral antibiotics.

D. M. Elston, MD

Twelve-Year Analysis of Severe Cases of Drug Reaction With Eosinophilia and Systemic Symptoms: A Cause of Unpredictable Multiorgan Failure
Eshki M, Allanore L, Musette P, et al (Bichat-Claude Bernard Hosp, Paris; Assistance Publique des Hôpitaux de Paris, Créteil; Charles Nicolle Hosp, Rouen; et al)
Arch Dermatol 145:67-72, 2009

Background.—Factors implicated in the severity of drug reaction with eosinophilia and systemic symptoms (DRESS) have not been identified. We retrospectively describe and analyze severe cases of DRESS defined by history of intensive care unit admission and death due to DRESS.

Observations.—Of 15 patients retrospectively recruited in France, 14 were admitted to the intensive care unit and 3 died. The culprit drugs were already known to cause or trigger DRESS: allopurinol, minocycline hydrochloride, anticonvulsants, sulfonamides, and antibiotics. Visceral involvement with severe manifestations responsible for intensive care unit admission or death was variable and often multiple (pneumonitis, hepatitis, renal failure, encephalitis, hemophagocytosis, cardiac failure, and pancytopenia) and resulted in multiorgan failure in 11 patients. These severe complications sometimes developed late in DRESS. Human herpesvirus 6 infection was demonstrated in 6 of 7 patients. In addition, human herpesvirus 6 infection was demonstrated in involved viscera in 2 patients.

Conclusions.—Severe DRESS is rare. Some specificities of visceral involvement were associated with allopurinol and minocycline. However, visceral involvement comprising multiorgan failure seemed to be unpredictable. Better knowledge of DRESS is necessary to propose specific and prompt treatment. Early demonstration of human herpesvirus 6 reactivation could be considered a prognostic factor for identifying patients at higher risk and, hence, needs to be evaluated.

▶ This retrospective study analyzed only severe cases of drug reaction with eosinophilia and systemic symptoms (DRESS), and found that minocycline along with allopurinol were associated with a higher risk. Considering the frequency of minocycline use for treatment of acne, this article is an important reminder as DRESS can be associated with significant morbidity, and sometimes mortality. This was illustrated in a 15-year-old girl that was prescribed minocycline for acne vulgaris and subsequently died 164 days after beginning of DRESS. Unfortunately, no definitive prognostic factors were identified during the course of this study. However, authors did support previous associations with human herpes virus 6 (HHV-6) infection. Due to the retrospective nature of the study, 8 out of 15 patients were not found to have HHV-6 PCR analyses. DRESS is clearly unpredictable and more research needs to be done to identify crucial prognostic factors that contribute to this potentially life-threatening drug reaction.

S. Bellew, DO
J. Q. Del Rosso, DO

Etanercept: Efficacy and safety
Jiménez-Puya R, Gómez-García F, Amorrich-Campos V, et al (Univ Hosp of Cordoba, Spain)
J Eur Acad Dermatol Venereol 23:402-405, 2009

Objective.—To evaluate the efficacy and safety of etanercept in the treatment of patients with moderate to severe plaque psoriasis.

Methods.—An observational, longitudinal, and retrospective study involving two groups of dose of treatment with etanercept (50 vs. 100 mg/week). The selected patients presented moderate to severe plaque psoriasis, and they had received treatment with the mentioned drug. A total of 58 patients were included in the study. The efficacy of the drug was evaluated by measuring the psoriasis area and severity index (PASI), body surface area (BSA) and physician's global assessment (PGA) in weeks 8, 16, 24, 32, 40 and 48.

Results.—A statistically significant improvement was observed in the PASI, BSA and PGA indexes after 24 and 48 weeks of therapy. As for PASI, and after 48 weeks of treatment, PASI 50, 75 and 90 were 100.0%, 92.3% and 69.2%, respectively. In our series, etanercept 50 mg/week reached the same results after 48 weeks as etanercept 100 mg/week, though the initial response was faster in the last group. The PASI, BSA and PGA indexes diminished significantly with the treatment, though without statistically significant differences between both groups. As for the safety, etanercept was well tolerated, and no serious adverse events were recorded. There were no cases of tuberculosis or opportunistic infections.

Conclusions.—Our study confirms the efficacy and safety outcomes of the clinical trials of etanercept in psoriasis with both doses of treatment. As for the safety, etanercept was well tolerated, and all the recorded adverse events coincided with the known potential side-effects of treatment.

▶ Etanercept is a dimeric competitive inhibitor at the receptor site that binds to both soluble and membrane-bound forms of tumor necrosis factor-α (TNF-α). It is among 3 anti-TNF agents (infliximab, adalimumab, and entanercept) currently FDA approved for treatment of moderate to severe psoriasis. This article compares the safety and efficacy of etanercept at 2 different doses (50 vs 100 mg/week). As stated, authors found no significant difference between the 2 dosing regimens. Although this study follows patients for 48 weeks, it is well known that psoriasis is a chronic condition that has periods of remission as well as exacerbations, and therefore additional longer term studies need to be investigated. To this end, there are established reports that combination therapy with an anti-TNF agent and phototherapy showed higher rates of response. Moreover, patients that experienced exacerbations following cessation of etanercept therapy found a recapturing of clinical response to adalimumab in one case report and in retreatment with etanercept 25 mg twice weekly in another case report. Lastly, although serious adverse events were not recorded in this retrospective study, clinicians should keep in mind the risk of infections, demyelinating disease, lupus-like syndromes, malignances, and congestive heart failure.

S. Bellew, DO
J. Q. Del Rosso, DO

Twenty years' experience of steroids in infantile hemangioma—
a developing country's perspective
Pandey A, Gangopadhyay AN, Gopal SC, et al (Banaras Hindu Univ, Varanasi,
India; et al)
J Pediatr Surg 44:688-694, 2009

Background.—Hemangioma is a common vascular tumor. Though it involutes spontaneously, results are unpredictable. Steroid therapy is an effective mode of its regression. We present our experience of largest series and possible recommendations for treatment.

Materials and Methods.—A total of 2398 patients were treated during the study period of 20 years. They were given oral prednisolone, intralesional triamcinolone, or combination of both as per the protocol and followed for the response. Response to the treatment was graded as excellent, good, poor, or no response.

Results.—The male-to-female ratio was 1:2.3. In 81% of patients, hemangioma was noticed within first month of life. The commonest site of involvement was head and neck (57%). The commonest clinical presentation was discoloration and swelling. Mean age and size were 8.43 ± 7.04 months and 23.64 ± 20.13 cm^2. Response rate was highest for superficial type using any modality of treatment. Patients younger than 1 year showed better response (90.3%) in comparison with children older than 1 year (80.8%). The specific complications occurring were infections in 249 (12.4%), cushingoid facies and growth delay in 62 (3.1%), and hypertension in 51 (2.5%) patients.

Conclusion.—Steroid therapy either oral or intralesional as per the requirement is an easy and safe modality. Results are good to satisfactory in most patients. The complications are minimal. If treatment is needed, it should be used as a first-line therapy, especially when cost is an important concern.

▶ This article summarizes the collective experience of one group in India over 10 years in treating hemangiomas of infancy (HOI). It confirms many of the principles that have been proven in American studies (increased incidence in females, prevalence of superficial type hemangioma, and response to treatments).

The authors concede that there is no control group in this study, which did not receive treatment; thus the effects of corticosteroid therapy cannot be compared with any treatment for any of the lesions, and most importantly for superficial small hemangiomas. In addition, multiple adverse effects were noted (ie, Cushingoid facies, growth delay) especially in those groups receiving oral steroids, and both oral and intralesional steroids, even though cortisol stimulation tests or other measures to assess hypothalamic-pituitary axis suppression were not performed. Therefore, we have no way of determining whether and with what frequency hypothalamic-pituitary axis suppression occurred in all groups.

K. Hook, MD
S. Fallon Friedlander, MD

Medications as Risk Factors of Stevens-Johnson Syndrome and Toxic Epidermal Necrolysis in Children: A Pooled Analysis

Levi N, Bastuji-Garin S, Mockenhaupt M, et al (Hôpital Henri Mondor Albert-Chenevier, Créteil, France; Univ Med Ctr, Freiburg, Germany; et al)
Pediatrics 123:e297-e304, 2009

Objective.—The aim of this study was to determine the relation of medications to the risk of Stevens-Johnson syndrome and toxic epidermal necrolysis in children <15 years of age.

Methods.—We conducted a pooled analysis by using data from 2 multi-center international case-control studies: the severe cutaneous adverse reaction (SCAR) study and the multinational severe cutaneous adverse reaction (EuroSCAR) study conducted in France, Germany, Italy, Portugal, the Netherlands, Austria, and Israel. We selected case subjects aged <15 years, hospitalized for Stevens-Johnson syndrome, Stevens-Johnson syndrome/toxic epidermal necrolysis-overlap, or toxic epidermal necrolysis, and age-, gender-, and country-matched hospital controls. Pooled crude odds ratios were estimated and adjusted for confounding by multivariate methods when numbers permitted.

Results.—Our study included 80 cases and 216 matched controls. Anti-infective sulfonamides, phenobarbital, carbamazepine, and lamotrigine were strongly associated with the risk of Stevens-Johnson syndrome or toxic epidermal necrolysis. Significant associations were highlighted in univariate analysis for valproic acid and nonsteroidal antiinflammatory drugs as a group and for acetaminophen (paracetamol) in multivariate analysis.

Conclusions.—We confirmed 4 previously highly suspected drug risk factors for Stevens-Johnson syndrome/toxic epidermal necrolysis in children: antiinfective sulfonamides, phenobarbital, carbamazepine, and lamotrigine. Among more unexpected risk factors, we suspect that aceta-minophen (paracetamol) use increases the risk of Stevens-Johnson syndrome or toxic epidermal necrolysis.

▶ This study pooled the data from 2 large case-control studies to evaluate the medication risk factors for Stevens-Johnson syndrome (SJS) and toxic epidermal necrolysis (TEN) in children less than 15 years of age. Controls consisted of patients of the same age, demographics, and gender that were hospitalized for acute conditions, including infection, trauma, and abdominal emergency. The homogeneity between the 2 studies was tested for each variable using the Cochran Q test with a significance of less than 10%. Univariate analysis was performed for all risk factors, and multivariate analysis was performed when at least 3 cases and controls were exposed and demonstrated univariate significance. The authors tried to account for protopathic bias by moving the index day (the probable onset of the disease) 3 days earlier for all the drugs that were significant in univariate analysis. The results of this thorough analysis demonstrated that anti-infective sulfonamides, phenobarbital, lamotrigine, and carbamazepine were independent risk factors with markedly elevated risk estimates. Additionally, valproic acid, nonsteroidal antiinflammatory drugs (NSAIDs), and acetaminophen were significantly associated with these diseases in children.

While the incidence and mortality rates of SJS and TEN are reported to be lower in children than in adults, these are still devastating diseases with significant morbidity and mortality rates and the potential for permanent adverse sequelae. This may be the first study to look at medication risk factors in SJS and TEN in children, and it is the hope of the authors that reporting such risk factors may increase our understanding of these disorders and lower their occurrence.

J. Levin, DO

J. Q. Del Rosso, DO

Different effects of pimecrolimus and betamethasone on the skin barrier in patients with atopic dermatitis

Jensen J-M, Pfeiffer S, Witt M, et al (Univ of Kiel, Germany; Microscopy Services, Flintbek, Germany, et al)
J Allergy Clin Immunol 123:1124-1133, 2009

Background.—Genetic defects leading to skin barrier dysfunction were recognized as risk factors for atopic dermatitis (AD). It is essential that drugs applied to patients with AD restore the impaired epidermal barrier to prevent sensitization by environmental allergens.

Objectives.—We investigated the effect of 2 common treatments, a calcineurin inhibitor and a corticosteroid, on the skin barrier.

Methods.—In a randomized study 15 patients with AD were treated on one upper limb with pimecrolimus and on the other with betamethasone twice daily for 3 weeks.

Results.—Stratum corneum hydration and transepidermal water loss, a marker of the inside-outside barrier, improved in both groups. Dye penetration, a marker of the outside-inside barrier, was also reduced in both drugs. Electron microscopic evaluation of barrier structure displayed prevalently ordered stratum corneum lipid layers and regular lamellar body extrusion in pimecrolimus-treated skin but inconsistent extracellular lipid bilayers and only partially filled lamellar bodies after betamethasone treatment. Both drugs normalized epidermal differentiation and reduced epidermal hyperproliferation. Betamethasone was superior in reducing clinical symptoms and epidermal proliferation; however, it led to epidermal thinning.

Conclusion.—The present study demonstrates that both betamethasone and pimecrolimus improve clinical and biophysical parameters and epidermal differentiation. Because pimecrolimus improved the epidermal barrier and did not cause atrophy, it might be more suitable for long-term treatment of AD.

▶ Although this double-blind, randomized study was small ($N = 15$), it represents an important step in the evaluation of epidermal barrier function and integrity after specific topical therapies for atopic dermatitis (AD). All subjects exhibited mild to moderate severity of AD. Both betamethasone valerate (BMV) and pimecrolimus (PIM) improved clinical parameters, restored disturbed epidermal differentiation (as evidenced by normalization of expression of filaggrin, involucrin, loricrin, and keratins) and marked reduction in transepidermal water loss. Importantly, presence of filaggrin mutation was not specifically addressed as part of the study inclusion or exclusion. A greater decrease in epidermal proliferation was noted with BMV, consistent with the atrophogenic potential associated with continued topical corticosteroid use. Presence of regular stratum corneum lipid bilayers were noted after treatment with PIM but not with BMV. Disturbed lamellar body extrusion was also noted with BMV but not with PIM. BMV exhibited both greater clinical improvement and decreased epidermal proliferation than PIM, however, PIM produced a superior ability to restore epidermal barrier structure. These findings support the use of topical corticosteroids for treatment of AD flares and topical calcineurin inhibitors as more suitable for longer courses of therapy.

J. Q. Del Rosso, DO

A Phase II, Open-Label Study of the Efficacy and Safety of Imiquimod in the Treatment of Superficial and Mixed Infantile Hemangioma

McCuaig CC, Dubois J, Powell J, et al (Univ of Montreal, Quebec, Canada)
Pediatr Dermatol 26:203-212, 2009

Objectives.—To explore the efficacy and safety of imiquimod 5% cream as a treatment for infantile hemangioma.

Design.—Phase II, open-label, noncomparative study of imiquimod applied during 16 weeks, with posttherapy follow-up 16 weeks later (8 months total).

Setting.—Outpatient pediatric tertiary care referral center in Quebec, Canada.

Participants.—Healthy infants up to 8.8 months of age with previously untreated, nonulcerated, proliferative superficial or mixed infantile hemangioma, excluding periorbital, or perineal localization, ≥ 100 cm^2 in size.

Intervention.—Topical imiquimod applied three to seven times per week for 16 weeks to infantile hemangioma.

Main Outcome Measures.—Lesion area, volume, depth (Doppler ultrasound), and color (erythema), serum drug, and interferon-alpha levels.

Results.—Sixteen infants (11 girls, 5 boys) with a mean age at entry of 4.1 months and mean lesion area of 32.89 cm ^{2}, and volume of 39.98 cm^3 were enrolled. Two participants discontinued treatment early, one for an adverse event (crying upon application), the other because of the lack of compliance. Local skin reactions were consistent with those reported in adults. Two cases had a decrease and three had an increase in lesion parameters; otherwise no meaningful changes in lesion area, volume, or depth were observed. At the 4-month posttreatment visit, 11 of 14 subjects had improvement in erythema (marginal homogeneity test $= 2.668$, $p = 0.008$). Measured serum drug and interferon-alpha levels were low or undetectable.

Conclusions.—Treatment of infants with infantile hemangioma with imiquimod up to seven times per week for 16 weeks was generally well tolerated with low systemic exposure. Improvement was observed in hemangioma coloration, but not lesion size, suggesting effects were limited to the superficial component.

▶ Imiquimod has been known to exhibit intrinsic proapoptotic activity and is an immune response modifier approved for the treatment of various dermatologic conditions. It is theorized that it has some antiangiogenic activity, which was the rationale for the treatment of infantile hemangioma (IH) in this study. This is a study of 16 infants treated with imiquimod 5% cream applied during 16 weeks with posttherapy follow-up 16 weeks later. Treated infants were otherwise healthy and were up to 8.8 months of age. Absorption through the skin after topical application is thought to be minimal, but the authors measured serum and urine levels of imiquimod to evaluate pharmacokinetics in infants. They also measured interferon alpha (IFNα) levels, basic fibroblast growth factor (bFGF), and vascular endothelial growth factor (VEGF) to observe the proangiogenic activity of imiquimod. No significant differences in the plasma and urinary levels of VEGF and in plasma bFGF were observed compared with baseline, but minor transitory increases in serum transaminases were observed in 7 of 14 subjects. The authors observed that surface erythema in IH lesions treated with imiquimod was significant, but there was no improvement in the area, surface elevation, depth, or volume of the IH lesions after 4 months of treatment or after 4 months of posttreatment. The strengths of this study were evaluation of the pharmacokinetic data and safety profile of imiquimod in infants and the depth of the IH lesions using Doppler ultrasound after topical imiquimod use. However, this study did not have a control group to compare results. The authors also felt that treatment should have been introduced earlier in the proliferative phase at the mean age of 4.1 months to more likely induce a major response to therapy. This factor should also be considered when treating a lesion that usually undergoes involution during its natural disease course.

G. K. Kim, DO

J. Q. Del Rosso, DO

Incidence of adverse cutaneous drug reactions in a Mexican sample: an exploratory study on their association to tumour necrosis factor alpha TNF2 allele

Charli-Joseph Y, Cruz-Fuentes C, Orozco-Topete R (Universidad Nacional Autónoma de México; Instituto Nacional de Psiquiatría Ramón de la Fuente Muñiz, México DF; Instituto Nacional de Ciencias Médicas y Nutrición Salvador Zubiran, México DF)
J Eur Acad Dermatol Venereol 23:788-792, 2009

Background.—Most adverse cutaneous drug reactions (ACDR) are mediated by delayed hypersensitivity (dh) with lymphocyte recruitment and inflammatory cytokines release, including tumour necrosis factor alpha (TNFα). Polymorphisms in the TNFα gene, such as the infrequent allele TNF2, predispose to certain inflammatory entities and enhance TNFα production. The incidence of the TNF2 allele is increased in British patients with severe ACDR, suggesting TNFα as a major contributor in the pathogenesis of ACDR.

Objective.—We designed a prospective study to analyse the epidemiology of ACDR in a third-level Mexican hospital and explore the possibility of a relationship between the TNF2 allele and ACDR-dh.

Methods.—A prospective study during 9 months allowed recognition of 34 ACDR-dh patients. The study included 33 paired patients, and 44 healthy volunteers. All subjects were genotyped for TNF2 by PCR DNA amplification and *NcoI* restriction endonuclease digestion.

Results.—Incidence of ACDR was 0.95%. The TNF2 allele was detected in 9.9% of the sample population with no significant differences between healthy controls, and patients with or without ACDR-dh. Only 3 of the 34 ACDR-dh subjects presented severe reactions, with 1 having the TNF2 allele. Comorbidity analysis showed significance only with autoimmune thyroid disease, consistent with reports on Chinese and Tunisian patients.

Conclusion.—ACDR incidence and TNF2/TNFA heterozygosity were lower in Mexican than in Caucasian patients. ACDR-dh patients showed no increased frequency in the TNF2 allele.

▶ Adverse cutaneous drug reactions (ACDR) involving the skin can range from a mild cutaneous eruptions to topic epidermal necrolysis (TEN). Serious ACDRs can lead to hospitalizations associated with high costs to the health care system. The aim of this study was to evaluate the susceptibility to develop ACDR and the role of tumor necrosis factor-α (TNF-α) with a case-control study to explore a plausible trend associated with promoter region polymorphism at the chromosome 6 allele over a 9-month period at a hospital in Mexico. There were 34 patients with ACDR due to delayed hypersensitivity reaction and 44 controls. Medication that precipitated an ACDR included trimethoprim-sulphamethoxazole (10.6%) and prednisone (8.5%). The most common reaction was an exanthematous eruption (35.5%), fixed drug eruption (15.1%), acneiform eruption (10.8%), and urticaria (8.6%), with an average of 13.47 days as the mean latency between drug administration and skin lesions. Frequency of polymorphism in ACDR patients was similar to that seen in controls. The only association between frequency of TNF2 allele and any of the comorbidities present in the population under study was with autoimmune thyroid disease. The authors concluded that in this study there was no association with TNF2 allele and ACDR in this population of Mexicans. They also found lower incidences of ACDR in this population of Mexicans compared with Caucasians, which could reflect genetic differences, which suggest ethnic susceptibility to ACDR. In conclusion, although in this study there was no correlation with TNF2 allele and ACDR, one must keep in mind that genetic polymorphism can vary between populations and that while this appears to be true in this Mexican population, results may differ in other populations.

G. K. Kim, DO

J. Q. Del Rosso, DO

A prospective clinical trial of open-label etanercept for the treatment of hidradenitis suppurativa

Lee RA, Dommasch E, Treat J, et al (Univ of Pennsylvania School of Medicine; et al)
J Am Acad Dermatol 60:565-573, 2009

Background.—Medical therapies for hidradenitis suppurativa (HS) are often ineffective. Tumor necrosis factor-α inhibitors may be a potential treatment for patients with moderate to severe HS.

Objectives.—We sought to evaluate the safety and efficacy of etanercept for patients with severe HS.

Methods.—We conducted a phase II clinical trial of etanercept (50 mg/wk subcutaneously) in patients with moderate to severe HS. Efficacy was measured using a Physician Global Assessment and several secondary physician- and patient-reported outcome measures. Responders were classified as those achieving at least a 50% reduction on the Physician Global Assessment score at week 12 compared with baseline.

Results.—Only 3 of the 15 patients who entered the study were classified as responders (response rate of 20%; 95% confidence interval: 4.3-48.1) based on the intention-to-treat analysis. Dermatology Life Quality Index scores improved slightly from a median of 19 to 15 ($P = .02$). Comparison of baseline with week-12 Physician Global Assessment scores, and secondary outcome measures of lesion counts and patient pain scores, failed to show statistically significant improvement. Etanercept was generally well tolerated; however, two patients discontinued the study as a result of skin infections at the site of hidradenitis lesions requiring oral antibiotics.

Limitations.—Lack of a control group and a small number of participants are limitations.

Conclusions.—Our study demonstrated minimal evidence of clinically significant efficacy of etanercept (50 mg/wk subcutaneously) in the treatment of hidradenitis. Future studies using higher doses of etanercept are indicated; however, patients need to be carefully monitored for infection and other adverse events. Randomized, controlled trials will be necessary to demonstrate the risk-to-benefit ratio of tumor necrosis factor-α inhibitors in the treatment of hidradenitis.

▶ Hidradenitis suppurativa (HS) is a debilitating inflammatory disease often refractory to currently available medical and surgical treatment modalities. In recent years, biologics have emerged as an alternative treatment option for consideration. Previous studies with etanercept seemed promising. However, the small number of patients involved along with short duration of follow-up, limited broad conclusions regarding the efficacy, and longevity of biologic agents for the general population suffering from HS. Similar limitations are echoed in this study, as only 10 of the 15 patients enrolled were able to complete the trial. It still remains debatable whether use of biologic agents is an effective treatment option for HS patients. Clearly more research needs to be done. If clinicians are considering use of tumor necrosis factor-α inhibitors as an alternative option for their HS patients, it is recommended that the patient's purified protein derivative skin test for tuberculosis and chest X-ray be checked before use. Patients also need to be closely monitored for adverse effects.

S. Bellew, DO
J. Q. Del Rosso, DO

12 Drug Development and Promotion

Skin and systemic pharmacokinetics of tacrolimus following topical application of tacrolimus ointment in adults with moderate to severe atopic dermatitis
Undre NA, Moloney FJ, Ahmadi S, et al (Astellas Pharma GmbH, Munich, Germany; Univ of Sydney, New South Wales, Australia; Beacon Consultant Clinic, Dublin, Ireland; et al)
Br J Dermatol 160:665-669, 2009

Background.—Systemic exposure to tacrolimus following topical application of tacrolimus ointment is minimal. There are, however, no data on the distribution of tacrolimus in the skin.

Objectives.—To assess the distribution of tacrolimus in the skin and the systemic pharmacokinetics of tacrolimus in adults with moderate to severe atopic dermatitis after first and repeated application of tacrolimus ointment.

Methods.—We investigated skin distribution of topically applied tacrolimus and systemic pharmacokinetics of percutaneously absorbed tacrolimus in adults with atopic dermatitis after topical application of tacrolimus $0 \cdot 1\%$ ointment twice daily for 2 weeks. Tacrolimus concentrations were assessed in full-thickness skin biopsies and blood samples.

Results.—Of 14 patients, 11 completed treatment and were analysed. Mean ± SD tacrolimus concentrations in the skin at 24 h after first and last ointment applications were 94 ± 20 and 595 ± 98 ng cm^{-3}, respectively. At 168 h after stopping treatment, values were 97% lower than at 24 h after last application. Tacrolimus concentration decreased with increasing skin depth. Systemic tacrolimus exposure after ointment application was low and highly variable, with 31% of samples below the limit of quantification ($0 \cdot 025$ ng mL^{-1}) and 94% below 1 ng mL^{-1}. Blood concentrations at 24 h after the first and last ointment applications were 750 and 1800 times lower, respectively, than those in skin. Physicians' assessments showed that tacrolimus ointment was effective and well tolerated.

Conclusions.—Tacrolimus was primarily partitioned in the skin, with minimal systemic absorption after topical application, in patients with atopic dermatitis.

▶ Undre et al conducted a single-center, open-label pharmacokinetics phase II study to assess the distribution of tacrolimus in the skin as well as the pharmacokinetics to determine systemic concentration and exposure after cutaneous application for moderate to severe atopic dermatitis. The study was initially comprised of 14 patients with twice daily application of tacrolimus ointment for 2 weeks. It was concluded that tacrolimus is primarily partitioned in the skin with minimal systemic exposure.

The study confirmed that tacrolimus is partitioned primarily in the skin with a subsequent decrease in cutaneous concentration after discontinuing treatment, in addition to proving minimal systemic absorption. Despite this, some questions remain regarding the study, especially about the small number of subjects. Of the 14 patients that began the study, only 11 finished the trial and were available for analysis. Further, while it was noted that 1 patient did not finish the study secondary to clinical ineffectiveness, would that percentage have changed had more patients been added to the study? Moreover, the length of the study was for 2 weeks, while treatment in the real world is generally for a longer duration.

Regardless, the authors were able to show that tacrolimus is primarily partitioned in the skin after the last topical treatment, and a progressive decrease in the amount of tacrolimus drug concentration is seen at 96 and 168 hours after the last application. Furthermore, at the first and last application, convincing evidence was provided that the tacrolimus concentration was 750 to 1500 times lower in the systemic circulation versus in the skin at the same time points. Future data involving additional patients and additional treatment duration would be an interesting follow-up to this study.

B. D. Michaels, DO

J. Q. Del Rosso, DO

Enhancement of bioavailability by lowering of fat content in topical formulations

Wirén K, Frithiof H, Sjöqvist C, et al (ACO Hud Nordic AB, Sweden; Uppsala Univ, Sweden)
Br J Dermatol 160:552-556, 2009

Background.—The cosmetic properties of topical formulations are important parameters for the adherence to treatment, where modern oil-in-water emulsions are considered more acceptable compared with ointments. After application of an emulsion to the skin, the concentration of active ingredients in the formulation residue on the skin will increase, due to evaporation of volatile ingredients.

Objectives.—The aim of the present study was to investigate the effect of changes in vehicle fatty content on the skin penetration of two active ingredients: benzyl nicotinate (BN) and betamethasone valerate (BV).

Methods.—Formulations containing 0.5% BN and 0.3% BV in vehicles with different lipid content (10–80%) were applied in a randomized and double-blind manner to the forearm of healthy volunteers. The changes in skin colour (erythema and blanching) were then monitored visually and with a new noninvasive instrument.

Results.—The BN formulation containing 10% fat induced erythema more rapidly and with higher intensity than the formulations with higher fat content. Increased efficacy was also observed from the low-fat content formulation of BV, which gave more blanching than the formulations with high fat content.

Conclusions.—The rate of penetration of the active ingredients was inversely related to the lipid content, i.e. simple changes of the cosmetic properties by modifications of the lipid content may affect the efficacy of a formulation.

▶ With recent studies demonstrating cream vehicles to be more efficacious than ointments, the objective of this study was to investigate the changes of vehicle fat content on the skin penetration of 2 active ingredients: benzyl nicotinate (BN) and betamethasone valerate (BV). This was done by measuring the induced erythema and induced blanching effect from the penetration of BN and BV respectively, via quantified changes in skin color. In agreement with recent studies, the authors found an inverse relationship between vehicle lipid content and skin response. In other words, BN and BV demonstrated a faster and increased penetration when dissolved in a low-lipid vehicle.

The results of this study lead us to consider 2 important points. First, that creams may be more efficacious than ointments. In other words, vehicles with low-lipid levels and high water content result in a higher concentration of active ingredient on the skin. This is explained by the evaporation of the volatile components of the vehicle after skin application. Second, that changing the lipid content of the vehicle while keeping the concentration of active ingredient constant may vary the efficacy of the formula.

This study was conducted on a small number of healthy subjects (12 subjects for BN and 16 subjects for BV), only 1 type of lipid vehicle was used (polar lipid dicaprylyl maleate), and both active ingredients were lipophilic (ie, have an oil-water partition coefficient greater than one). Further investigations are required with increased number of subjects and with varying active ingredient and vehicle compounds. It should also be noted that subjects in this study were only required to discontinue caffeine and tobacco use as well as any topical products 1 hour before experimentation when the standard for percutaneous absorption experimentation is generally 24 hours. Yet, overall the study was well designed and the results may be significant. It is the authors' hope that the use of low-lipid vehicles such as creams and solutions will not only increase the efficacy of applied compounds but also increase patient compliance with topical medications.

J. Levin, DO

J. Q. Del Rosso, DO

Hematologic Safety of Dapsone Gel, 5%, for Topical Treatment of Acne Vulgaris

Piette WW, Taylor S, Pariser D, et al (John H. Stroger Jr Hosp of Cook County, Chicago, IL; Society Hill Dermatology, Philadelphia, PA; Virginia Clinical Res Inc, Norfolk; et al)

Arch Dermatol 144:1564-1570, 2008

Objective.—To evaluate the risk of hemolysis in subjects with glucose-6-phosphate dehydrogenase (G6PD) deficiency who were treated for acne vulgaris with either dapsone gel, 5% (dapsone gel), or vehicle gel.

Design.—Double-blind, randomized, vehicle-controlled, crossover study.

Setting.—Referral centers and private practice.

Participants.—Sixty-four subjects 12 years or older with G6PD deficiency and acne vulgaris.

Intervention.—Subjects were equally randomized to 1 of 2 sequences of 12-week treatment periods (vehicle followed by dapsone gel or dapsone gel followed by vehicle). The washout period was 2 weeks. Treatments were applied twice daily to the face and to other acne-affected areas of the neck, upper chest, upper back, and shoulders as required.

Main Outcome Measures.—Results of clinical chemical analysis and hematology values; plasma dapsone and N-acetyl dapsone concentrations; spontaneous reports of adverse events.

Results.—A 0.32-g/dL decrease in hemoglobin concentration occurred from baseline to 2 weeks during dapsone gel treatment. This was not accompanied by changes in other laboratory parameters, including reticulocytes, haptoglobin, bilirubin, and lactate dehydrogenase levels, and was not apparent at 12 weeks as treatment continued. The number of subjects with a 1-g/dL drop in hemoglobin concentration was similar between treatment groups at both week 2 and week 12. The largest drops in hemoglobin concentration were 1.7 g/dL in the vehicle gel treatment group and 1.5 g/dL in the dapsone gel treatment group. No clinical signs or symptoms of hemolytic anemia were noted.

Conclusions.—After treatment with dapsone gel, 5%, no clinical or laboratory evidence of drug-induced hemolytic anemia was noted in G6PD-deficient subjects with acne vulgaris.

Trial Registration.—clinicaltrials.gov Identifier: NCT00243542.

▶ This article evaluates the safety profile of topical dapsone gel 5% for the treatment of acne vulgaris. One of the known serious adverse effects of oral dapsone is drug-induced hemolytic anemia. The goal of this study was to evaluate the risk of developing hemolytic anemia in patients with glucose-6-phosphate dehydrogenase (G6PD) deficiency when using topical dapsone for treatment of acne vulgaris, given that patients with G6PD deficiency are more sensitive to developing hemolytic anemia. Given the requirement of both G6PD deficiency and acne vulgaris, the sample size of 64 patients is reasonable to extrapolate the conclusions to other similar patients.

The significance of this article is that even in patients with G6PD deficiency treated with topical dapsone, there was no clinical or laboratory evidence of drug-induced hemolytic anemia. With such information, it can be concluded that the risk of hemolytic anemia is remote, and thus the use of topical dapsone in the treatment of acne vulgaris does not warrant routine baseline G6PD testing. Overall, the article provides important data regarding the use of topical dapsone for the treatment of acne vulgaris.

B. D. Michaels, DO
J. Q. Del Rosso, DO

13 Practice Management and Managed Care

Recognition of skin malignancy by general practitioners: observational study using data from a population-based randomised controlled trial
Pockney P, Primrose J, George S, et al (Southampton General Hosp, UK; et al)
Br J Cancer 100:24-27, 2009

Skin malignancy is an important cause of mortality in the United Kingdom and is rising in incidence every year. Most skin cancer presents in primary care, and an important determinant of outcome is initial recognition and management of the lesion. Here we present an observational study of interobserver agreement using data from a population-based randomised controlled trial of minor surgery. Trial participants comprised patients presenting in primary care and needing minor surgery in whom recruiting doctors felt to be able to offer treatment themselves or to be able to refer to a colleague in primary care. They are thus relatively unselected. The skin procedures undertaken in the randomised controlled trial generated 491 lesions with a traceable histology report: 36 lesions (7%) from 33 individuals were malignant or pre-malignant. Chance-corrected agreement (κ) between general practitioner (GP) diagnosis of malignancy and histology was 0.45 (0.36–0.54) for lesions and 0.41 (0.32–0.51) for individuals affected with malignancy. Sensitivity of GPs for the detection of malignant lesions was 66.7% (95% confidence interval (CI), 50.3–79.8) for lesions and 63.6% (95% CI, 46.7–77.8) for individuals affected with malignancy. The safety of patients is of paramount importance and it is unsafe to leave the diagnosis and treatment of potential skin malignancy in the hands of doctors who have limited training and experience. However, the capacity to undertake all of the minor surgical demand works demanded in hospitals does not exist. If the capacity to undertake it is present in primary care, then the increased costs associated with enhanced training for general medical practitioners (GPs) must be borne.

▶ The concept behind this study was good to demonstrate that general practitioners (GPs) need enhanced training in dermatology to recognize skin malignancies because many perform minor dermatological surgery. This study used data collected on histological specimens to compare the quality of minor surgery performed by GPs and hospital doctors in one region of the United

Kingdom. In the United States (US), the majority of the minor dermatological surgeries are performed in private practice setting. This article does reference a study done in the US demonstrating the same conclusion that primary care physicians (PCPs) need to have improved diagnostic skills related to dermatology.[1] As increasing number of PCPs are performing biopsies and cryosurgery, they need to be properly educated and trained to not only detect malignant skin lesions but to also be able to perform appropriate dermatological procedure in diagnosing skin malignancies.

S. B. Momin, DO

J. Q. Del Rosso, DO

Reference

1. Whited JD, Hall RP, Simel DL, Horner RD. Primary care clinicians' performance for detecting actinic keratoses and skin cancer. *Arch Intern Med.* 1997;157: 985-990.

The relative ease of obtaining a dermatologic appointment in Boston: How methods drive results

Weingold DH, Lack MD, Yanowitz KL (Arkansas State Univ, Jonesboro)
J Am Acad Dermatol 60:944-948, 2009

Background.—Recent reports have indicated long wait times for dermatologic appointments even for changing moles.

Objective.—Our objective was to determine the wait time for a person willing to make multiple calls and accept an appointment from any dermatologist at any satellite location for a changing mole from a dermatologist who advertised in a Boston, MA, telephone book.

Methods.—We telephoned each practice listed in a Boston, MA, telephone book.

Results.—Patients making one call to each dermatologic practice on average obtained an appointment in 18 days. Patients calling two practices were offered an appointment on average in 7 days. Patients calling 3 practices were also offered an appointment in 1 week.

Limitations.—We only telephoned practices listed in a Boston, MA, telephone book and we only surveyed one urban area.

Conclusions.—These results suggest that a reasonable concerned patient who was willing to make multiple calls to different providers in Boston, MA, can be seen in a timely fashion.

▶ The Boston, MA, area has traditionally been considered one in which a dermatology appointment is difficult to obtain. A previous study has documented a 70-day wait time for patients seeking to see a dermatologist for a changing mole in that city's metropolitan region.[1] The results of this study contrast sharply with those previously reported, likely a reflection of the different methodologies used in the 2 studies. A commentary by Feldman and

Resneck that accompanied this article addressed the problem of how methods drive results and how we can use data generated by studies such as those discussed here to determine whether there is in fact a shortage (or oversupply) of dermatologists.[2] Feldman and Resneck addressed many of the variables that are difficult to quantify, not the least of which is the fact that most patients do not choose their dermatologist from the telephone book but from a list of physicians provided by their insurance provider. The 2007 American Academy of Dermatology Practice Profile data suggest that the average wait time for a dermatology visit is approximately 1 month.[3] This (in this reviewer's opinion) is still too long and forces patients to seek care from less well-trained individuals, some of whom are nonphysicians. It is in our interest and in the interest of our patients that any health care reform program assures that all patients have access to expert specialist care, including care for skin disease.

B. H. Thiers, MD

References

1. Tsang MW, Resneck JS Jr. Even patients with changing moles face long dermatology appointment wait-times: a study of simulated patient calls to dermatologists. *J Am Acad Dermatol.* 2006;55:54-58.
2. Feldman SR, Resneck JS Jr. Commentary: The relative ease of obtaining a dermatologic appointment in Boston. how methods drive results. *J Am Acad Dermatol.* 2009;60:949-950.
3. *Practice Profile Surveys (database provided to authors).* Schaumburg, IL: American Academy of Dermatology; 2007.

14 Miscellaneous Topics in Clinical Dermatology

Efficacy of Graduated Compression Stockings for an Additional 3 Weeks after Sclerotherapy Treatment of Reticular and Telangiectatic Leg Veins
Nootheti PK, Cadag KM, Magpantay A, et al (Dermatology/Cosmetic Laser Associates of La Jolla, Inc, CA)
Dermatol Surg 35:53-58, 2009

Background.—Sclerotherapy with post-treatment graduated compression remains the criterion standard for treating lower leg telangiectatic, reticular, and varicose veins, but the optimal duration for that postsclerotherapy compression is unknown.

Objective.—To determine whether 3 weeks of additional graduated compression with Class I compression stockings (20–30 mmHg) improves efficacy when used immediately after 1 week of Class II (30–40 mmHg) graduated compression stockings.

Methods.—Twenty-nine patients with reticular or telangiectatic leg veins were treated with sclerotherapy; one leg was assigned to wear Class II compression stocking for 1 week only, and the contralateral leg was assigned an additional 3 weeks of Class I graduated compression stocking.

Results and Conclusions.—Postsclerotherapy pigmentation and bruising was significantly less with the addition of 3 weeks of Class I graduated compression stockings.

▶ According to the results of this study, the additional use of class I compression stockings for 3 weeks (after 1 week of wearing class II compression stockings) may hasten the disappearance of postsclerotherapy pigmentation and bruising. The results of decreased pigmentation and bruising were subjectively assessed and scored by a physician and the patient, respectively. The authors found no statistical significance in the overall disappearance of leg veins or degree of superficial thrombophlebitis after wearing class I stockings for an additional 3 weeks.

Limitations of this study include the small sample size of patients tested as well as the subjective nature of evaluating and scoring the cosmetic improvement.

It should be noted that the improvement in hyperpigmentation and bruising seen in this study is likely only a temporary improvement, and the overall cosmetic result may have been equivalent if subjects were followed over a longer time period. If the final cosmetic result is indeed equivalent, then the recommendation for use of these highly uncomfortable and expensive stockings for 3 additional weeks is controversial.

J. Levin, DO
J. Q. Del Rosso, DO

Successful treatment of earlobe keloids in the pediatric population

Hamrick M, Boswell W, Carney D (Memorial Health Univ Med Ctr, Savannah, GA)
J Pediatr Surg 44:286-288, 2009

Background.—Keloid scars present a difficult treatment challenge. Recently, intralesional steroid injection has become a common treatment modality. Although this has become a proven treatment technique, there is no standard injection protocol to which treating physicians commonly adhere. We hypothesize that timing of steroid injection may improve outcomes using this treatment technique in combination with lesion excision.

Methods.—Fifteen patients with 16 earlobe keloids were treated using a standard steroid injection protocol with Kenalog (Bristol-Myers Squibb, New York, NY), in combination with lesion excision. Strict follow-up was enforced, with repeat injections as needed at any sign of abnormal scar formation postoperatively.

Results.—Of 16 lesions, 15 (94%) were treated successfully with no sign of lesion recurrence at 6 months of follow-up. A single lesion was lost to follow-up and presented 18 months postoperatively with recurrence. This lesion was subsequently retreated successfully.

Conclusions.—Kenalog injection in combination with excision is a well-tolerated and effective treatment of earlobe keloids in the pediatric population. We feel that timing of injection and adherence to a strict follow-up regimen is crucial to success.

▶ This small case study demonstrates success of using intralesional triamcinolone (Kenalog) injection (ILK) in combination with excision for treatment of keloid and reasons for its effectiveness. This article defines success as minimal scar formation with no evidence for scarring extending outside of the borders of the surgical incision at 6-month follow-up, but it does not discuss if there was hypertrophic scar formation in any of the patients. Although a small study size and no control group, this study does provide a good injection protocol to follow when treating keloid in the pediatric or adult population. The strength of intralesional triamcinolone injection was noted preoperatively, but there is no documentation of the strength used intraoperatively and postoperatively.

S. B. Momin, DO

J. Q. Del Rosso, DO

Effectiveness of Vitamin B_{12} in Treating Recurrent Aphthous Stomatitis: A Randomized, Double-Blind, Placebo-Controlled Trial

Volkov I, Rudoy I, Freud T, et al (Ben-Gurion Univ of the Negev Beer-Sheva, Israel)

J Am Board Fam Med 22:9-16, 2009

Background.—The frequency of recurrent aphthous stomatitis (RAS), the most common oral mucosa lesions seen in primary care, is up to 25% in the general population. However, there has been no optimal therapeutic approach. Our objective was to confirm our previous clinical observation of the beneficial treatment of RAS with vitamin B_{12}.

Methods.—A randomized, double-blind, placebo-controlled trial was done using primary care patients. A sublingual dose of 1000 mcg of vitamin B_{12} was used in patients in the intervention group for 6 months.

Results.—In total, 58 patients suffering from RAS participated in the study: 31 were included in the intervention group and 27 were included in control group. All parameters of RAS among patients in the intervention group were recorded and compared with the control group. The duration of outbreaks, the number of ulcers, and the level of pain were reduced significantly ($P < .05$) at 5 and 6 months of treatment with vitamin B_{12}, regardless of initial vitamin B_{12} levels in the blood. During the last month of treatment a significant number of participants in the intervention group reached "no aphthous ulcers status" (74.1% vs 32.0%; $P < .01$).

Conclusion.—Vitamin B_{12} treatment, which is simple, inexpensive, and low-risk, seems to be effective for patients suffering from RAS, regardless of the serum vitamin B_{12} level.

▶ Patients older than 18 years of age and who had been suffering from recurrent aphthous stomatitis (RAS) for at least 1 year, and with a frequency of at least 1 outbreak every 2 months were included in this randomized double-blinded placebo-controlled study. The patients took either 1000 mcg of vitamin B12 or placebo daily for 6 months with follow-up every month. The average duration of RAS episode (number of days) and the average number of RAS lesions per month decreased in both groups during the first 4 months of treatment. However, in the active (intervention) group, it continued to decrease in months 5 and 6. The subjective level of pain decreased throughout the study period in the active group while in the placebo group, a decline in reported pain level was noted only during the first 3 months with the pain level increasing in the last 3 months. More than 74.1% of patients in the active group were free from RAS lesions at the end of the treatment period compared with 32% of patients in the placebo group. Although this study was comprised of a small sample size, vitamin B12 does appear to provide an inexpensive, effective treatment for patients suffering from RAS either alone or as adjuvant therapy.

S. B. Momin, DO

J. Q. Del Rosso, DO

Density of Indoor Tanning Facilities in 116 Large U.S. Cities
Hoerster KD, Garrow RL, Mayer JA, et al (San Diego State Univ/Univ of California, San Diego, CA)
Am J Prev Med 36:243-246, 2009

Background.—U.S. adolescents and young adults are using indoor tanning at high rates, even though it has been linked to both melanoma and squamous cell cancer. Because the availability of commercial indoor tanning facilities may influence use, data are needed on the number and density of such facilities.

Methods.—In March 2006, commercial indoor tanning facilities in 116 large U.S. cities were identified, and the number and density (per 100,000 population) were computed for each city. Bivariate and multivariate analyses conducted in 2008 tested the association between tanning-facility density and selected geographic, climatologic, demographic, and legislative variables.

Results.—Mean facility number and density across cities were 41.8 (SD = 30.8) and 11.8 (SD = 6.0), respectively. In multivariate analysis, cities with higher percentages of whites and lower ultraviolet (UV) index scores had significantly higher facility densities than those with lower percentages of whites and higher UV index scores.

Conclusions.—These data indicate that commercial indoor tanning is widely available in the urban U.S., and this availability may help explain the high usage of indoor tanning.

▶ The widespread accessibility of indoor tanning facilities is a cause of concern, and many countries around the world are now regulating or considering regulation of their availability to minors. News reports in early 2009 indicate that Australia and Germany are at the forefront of this movement.

In terms of practical application of this article for the clinician, the article provides very limited useful information that can be incorporated into a practice setting. Although limited, the methodologies and conclusions of the article are best directed (and most useful) as a baseline for state, regional, and national organizations lobbying for more stringent regulation of the industry. Its premise is best used for incorporation into programs such as public service campaigns and community screening efforts.

On a very limited basis, the article may provide a clinician with some knowledge that these facilities are possibly more prevalent in their areas than they were aware of, and this may direct a more focused effort and resources to activities such as skin screenings and community education programs.

The article drew on previous studies effectively but then incorporated some serious weaknesses in its own methodologies. The ability to convert this data to small and midsized cities does not exist, and the sources from which they collected their data could not be easily validated and may not have been the most accurate available.

The widespread availability and lack of adequate regulation and monitoring is frightening. A coordinated effort by public health officials, preventative medical experts, and dermatologists is needed to counteract this frightening trend.

R. I. Ceilley, MD

Military Aeromedical Evacuations From Central and Southwest Asia for Ill-Defined Dermatologic Diseases

McGraw TA, Norton SA (Uniformed Services Univ of the Health Sciences, Bethesda, MD)
Arch Dermatol 145:165-170, 2009

Objectives.—To determine the diagnoses of US military patients medically evacuated from Central and Southwest Asia for ill-defined dermatologic diseases, to compare these diagnoses with data from earlier military conflicts, and to identify ways to reduce the number of dermatologic evacuations of military personnel from the combat zone.

Design.—We evaluated the preevacuation and postevacuation diagnoses of military personnel who were evacuated from Central and Southwest Asia for ill-defined dermatologic conditions. Outside the combat zone, these individuals were examined by dermatologists who provided a diagnosis regarded as correct for the purposes of this study. We excluded patients with precise pre-evacuation diagnoses, battle-related cutaneous injuries, and incomplete identifying data.

Setting.—The geographic area of responsibility for the US Central Command, including Iraq and Afghanistan. Data from January 1, 2003, through December 31, 2006, were obtained from aeromedical evacuation records and the military's electronic medical records system.

Patients.—A total of 170 patients evacuated from the combat zone for ill-defined dermatologic diseases, such as skin disorder, not otherwise specified (*International Classification of Diseases, Ninth Revision, Clinical Modification* code 709.9).

Main Outcome Measures.—The postevacuation diagnosis assigned, in nearly all cases, by a board-certified dermatologist.

Results.—Dermatitis, benign melanocytic nevus, malignant neoplasms, benign neoplasms, urticaria, and a group of nonspecific diagnoses were the most common post-evacuation diagnoses.

Conclusions.—We propose that thorough predeployment identification of individuals with chronic skin diseases, emphasis of preventive measures, and development of treatment plans will reduce the number of dermatologic evacuations. Improving diagnostic accuracy and treatment plans via teledermatology may also reduce evacuations. The most common dermatologic diseases leading to evacuations are similar to those from 20th century wars.

▶ Dermatologic conditions become more prevalent in hot and humid environments and account for more than half of the man-days lost during military operations. The most dramatic example of this was during the Vietnam War, when approximately half of the United States force in the Mekong delta region was immobilized because of a highly inflammatory zoonotic dermatophyte infection. Evacuation is reasonable when the affected individual cannot function or contribute to his unit, or when the individual is at risk because the skin condition makes it impossible to wear protective gear.

The study by McGraw and Norton sought to determine the conditions that led to aeromedical evacuations from the Gulf region. If ever there was an argument for the cost-effectiveness of telemedicine, this is it. In many cases, the cause for evacuation was not the seriousness or lack of response to treatment, but rather the uncertainty of diagnosis. It would be premature to say that telemedicine will solve all of these ills. Front line medicine presents a host of challenges, including lack of availability of medications, difficulty with compliance with treatment regimens, continued environmental exposure, and potential loss of biopsy specimens during transport.

Improvements can be achieved through careful predeployment screening and preventive measures, especially those aimed at dermatophytosis, immersion foot, and other environmental injuries.

D. M. Elston, MD

Nephrogenic Systemic Fibrosis: Late Skin Manifestations
Bangsgaard N, Marckmann P, Rossen K, et al (Univ Hosp of Copenhagen Gentofte, Hellerup, Denmark; Univ Hosp of Copenhagen Herlev, Denmark; et al)
Arch Dermatol 145:183-187, 2009

Background.—Nephrogenic systemic fibrosis (NSF) is a serious disease that occurs in patients with severe renal disease and is believed to be caused by gadolinium-containing contrast agents. A detailed description of the late skin manifestations of NSF is important to help dermatologists and nephrologists recognize the disease.

Observations.—We studied 17 patients with NSF late in the disease. All patients showed epidermal atrophy and hairlessness of the affected regions, primarily the lower legs. Affected areas were symmetrically distributed and hyperpigmented in most cases. Eleven patients showed confluent dermal plaques with thickening and hardening. In contrast, 3 patients presented with wrinkled, redundant skin as seen in cutis laxa. Patients with NSF had significantly poorer scores than control patients on the Daily Life Quality Index (mean [SD], 11. 4 [7.4] vs 1.5 [2. 3]; $P < .001$).

Conclusions.—This descriptive case series of patients with NSF gives a detailed clinical picture of the skin manifestations late in the disease. It demonstrates that the clinical picture in the late stage has a varied presentation and that NSF has a significant effect on the quality of life.

▶ This article is a good review of both the objective and subjective impact of nephrogenic systemic fibrosis (NSF). Dermatologists should become familiar with the assessment of patient profiles and cutaneous manifestations of the disease, particularly the differential diagnosis of scleroderma, scleromyxedema, and other disorders of fibrosis in comparison to NSF. These clinical findings of NSF, although more pronounced at late stages, are well described in the tables of the article and are often overlooked by clinicians unfamiliar with the disease.

In contrast to description of the late stage manifestations, there is suggestion of the correlation of serum procollagen III peptide to early onset disease, which although potentially useful as a marker, has little impact on prognostic features of NSF given its severity and poor treatment options.

This is a good overview for dermatologists of all levels of experience to familiarize or expand their understanding of a rare but significant disease described as potentially iatrogenic, yet lacking a remedy. Awareness of the presentation profiles might help provide patients with quality of life improvements if disease resolution may not yet be available.

N. Bhatia, MD

The Spectrum of Skin Disease Among Indian Children

Sardana K, Mahajan S, Sarkar R, et al (Maulana Azad Med College and Lok Nayak Hosp, Delhi, India; Lady Hardinge Med College, Delhi, India)
Pediatr Dermatol 26:6-13, 2009

Skin diseases in children are encountered frequently and their characterization is essential for the preparation of academic, research and health plans. A retrospective study was designed to evaluate the epidemiologic features of pediatric dermatoses in India. The setting was a tertiary care referral center in India (Kalawati Saran Children's Hospital, New Delhi) during January 1997 to December 2003. A total of 30,078 children less than 12 years of age with 32,341 new dermatoses were recorded, with a male to female ratio of 1.07:1. Most of the disease was seen in the 1- to 5-year age group (44.94%). The most common skin diseases were infections and infestations (47.15%) consisting of bacterial infections (58.09%) and scabies (21.54%), followed by eczemas (26.95%), infantile seborrheic dermatitis, scabies, and pityriasis alba. Other unique dermatoses in our settings were papular uticaria (3.59%), miliaria (5.46%), postinflammatory pigmentary abnormalities (1.68%), and nutritional deficiency dermatoses (0.45%). A majority of patients were diagnosed clinically and special diagnostic tests were conducted in 2.6% of patients. The most common diagnostic test used was KOH mount (59.2%), followed by skin biopsy (39%). Nearly 90% of patients were seen without any referral and in the remaining, a majority were referred by pediatricians (75%). A majority of patients were diagnosed to have infection followed by dermatitis in our setting.

▶ Sardana et al designed one of the largest retrospective studies to evaluate common skin dermatoses in Indian children and to compare the pattern of dermatoses among patients grouped into 3 categories: infants, preschool children, and school children. This is a very well referenced article and provides comparative results from many studies, including other tropical countries and countries from the west. This article and its references are excellent for primary care physicians and pediatricians to review and become aware of the common skin diseases seen in children. Interestingly, infections and infestations comprised almost half of the cases.

S. B. Momin, DO

J. Q. Del Rosso, DO

Lipodermatosclerosis: a clinicopathologic study of 17 cases and differential diagnosis from erythema nodosum

Huang T-M, Lee JY-Y (Natl Cheng Kung Univ Med College and Hosp, Tainan, Taiwan)
J Cutan Pathol 36:453-460, 2009

Background.—The clinical manifestations of lipodermatosclerosis (LDS) may mimic cellulitis and various panniculitides.

Methods.—To better characterize the histopathologic changes of LDS, we reviewed the clinicopathologic findings of 26 cases with a pathologic diagnosis consistent with LDS. A final diagnosis of LDS was made in 17 cases based on the clinicopathological correlation. As some cases manifested erythema nodosum (EN)-like lesions, 14 specimens of EN were reviewed to identify features for differential diagnosis.

Results.—Microscopically, the acute LDS lesions were characterized by patchy hemorrhage, ischemic fat necrosis with lipophages or hyalinization in the fat lobules. As the disease progressed to the subacute and chronic stages, lipomembranous or membranocystic fat necrosis, septal fibrosis and background venous stasis in the dermis became more pronounced. In contrast, EN typically displayed minimal venous stasis and membranocystic fat necrosis.

Conclusions.—LDS may manifest as EN-like lesions. Therefore LDS should be included in the differential diagnosis of EN. Clinicopathologic correlation is essential for diagnosis. Differentiating the acute LDS from the early EN is more difficult. A constellation of the findings of septal/lobular panniculitis, hemorrhage in the subcutaneous tissue, and lipophages and/or ischemic fat necrosis in the fat lobules favors the diagnosis of acute LDS. Huang T-M, Lee JY-Y. Lipodermatosclerosis: a clinicopathologic study of 17 cases and differential diagnosis from erythema nodosum.

▶ This is a good review article to differentiate lipodermatosclerosis (LDS) from erythema nodosum (EN). LDS is a fibrosing septo-lobular panniculitis with fat necrosis associated with venous stasis. Clinically, as the disease progresses, there are varicosities, venous ulcers, mottled hyperpigmentation, and sclerosis leading to an inverted champagne bottle appearance of the lower legs. Histologically, the early stage of LDS is characterized by septal lymphocytic infiltrate, ischemic necrosis, and lobular hemorrhage. The intermediate stage shows stasis changes with perivascular lymphocytic infiltrate in the dermis, lipophagic fat necrosis of the adipose lobules, and increasing fibrosis. The late stage of LDS is characterized by stasis changes, dermal atrophy, subcutaneous fibrosis, extensive fat microcysts, and membranous fat necrosis. Clinically, EN presents with bilateral, symmetrical, tender nodules, and plaques on lower legs, mainly the anterior tibial region. Histologically, venous stasis is minimal in EN and the panniculitis is primarily septal with little or no ischemic fat necrosis in the lobules. There is more prominent granulomatous infiltrate with aggregates of histiocytes forming Miescher's radial granuloma.

S. B. Momin, DO

J. Q. Del Rosso, DO

Lack of efficacy of topical latanoprost and bimatoprost ophthalmic solutions in promoting eyelash growth in patients with alopecia areata
Roseborough I, Lee H, Chwalek J, et al (Univ of Iowa; Kaiser Permanente Med Group, Richmond, CA; Univ of Maryland, Baltimore; et al)
J Am Acad Dermatol 60:705-706, 2009

Background.—Treatments have been developed for regrowing scalp and eyebrow hair in persons with alopecia areata (AA), but not for regrowing eyelashes. Latanoprost and bimatoprost reduce intraocular pressure in open-angle glaucoma and have the side effect of eyelash hypertrichosis. The efficacy of these agents in treating eyelash regrowth in patients with AA was reported in a research letter published in the *Journal of the American Academy of Dermatology*.

Methods.—Eleven adult patients with AA were randomly assigned to receive either latanoprost or bimatoprost. Medication was applied using a cotton-wrapped applicator directly to the upper and lower eyelid margins of one eye once a day; the contralateral eye served as a control. Patients were seen by a dermatologist at four visits, 4 weeks apart. At each visit eyelid margins were checked for lash growth, and iris color or periorbital discoloration was noted. Slit lamp examination, intraocular pressure measurements, and photographs were also obtained every 8 weeks. Schirmer examination test strips photographed on the eyelid margin documented eyelash length.

Results.—Although the cutaneous applications were well tolerated, none of the patients experienced appreciable regrowth of their eyelashes. Iris color, periorbital color, and intraocular pressure showed no significant change.

Conclusions.—The prostaglandin analogues did not stimulate appreciable eyelash regrowth in these patients with AA. Such lack of regrowth may be caused by insufficient stimulation or blockage of an essential hair growth mediator. It was hypothesized that ocular instillation may be a more effective way to apply prostaglandin analogues to stimulate eyelash regrowth.

▶ Latanoprost and bimatoprost are prostaglandin F2-α analogues, both of which reduce intraocular pressure in patients with open-angle glaucoma. A 16-week randomized, investigator masked, controlled study was done to evaluate the efficacy of these agents in promoting eyelash growth in alopecia areata patients with greater than 50% bilateral eyelash loss for 6 months or longer. The patients applied either latanoprost or bimatoprost solution to the affected upper and lower eyelid margins of one eye only, once daily. The untreated contralateral eye served as the control. Eyelash length was estimated using Schirmer exam test strips photographed on the eyelid margin. Eleven patients completed the study and no eyelash regrowth was appreciated. The same concentration was used as in the management of glaucoma.

Latanoprost was first documented to stimulate hair growth in 1997, and mean increase in eyelash length of the lower eyelid was 19.5% in the treated eye. Two patients demonstrated an increase in the number of eyelashes, but there was no measurable eyelash length change.[1]

The suggested mechanism of minoxidil is through its effect of prostaglandin E2 synthesis. It is reasonable to assume other prostaglandin analogs would provide positive results in stimulating hair growth. However, latanoprost and bimatoprost were not efficacious in promoting eyelash growth in patients whose eyelash regions are affected by alopecia areata.

S. B. Momin, DO

J. Q. Del Rosso, DO

Reference

1. Johnstone M. Hypertrichosis and increase pigmentation of eyelashes and adjacent hair in the region of the ipsilateral eyelids of patients treated with unilateral topical lantanoprost. *Am J Opthalmol.* 1997;124:544-547.

Sensitive skin in Europe

Misery L, Boussetta S, Nocera T, et al (Univ of Western Brittany, Brest, France; Dept of Public Health, Pierre Fabre, France; Eau Thermale Avène, France)
J Eur Acad Dermatol Venereol 23:376-381, 2009

Introduction.—Sensitive skin appears as a very frequent condition, but there is no comparative data between countries.

Objectives.—To perform an epidemiological approach to skin sensitivity in different European countries.

Methods.—An opinion poll was conducted in eight European countries: Belgium, France, Germany, Greece, Italy, Portugal, Spain and Switzerland. This sample (4506 persons) was drawn from a representative sample of each population aged 15 years or older.

Results.—Sensitive or very sensitive skin was declared by 38.4% and slightly or not sensitive skin by 61.6%. Women declared more sensitive skin than men. A dermatological disease was declared by 31.2% of people with very sensitive skin, 17.6% of those with sensitive skin, 8.7% of those with slightly sensitive skin and 3.7% of those who do not have sensitive skin. A history of childhood atopic dermatitis was more frequent in patients with sensitive or very sensitive skin. The interviewees who declared that they had dry or oily skin also reported significantly more frequently sensitive or very sensitive skin than those with normal skin. Sensitive and very sensitive skins were clearly more frequent in Italy and France.

Discussion.—This study is the first study that compares skin sensitivity in European countries. Prevalence is high, but significant differences are noted between these countries. Dermatological antecedents (or treatments?) could be involved in the occurrence of skin sensitivity.

▶ The aim of this study was to compare patient declared sensitive skin epidemiology data among 8 European countries. Interviewers not only responded to questions about the presence of sensitive skin, but also were then asked about the occurrence of sensitive skin symptoms such as prickling, burning, flushing, and irritation.

The results of this study suggest that prevalence of sensitive skin varies according to country. The prevalence of self-declared sensitive skin was highest in Italy and France. The authors hypothesize that cultural factors may play a larger role than ethnic factors as the European population is crossbred. The authors also considered that the people in Italy and France may be generally more aware of sensitive skin as numerous media dollars are dedicated to promotion of beauty and skin care in these countries.

By design the authors of this survey were assessing the prevalence of sensitive skin in differing environments rather than ethnicity. For example, just because an interviewer lives in Italy does not mean that they themselves have Italian heritage. It would have been interesting to gather ancestry data in addition to the other data collected in this study to determine if a correlation exists between heritage and the presence of sensitive skin. Additionally, environments within the European countries themselves vary greatly from city to city. Perhaps generalizing a European country as a whole is too broad an approach for such a survey.

It should be noted that the determinations of sensitive skin versus nonsensitive skin where made by the patients and not by physicians, other qualified health professionals, or by standardized criteria. Therefore, the data presented in this study could be severely overestimated or underestimated.

J. Levin, DO

J. Q. Del Rosso, DO

Dystrophic Calcification in Chronic Leg Ulcers—A Clinicopathologic Study

Wollina U, Hasenöhrl K, Köstler E, et al (Dept of Dermatology and Allergology, Dresden, Germany; et al)
Dermatol Surg 35:457-461, 2009

Background.—Dystrophic calcification (DC) is a risk factor for conservative treatment failure in chronic leg ulcers of various pathologies.

Patients and Methods.—We performed a retrospective noncontrolled trial of 212 patients with 362 chronic leg ulcers who underwent ulcer shave excision with subsequent skin grafting. The ulcers existed for at least 3 months, and no healing was achieved with good ulcer care. Tissue was subjected to histopathology (hematoxylin-eosin and van Kossa stains).

Results.—DC was evident in 39 patients (18%). Metaplastic subcutaneous bone formation was observed in 15 patients (7%). Clinical symptoms associated with DC were resistance to good ulcer care, pain, and ineffective effects of compression therapy (in venous ulcers). Ulcers were treated with deep dermatome shaving of the ulcer bed and surgical removal of DC. In the same setting, defects were closed using mesh graft transplantation. The procedure achieved a complete take rate in 80% and a significant decrease of pain in 95% of cases. When comparing the take rates in patients with and without DC, DC had a negative effect on outcome (take rate: 91% without DC vs 80% with DC, $p < .05$).

Conclusions.—DC is resistant to conservative treatment. The first-line treatment is deep ulcer dermatome shaving and complete removal of calcifications whenever possible.

▶ The aim or objective of this article is very hard to interpret. We, the reviewers, were not sure if the authors were trying to provide retrospective evidence that ulcers with dystrophic calcification (DC) are harder to treat or if the authors were trying to determine the best therapy for those with DC positive ulcers.

In any case, the conclusion of this article seems to be that patients who suffer from chronic legs ulcers with DC typically do not respond well to conservative treatment such as application of hydrogel dressings, and the best method of treatment may be deep dermatome shaving of the ulcer bed with surgical removal of DC combined with split-skin grafting. However, the authors note that even this technique has less of a success rate than in those leg ulcer cases that do not exhibit DC.

While these specific conclusions were made, there was no actual data presented comparing conservative treatment failure for leg ulcers without DC versus leg ulcers with DC. More scientifically accumulated data would be helpful to understand the impact of DC on ulcer treatment.

In conclusion, this study is limited by its unclear objective, the retrospective nature of the study, lack of sound scientific methodology, and absence of comparison with control.

J. Levin, DO

J. Q. Del Rosso, DO

Impact of neurofibromatosis 1 upon quality of life in childhood: a cross-sectional study of 79 cases
Wolkenstein P, Rodriguez D, Ferkal S, et al (Paris 12 Univ, Créteil, France; Paris 6 Univ, France; Clinical Investigation Centre, Créteil, France; et al)
Br J Dermatol 160:844-848, 2009

Background.—Neurofibromatosis 1 (NF1) has a significant impact on quality of life (QoL).

Objectives.—To evaluate QoL in NF1 according to phenotype from the viewpoint of children and proxy.

Methods.—One hundred and forty families with a child aged between 8 and 16 years, seen consecutively at the National Academic Paediatric Referral Centre for NF1 for a phenotype evaluation, were contacted by mail. Families agreeing to participate were sent two questionnaires, the DISABKIDS for children and proxy and the cartoon version of the Children's Dermatology Life Quality Index (CDLQI). QoL scores were compared with those in other major diseases and were analysed according to age, gender and phenotype.

Results.—Eighty families agreed to participate, and 79 returned the questionnaires. Using DISABKIDS, NF1 had a higher impact on health-related QoL than asthma (mean ± SD $75·18 ± 18·22$ vs. $79·78 ± 13·41$; $P = 0·005$). The total score was more altered when assessed by proxy than by children ($71·20 ± 17·94$ vs. $75·18 ± 18·22$; $P = 0·002$). Orthopaedic manifestations, learning disabilities and presence of at least two plexiform neurofibromas were independently associated with a higher impact ($P < 0·01$). The CDLQI score was slightly altered ($11·3\%$). Dermatological signs, such as café-au-lait spots and freckling, did not have a significant impact.

Conclusions.—Orthopaedic manifestations, learning disabilities and plexiform neurofibromas are the main complications impacting on QoL during childhood NF1. QoL could be considered as an endpoint for intervention studies in this context.

▶ This study explored the impact of neurofibromatosis (NF1) on quality of life (QoL) during childhood with a specific interest on influence of phenotype (including dermatological changes) from the viewpoint of proxy and patients. This well designed and executed study demonstrated the strong impact of NF-1 on QoL of children and their families. This impact was higher than some other chronic diseases such as asthma, but lower than diseases such as psoriasis or diffuse eczema. As expected, the authors determined that the presence of certain phenotypes more significantly impacted QoL than others.

The authors suggest the need for additional support for children with NF-1 with a poor QoL. This is because children with NF-1 are characterized by behavioral and developmental problems during adulthood, likely as a result of QoL and self-esteem issues related to the disease. Social support and family functioning are reported to be strongly associated with increased psychological well-being. Strategies that enhance self-esteem at a young age may be able to prevent the development of these behavior problems and help academic functioning. The results of this study suggest that those children that possess phenotypic markers associated with poor QoL should be given special attention and offered support at an early age.

This study has several limitations that are well summarized by the authors. First, their population was hospital based, which could have possibly led to an overestimation of the severity of the disease when compared with the general population. Second, the QoL questionnaires were not specifically designed for children with NF-1, a disadvantage for accuracy, but an advantage for comparison with other chronic diseases. Third, the authors chose children with other chronic diseases in various European cultures as controls, thereby introducing a potential cultural bias. Further studies should be conducted to confirm these findings in other settings and countries.

J. Levin, DO

J. Del Rosso, DO

Efficacy and safety of tacrolimus ointment 0·1% vs. betamethasone 17-valerate 0·1% in the treatment of chronic paronychia: an unblinded randomized study
Rigopoulos D, Gregoriou S, Belyayeva E, et al (Univ of Athens, Greece)
Br J Dermatol 160:858-860, 2009

Background.—Recent studies have established the pivotal role of irritants and allergens in development of chronic paronychia and the significant improvement with corticosteroid therapy.

Objectives.—The objective of this randomized, unblinded, comparative study was to compare the efficacy of tacrolimus ointment 0·1% vs. betamethasone 17-valerate 0·1% in the treatment of chronic paronychia.

Methods.—Forty-five patients with chronic paronychia were randomized 1 : 1 : 1 to apply twice daily either betamethasone 17-valerate 0·1% or tacrolimus 0·1% ointment or emollient. Protective measures were counselled to all patients. Treatment duration was 3 weeks and patients were followed for an additional 6 weeks.

Results.—Eight patients in the betamethasone group were considered as cured, two as improved and four as nonresponders at the end of the treatment period. Thirteen patients in the tacrolimus group were considered as cured and one as improved at the end of the treatment period. Nine patients in the emollient group were considered as stable and six failed to respond. Both betamethasone and tacrolimus groups presented statistically significantly greater cure or improvement rates when compared with the emollient group ($P < 0·001$).

Conclusions.—Tacrolimus ointment appears to be a more efficacious agent than betamethasone 17-valerate or placebo for the treatment of chronic paronychia.

▶ Recent studies have shown that inflammation, allergens, and irritants play a role in chronic paronychia. Topical corticosteroids have been shown in some studies to be an effective treatment. The authors surmised that tacrolimus may also be effective due to its anti-inflammatory properties. This study compared the efficacy of tacrolimus ointment and betamethasone 17-valerate ointment with an emollient placebo in the treatment of chronic paronychia. Patients with a positive potassium hydroxide preparation or fungal culture were excluded from the study, as *Candida* spp have been shown in past studies to contribute to chronic paronychia, although the exact role of the presence of these yeast organisms is unclear. Both topical betamethasone and topical tacrolimus resulted in a significantly greater cure rate when compared with the emollient group ($P < .001$). Tacrolimus appeared to have a greater cure rate compared with betamethasone, but statistics for this comparison were not reported or discussed in this article. Interestingly, the authors chose to use an ointment form of the study drugs, but a cream-based emollient for the placebo comparison. It is possible that this difference contributed to the benefit of the ointment-based drugs over placebo? Furthermore, while the authors conclude that tacrolimus is more efficacious than betamethasone in treating chronic paronychia, they do not provide results from any statistical evaluations to support this statement. A larger study may be necessary to show a significant difference between these 2 treatments.

J. Moore, MD
P. Rich, MD

Changes in hands microbiota associated with skin damage because of hand hygiene procedures on the health care workers

Rocha LA, Ferreira de Almeida E Borges L, Gontijo Filho PP (The Imunologia e Parasitologia Aplicadas, Programa de Pós Graduaçãxo em Imunologia e Parasitologia Aplicadas; Área de Imunologia, Microbiologia e Parasitologia, Instituto de Ciências Biomédicas, Universidade Federal de Uberlândia, Minas Gerais, Brazil)
Am J Infect Control 37:155-159, 2009

Background.—The purpose of this study was evaluating the microbial flora of nurses' healthy (n = 30) and damaged hand (n = 30) by frequent handwashing and/or wearing of gloves.

Methods.—Hand cultures were obtained both before and after washing hands with nonantimicrobial soap, through the sterile polyethylene bag method.

Results.—The bacteria counts of the hands of professionals with damaged hands were higher than those with healthy hands, and those with damaged hands presented higher frequency of *Staphylococcus aureus*, 16.7% versus 10%; gram-negative bacteria, 20% versus 6.7%; and yeast, 26.7% versus 20%, respectively, as well as the sum of these microorganisms. The presence of *Staphylococcus haemolyticus* was only seen in nurses with damaged hands ($P = .02$), and enterococci were not recovered from the hands of any volunteer. The presence of antimicrobial-resistant *S aureus* and gram-negative bacteria was also greater among damaged hands.

Conclusion.—The irritation caused on the skin by frequent washing and/or wearing of gloves is associated with changes in hands microbial flora, and their potential risks should be considered when institutions/users are selecting products/formulations to assure hands skin health and consequent compliance with their own hygiene procedures.

▶ The hand has long been recognized as an important vector in the transmission of pathogens in health care settings be it the operating theater, newborn nursery, or in-patient floor. Frequent hand washing between patient contact, use of antimicrobial cleansers, alcohol-based hand rubs and gloves are important preventive measures that can lead to damaged skin. This study confirms results from previous studies and demonstrates that damaged skin is associated with increased numbers of microorganisms and higher carriage rates of potential pathogens. The method of recovery of microorganisms from the hand is known as the "glove juice" test and involves placing the hand in a sterile bag containing a nonionic detergent to facilitate removal of organisms and to disperse macro colonies into colony-forming units on general and selective media. This permits quantitative and qualitative analyses. This method also samples the subungual spaces, which are rich sources of numerous species of microorganisms that can find their way into the surgeon's glove and potentially to the operative field if there is glove breakage. The microbial flora of the hand is also influenced by factors other than irritation by detergents and gloves eg, individuals with atopic dermatitis have a high carriage rate of *S aureus* on their hands even when hands are clinically normal in appearance.[1-3]

J. Leyden, MD

References

1. Leyden JJ, McGinley KJ, Kates SG, Myung KB. Subungual bacteria of the hand: contribution to the glove juice test; efficacy of antimicrobial detergents. *J Inf Control & Hospital Epidem.* 1989;10:451-454.
2. McGinly KJ, Larson EI, Leyden JJ. Composition and density of the microflora in the subungual space. *J Clin Micro.* 1988;26:950-953.
3. Willliams JV, Vowels B, Honig P, Leyden JJ. Staphylococcus aureus isolation from the lesions, the hands, and anterior nares of patients with atopic dermatitis. *J Emer Med.* 1999;17:207-211.

Similar Deficiencies in Procedural Dermatology and Dermatopathology Fellow Evaluation Despite Different Periods of ACGME Accreditation: Results of a National Survey
Freeman SR, Nelson C, Lundahl K, et al (Univ of Colorado at Denver; Univ of Nevada School of Medicine, Reno)
Dermatol Surg 34:873-876, 2008

Background.—Fellow evaluation is required by the Accreditation Council for Graduate Medical Education (ACGME). Procedural dermatology fellowship accreditation by the ACGME began in 2003 while dermatopathology accreditation began in 1976.

Objective.—The objective was to compare fellow evaluation rigor between ACGME-accredited procedural dermatology and dermatopathology fellowships.

Methods.—Questionnaires were mailed to fellowship directors of the ACGME-accredited (2006–2007) procedural dermatology and dermatopathology fellowship programs. Information was collected regarding evaluation form development, delivery, and collection.

Results.—The response rates were 74% (25/34) and 53% (24/45) for procedural and dermatopathology fellowship programs, respectively. Sixteen percent (4/25) of procedural dermatology and 25% (6/24) of dermatopathology programs do not evaluate fellows. Fifty percent or less of program (4/8 procedural dermatology and 3/7 dermatopathology) evaluation forms address all six core competencies required by the ACGME.

Conclusion.—Procedural fellowships are evaluating fellows as rigorously as the more established dermatopathology fellowships. Both show room for improvement because one in five programs reported not evaluating fellows and roughly half of the evaluation forms provided do not address the six ACGME core competencies.

▶ In academic medicine the evaluation of fellows and residents are important factors that Accreditation Council for Graduate Medical Education (ACGME) programs must do; 6 core competencies are included.

This article points out that the similar evaluation of the dermatological procedure program and dermatopathological fellows suffers from a lack of core competency evaluations of a standardized evaluation. Fellowship programs could be improved with a more standardized evaluation of these 6 core competencies. The requirement for evaluation of core competency was only 39% in dermatopathology and 38% in procedural fellowship evaluation. There was less than 50% of program evaluation in all 6 core competencies.

Although the fellowship program in procedural dermatology is relatively new, it is rapidly growing in number. These are postresidency fellow positions. The requirements from the ACGME are that all fellows are evaluated; there were 15% (4/25) procedural programs and 25% (6/24) dermatopathology programs that did not evaluate fellows. These data are based on a voluntary small survey population.

L. Cleaver, DO

The Cross-Section Trichometer: A New Device for Measuring Hair Quantity, Hair Loss, and Hair Growth

Cohen B (Univ of Miami, Coral Gables, FL)
Dermatol Surg 34:900-910, 2008

Background.—Office physicians are unable to measure hair quantity, hair loss, and hair growth in a simple and meaningful manner. One solution is to measure the cross-sectional area of a bundle of hair that is growing within a premeasured cross-section of scalp.

Objective.—The objective was to design a mechanical device that precisely measures the cross-sectional area of a bundle of hair and design a device that can precisely delineate an area of scalp. It was assumed that density and diameter changes are evidenced by changes in the bundle cross-sectional area and that growth and loss are the result of density and diameter changes. These assumptions were confirmed using various sized bundles of known diameter non-hair filaments.

Materials and Methods.—Bundles of hair and surgical silk fibers were tested using a mechanical device that compressed the bundle and measured its cross-sectional area. Balding patients were categorized according to their observed severity of the loss. Bundles of their uncut hair from 4-cm^2 scalp sites were measured and the values were compared to the patient's category of hair loss severity.

Results.—In patients with balding, there was a direct correlation between the bundle's cross-sectional area and the observed severity of the loss. The cross-sectional area was expressed as square millimeters of hair per square centimeter of skin × 100 (mm^2/cm^2 × 100) and named the trichometric index (TI). Using surgical silk fibers, there was a direct correlation between the bundle's cross-sectional area and the number of filaments, the diameter of the filaments, and the dry weight of the filament bundle. Using aggregates of cut human hair, there was a direct correlation between the cross-sectional area and the dry weight of the bundle.

Conclusion.—This prototype device shows promise as a diagnostic instrument for measuring changes in hair quantity (mass), hair diameter, and hair density, as evidenced by preliminary studies using silk sutures, cut human hair, and patients with various degrees of balding. Formal clinical studies are needed. Although the device itself showed a high degree of precision, the accuracy and reproducibility of the measurements can be compromised if the sampling method is not carefully performed using magnification. The device is intended for use on uncut hair that is more than 1 inch in length.

▶ Visual inspection and physician global assessment are notoriously problematic in the assessment of hair density. In clinical trials, where objective measurements are critical, the gold standard has been standardized photography, or Vera Price's method of harvesting and weighing defatted hair from a defined area of the scalp. The latter method has the advantage of allowing quantitative comparisons, but is labor-intensive and difficult to perform. The author's method of measuring the cross-sectional area of a bundle of hair also allows for quantitative comparisons and is easier to perform.

The method was studied on surgical silk fibers and needs to be validated in clinical studies. It has the advantage of measuring both density and diameter, but cannot distinguish between changes in the two. Issues of compressibility and shaft fracture will have to be investigated, but this is a promising tool that is likely to be adopted widely.

D. M. Elston, MD

A survey of the quality and accuracy of information leaflets about skin cancer and sun-protective behaviour available from UK general practices and community pharmacies
Nicholls S, Hankins M, Hooley C, et al (Brighton and Sussex Med School, Brighton, UK)
J Eur Acad Dermatol Venereol 23:566-569, 2009

Background.—Better information promotes sun protection behaviour and is associated with earlier presentation and survival for malignant melanoma.

Aim.—To assess the quality of patient information leaflets about skin cancer and sun-protective behaviour available from general practices and community pharmacies.

Design of Study.—A structured review of patient information leaflets.

Setting.—All community pharmacies and general practices in one Primary Care Trust were invited to supply leaflets.

Methods.—Readability was assessed using the SMOG scoring system. Presentation and content were reviewed using the Ensuring Quality Information for Patients (EQIP) guidelines. Three consultant dermatologists assessed each leaflet for accuracy.

Results.—Thirty-one different patient information leaflets were returned. Thirteen (42%) were published in the previous 2 years, but 10 (32%) were over 5 years old. Nine (29%) leaflets were produced by the NHS or Health Education Authority, and 8 (27%) were linked to a commercial organization. One leaflet had readability in the primary education range (SMOG score = 6), and none with the recommended range for health education material (SMOG score ≤ 5). Two leaflets (6%) were in the highest quartile of EQIP score for presentation and content. Five leaflets (17%) had a major inaccuracy such as over-reliance on sun screen products instead of shade and clothing.

Conclusions.—Leaflets were of variable quality in presentation and content. All required a reading age higher than recommended. All leaflets with major inaccuracies had links with commercial organizations. This study raises important issues about the potential conflict between marketing and health messages in the way sun creams are promoted.

▶ Providing patient education is critically important in changing behavior of patients. This is especially true in trying to modify the patient's behavior in regards to their sun protection, potential for evaluation of serious skin lesions, and prevention of both melanoma and nonmelanoma skin cancers.

This short study examines the quality and accuracy of information about skin cancer and sun protection available in the United Kingdom's general practice and community pharmacies. This article is a rating of the collection of various literature used and distributed to patients. A sampling of leaflets in the area of community pharmacies and general practices in the Brighton and Holt areas in the United Kingdom were reviewed. Thirty-one were analyzed and reviewed for content, accuracy, readability, and were summarized and critically acclaimed. The importance of this is for us to review our current literature. General practices and information provided by dermatologists needs to be updated continuously and we need to have the information to be readable. It was estimated that the general public in England is at an 11-year-old reading level. Defects and major inaccuracies of the leaflets were reviewed. It is a necessity to continuously review our own information that is used and distributed so that it is accurate, up-to-date, and useful information for our patients.

L. Cleaver, DO

Wet dressings used with topical corticosteroids for pruritic dermatoses: A retrospective study

Bingham LG, Noble JW, Davis MDP (Mayo Clinic, Rochester, MN)
J Am Acad Dermatol 60:792-800, 2009

Background.—Wet dressings are a mainstay for initial management of pruritic adult dermatoses at Mayo Clinic, yet few recent reports describe their effectiveness for pruritic conditions other than atopic dermatitis in children.

Objective.—To examine the effectiveness of wet dressings for pruritic dermatoses.

Methods.—This is a retrospective study of adult patients admitted to our inpatient dermatology service between January 1, 2004, and August 31, 2007, treated with wet dressings and topical corticosteroids. Improvement was evaluated 1 day after admission and at dismissal.

Results.—Three hundred thirty-one patients with pruritus (54 unique diagnoses) had 391 admissions. Improvement was reported for 146 (94%) of 156 admissions at 1 day after admission and for 351 (98%) of 357 admissions at dismissal.

Limitations.—Retrospective nature of study.

Conclusions.—Wet dressings effectively alleviate recalcitrant pruritic dermatoses in adults. The lack of published reports on this treatment method suggests that wet dressings are underused.

▶ Wet dressings were historically used since the last century for wound care and treatment of inflamed skin. However, authors state that lack of recent reports on efficacy of wet dressings indicate that it is an underused treatment modality. This retrospective study looked at 331 patients with severe pruritus successfully treated with wet dressings in conjunction with topical corticosteroids. The wet dressing instructions for home (Table 4 in the original article) are the most beneficial piece of information in this article for clinicians practicing in outpatient settings. However, there are limitations to this study, which includes those that are inherent to retrospective studies as stated by the authors. Results were limited by missing data in medical records, and only one institution was evaluated. Therefore, results may not by generalizable to other settings. In addition, patients were treated as inpatients and therefore, methods or results may not be applicable or practical in the outpatient setting. In summary, clinicians should consider the option of using wet dressing therapy for management of pruritic dermatoses where potentially applicable.

S. Bellew, DO
J. Q. Del Rosso, DO

Audit of dermatological content of U.K. undergraduate curricula
Davies E, Burge S (Churchill Hosp, Oxford, UK)
Br J Dermatol 160:999-1005, 2009

Background.—Recommendations for the dermatology content (learning outcomes) of the core undergraduate curriculum were sent to all U.K. medical schools in June 2006.

Objective.—To carry out an audit of the content of the core curriculum in each U.K. medical school against the recommendations for a core undergraduate dermatology curriculum (the criteria) published by the British Association of Dermatologists, to identify areas of good practice and to gather evidence for developing the learning and teaching of dermatology.

Methods.—A questionnaire was circulated to the dermatology teaching leads of all U.K. medical schools (29) and one Irish medical school. Questions which the teaching leads were unable to answer were sent to the relevant deans and responses incorporated into the results. All curricula should include the essential learning outcomes that focus on clinical skills; as this was an audit to benchmark current practice, we did not set standards for the other recommendations for a core curriculum.

Results.—Replies were received from teaching leads in 29 of the 30 medical schools and from 16 of the deans. Essential clinical skills such as taking a dermatological history and examining the skin were included in the curricula of most, but not all, medical schools. Areas of good practice include teaching on tumours, acne and psoriasis, but we found some surprising omissions including the diagnosis of meningococcaemia. Our data suggest that some students have little exposure to dermatology, but dermatology teaching takes place in secondary care in all medical schools. Knowledge-based assessments are used by 27 medical schools.

Conclusions.—Curricula should be strengthened so that the recommended learning outcomes feature in the core curricula of all medical schools. Teaching leads in all specialties, including those in the community, should communicate so that learning and teaching are integrated horizontally and vertically. The results should provide a baseline for future audits.

▶ This study sought to compare the core curriculum for teaching dermatology in UK medical schools with the one recommended by the British Association of Dermatologists. The authors hoped to identify areas of good practice and to gather evidence for developing a sound teaching program for the specialty. The method used was a questionnaire designed to determine how many of the recommended learning outcomes were included in the core curriculum of each medical school. Not surprisingly, the authors found that the time allocated to dermatology teaching varied widely across the different medical schools. There was great variation in the number of lectures given (0-39) and the minimum number of clinics that a student was expected to attend (0-18). Clearly, as in the United States, some students in the UK have little exposure to dermatology, a disappointing finding considering that, at least in the UK, 10% to 15% of general practitioner consultations involved a dermatologic problem. Some areas received more emphasis than others: teaching of tumors, acne, atopic dermatitis, and psoriasis, as well as the structure and function of the skin, appeared to be adequate. Other important topics such as wound healing and the recognition of skin signs of systemic disease receive less attention. Certain aspects of the "art" of dermatology, such as describing skin lesions, exploring a patient's concerns, and providing parents advice about dealing with children with eczema, were omitted from some teaching programs.

B. H. Thiers, MD

Nodular fasciitis: a sarcomatous impersonator

Tomita S, Thompson K, Carver T, et al (Naval Med Ctr San Diego, CA)
J Pediatr Surg 44:E17-E19, 2009

Reports of nodular fasciitis among adults are common; however, this condition is relatively rare in the pediatric population. Its clinical and histologic characteristics are similar to malignancies such as sarcoma; thus, it is prudent for the clinician caring for children and adolescents to be aware of the possibility of its occurrence. Nodular fasciitis is a benign mesenchymal tumor. Often presenting as a rapidly enlarging soft tissue mass, clinically, it can easily be mistaken as a sarcoma or other malignancy during clinical evaluation. In addition, the pathologist may recognize its high cellularity, high mitotic index, and infiltrative borders, which, as a result, may lead to erroneous diagnosis as a malignancy. Although more frequently seen in adults, it does occur in the pediatric population and should be considered during evaluation and treatment of soft tissue masses in children and adolescents.

▶ This article presents 3 pediatric cases of nodular fasciitis, which is relatively uncommon, but more common in adults. It can be injury related but in these 3 cases described, there was no history of injury. This article also mentions that this benign mesenchymal tumor can present as a rapidly enlarging mass, and is commonly mistaken as a malignancy histologically and clinically (especially sarcoma). This article concludes that nodular fasciitis should be considered in the differential diagnosis in a pediatric patient presenting with soft tissue mass.

S. B. Momin, DO
J. Q. Del Rosso, DO

Acrodermatitis Enteropathica-Like Eruption in Metabolic Disorders: Acrodermatitis Dysmetabolica Is Proposed as a Better Term

Tabanlioğlu D, Ersoy-Evans S, Karaduman A (Hacettepe Univ, Ankara, Turkey)
Pediatr Dermatol 26:150-154, 2009

Background.—Acrodermatitis acidemica is a recently proposed term for the rash that is similar to acrodermatitis enteropathica, which is encountered in organic acidemias. However, acrodermatitis enteropathica-like eruption may be seen in metabolic disorders other than organic acidemias.

Objective.—The aim of this study was to evaluate the clinical features of acrodermatitis enteropathica-like eruption secondary to metabolic disorders.

Methods.—Clinical and demographic features of 12 patients with acrodermatitis enteropathica-like eruption were prospectively evaluated between 2004 and 2006 in this single-center study.

Results.—Among the 12 patients, underlying metabolic disorders included maple syrup urine disease ($n = 5$), methylmalonic acidemia ($n = 3$), phenylketonuria ($n = 2$), ornithine transcarbamylase deficiency ($n = 1$), and propionic acidemia ($n = 1$). Mean age at first presentation was 29.9 months. Mean duration of acrodermatitis enteropathica-like eruption at the time of presentation was 25.2 days. The diaper area was involved in all presentations. Plasma zinc level was measured in 62.5% ($n = 10$) of the presentations and all had normal levels. All phenylketonuria cases had a low plasma phenylalanine level, and a low plasma isoleucine level was observed in the propionic acidemia case and all maple syrup urine disease cases. The rash responded dramatically to appropriate diet management in all cases.

Conclusion.—In this study, acrodermatitis enteropathica-like eruption was noted in various metabolic disorders, including organic acidemias. We suggest that acrodermatitis dysmetabolica might be a better term for acrodermatitis enteropathica-like eruption occurring secondary to metabolic disorders other than acquired zinc deficiency.

▶ Acrodermatitis enteropathica was first described as an autosomal recessive disorder associated with zinc deficiency. Characteristic findings include acral and periorificial dermatitis, alopecia, and diarrhea. Further studies revealed similar clinical findings in patients that were lacking essential amino acids and fatty acids unrelated to zinc deficiency. These groups of disorders were subsequently called acrodermatitis enteropathica-like eruptions (AELE). Other suggestions for a more descriptive terminology has been made such as acrodermatitis acidemica; however, studies show that AELE is also found with metabolic disorders other than organic acidemias. This study proposes the newer term of acrodermatitis dysmetabolica to encompass AELE that are secondary to metabolic disorders in general. To this end, 12 AELE patients were prospectively studied. Although clinically the presentations were highly suggestive of AELE, this was not confirmed by histopathologic examination. This may be a limitation as patients are ideally diagnosed by a combination of clinical suspicion, dietary survey, laboratory tests, and histopathological findings of characteristic skin lesions. Nevertheless, acrodermatitis dysmetabolica seems to be a very appropriate term in AELE cases where the presentation is secondary to metabolic disorders without association with zinc deficiency.

S. Bellew, DO

J. Q. Del Rosso, DO

The current state of dermatopathology education: a survey of the association of professors of dermatology
Hinshaw M, Hsu P, Lee L-Y, et al (Univ of Wisconsin School of Public Health, Madison; Univ of Wisconsin-Madison; et al)
J Cutaneous Pathol 36:620-628, 2009

Background.—Dermatology training programs develop program specific dermatopathology (DP) curricula. We summarize the current state of DP education in dermatology residency programs and identify opportunities for DP education resource development.

Methods.—A 27-question survey was emailed to members of the Association of Professors of Dermatology (APD).

Results.—Fifty-two of 109 programs responded for a response rate of 48%. Results were calculated using a non-response adjustment. Thirty per cent of the overall education time during residency is spent in DP-specific education. Lever and Weedon are the texts most often cited as primary texts utilized for DP education. Three-quarters of programs have third year residents spend three or more weeks on the DP service. The majority of dermatology residency programs have a specific DP service rotation at some point during residency.

Conclusions.—The majority of training programs use a variety of resources and mechanisms for teaching DP to dermatology residents. Some programs list barriers to DP education including lack of cases, microscopes, resident education time for DP-related teaching and availability of educators. We conclude that a greater depth and breadth of resources for DP education would be of benefit to dermatology residency programs.

▶ This article sought to investigate, by means of a survey instrument sent to 174 e-mail addresses possessed by the Association of Professors of Dermatology, and representing the 109 American dermatology residency programs, the means by which dermatopathology was taught to trainees. With a response rate of about 50%, the authors found that about 30% of total educational hours (7 hours on average) are devoted to the study of dermatopathology, and this number is in general agreement with other historic assessments. Interestingly, programs in the southern United States reported spending nearly twice as much time (13 hours) on dermatopathology education than did the other geographic areas of the United States. This is particularly interesting as it is well accepted that more dermatologists read their own slides as one moves west across the country, and yet this is not the area of the country where programs report spending the greatest amount of time in dermatopathology education.

W. A. High, MD, JD, MEng

Vitamin D and sun protection: The impact of mixed public health messages in Australia

Youl PH, Janda M, Kimlin M (Viertel Centre for Res in Cancer Control, Brisbane, Queensland, Australia; Queensland Univ of Technology, Brisbane, Australia)

Int J Cancer 124:1963-1970, 2009

Exposure of the skin to sunlight can cause skin cancer and is also necessary for cutaneous Vitamin D production. Media reports have highlighted the purported health benefits of Vitamin D. Our aim was to examine attitudes and behaviours related to sun protection and Vitamin D. A cross-sectional study of 2,001 residents in Queensland, Australia, aged 20–70 years was undertaken. Information collected included the following: skin cancer risk factors; perceptions about levels of sun exposure required to maintain Vitamin D; belief that sun protection increases risk of Vitamin D deficiency; intention, and actual change in sun protection practices for adults and children. Multivariate models examined predictors of attitudinal and behavioural change. One-third (32%) believed a fair-skinned adult, and 31% thought a child required at least 30 min/day in summer sun to maintain Vitamin D levels. Reductions in sun protection were reported by 21% of adults and 14% of children. Factors associated with the belief that sun protection may result in not obtaining enough Vitamin D included age of $\geq$60 years (OR = 1.35, 95% CI 1.09–1.66) and having skin that tanned easily (OR = 1.96, 95% CI 1.38–2.78). Participants from low-income households, and those who frequently used sun-protective clothing were more likely to have reduced sun protection practices (OR = 1.33, 95% CI 1.10–1.73 and OR = 1.73, 95% CI 1.36–2.20, respectively). This study provides evidence of reductions in sun protection practices in a population living in a high UV environment. There is an urgent need to refocus messages regarding sun exposure and for continued sun protection practices.

▶ Marks et al demonstrated that in 113 patients, vitamin D insufficiency or deficiency was not induced when SPF-17 sunscreen was used at levels sufficient to prevent actinic keratoses, along with avoidance of sun exposure at midday and wearing appropriate sun protective clothing and hats.[1]

In another study by Davie et al, 5% of the skin surface with suberythemogenic exposure produced mean serum 25 (OH) vitamin D levels above deficient range in the elderly patients, and the conclusion was drawn that younger individuals will likely have higher levels. The face and dorsal hands have > 5% total body surface area.[2]

This is an excellent article demonstrating why there is an important need to refocus patient education regarding sun exposure and the need to continue sun protective behaviors. Media, health care professionals, schools, etc should be taking an active role in educating the public regarding sun protection and vitamin D. If the health professionals did not agree about the relationship between vitamin D and sun protection, then that will continue to give the public mixed messages.

S. B. Momin, DO

J. Q. Del Rosso, DO

References

1. Marks R, Foley PA, Jolley D, Knight KR, Harrison J, Thompson SC. The effect of regular sunscreen use on vitamin D levels in an Australian population; Results of a randomized controlled trial. *Arch Dermatol.* 1995;131:415-421.
2. Davie MW, Lawson DE, Emberson C, Barnes JL, Roberts GE, Barnes ND. Vitamin D from skin:contribution to vitamin D status compared with oral vitamin D in normal and anticonvulsant-treated subjects. *Clin Sci (Colch).* 1982;63:461-472.

Adoption of Western Culture by Californian Asian Americans: Attitudes and Practices Promoting Sun Exposure

Gorell E, Lee C, Muñoz C, et al (Stanford Univ School of Medicine, CA)
Arch Dermatol 145:552-556, 2009

Objective.—To investigate whether the adoption of Western culture is associated with attitudes and practices promoting sun exposure among Asian Americans.

Design.—Survey conducted from November 28, 2007, to January 28, 2008.

Setting.—Primarily northern California community groups via online survey.

Participants.—Adult volunteers who self-identified as Asian American.

Main Outcome Measures.—Results based on 546 questionnaires returned.

Results.—The overall response rate was 74.4%. Multivariate regression analysis controlling for age and skin type showed that westernization (as determined by generation in the United States, location raised, or self-rated acculturation) was associated with attitudes and behaviors promoting sun exposure (including the belief that having a tan is attractive, negative attitudes toward use of sunscreen and sun protective clothing, and increased weekend sun exposure, lying out to get a tan, and tanning bed use) at a level of $P < .05$.

Conclusions.—Our data suggest that adoption of Western culture may be associated with attitudes and behaviors promoting sun exposure among Asian Americans. This group should be targeted by dermatologists for increased education regarding sun protection, solar damage, and skin cancer prevention and detection.

▶ The incidence of skin cancer in the United States is rising. Concurrently, the United States census bureau projects that the Asian population will triple in the next 50 years. With an overall rise in skin cancer and anticipated increases in the Asian population, clinicians and patients alike must focus efforts to obtain better understanding of skin cancer in this minority population. Unfortunately, there is limited information available. Authors of this article explored the connection between westernization of the Asian Americans in California and increased practices of sun exposure ultimately placing them at risk for developing skin cancer.

This study relied upon the self-identification of the subject's ethnic background. The Asian population is a heterogeneous group. Therefore, there may be significant differences in attitude or beliefs between a self-identified Asian with mixed ethnicity, versus one who was born in Asia and subsequently immigrated to the United States. Further, this study is limited to the state of California where the beach culture of sunbathing is commonplace, and results therefore cannot be generalized to all Asian Americans in the United States. In addition, as the authors state, self-reported data is at risk for recall and sampling biases.

S. Bellew, DO
J. Q. Del Rosso, DO

Cutaneous sarcoidosis: a histopathological study

Cardoso JC, Cravo M, Reis JP, et al (Coimbra Univ Hosp, Portugal)
J Eur Acad Dermatol Venereol 23:678-682, 2009

Background.—Sarcoidosis is a granulomatous disease of uncertain aetiology in which the skin is frequently involved. Naked sarcoidal granulomas are the characteristic histological feature in specific lesions of sarcoidosis.

Objective.—This study aims to describe the histological findings in a population of patients with cutaneous sarcoidosis.

Materials and Methods.—This study is a retrospective analysis of 31 biopsies of specific lesions of cutaneous sarcoidosis, corresponding to 30 patients.

Results.—Typical naked granuloma was found in the majority of cases (71%). In 9 cases (29%), granulomas had a significant number of lymphocytes. Necrosis was found in two cases (6%). Periadnexal distribution (mostly perisudoral) was found in 32% of cases. Interstitial distribution of granulomas was observed in five cases (16%). Foreign material was detected in 13% of cases (without the use of polarized light microscopy). Epidermal changes were found in 55% of cases, with atrophy and parakeratosis being the most frequent alterations.

Conclusions.—Although typical naked sarcoid granulomas are the most common features of cutaneous sarcoidosis, the dermatopathologist must be aware of possible atypical findings, which are more common than previously expected, because of the differential diagnosis with other causes of cutaneous granulomas, namely infectious diseases.

▶ Sarcoidosis is a multisystem disease with variable clinical findings. Multiple organs can be involved including lungs, lymph nodes, skin, and eyes. Cutaneous findings are present in 25% of the cases. Thirty-one biopsies from 30 patients were obtained to identify main histologic features and highlighting some atypical histologic findings. Common findings in decreasing order of frequency on hematoxylin and eosin (H & E) stain are as follows: typical naked or sarcoid granulomas, epidermal changes, including atrophy and parakeratosis, periadnexal distribution, predominantly lymphocytic infiltrate, interstitial distribution of granulomas, foreign material, and necrosis. The frequency of atypical findings remind us to consider the possibility of foreign material in sarcoidosis, and although nonspecific, histologic epidermal changes may appear more frequently than originally thought in sarcoidosis. A larger study involving a greater number of biopsies and perhaps the use of polarized light microscopy may be needed to support present findings.

S. Bellew, DO

J. Q. Del Rosso, DO

A randomized, double-blinded, placebo-controlled trial of pseudocatalase cream and narrowband ultraviolet B in the treatment of vitiligo
Bakis-Petsoglou S, Le Guay JL, Wittal R (Skin & Cancer Foundation Australia, Darlinghurst, Sydney)
Br J Dermatol 161:910-917, 2009

Background.—Pseudocatalase cream in conjunction with narrowband ultraviolet B (NB-UVB) has previously been reported to result in repigmentation of vitiliginous skin.

Objectives.—The purpose of this 24-week, double-blind, placebo-controlled, randomized, single-centre trial was to assess the efficacy of pseudocatalase cream and NB-UVB vs. placebo and NB-UVB for the treatment of vitiligo.

Methods.—Patients with active vitiligo on their face and/or hands applied either pseudocatalase cream or placebo to their whole body, twice daily for 24 weeks. NB-UVB therapy was administered three times a week for the duration of the trial. Efficacy was assessed primarily by digital image analysis of photographs.

Results.—Thirty-two patients were randomized to either the pseudocatalase arm (n = 14) or placebo (n = 18). Between-group analysis did not show a statistically significant improvement in percentage area affected in the pseudocatalase cream group when compared with placebo.

However, a statistically significant improvement was found within each group by week 12, which was maintained throughout the study.

Conclusions.—NB-UVB treatment is a moderately effective treatment for vitiligo. Pseudocatalase cream does not appear to add any incremental benefit to NB-UVB alone.

▶ Vitiligo is an acquired disorder of skin depigmentation that is often very difficult to treat. Therapeutic response is variable and dependent somewhat on the site involved. It has been shown that pseudocatalase cream in conjunction with narrow band ultraviolet B (NB-UVB) exposure results in repigmentation on the face and dorsum of the hands after 2 to 4 months of depigmentation. It has been previously suggested that pseudocatalase with calcium treatments replaces low catalase and calcium levels known to exist in patients with vitiligo. NB-UVB radiation is also used to activate the pseudocatalase cream. This is a randomized, double-blind, placebo-controlled trial of 32 vitiligo patients with active vitiligo on their face and the dorsal of hands treated with pseudocatalase cream plus NB-UVB compared with placebo plus NB-UVB. Those that had received systemic therapy or radiation therapy in the last 2 months or used topical therapy within 2 weeks were excluded. Patients were randomized into the pseudocatalase ($n = 14$) or placebo cream ($n = 18$) group. Both groups received NB-UVB therapy between 10 to 30 minutes after application of the cream 3 times a week for the entire duration of the study. A thin layer of the pseudocatalase cream was applied to the entire body twice a day for 24 weeks. Repigmentation, compliance and treatment safety, and tolerability were reassessed by both patient and investigators at 12 weeks and 24 weeks with photographs taken. Patients were also asked about compliance and their treatment cream at each visit. Most patients were >75% compliant. This trial did not find a significantly increased repigmentation rate of the hand and face in the pseudocatalase group compared with placebo ($P > .02$), with both groups receiving NB-UVB. Both groups showed significant repigmentation from baseline especially in the face ($P < .02$). This improvement within each group was observed by week 12, which was maintained throughout the study. This phenomenon could be due to NB-UVB therapy in both the treatment and placebo group. Limitations include a small sample size. To add, the face and the hands are areas known to be poorly responsive to treatment. Other limitations were that patients were only 75% compliant with therapy. Included in the intent to treat (ITT) analysis was anyone that had used at least one dose of study medication or had at least one NB-UVB treatment with at least one posttreatment efficacy measurement. Additionally, the "endpoint" analysis for the ITT group was performed using the last available observation carried forward for each patient where data was missing. This study demonstrated that NB-UVB treatment alone is a moderately effective treatment for vitiligo. In conclusion, authors suggest that pseudocatalase cream plus NB-UVB does not appear to have a benefit for vitiligo compared with NB-UVB alone.

J. Q. Del Rosso, DO
G. K. Kim, DO

Assessing the Value of Supportive Skin Care: Development and Validation of an Instrument for Evaluating Patient-Relevant Benefit
Augustin M, Schäfer I, Rabini S, et al (Hamburg-Eppendorf Univ Hosp; Bayer Vital GmbH, Leverkusen, Germany)
Dermatology 218:255-259, 2009

Background.—Supportive skin care for irritated and inflamed skin is one of the most important measures in the prevention and treatment of eczema and sensitive skin.

Objectives.—To develop and validate an instrument for the evaluation of patient-relevant benefit in the supportive care of irritated skin with non-pharmacological topical agents.

Methods.—Patient-defined treatment objectives and benefits of supportive skin care were determined in an open survey of patients with irritated skin. A pilot questionnaire was constructed according to the Patient Benefit Index (PBI). The questionnaire was tested for feasibility and validity in 1,886 patients with various irritated skin conditions.

Results.—From a total of 90 characteristics of basic therapy benefit, a 23-item questionnaire was constructed. This questionnaire ('PBI-k') proved to be feasible, reliable and was associated with a high level of patient acceptance in the surveillance field. The questionnaire showed good internal consistency, distribution characteristics and convergent validity with patient satisfaction.

Conclusion.—The PBI-k is the first specific instrument developed for the evaluation of patient-defined benefit in supportive skin care with nonpharmacological topical agents. Feasibility and psychometric properties make this questionnaire suitable for application in studies involving patients with irritated, sensitive skin.

▶ Until now, there has been a lack of instruments for the assessment of patient-relevant benefit in the prophylactic treatment of dermatologic conditions and in the evaluation of supportive skin care with nonpharmacologic agents. The authors in this study may be the first to develop a way to evaluate patient-defined benefit in this setting.

The instrument itself is a prospective, noninterventional, single-arm postmarketing surveillance study. The open survey lists 23 particularly relevant treatment benefits, individual therapy needs, and treatment goals that the patient ranks in order of importance before beginning treatment. At the end of treatment (or in the course of treatment), the subject is questioned about the extent to which his individually selective benefits were achieved. Finally, the preferences determined before therapy and the benefits achieved after therapy are incorporated into a weighted index value, which is the patient benefit index (PBI). Therefore, the construct of this patient benefit was developed on the basis of goal oriented outcome measurement.

The survey itself critically evaluated for feasibility, internal consistency, distributional characteristics, and construct validity and received very high results in each assessment/measurement.

This survey offers the opportunity to assess the specific characteristics of irritated skin with higher specificity and greater sensitivity than the usual quality of life questionnaires available. An advantage of this survey is incorporation of both the patient defined importance of treatment and the resulting benefits. The results of the survey itself demonstrated a very broad range in the patient defined importance of treatment, but also found consistency between meeting patient needs and patient satisfaction. This instrument represents an excellent way to assess patient relevant benefit for supportive skin care.

J. Levin, DO

J. Q. Del Rosso, DO

Adolescents with Skin Disease Have Specific Quality of Life Issues
Golics CJ, Basra MKA, Finlay AY, et al (Cardiff Univ, UK)
Dermatology 218:357-366, 2009

Background.—Adolescence is a period of life with its own unique characteristics.

Objectives.—To provide an in-depth understanding of the impact of skin disease on different aspects of adolescents' health-related quality of life (HRQoL).

Methods.—Semi-structured qualitative interviews were conducted with a sample of dermatology patients between 12 and 19 years of age, attending the dermatology outpatient clinic of a secondary referral centre. Participants were invited to talk in detail about all the ways their lives had been affected by their skin disease. Interviews were transcribed verbatim.

Results.—Thirty-two adolescents (males = 10, females = 22) with a mean age of 15.7 years (range = 12–18 years) participated in the interviews. Twenty-eight HRQoL themes adversely affected by skin diseases were identified from the interviews which were grouped under 6 main HRQoL domains – psychological impact (91% of patients), physical impact (81%), social impact (81%), impact on lifestyle (63%), need for support (41%) and education and employment (34%). The number of HRQoL themes affected in each individual varied between 1 and 23 (mean = 8.1).

Conclusions.—The results of this study revealed the extent and nature of the impact of skin diseases on adolescents' HRQoL. A number of issues identified were specific to adolescents, highlighting the need for specific HRQoL assessment.

▶ Skin conditions are common in the adolescent years and can have a significant effect on an individual's quality of life. This is a study of 32 adolescent patients between 12 to 19 years of age that have been attending the dermatology outpatient clinic of a secondary referral center. Patients were invited to talk in detail about how their skin conditions have affected their lives. There were 28 health related quality of life (HRQoL) themes adversely affected by skin conditions. These were divided into 6 domains: psychological impact, physical impact, social impact, impact on lifestyle, need for support, and education and employment. Patients were interviewed and transcription of answers was taken verbatim. The 3 main skin diseases that caused the most impairment of HRQoL in young patients were eczema, psoriasis, and acne. Individuals with concomitant medical or psychiatric illness were excluded. The physical domain was divided into 2 subdomains—disease-related impact and treatment-related impact. The psychological impact of skin disease on adolescents was expressed by most patients in this study. Bullying and being judged by others affected 41% of subjects interviewed. Effects on self-esteem were common among 47% of patients because they were constantly worrying about their skin. Physical impacts like itching and pain were the most frequently mentioned sensation in 38% of patients. Researchers also noted that 25% of subjects experienced decreased confidence around the opposite sex as a result of their skin condition. There were some limitations to this study, which included interviewer bias. The sample size was also small, and 91% of patients were Caucasian. The quality of life issues may differ for different ethnicities, which should be further researched. Another limitation was that patients included in this study had more advanced skin conditions because this was a secondary referral center; therefore, their quality of life could have been more adversely affected. Furthermore, this study did not include a control group for comparison. However, there is a limited amount of research on the HRQoL on adolescence, and this study was an informative incite on the emotional and social impact of skin conditions in this age group. In conclusion, the results of this study revealed the nature and extent of the impact of skin diseases on adolescents and highlighted the importance of viewing this age group with unique emotional and social needs.

G. K. Kim, DO

J. Q. Del Rosso, DO

DERMATOLOGIC SURGERY AND CUTANEOUS ONCOLOGY

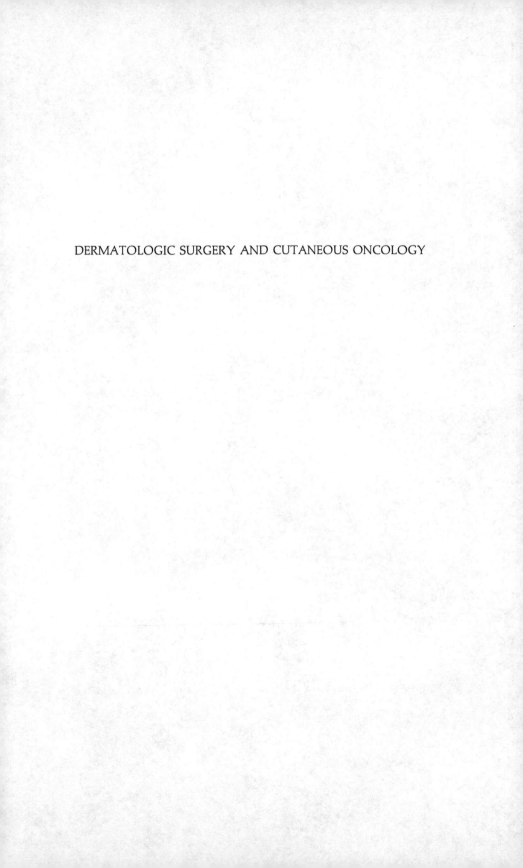

15 Nonmelanoma Skin Cancer

Sequential effects of photodynamic treatment of basal cell carcinoma

Prignano F, Lotti T, Spallanzani A, et al (Univ of Florence, Italy)
J Cutan Pathol 36:409-416, 2009

Background.—Photodynamic therapy (PDT) of superficial basal cell carcinoma (SBCC) acts as a biological response modifier or killing target cells, but sequential biological effects have not been reported in depth in humans.

Methods.—In 15 patients with SBCC treated with aminolevulinic acid (ALA)-PDT, inflammatory infiltrate, apoptosis phenomena and tumor-derived molecules were investigated on biopsies at baseline, and after 15 min and 4, 24, 48 and 72 h, by immunohistochemistry and ultrastructure.

Results.—Early apoptosis of keratinocytes was already observed at 15 min, while late apoptotic markers were maximally found at 24 h. Baseline mast cells tended to slightly increase up to 72 h; polymorphonuclear phagocytes significantly increased at 4 h but decreased at 24/48/72 h; on the contrary, lymphocytes and macrophages gradually increased starting at baseline. At baseline, SBCC cells expressed stem cell factor in all cases, and granulocyte-monocyte colony-stimulating factor, basic fibroblastic growth factor, interleukin (IL)-8 and vascular endothelial growth factor in most cases. IL-6 and monocyte chemoattractant protein-1 were poorly expressed, and transforming growth factor-beta was absent.

Conclusions.—We show a clear time-dependent profile of apoptotic markers and inflammatory infiltrate composition in SBCC after ALA-PDT. SBCC cells express cytokines and chemotactic molecules that are likely related to the recruitment of inflammatory cells.

▶ In this very well-written and well-performed clinical evaluation, 15 patients with superficial basal cell carcinomas (BCCS) were biopsied at baseline and after photodynamic therapy (PDT) with 5-aminolevulinic acid (ALA) at 15 minutes, and at 4, 24, 48, and 72 hours by immunohistochemistry and ultrastucture analysis. The study examined the inflammatory infiltrate, the apoptosis phenomena created, and the tumor-derived molecules generated following ALA-PDT.

In this study, the authors found that cancer cells undergo apoptotic modifications at 15 minutes after PDT, while late signs of apoptosis reach their highest values at 24 hours and, conversely, Bcl-2 antiapoptotic molecules rapidly decrease. PDT also represents a proinflammatory event inducing both innate and adaptive immune responses, which contribute to tumor cell killing. Polymorphonuclear leukocytes are the major component of the early infiltrate at 4 hours, followed by T lymphocytes at 24 to 48 hours, while macrophages increase late (48-72 hours). Mast cells, which are predominant at baseline, only slightly increase over time. Cytokines and chemotactic molecules (interleukin [IL]-8, granulocyte-monocyte colony-stimulating factor [GM-CSF], basic fibroblastic growth factor [bFGF], vascular endothelial growth factor [VEGF], stem cell factor [SCF], and IL-6) are also expressed at baseline in the cancer cells, which are capable of exerting chemotactic activity on the inflammatory infiltrate.

The authors conclude that there is a clear sequential profile of inflammation in BCCs treated with ALA-PDT, according to the expression of cytokines and immunogenic molecules on tumor cells. The further recruitment of inflammatory cells appears to be an important effect of ALA-PDT treatment, in addition to them killing off target cells because of apoptosis.

It's nice to see science behind the clinical effects we observe in our everyday clinical practices. This helps further define why PDT is effective in the treatment of BCC, and why PDT is effective for treatment of these lesions.

M. H. Gold, MD

Anatomic Location and Histopathologic Subtype of Basal Cell Carcinomas in Adults Younger than 40 or 90 and Older: Any difference?
Betti R, Radaelli G, Mussino F, et al (Univ of Milan, Italy; et al)
Dermatol Surg 35:201-206, 2009

Background.—Differences in age, site, and histopathologic subtype exist in basal cell carcinoma (BCC).

Objective.—To compare the distribution of BCCs in patients younger than 40 with that of those aged 90 and older according to sex, site, and subtype.

Methods & Materials.—One hundred seventy-five BCCs were examined. The site was classified as head and neck, trunk, or limbs and the subtype as nodular, superficial, or morpheic-infiltrative.

Results.—Younger exhibited a lower prevalence of BCCs on the head and neck (36.0% vs 57.3%, $p < .01$) and a higher prevalence on the trunk (59.3% vs 31.5%, $p < .01$) and of superficial BCCs (43.0% vs 31.5%, $p < .05$) than older patients. Site was associated with subtype in younger ($p < .001$) and older ($p = .004$) patients. Superficial BCCs were mostly on the trunk ($p < .001$), with a higher prevalence in younger patients (86.5% vs 62.5%, $p < .05$). Morpheic BCCs were mostly on the head and neck ($p < .001$), and prevalence did not differ between age groups. Nodular BCCs were mostly on the head and neck in older patients

($p = .011$). Subtype was independently associated with site ($p = .005$) but not with age or sex.

Conclusion.—A different distribution of site and subtype occurs in younger and older patients. Subtype is associated with site independent of age and sex. These findings suggest that, at least in some patients, the anatomic location of BCC may favor the development of a particular subtype.

▶ The objective of this article was to compare the distribution and histopathologic subtype of basal cell carcinoma (BCC) in adults younger than 40 with adults 90 and older. The article does meet its objective. The results of the study were as expected that younger patients get more superficial BCC on the trunk while older patients are more prone to nodular BCC in the head and neck region. The study points out one interesting fact that incidence of nonmelanoma skin cancer is rising among younger patients, and thus it is important to target and educate them on sun protection and skin cancer prevention.

The article does have some limitations. The effect of ultraviolet exposure on the type of BCC was not assessed. Also, it is interesting to note that extensively sun exposed areas such as limbs had the fewest number of BCC.

S. Bhambri, DO

J. Q. Del Rosso, DO

Detection of basal cell carcinomas in Mohs excisions with fluorescence confocal mosaicing microscopy
Karen JK, Gareau DS, Dusza SW, et al (Memorial Sloan-Kettering Cancer Ctr, NY)
Br J Dermatol 160:1242-1250, 2009

Background.—High-resolution real-time imaging of human skin is possible with a confocal microscope either *in vivo* or in freshly excised tissue *ex vivo*. Nuclear and cellular morphology is observed in thin optical sections, similar to that in conventional histology. Contrast agents such as acridine orange in fluorescence and acetic acid in reflectance have been used in *ex vivo* imaging to enhance nuclear contrast.

Objectives.—To evaluate the sensitivity and specificity of *ex vivo* real-time imaging with fluorescence confocal mosaicing microscopy, using acridine orange, for the detection of residual basal cell carcinoma (BCC) in Mohs fresh tissue excisions.

Methods.—Forty-eight discarded skin excisions were collected following completion of Mohs surgery, consisting of excisions with and without residual BCC of all major subtypes. The tissue was stained with acridine orange and imaged with a fluorescent confocal mosaicing microscope. Confocal mosaics were matched to the corresponding haematoxylin and eosin-stained Mohs frozen sections. Each mosaic was divided into subsections, resulting in 149 submosaics for study. Two Mohs surgeons, who were blinded to the cases, independently assessed confocal submosaics and recorded the presence or absence of BCC, location, and histological subtype(s). Assessment of confocal mosaics was by comparison with corresponding Mohs surgery maps.

Results.—The overall sensitivity and specificity of detecting residual BCC was 96·6% and 89·2%, respectively. The positive predictive value was 92·3% and the negative predictive value 94·7%. Very good correlation was observed between confocal mosaics and matched Mohs frozen sections for benign and malignant skin structures, overall tumour burden and location, and identification of all major histological subtypes of BCC.

Conclusions.—Fluorescent confocal mosaicing microscopy using acridine orange enables detection of residual BCC of all subtypes in Mohs fresh tissue excisions with high accuracy. This observation is an important step towards the long-term clinical goal of using a noninvasive imaging modality for potential real-time surgical pathology-at-the-bedside for skin and other tissues.

▶ This was a study to evaluate the sensitivity and specificity of ex vivo real-time imaging with fluorescence confocal mosaicing microscopy, using acridine orange, for the detection of residual basal cell carcinoma (BCC) in Mohs fresh tissue excisions. The intent was as a step toward the long-term clinical goal of using a noninvasive imaging modality for potential real-time surgical pathology-at-the-bedside for skin and other tissues. Confocal mosaics stained with acridine orange were matched to the corresponding hematoxylin and eosin-stained Mohs frozen sections and showed an overall sensitivity and specificity of detecting residual BCC of 96.6% and 89.2%, respectively.

It was a well planned and executed study that has provided valuable information. As the authors themselves acknowledge, in order for real time confocal imaging to have clinical use, the applicability of confocal microscopy in tumors other than BCC has to be better explored. A reproducible contrast protocol with consistent image quality and interpretation will be needed as well as more efficient and cost-effective image acquisition technology. Yet, more importantly this was a small study with a limited number of observers and reviewers, and the challenges are much greater in dealing with excised tissues with variable thickness, size, and contour when the specimens will entail those that are freshly excised as opposed to dealing with residual tissue that has already been partially manipulated.

Nevertheless, this was a creative approach that deserves a gander by anyone treating cancer, and I look forward to further larger studies by this group of investigators.

A. Torres, MD, JD

Clinical Outcome of Surgical Treatment for Periorbital Basal Cell Carcinoma

Kakudo N, Ogawa Y, Suzuki K, et al (Kansai Med Univ, Osaka, Japan; Otowa Kinen Hosp, Kyoto, Japan)
Ann Plast Surg 63:531-535, 2009

Basal cell carcinoma (BCC) has a predilection for the periorbital region, which is a special, prominent, cosmetic, functional area to protect the eyeball. For squamous cell carcinoma and melanoma, extensive resection with reconstruction is performed. In contrast, for BCC, resection is often confined to a small to medium-sized area, necessitating higher-quality reconstructive surgery.

We analyze the surgical outcomes of treatment for periorbital BCC, and evaluate reconstruction method after resection.

Forty-nine patients with periorbital BCC had surgery in our hospital over 20 years. Age, gender of the patients, and size, localization, and histology of the tumor, and surgical procedures, and their early and late complications were analyzed retrospectively.

BCC was most frequently occurred in the lower lid (55%), followed by inner canthus (19%), upper lid (17%), and outer canthus (9%). The histologic classifications were solid (80%), morphea (7%), mix (7%), superficial (2%), keratotic (2%), and adenoid (2%). Recurrence of the tumor was observed in 2 advanced cases in patients treated with resection of the tumor including surrounding tissue 5 mm from the margin. A rotation advancement cheek flap procedure was most frequently applied. Horizontal shift of the skin was most effective to prevent postoperative lagophthalmos.

BCC occurred most frequently in the lower lid within the periorbital area. Rotation advancement of cheek flap with horizontal shift of the skin is most effective procedure in both appearance and function of the eyelid.

▶ Basal cell carcinoma (BCC) is a common malignancy that can occur quite often in the periorbital region. This is a retrospective cohort study analyzing surgical outcomes and reconstruction methods in 49 periorbital BCC cases at Kansai Medical University Hospital from 1988 to 2007. Authors retrospectively analyzed patient age, gender, size of tumor, location of tumor, histology of tumor, surgical procedure, and postsurgical complications. Tumor was frequently in the lower eyelid (55%), inner canthus (19%), upper eyelid (17%), and outer canthus (9%). The most frequent type of BCCs seen were the solid (nodular) type BCC (80%) and morpheaform type BCC (7%). Results revealed that tumor size was smaller than 15 mm in 83% of the cases. Complications included bleeding (2/49) and swelling (1/49). The authors also noted that there was a slightly higher incidence of BCC involving the eyelid in males (1:0.88). Eyelid BCC was also found mostly in the elderly population during the sixth to seventh decade in life. This facility resects eyelid BCCs routinely with a 5 mm margin; therefore, a 15 mm defect (excision around a 5 mm lesion) was produced. Reconstruction was required for repair in this study. For the upper eyelid and outer canthus, horizontal VY plasty from the outer sides was indicated in 4 cases followed by Mustarde flap in 2 cases. A rotational cheek advancement flap was used for repair in 17 cases. Recurrence was observed in 4% of the group after 5 years. Since the eyelid area may need reconstruction, it is essential to try to avoid ectropion especially with surgery involving the lower eyelid. If there is a larger skin defect, a flap reconstruction may be considered. The authors also noted that a rotational cheek advancement with horizontal shift of the skin was the most effective procedure for the eyelid both in terms of function, avoidance of ectropion, and for aesthetics.

G. K. Kim, DO

J. Q. Del Rosso, DO

Elevated frequency of p53 genetic mutations and AgNOR values in squamous cell carcinoma

Bukhari MH, Niazi S, Khaleel ME, et al (King Edward Med Univ, Lahore, Punjab, Pakistan; et al)
J Cutan Pathol 36:220-228, 2009

Background.—Epidermal squamous cell carcinoma (SCC) is a common malignancy in Pakistan. We hypothesize that it is characterized by higher frequency of p53 genetic mutations and increased AgNOR values compared with squamous cell papilloma (SCP) and basal cell carcinoma (BCC).

Experimental Design.—To test our hypothesis, 140 skin biopsies (including 20 normal skin, 20 SCP, 20 BCC and 80 SCC samples of various grades) were examined for p53 mutations using immunohistochemistry (IHC) and polymerase chain reaction (PCR). AgNOR staining was used for histological determination of AgNOR index.

Results.—Both markers were undetectable in normal skin and were low in SCP. They were upregulated in BCC and SCC. PCR experiments revealed p53 mutations in 70% and 96.25% of BCC and SCC, respectively. Higher AgNOR values were seen in SCC than in BCC (mean AgNOR count = 5.81 ± 31 and 8.36 ± 19; percentage of AgNOR was 43.5% and 53% in BCC and SCC, respectively). Finally, p53 IHC score was found to be related to the AgNOR index in the histological grading of BCC and SCC ($r = +0.983$, $p < 0.0001$).

Conclusion.—Our results suggest that a higher frequency of p53 genetic mutations and increased AgNOR values exist in SCC compared with BCC and SCP. 'Consequently, SCC patients may have poorer prognosis'.

► It is widely accepted that mutations of the p53 tumor suppressor gene contribute to the pathogenesis of many malignancies, including those of the skin. A growing body of literature in dermatology is devoted to the detection and characterization of such mutations, particularly in squamous cell and basal cell carcinomas. p53 mutations, including the so-called ultraviolet (UV) signature mutations, have been demonstrated not only in malignant lesions but also in sun-damaged skin and premalignant conditions. Efforts have been made to correlate emergence and type of mutation with tumor aggressiveness and metastatic potential. Previous studies have yielded broadly similar results, although some differences in frequency of p53 mutations within tumor categories were reported; this was most likely attributable to differences in study design, including sample size and breadth of screening for mutations. In this study, Bukhari et al investigated not only p53 expression and mutation but also cell proliferative status in human skin tumors derived from a relatively small patient population. A semiquantitative method was used to examine p53 expression, and a single-point mutation in exon 7 was selected for evaluation of frequency of p53 gene mutation in this population. The argyrophilic nucleolar organizer region (Ag-NOR) technique, which uses a silver nuclear stain, was used to derive an index of cell proliferation. The major findings were perhaps not surprising: both p53 expression and mutation were detected in a high percentage of patients with either basal cell or epidermal squamous cell carcinoma, with significantly increased proportions of positive cells found in those patients with more advanced disease. Twenty patients with squamous cell papilloma were also included in this study, with interesting results. Although p53 expression was detected by immunohistology in 80% of samples from this group (albeit at a low level), no p53 mutation was found in any sample. This is an important finding, because p53 expression is frequently considered a marker of mutation, which is clearly not always the case.

G. M. P. Galbraith, MD

Adenosquamous carcinoma: a report of nine cases with p63 and cytokeratin 5/6 staining
Ko CJ, Leffell DJ, McNiff JM (Yale Univ School of Medicine, New Haven, CT)
J Cutan Pathol 36:448-452, 2009

Adenosquamous carcinoma, a rare tumor of the skin with few reported cases in the literature, has not been studied with p63, cytokeratin 5/6 and cytokeratin 7. We stained nine such tumors with these markers. Histologically, the tumors showed superficial, atypical islands of keratinocytes in close association with islands displaying glandular differentiation. Clinically, lesions favored the head and trunk, and a subset of cases showed aggressive behavior. All tumors marked with p63 and cytokeratin 5/6, substantiating that diffuse positivity with these stains is supportive of a primary cutaneous origin. Six tumors stained focally in luminal areas with cytokeratin 7. Recognition of adenosquamous carcinoma is important for appropriate therapy, and stains for p63 and cytokeratin 5/6 may be helpful in ruling out metastatic adenocarcinoma.

▶ Adenosquamous carcinoma of the skin is a rare tumor. The objective of the article was to examine the positivity of these tumors with p63 and cytokeratin 5/6. The study size was small with 9 patients, but it must be kept in mind that these tumors are rare. Approximately 15 years of data was analyzed with 9 cases identified. Majority of cases (8/9) were seen in patients over age 70, and the most common location was the head (5/9). All cases were positive for p63 and cytokeratin 5/6. The positivity of adenosquamous carcinoma for p63 and cytokeratin 5/6 may help differentiate primary from metastatic origin, which may in turn change the treatment options.

S. Bhambri, DO

J. Q. Del Rosso, DO

Clinical and histological findings in re-excision of incompletely excised cutaneous squamous cell carcinoma

Bovill ES, Cullen KW, Barrett W, et al (Frenchay Hosp, Bristol, UK; Queen Victoria Hosp, West Sussex, UK)
J Plast Reconstr Aesthet Surg 62:457-461, 2009

Background.—Current guidelines mandate treatment of primary cutaneous squamous cell carcinoma (SCC) through to completion, including the demonstration of a margin of normal tissue, with surgical excision as the treatment of choice. Histologically incomplete excisions of all cutaneous SCC are preferably treated by surgical re-excision. The yield of performing further resection of scar tissue in patients with incompletely excised SCCs has not been previously evaluated.

Methods.—A retrospective audit was conducted of 676 consecutive patients with surgically managed SCCs treated in our unit during 2005–2006.

Results.—One hundred and nineteen (17.6%) tumours were incompletely excised, of which 84 underwent further excision. Routine histological examination revealed residual SCC in 24 (28.6%) of these specimens. Logistic regression analysis revealed tumour diameter and Breslow thickness to contribute independently to residual SCC ($P < 0.001$). A lengthier delay between initial excision and re-excision predicted less residual tumour ($P < 0.005$). Although the positive re-excision group tended towards a higher mean age (79 ± 9 vs 74 ± 12), with more head and neck lesions (79 vs 66%), logistic regression revealed no independent influence of age, gender, histological grade or anatomical site of the original lesion.

Conclusion.—In our series, 28.6% of incompletely excised primary cutaneous SCCs showed residual tumour in re-excision specimens. Factors associated with residual tumour were similar to characteristics of high risk SCCs; larger lesions in particular are more likely to result in residual SCC at re-excision and may benefit from greater excision margins at the time of original resection. It is possible that regression of remaining tumour cells may contribute to our time-dependent findings and this warrants further research.

▶ Bovill et al performed a retrospective analysis to evaluate the yield of performing re-excision of incompletely excised squamous cell carcinomas (SCCs) using clinical and histological findings. One of the conclusions made in this article was that gender did not show an independent influence on re-excision findings. This is an irrelevant conclusion because the main cause of SCC is chronic UV radiation. Positive residual SCC in the re-excision group tended toward a higher mean age. There was no clinical significance when compared with the negative re-excision patients. Larger primary tumors predicted to have residual SCC on re-excision. This is a known risk factor for residual tumors and does not provide any new information. Interestingly, histological grade had no influence on the presence of residual SCC; however, this is not surprising as histologic grade may not necessarily correlate with subclinical tumor extension.

A lengthier delay between initial excision and re-excision predicted less residual tumor. A large proportion of residual SCC in the re-excised specimens were from the high-risk head and neck region. Unfortunately, the article does not mention what surgical margins were used for re-excision. The authors did acknowledge that Mohs micrographic surgery offers the best cure rate. Overall, this article does not offer any new clinical information to the reader.

S. B. Momin, DO

J. Q. Del Rosso, DO

Sentinel lymph-node biopsy in patients with squamous cell carcinoma of the penis
Jensen JB, Jensen KM-E, Ulhøi BP, et al (Inst of Pathology; Aarhus Univ Hosp and Aarhus Sygehus NBG, Skejby, Denmark)
BJU Int 103:1199-1203, 2009

Objectives.—To evaluate a single-centre experience with sentinel lymph-node biopsy (SLNB) as a staging procedure in patients with squamous cell carcinoma (SCC) of the penis.

Patients and Methods.—The study included 60 patients with SCC of the penis, who had SLNB in all groins where no palpable nodes were found, and in groins with palpable nodes with negative fine-needle aspiration cytology. Lymphoscintigraphy and intraoperative lymph node detection was done using ^{99m}Tc-nanocolloid and no use of blue dye.

Results.—In all, there were 97 SLNB procedures in 52 patients; 20 (20.6%) of the SLNB were positive for nodal metastases. Two negative SLNB proved to be false-negative during the observation period. The false negative-rate was 9%, the sensitivity 91% and the negative predictive value 97.5%. Minor early complications occurred after 4% of the SLNB procedures. No major or late complications were recorded.

Conclusions.—SLNB is minimally invasive and can be used as a safe and reliable staging procedure in patients with SCC of the penis. Thus standard lymph-node dissection can be avoided in most patients.

▶ While dermatologists may evaluate, biopsy, and even do the primary excision of squamous cell carcinoma of the penis, further workup would be referred to our urology or surgical oncology colleagues. This important study helps to establish the use and the minimal morbidity provided by sentinel lymph node biopsy (SLNB) for squamous cell carcinoma of the penis with or without clinical evidence of metastatic disease. The study highlights the common controversies of SLN biopsies used for melanoma. Such an approach assumes a lymphatic route of spread for the cancer. This assumption is supported by the 2 groups of patients who had similar survival characteristics. These 2 groups were patients with metastatic disease confined to the SLN (followed by a regional lymph node dissection) and those where metastatic disease was present.

SLNB is a technique sensitive procedure so that accuracy and efficiency with the procedure increases with an institution's experience in performing the procedure. In this series, false-negative SLNs were encountered early in the chronological case numbers. Pathological interpretation is not quite as difficult with squamous cell carcinoma in lymph nodes as it is with melanoma in an SLN because normal nevus cells can occur in SLN. Even these normal nevus cells sometimes have partial staining with melanoma markers making interpretation even more difficult.

It is encouraging that no major late complications (with a 3-year follow-up) were noted. This minimally invasive but technically challenging procedure can be helpful in avoiding radical ilio-inguinal (RIL) lymph node dissection in most patients. Unfortunately, this study only reported the degree of tumor differentiation and it's correlation with node positivity. A review of their data looking at other factors such as in situ disease, duration, ulceration, thickness, and locations is warranted. Further studies are needed to see which patients will receive the most benefit from SLNB.

R. I. Ceilley, MD
A. K. Bean, MD

Metastatic Cutaneous Squamous Cell Carcinoma of the Head and Neck: The Immunosuppression, Treatment, Extranodal Spread, and Margin Status (ITEM) Prognostic Score to Predict Outcome and the Need to Improve Survival
Oddone N, Morgan GJ, Palme CE, et al (Univ of Sydney, Australia)
Cancer 115:1883-1891, 2009

Background.—The authors propose a prognostic score model using a prospective study of patients with regional metastatic cutaneous squamous cell carcinoma of the head and neck.

Methods.—Two-hundred fifty patients were analyzed using a competing risks model to identify risk factors for survival. A risk score was obtained using the significant coefficients from the regression model, and cutoff points were determined that separated the score into 3 risk groups (low risk, moderate risk, and high risk).

Results.—At a median follow-up of 54 months (range, 1.3-212 months) 70 of 250 patients (28%) developed recurrent disease: Most were regional recurrences (51 of 70 patients; 73%) in the treated lymph node basin. After regional recurrence, a majority (73%) died of disease. The following 4 variables were associated significantly with survival: immunosuppression (hazard ratio [HR], 3.13; 95% confidence interval [CI], 1.39-7.05), treatment (HR, 0.32; 95% Cl, 0.16-0.66), extranodal spread (HR, 9.92; 95% CI, 1.28-77.09), and margin status (HR, 1.85; 95% CI, 1.85-3.369); and those 4 variables (immuosuppression, treatment, extranodal spread, and margin status) were used to calculate the ITEM score. The 5-year risk of dying from disease for patients with high-risk (>3.0), moderate-risk (>2.6-3.0), and low-risk (≤2.6) ITEM scores were 56%, 24%, and 6%, respectively. Fifty-six of 250 patients (22%) died from another cause.

Conclusions.—Patients who underwent surgery and received adjuvant radiotherapy had a better outcome compared with patients who underwent surgery alone. Patients who had moderate- or high-risk ITEM scores, usually because of extranodal spread and involved excision margins, had a poor outcome. The authors recommend considering these patients for inclusion in adjuvant chemoradiotherapy trials.

▶ Squamous cell carcinoma (SCC) is the second most common cutaneous malignancy seen in dermatology practice. The purpose of this study was to come up with a score model, which would then correlate into mortality rate in patients with regional metastatic cutaneous SCC of the head and neck. The study size was adequate given the nature of the cancer. The authors looked at 4 variables: immuosuppression, treatment, extranodal spread, and margin status in calculating the Immunosuppression, Treatment, Extranodal spread, and Margin status (ITEM) score. Higher ITEM scores correlated with higher mortality. The authors also compared outcomes in patients treated with surgery alone versus patients treated with surgery and adjuvant chemotherapy. Outcomes were better when surgery was combined with radiation. One weakness of this study was the disparity in the number of patients assigned to surgery or combination treatment. Only 28 patients were treated with surgery alone compared with 222 who received combination treatment.

S. Bhambri, DO
J. Q. Del Rosso, DO

A case-control study of cutaneous squamous cell carcinoma among Caucasian organ transplant recipients: The role of antibodies against human papillomavirus and other risk factors

Casabonne D, Lally A, Mitchell L, et al (Univ of Oxford, Headington, UK; Oxford Radcliffe Hosps, UK; Univ of London, UK; et al)
Int J Cancer 125:1935-1945, 2009

A case-control study was conducted in 140 people with histology proven cutaneous squamous cell carcinoma (SCC) and 454 controls, nested within 2 cohorts of organ transplant recipients (OTR) recruited in London and Oxford between 2002 and 2006. All participants had a skin examination, completed a questionnaire and had serum tested for antibodies against the L1 antigen of 34 HPV types using Luminex technology. SCC was more common in men than women (odds ratio [OR] = 1.7, 95% confidence interval [CI]: 1.1–2.8, $p = 0.02$) and in people with susceptibility to burn easily (OR = 3.0, 95%CI: 1.9–4.8; $p < 0.001$). The risk increased with increasing age (p-trend < 0.001), increasing time since transplant (p-trend < 0.001), increasing self-reported number of sunburns as a child (p-trend < 0.001) and with the presence of viral warts ($p < 0.001$). As expected, antibodies against HPV 16 were associated with a self-reported history of an abnormal cervical smear among women (OR 5.1, 95% CI: 2.6–10.2) and antibodies against HPV 6 were associated with a self-reported history of genital warts (OR 4.0, 95%CI: 2.2–7.2). However, no clear associations between any of the HPV types examined (including cutaneous betaHPVs) and SCC were identified. For example, the seroprevalence of HPV 5 was 15% among cases and 9% among controls ($p = 0.09$) and the seroprevalence of HPV 8 was 23% among cases and 21% among controls ($p = 0.6$). Nor was seropositivity to multiple types associated with SCC. These serological data do not provide evidence for a role for HPV in the aetiology of cutaneous SCC among OTR in two UK-based populations.

► Several interesting points are brought up in this article, the most important being the numbers of squamous cell carcinomas (SCC) that are found when screening is scheduled and preventative (the London group) as compared with those discovered upon referral or upon self-screening (the Oxford group). Cutaneous SCC is the #1 enemy for an organ transplant recipient (OTR) patient and without an understanding of the severity as well as stressing the need for regular skin surveillance, the patient's risks will significantly increase.

Although the mechanisms of epidermal dysplasia induced by human papillomavirus (HPV) are well-established, this study did not demonstrate a clear link to cutaneous SCC in the immunosuppressed population. We know that OTR patients develop atypical verrucal keratoses, actinic keratoses, and SCC at higher rates than immunocompetent population and that the risk factors (cumulative solar exposure, gender, and age) for both groups are significant, the correlation of HPV and SCC based on serology and subtyping cannot be established akin to HPV 16 to 18 and cervical carcinoma. Nevertheless, this magnifies the necessity for routine screening, aggressive combination therapies directed against verrucal keratoses, and lower threshold for biopsies of atypical lesions in the organ transplant patient.

N. Bhatia, MD

Merkel cell carcinoma of the skin: pathological and molecular evidence for a causative role of MCV in oncogenesis

Sastre-Garau X, Peter M, Avril M-F, et al (Institut Curie, Paris, France; Hôpital Cochin-APHP, Paris, France; Faculté de Médecine, Université René Descartes, Paris, France; et al)

J Pathol 218:48-56, 2009

Merkel cell carcinoma (MCC), a skin tumour with neuroendocrine features, was recently found to be associated with a new type of human polyomavirus, called Merkel cell virus (MCV). We investigated the specificity of this association as well as a causal role of MCV in oncogenesis. DNA and RNA from ten cases of MCC were analysed using PCR and RT-PCR. DNA from 1241 specimens of a wide range of human tumours was also analysed. The DIPS technique was used to identify the integration locus of viral DNA sequences. Array CGH was performed to analyse structural alterations of the cell genome. MCV DNA sequences were found in all ten cases of MCC and in none of the 1241 specimens of other tumour types. Clonal integration of MCV into the host genome was seen in all MCC cases and was checked by FISH in one case. A recurrent pattern of conserved viral sequences which encompassed the replication origin, the small tumour (ST), and the 5′ part of the large tumour (LT) antigen DNA sequences was observed. Both ST and LT viral sequences were found to be significantly expressed in all MCCs. Neither recurrent site of integration nor alteration of cellular genes located near the viral sequences was observed. The tight association of MCV with MCC, the clonal pattern of MCV integration, and the expression of the viral oncoproteins strongly support a causative role for MCV in the tumour process. This information will help the development of novel approaches for the assessment and therapy of MCC and biologically related tumours.

▶ Merkel cell carcinoma (MCC) has been on the rise in the past 15 years due to the increase in the aging population on sun exposed areas. In the past, MCC has been believed to derive from Merkel neuroendocrine epidermal cells, but the histogenesis of the tumor is still uncertain. A new type of human polyomavirus has recently been identified called Merkel cell polyomavirus (MCV or MCPyV) in the pathogenesis of MCC, but a definitive causative role has not been established. This is a study evaluating 10 cases of MCC using polymerase chain reaction (PCR) and investigating the specificity of this association as well as a causal role of MCV in oncogenesis. To analyze the specificity of MCV association with MCC, authors analyzed more than 1200 various tumor specimens, including melanoma and basal cell carcinoma. MCV DNA sequences were found to be integrated into the host genome in all MCC cases. A single integration site was detected in both primary and metastatic MCC, indicating that integration took place before clonal expansion of carcinoma cells. No specific translocation has been identified in cytogenic studies, but comparative genomic hybridization showed recurrent imbalances affecting whole chromosomes in the genomic profile of MCC. There was also an expression of viral oncoprotein similar to high-risk human papillomaviruses in uterine and cervical neoplasms. In conclusion, there is a need for further virological studies associated with MCV in the pathogenesis of MCC development for the assessment, prevention, and for the design of specific future therapies.

G. K. Kim, DO
J. Q. Del Rosso, DO

Clinical course and prognostic factors of Merkel cell carcinoma of the skin

Güler-Nizam E, Leiter U, Metzler G, et al (Eberhard-Karls-Univ, Germany)
Br J Dermatol 161:90-94, 2009

Background.—Merkel cell carcinoma (MCC) is a rare neuroendocrine malignancy of the skin first described by Toker as 'trabecular carcinoma of the skin' in 1972. To date, the origin of the tumour cells still remains unclear.

Objectives.—The present study analyses prognostic factors of MCC.

Patients and Methods.—The medical records of 57 patients with MCC treated between 1988 and 2006 at the Department of Dermatology in Tübingen were reviewed.

Results.—We identified 26 (45·6%) male and 31 (54·4%) female patients with MCC; the age at diagnosis ranged from 26 to 97 years (median 71 years). Primary tumours were located mainly on the head and neck areas (27 cases, 47·4%) and upper extremities (14 cases, 24·6%); 11 tumours were found on the lower extremities (19·3%) and four lesions on the chest (7%); one patient had an unknown primary location. Forty-five (78·9%) patients were diagnosed at stage I of the disease, 11 (19·3%) at stage II, and one patient (1·8%) at stage III at initial presentation. Stage of the disease and age at initial presentation were statistically significant with regard to overall ($P < 0·0001$; $P = 0·0327$) and tumour-specific survival ($P < 0·0001$; $P = 0·0156$). Use of the Cox regression model revealed initial stage of the disease as the only significant factor in the multivariate analysis. Radiotherapy applied promptly after excision of the primary tumour extended the time to progression significantly ($P = 0·0376$) but did not prolong overall or tumour-specific survival. Other parameters such as sex, site of tumour, sentinel node biopsy, excision margins, skin and noncutaneous malignancies were found to be not significant.

Conclusions.—Currently, early recognition of the disease seems to be the only method of ensuring overall survival. However, evidence-based treatment modalities are still urgently needed.

▶ The stage of the disease and age at initial presentation are the parameters that were found to have a statistically significant correlation with tumor specific and overall survival with Merkel cell carcinoma (MCC). The sample size of this study is small, but relative to the low incidence of MCC, it is a good sample size. This study did not find sex, tumor site, excision margins, and other noncutaneous malignancies to be prognostically significant in terms of survival rates. The high incidence of other malignancies may be due to the elderly population itself. In this study, the median margin was low due to the method of 3D-histology that was used. Another conclusion drawn was that the benefit on survival with performing sentinel lymph node biopsy remains unclear. Although it has been suggested that postoperative radiation treatment (RTX) of the primary site and draining lymph nodes reduces local recurrence rate, the high risk of distant metastases remains. This study found a significant difference in recurrence-free survival for patients treated with RTX after surgery but did not see significant prolongation in the tumor specific and overall survival.

S. B. Momin, DO
J. Q. Del Rosso, DO

Clinical Factors Associated With Merkel Cell Polyomavirus Infection in Merkel Cell Carcinoma

Sihto H, Kukko H, Koljonen V, et al (Laboratory of Molecular Oncology, Biomedicum, Helsinki, Finland; Helsinki Univ Central Hosp, Finland; et al)
J Natl Cancer Inst 101:938-945, 2009

Background.—Merkel cell carcinoma is a rare malignancy of the skin. Integration of Merkel cell polyomavirus (MCPyV) DNA to the tumor genome is frequent in these cancers. The clinical consequences of MCPyV infection are unknown.

Methods.—We analyzed formalin-fixed paraffin-embedded Merkel cell carcinoma tissue samples from 114 of 207 patients diagnosed with Merkel cell carcinoma in Finland from 1979 to 2004 for the presence of MCPyV DNA with the use of polymerase chain reaction (PCR), quantitative PCR, and DNA sequencing and examined associations between tumor MCPyV DNA status and histopathologic factors and survival. The median follow-up time after Merkel cell carcinoma diagnosis for subjects who were alive was 9.9 years (range $= 4.9$–21.9 years). All P values are two-sided.

Results.—MCPyV DNA was present in 91 carcinomas (79.8%). Compared with MCPyV DNA–negative cancers, MCPyV DNA–positive cancers were more often located in a limb (40.7% vs 8.7%, $P = .015$) and less frequent in patients who had regional nodal metastases at diagnosis (6.6% vs 21.7%, $P = .043$). Patients with MCPyV DNA–positive tumors had better overall survival than those with MCPyV DNA–negative tumors (5-year survival: 45.0% vs 13.0%, respectively; $P < .001$, two-sided log-rank test).

Conclusions.—MCPyV infection is associated with clinical outcomes in patients with Merkel cell carcinoma. These findings lend support to the hypothesis that viral infection is frequently associated with the pathogenesis of Merkel cell carcinoma.

▶ The association of Merkel cell polyomavirus (MCPyV) and Merkel cell carcinoma was one of the most interesting observations of virus-related oncogenesis to impact dermatology and dermatopathology in recent memory. In fact, it is akin to the discovery of the association of human herpes virus 8 (HHV-8) and Kaposi's sarcoma (KS) a number of years ago.

The only caveat to this is that the association may not be quite as tight as that of HHV-8 and KS, because certainly not all studies are in agreement with regard to the degree of the association. In fact, using PCR-based methods, various studies have found MCPyV in 24% to 89% of Merkel cell carcinomas examined. In this study, MCPyV was detected in 79.8% of cases (bringing closer to the upper end of the current range of data), but importantly 45% of all possible cases in the Finnish Cancer Registry were excluded, usually for lack of paraffin-embedded tissue to study.

It seems apparent that Merkel cell carcinoma could be a tumor for which multiple final pathways, and/or insults, converge to yield the malignancy. Is this really that much different from other malignant processes? For example, cervical cancer is certainly highly associated with certain forms of human papillomavirus (HPV) infection, but it is also impacted by other events, like cigarette smoking, and finally, certain cases, albeit a small number, may be uninvolved with HPV at all.

Finally, the authors attempt to identify whether or not infection with MCPyV impacts the clinical characteristics or the prognosis of Merkel cell carcinoma. MCPyV-positive cancers more often affected the limb, less often had regional metastasis at the time of diagnosis, and had a better overall survival. In my mind, these differences, which were statistically significant also suggest that there may be various subcategories of Merkel cell carcinoma that we previously lumped together for lack of ability to discriminate otherwise. It is even conceivable that testing for the presence of MCPyV may become a standard means of determining prognosis and/or customizing treatment.

W. A. High, MD, JD, MEng

Merkel cell polyomavirus sequences are frequently detected in nonmelanoma skin cancer of immunosuppressed patients

Kassem A, Technau K, Kurz AK, et al (Univ Hosp Freiburg, Germany; et al)
Int J Cancer 125:356-361, 2009

Recently, a new human polyoma virus has been identified in Merkel cell carcinomas (MCC). MCC is a highly aggressive neuroendocrine nonmelanoma skin cancer (NMSC) associated with immunosuppression. Clonal integration of this virus which was termed Merkel cell polyoma virus (MCPyV) was reported in a number of MCC. Squamous cell carcinoma (SCC) and basal cell carcinoma (BCC) are also NMSC and are the most frequent cancers in the setting of immunosuppression. A unique group of 56 NMSC from 11 immunosuppressed patients and 147 NMSC of 125 immunocompetent patients was tested for MCPyV by DNA PCR, targeting the Large T Antigen and the structural Viral Protein 1. NMSC included SCC, BCC and Bowen's disease (BD). In addition, normal skin and 89 colorectal cancers were tested. MCPyV specific sequences were significantly more frequently found in NMSC of immunosuppressed patients compared to immunocompetent patients ($p < 0.001$). In particular BD and BCC revealed a significant increased association of MCPyV of immunosuppressed patients ($p = 0.002$ and $p = 0.006$). Forty-seven of 147 (32%) sporadic NMSC were MCPyV positive. Interestingly, 37.5% (36/96) of sporadic BCC of immunocompetent patients were MCPyV positive. No MCPyV was detected within normal skin and only 3 out of 89 of additionally tested colorectal cancers were MCPyV positive. Our data show that MCPyV is a frequently reactivated virus in immunocompromized patients. How MCPyV contributes to the pathogenesis of NMSC, *i.e.*, BD, SCC and BCC, in immunosuppressed patients and in addition, potentially to the pathogenesis of a subset of sporadic BCC needs further investigations.

▶ Merkel cell carcinoma (MCC) is a rare but aggressive malignant neuroendocrine skin cancer, usually affecting the elderly and immunosuppressed. Past studies have identified a new human polyoma virus named Merkel cell polyoma virus (MCPyV) possibly related to the pathogenesis of nonmelanoma skin cancers (NMSC). This is a study of 56 NMSC of 22 immunosuppressed patients, including Bowen's disease (BD), squamous cell carcinoma (SCC), and basal cell carcinoma (BCC), evaluating for the presence of MCPyV as compared with sporadic BCC ($n = 96$), sporadic BD ($n = 30$), and sporadic SCC ($n = 30$) cases. There were 147 NMSC involving 125 immunocompetent patients tested for MCPyV by DNA polymerase chain reaction (PCR), targeting the Large T antigen (LT3), and the structural Viral Protein 1 (VP1). Also, the authors tested normal skin and 89 colorectal cancers and compared the results. MCPyV PCR products were found in 32% of the sporadic NMSC seen in the immunocompetent patients. In contrast, 62% of NMSC of the immunosuppressed patients were positive for MCPyV by either LT3 or VP1 by PCR. The prevalence of MCPyV compared with NMSC in immunocompetent patients was significantly increased ($P < .001$; 1.9-fold). The number of tumors positive for both LT3 and VP1 was significantly increased also ($P < .001$; 4.2-fold) in the NMSC of the immunosuppressed patients. Thirteen of the 18 (72.2%) immunosuppressed patients tested positive for MCPyV sequences either by LT3 or VP1. Compared with BCC of immunocompetent patients, MCPyV sequences were found more frequently in BCC found in the immunosuppressed patients (0.006), with 50% revealing products for LT3 and VP1 ($P < .001$). The number of MCPyV positive SCC cases was 2-fold higher in the immunosuppressed patients ($P = .043$). There was a striking difference with 69% of the BD group positive for MCPyV in the immunosuppressed study arm compared with 17.4% in the immunocompetent study arm ($P = .002$). All cases were positive for either LT3 or VP1 but not for both in immunocompetent patients. No MCPyV was detected in normal skin and 3 of 89 colorectal cancers were MCPyV positive. MCPyV was 4.3-fold more frequent in the NMSC of immunosuppressed patients ($P < .0001$). This could be due to enhanced viral replication correlated with a reduced capability to contain viral proliferation in the immunosuppressed patients. The MCPyV positivity in BD of immunosuppressed patients may reflect viral replication in a precursor lesion of invasive SCC in patients. Although it has been well described that certain immunosuppressive treatments may affect the frequency of NMSC, this study did not report which immunosuppressive medications were used by each patient. Another limitation was that this study did not correlate MCPyV and histological subtypes of NMSC. This study may possibly suggest reactivation of latent MCPyV contributing to NMSC development, especially in immunocompromised patients. Additionally, presence of MCPyV in immunocompetent patients suggests that there may be a localized immunocompromised response associated with actinic damage. However, this doesn't explain the differences in NMSC rates between populations. Future studies are needed with matched NMSC cases compared with normal skin in both the diverse immunosuppressed and immunocompetent patient groups.

G. K. Kim, DO

J. Q. Del Rosso, DO

Prevalence of Merkel cell polyomavirus in Merkel cell carcinoma
Duncavage EJ, Zehnbauer BA, Pfeifer JD (Washington Univ Med Ctr, St Louis, MO)
Mod Pathol 22:516-521, 2009

It has recently been shown that Merkel cell carcinoma, a rare and often lethal cutaneous malignancy, frequently harbors a novel clonally integrated polyomavirus aptly named Merkel cell polyomavirus. We aimed to study the prevalence of Merkel cell polyomavirus in cases of Merkel cell carcinoma, using specimens from formalin-fixed, paraffin-embedded tissue blocks. In our archives we identified 41 cases of Merkel cell carcinoma (from 29 different patients). Of these, 20 cases were primary cutaneous tumors, 4 were local recurrences, and 17 were metastases. PCR using two previously published primer sets, LT1 (440 bp amplicon) and LT3 (308 bp amplicon), as well as a novel primer set MCVPS1 (109 bp amplicon), was performed on all cases. Selected PCR products were sequenced to confirm amplicon identity. In addition, the MCVPS1 products were digested with *Bam*H1, yielding an 83 bp product. Amplifiable DNA was recovered in all 41 study cases. The detection rate of Merkel cell polyomavirus for each of the three primer sets was 22 of 29 patients (76%) for MCVPS1, 12 of 29 (41%) for LT3, and 8 of 29 (28%) for LT1. The variation between primer set detection rates was largely due to poor DNA quality, as supported by poor amplification of the higher molecular weight markers in size control ladder products and the fact that all cases that were positive by LT1 and LT3 were positive by MCVPS1. Our findings provide further evidence to link Merkel cell polyomavirus with a possible role in the oncogenesis of Merkel cell carcinoma. On a more practical level, our paraffin-optimized primer set may be used as an ancillary test to confirm the diagnosis of Merkel cell carcinoma in the clinical setting or for screening other rare tumor types for the causative virus, especially those tumor types that are underrepresented in frozen tissue repositories.

▶ Merkel cell carcinoma was recently shown to harbor a novel polyomavirus named the Merkel polyomavirus. The aim of this study was to determine the prevalence of Merkel polyomavirus in formalin-fixed paraffin specimens of Merkel cell carcinoma using 3 different polymerase chain reaction (PCR) primer sets (LT1, LT3, and MCVPS1). The detection rate of Merkel polyomavirus was the largest for the MCVPS1 primer set—22 of 29 patients (76%). However, all cases that were detected by the LT1 and LT3 primers were also positive by the MCVPS1 primer set. The MCVP1 primer set is the smallest of the 3 amplicons, and an increased efficacy of smaller amplicons is expected when using formalin-fixed tissue.

The demonstration of Merkel cell polyomavirus in 76% (22 of 29) of unique cases of Merkel cell carcinoma provides support for a link between Merkel polyomavirus and the oncogenesis of Merkel cell carcinoma. Importantly, a formal cause and effect link has not been definitively established, and further investigation is needed to understand the function of Merkel cell polyomavirus in the development of Merkel cell carcinoma.

This study was excellently designed with good controls (none of the 40 control DNA samples showed evidence of Merkel cell polyomavirus by the MCVPS1 primer set) and with an adequate comparison of 3 primer sets (MCVPS1, LT1, and LT3) for the detection of Merkel polyomavirus in formalin-fixed specimens of Merkel cell carcinoma. The major limitations of this study stem from the small number of cases of Merkel carcinoma; however, the relative rarity of this cutaneous malignancy makes it difficult to accrue large numbers of study subjects. Another important consideration is that any detection method, even the highly sensitive PCR, is not 100% sensitive and specific.

J. Levin, DO
J. Q. Del Rosso, DO

Imiquimod 5% Cream as Adjunctive Therapy for Primary, Solitary, Nodular Nasal Basal Cell Carcinomas Before Mohs Micrographic Surgery: A Randomized, Double Blind, Vehicle-Controlled Study
Butler DF, Parekh PK, Lenis A (Texas A&M Univ College of Medicine, Temple)
Dermatol Surg 35:24-29, 2009

Background.—Imiquimod 5% cream is currently approved for treatment of nonfacial, superficial basal cell carcinomas (BCCs). Topical imiquimod might be a reasonable candidate for adjunctive therapy of nodular, nasal BCCs before Mohs surgery.

Objective.—To observe the effectiveness of imiquimod 5% cream in reducing the number of Mohs stages, defect size, cost of Mohs surgery, and reconstruction.

Methods.—Patients applied the study medication nightly for 6 weeks with occlusion followed by a 4-week rest period before Mohs surgery was performed.

Results.—No differences were demonstrated in the number of Mohs stages, defect sizes, or costs between the two groups, possibly because of our small sample size. Only five of 12 patients (42%) in the treatment group were found histologically clear of tumor (complete responders).

Conclusion.—Imiquimod 5% cream was not helpful as an adjunctive treatment of nodular, nasal BCCs before Mohs surgery, but a larger study might show a benefit. Clearance of nodular, nasal BCCs treated with imiquimod prior to Mohs surgery was less than described in previous studies. Nasal BCCs may be more resistant to imiquimod treatment. Local inflammatory reactions limit imiquimod's usefulness in this setting. Histologic assessment of nasal BCCs treated with imiquimod is recommended.

▶ Basal cell carcinoma (BCC) is the most common cutaneous malignancy. This study looked at patients with only nodular BCCs, and the goal was to determine if pretreating patients with imiquimod 5% had any effect on the number of Mohs stages and defect size, among other things. The weakness of this study was the small size with 31 patients included and the location of nodular BCCs. There was a lack of variety in terms of anatomic location with all BCCs located on the same anatomic region, the nose. Complete response to imiquimod was seen in 42% (5 of 12) of patients. The authors suggested that nodular BCC on the nose may be more resistant to imiquimod therapy. Nodular BCC is not an approved indication for imiquimod therapy, although its use has been reported.[1] Cure rates using imiquimod for nodular BCC are lower and less consistent than those observed with treatment of superficial BCC, and are markedly lower than those achieved using surgical excisional modalities.[1] Therefore, the use of topical imiquimod for treatment of nodular BCC is not a primary option and is applicable only in selected cases based on patient-specific factors. Importantly, based on results from this study, pretreatment of nodular BCC on the nose with imiquimod was not consistently effective in reducing the number of Mohs stages or post-Mohs defect size.

S. Bhambri, DO

J. Q. Del Rosso, DO

Reference

1. Telfer NR, Colver GB, Bowers PW. Guidelines for the management of basal cell carcinoma. British Association of Dermatologists. *Br J Dermatol.* 1999;141: 415-423.

Nonmelanoma Skin Cancers of the Ear: Correlation Between Subanatomic Location and Post-Mohs Micrographic Surgery Defect Size
Duffy KL, McKenna JK, Hadley ML, et al (Univ of Utah, Salt Lake City; Peoria Ambulatory Surgery Ctr, IL)
Dermatol Surg 35:30-33, 2009

Background.—Nonmelanoma skin cancer (NMSC) of the ear can result in large defects with significant morbidity.

Objective.—To determine whether subanatomic location of NMSCs, based on ease of visualization of the ear, correlated with post-Mohs micrographic surgery (MMS) defect size.

Methods.—A retrospective chart review of 142 post-MMS ear lesions was performed and categorized according to subanatomic location: the helix, antihelix, and tragus (Location 1); retroauricular (Location 2); and conchal bowl, scapha, and triangular fossa (Location 3).

Results.—The average defect sizes were 2.50 cm^2(Location 1), 5.76 cm^2 (Location 2), and 4.03 cm^2 (Location 3). Tumors in Location 1 were significantly smaller than those occurring in Location 2 ($P < .001$) and Location 3 ($P < .01$), but a significant difference in size was not seen between Locations 2 and 3 ($P = .16$). As a control group, we randomly selected 50 NMSC cases from the nose and found the average defect size of nose NMSCs to be 1.58 cm^2.

Conclusions.—MMS defects of the ear are larger in nonvisible parts of the ear. As a group, MMS defects on the ear were larger than those on the nose.

► The article examines whether subanatomic location of nonmelanoma skin cancer correlates with the postMohs micrographic surgery (MMS) defect size. The study size was small with 142 patients. The authors divided the ear into 3 subanatomic locations. The postMMS defect size was noted to be larger in the retroauricular areas than the other 2 locations. It was postulated that this could be because skin cancers in the retroauricular areas are not easily visualized by patients and are in an area not routinely checked by many clinicians. The clear weakness of this study is its small size. Nonmelanoma skin cancers are most common cutaneous malignancy. The ear represents a common location, therefore the study size should have been larger. However, it is an interesting finding and physicians should not neglect the posterior ear region during skin examination.

S. Bhambri, DO

J. Q. Del Rosso, DO

Second primary cancers in patients with skin cancer: a population-based study in Northern Ireland
Cantwell MM, Murray LJ, Catney D, et al (Queen's Univ Belfast, Northern Ireland; et al)
Br J Cancer 100:174-177, 2009

Among all 14 500 incident cases of basal cell carcinoma (BCC), 6405 squamous cell carcinomas (SCC) and 1839 melanomas reported to the Northern Ireland Cancer Registry between 1993 and 2002, compared with the general population, risk of new primaries after BCC or SCC was increased by 9 and 57%, respectively. The subsequent risk of cancer, overall, was more than double after melanoma.

▶ Individuals with skin cancer are at higher risk of developing another malignancy. Authors looked at subsequent risk for any cancer in patients with basal cell carcinoma (BCC), squamous cell carcinoma (SCC), or melanoma. The study size was large with more than 20 000 patients. One limitation of the study is that the mean follow-up was only 4 years. Having a cutaneous malignancy (BCC, SCC, or melanoma) did put patients at a higher risk for developing another primary carcinoma. Authors were able to show that having a SCC put patients at a higher risk for developing melanoma. Also, the study population was mainly whites in Northern Ireland. This would serve as a limitation in applying the data to other regions or other racial groups.

S. Bhambri, DO

J. Q. Del Rosso, DO

Food intake, dietary patterns, and actinic keratoses of the skin: a longitudinal study
Hughes MCB, Williams GM, Fourtanier A, et al (Queensland Inst of Med Res, Brisbane, Australia; Univ of Queensland, Australia; L'Oréal Recherche, Paris, France)
Am J Clin Nutr 89:1246-1255, 2009

Background.—Actinic keratoses (AKs) are premalignant actinic tumors of the skin. Evaluation of the role of diet in their development is lacking.

Objective.—The objective was to determine whether intake of certain food groups or dietary patterns retard the occurrence of AKs over a 4.5-y period.

Design.—In a community-based study of skin cancer in Queensland, Australia, food intake of 1119 adults was assessed in 1992, 1994, and 1996 by using a validated food-frequency questionnaire. Dermatologists counted prevalent AKs during full-body skin examinations in 1992 and 1996. The relative ratio (RR) of AK counts in 1996 relative to 1992 was compared across increasing intakes of 26 food groups, and for 3 dietary patterns identified by principal components analysis, with the use of generalized linear models with negative binomial distribution, allowing for repeated measures. All analyses were adjusted for confounding factors, including skin color and sun exposure indexes.

Results.—AK acquisition decreased by 28% (RR: 0.72; 95% CI: 0.55, 0.95) among the highest consumers of oily fish (average of one serving every 5 d) compared with those with minimal intake. Similarly, the rate of acquisition of AKs was reduced by 27% (RR: 0.73; 95% CI: 0.54, 0.99) in those with the highest consumption of wine (average of half a glass a day in this study population). There was no consistent association of dietary pattern with AK acquisition.

Conclusion.—Moderate intake of oily fish and of wine may decrease the acquisition of AKs and thus complement sun protection measures in the control of actinic skin tumors.

▶ In the typical patient assessment for risks of development of skin cancer and actinic keratoses (AK), the role of diet and alcohol consumption is often overlooked in favor of history of solar exposure, artificial tanning, and sunscreen use. This article provides an overview of how moderate consumption of wine and oily fish over time may provide a protective effect in patients at high risk for AK development in conjunction with sunblock, ultraviolet (UV) protective clothing, and other measures. Some of these benefits may result from the direct effects of omega-3 fatty acids found in oily fish, on the immune mechanisms of the skin itself, as well as those food sources of vitamin D and antioxidants found in fish.

Several publications have attempted to provide a correlation between diet and prevention of onset of skin cancer and actinic keratoses. One study involved 76 patients for a 2-year period and suggested a low-fat diet may be beneficial in skin cancer prevention.[1] Another similar study was completed over a 2-year duration with a smaller population.[2] Both investigations looked at lowering dietary fat and should be compared with this evaluation studying beneficial fats and low intakes of wine.

It is important to note that this study was performed over 5 years and involved a large study population in Australia where UV protection and skin cancer awareness are part of daily life. In comparison with other countries, where these patterns may not be observed as readily, there should be consideration of average dietary fat intake, sunscreen use, and patient compliance with overall health prevention measures.

N. Bhatia, MD

References

1. Black HS, Herd JA, Goldberg LH, et al. Effect of a low-fat diet on the incidence of actinic keratosis. *N Engl J Med.* 1994;330:1272-1275.
2. Jaax S, Scott LW, Wolf JE, Thornby JI, Black HS. General guidelines for a low-fat diet effective in the management and prevention of nonmelanoma skin cancer. *Nutr Cancer.* 1997;27:150-156.

Bowen's Disease: A Four-Year Retrospective Review of Epidemiology and Treatment at a University Center

Hansen JP, Drake AL, Walling HW (Univ of Iowa)
Dermatol Surg 34:878-883, 2008

Background.—Cutaneous squamous cell carcinoma (SCC) in situ (Bowen's disease; BD) is a common intraepidermal malignancy. The aim of this study was to characterize the demographics, distribution, treatment, and recurrence risk of BD in a university population.

Methods.—A retrospective survey of histologically confirmed BD diagnosed between January 1999 and January 2003.

Results.—A total of 299 patients (193 men, 106 women) with 406 cases of BD were identified. The most common sites were the upper extremities (27%), ears (15%), and cheeks (11%). Men were significantly more likely to have SCC in situ on the scalp, ear, and anterior trunk, while the cheek, nose, and lower legs were significantly more common sites among women ($p < .05$). An office-based procedural treatment was performed in 92% of cases. Elliptical excision was the most common treatment modality (27%) followed by Mohs micrographic surgery (MMS; 20%) and then shave excision (19%). Histologic recurrence was seen in 15 of 406 cases (4%), one of which recurred as invasive SCC. Cryotherapy was associated with the highest recurrence rate (5-year recurrence of 13.4%), followed by topical 5-fluorouracil (9%) and shave excision (9%). Curettage and fulguration (6.5%), MMS (6.3%), and elliptical excision (5.5%) had lower 5-year recurrence rates.

Limitations.—Our experience at a single institution in the midwestern United States may not be reflective of a wider population.

Conclusion.—The most common locations for BD were in areas with high sun exposure. Multiple treatment options are available and recurrence is uncommon. Margin control surgery should be considered for tumors in high-risk areas.

▶ Bowen's disease is encountered frequently by dermatologists. The goal of this study was to look at the distribution, treatment, and recurrence in a specific population at the University of Iowa.

The study is well conducted, and the article is well referenced. The study size was adequate to determine reasonable conclusions with 406 Bowen's disease tumors. Sun exposed areas such as head and neck and extremities were most commonly involved. Treatment modalities and recurrences were thoroughly reviewed. Cryotherapy was associated with the highest recurrence risk. Mohs micrographic surgery (MMS) was performed in 92% of cases on lesions above the neck. Elliptical excisions had lower recurrence rate (5.5%) versus MMS (6.3%), but this difference was not statistically significant. Furthermore as authors note, a greater proportion of tumors treated with MMS were located at anatomically challenging sites such as ear and nose. Overall recurrence rate seen in this study is within rates reported by other studies.[1,2]

S. Bhambri, DO

J. Q. Del Rosso, DO

References

1. Kossard K, Rosen R. Cutaneous Bowen's disease. *J Am Acad Dermatol.* 1992;27: 406-410.
2. Leibovitch I, Huigol SC, Selva D, Richards S, Paver R. Cutaneous squamous carcinoma in situ (Bowen's disease): treatment with Mohs micrographic surgery. *J Am Acad Dermatol.* 2005;52:997-1002.

Occurrence of Nonmelanoma Skin Cancers on the Hands After UV Nail Light Exposure

MacFarlane DF, Alonso CA (The Univ of Texas, M. D. Anderson Cancer Ctr, Houston; The Univ of Texas Med School, Houston)
Arch Dermatol 145:447-449, 2009

Background.—Exposure to tanning beds, which contain mostly high-dose UV-A emitters, is a known cause of photoaging. Evidence is also accumulating for an association between tanning bed use and the development of skin cancer. Another source of high-dose UV-A is UV nail lights, available for use in the home and in beauty salons.

Observations.—Two healthy middle-aged women with no personal or family history of skin cancer developed nonmelanoma skin cancers on the dorsum of their hands. Both women report previous exposure to UV nail lights.

Conclusions.—It appears that exposure to UV nail lights is a risk factor for the development of skin cancer; however, this observation warrants further investigation. In addition, awareness of this possible association may help physicians identify more skin cancers and better educate their patients.

▶ This is a valuable case report series providing another source of documentation that artificial ultraviolet (UV) light can be a major risk factor for development of skin cancer. The public is not aware of UV nail light exposure compared with use of tanning beds and their potential consequences. Physicians and the public need to be made aware that any chronic use of UV light puts one at risk of skin cancer. Physicians should inquire during history taking if the patient is currently using or has used artificial UV lights of any type. It is also suggested to include questions about use of artificial light sources in patient history questionnaires.

S. B. Momin, DO

J. Q. Del Rosso, DO

Non-Melanoma Skin Cancer Incidence and Risk Factors After Kidney Transplantation: A Canadian Experience
Comeau S, Jensen L, Cockfield SM, et al (Univ of Alberta, Edmonton, Canada)
Transplantation 86:535-541, 2008

Background.—Non-melanoma skin cancer (NMSC) after kidney transplantation is common and can result in significant morbidity and mortality. Incidence and risk factors for NMSC can vary between geographic locations and there is no literature describing the incidence or risk factors for NMSC in Canada.

Methods.—The purpose of this retrospective cohort study was to determine the incidence of NMSC, the time of development of NMSC, and risk factors (including sun exposure history) for NMSC in kidney transplant recipients between 1990 and 2003 in our center (n = 926).

Results.—We observed a 9.7% incidence of NMSC lesions after kidney transplant with a median time of development of a first NMSC lesion of 4 years. Risk factors for NMSC (multivariate analysis) include older men (>45 years), a history of posttransplant warts, and longer duration of residence in a northern climate.

Conclusion.—We conclude that NMSC is common after kidney transplantation in a northern climate and these individuals require disease prevention-specific education, more vigilant surveillance and early referral and treatment.

▶ Organ transplant recipients (OTRs) present a challenge for the dermatologist in that the usual risk factors for skin cancer such as age, skin type, cumulative solar exposure, and gender are compounded by the influence of immunosuppression. However, OTRs who live in northern areas are not exempt from the risks of skin cancer compared with patients who live in southern climates, or warmer areas where solar exposure history may be more significant.

In this study, the authors report an incidence of nearly 10% of skin cancer in the renal transplant patients, which developed anywhere from 4 to 9 years posttransplant. Affected patients presented primarily with Fitzpatrick skin types I or II and were over age 45 years. In addition, the OTRs who had skin cancer also had a high percentage of warts, sunburns, and low compliance with sunscreens, all risk factors that are also to be taken into account with the immunocompetent patient.

This article serves as a good reminder to clinicians that patients in northern colder climates that have high risk factors for skin cancer are no different than those in the warmer climates, and that sunscreens and regular surveillance should not be overlooked or minimized.

N. Bhatia, MD

Photodynamic therapy of actinic keratoses with 8% and 16% methyl aminolaevulinate and home-based daylight exposure: a double-blinded randomized clinical trial
Wiegell SR, Hædersdal M, Eriksen P, et al (Univ of Copenhagen, Denmark; Danish Meteorological Inst, Copenhagen, Demark)
Br J Dermatol 160:1308-1314, 2009

Background.—Photodynamic therapy (PDT) is an effective but time-consuming and often painful treatment for actinic keratosis (AK). Home-based daylight–PDT has the potential to facilitate treatment procedure and to reduce associated pain due to continuous activation of small amounts of porphyrins. Moreover, a reduced methyl aminolaevulinate (MAL) concentration may reduce associated inflammation, making the treatment more tolerable for the patients.

Objectives.—To compare response rates and adverse effects after PDT using conventional 16% and 8% MAL with home-based daylight exposure in treatment of AK.

Methods.—Thirty patients with mostly thin-grade AK of the face or scalp were treated with 16% and 8% MAL–PDT in two symmetrical areas after application of sunscreen. Immediately after, patients left the hospital with instructions to spend the remaining day outside at home in daylight. Patients scored pain during treatment and light exposure was monitored with an electronic wristwatch dosimeter.

Results.—The complete response rate after 3 months was 76·9% for 16% MAL and 79·5% for 8% MAL ($P = 0·37$). Patients spent a mean of 244 min outdoors and received a mean effective light dose of $30\,J\,cm^{-2}$. Light doses of $8\text{–}70\,J\,cm^{-2}$ induced similar response rates ($P = 0·25$). Patients experienced mild to moderate pain during daylight exposure (mean maximal pain score of 3·7). No differences in pain scores and erythema were seen between the areas treated with 16% MAL and with 8% MAL.

Conclusions.—Home-based daylight-mediated MAL–PDT was an effective and well-tolerated treatment for AK. No differences in response rates or adverse events were found between the areas treated with 16% MAL and with 8% MAL.

▶ This study demonstrated that home-based daylight-mediated photodynamic therapy (PDT) was effective and safe for the treatment of actinic keratoses (AKs), with the use of both 8% and 16% methyl aminolaevulinate (MAL) in a well designed, double-blind, randomized clinical trial. The results of this experiment were very consistent despite the significant variation in the time between the application of MAL and exposure to daylight, and length of time each subject was exposed to daylight, and the weather conditions of the day.

The major limitation of this study was the number of subjects involved and the inability to monitor patient behavior at home.

Despite the significant success rates achieved in this study, it seems important to compare response rate of the at home therapy to the response rate of the equivalent in office therapy to make sure that by offering at home treatment, we are not sacrificing positive therapeutic outcomes.

J. Levin, DO

J. Q. Del Rosso, DO

Frequency of sensitization to methyl aminolaevulinate after photodynamic therapy
Korshøj S, Sølvsten H, Erlandsen M, et al (Aarhus Univ Hosp, Denmark; Univ of Aarhus, Denmark)
Contact Dermatitis 60:320-324, 2009

Background.—Allergic contact dermatitis to methyl aminolaevulinate (Metvix™) after topical application in photodynamic therapy (PDT) has previously been described in case reports.

Objective.—To compare the frequency of sensitization to Metvix® cream in a group of patients previously treated at least five times with Metvix-PDT with the frequency observed in an unexposed control group.

Methods.—Twenty patients treated five times or more with Metvix-PDT and 60 controls with no prior exposure to Metvix® were patch tested with Metvix® cream and Metvix® placebo cream. Subsequently, the patients were interviewed to determine the relevance of a positive patch test reaction to Metvix®.

Results.—Of 20 patients treated with Metvix-PDT, 7 were sensitized to Metvix® cream, giving a sensation risk of 35%. In the control group, 1 of 60 became sensitized after a single exposure to Metvix® cream (1.7%). There was no reaction to the placebo cream. The positive patch tests to Metvix® were considered relevant in four of seven patients (57%).

Conclusions.—This study demonstrates a considerable risk of sensitization after Metvix-PDT. We suggest that the patients are interviewed to detect late or persistent local reactions after PDT. These reactions are often considered to be local infections but may represent allergic contact dermatitis, and therefore, patients should be offered patch testing with Metvix® cream.

▶ This Food and Drug Administration (FDA) approved product is widely used in Europe for actinic keratosis, Bowen's disease, and superficial basal cell carcinoma. Contact sensitization to Metvix cream has been described. However, in this article patients with at least 5 previous treatments with Metvix-photodynamic therapy (PDT) showed a surprising 35% risk of sensitization in the treatment

TABLE 2.—Metvix Patch Test Results[a]

	n	Positive Proportion [% (95% exact CI)]	Total (N)
Metvix group	7	35 (15–59)	20
Control group	1	1.7 (0.0–8.9)	60
Total	8		80

CI, confidence interval.
[a]P < 0.0001 Fisher's exact test.

group (Table 2). This is a cause for concern and should alert us to be vigilant of this side effect in patients receiving multiple treatments with this product. Contact dermatitis with 5-aminolaevulinic acid (5-ALA) is an unusual event, and there is no cross allergy between 5-ALA and Metvix.

E. A. Tanghetti, MD

Actinic Keratoses: Natural History and Risk of Malignant Transformation in the Veterans Affairs Topical Tretinoin Chemoprevention Trial

Criscione VD, for the Department of veteran Affairs Topical Tretinoin Chemoprevention Trial Group, et al (Veterans Affairs Med Ctr, Providence, RI; et al)
Cancer 115:2523-2530, 2009

Background.—Actinic keratoses (AKs) are established as direct precursors of squamous cell carcinoma (SCC), but there is significant controversy regarding the rate at which AKs progress to SCC. The authors of this report studied a high-risk population to estimate the risk of progression of AK to SCC and to basal cell carcinoma (BCC) and the risk of spontaneous regression of untreated AKs.

Methods.—Data were obtained from participants in the Department of Veterans Affairs Topical Tretinoin Chemoprevention Trial. Participants were examined every 6 months for up to 6 years. At each examination, the locations on the face and ears of clinically diagnosed AKs and lesions scheduled for biopsy were marked, and high-resolution digital photographs were taken. These photographs were used later to map and track the presence, absence, or biopsy of each AK across visits.

Results.—In total, 7784 AKs were identified on the face and ears of 169 participants The risk of progression of AK to primary SCC (invasive or in situ) was 0.60% at 1 year and 2.57% at 4 years. Approximately 65% of all primary SCCs and 36% of all primary BCCs diagnosed in the study cohort arose in lesions that previously were diagnosed clinically as AKs. The majority of AKs (55%) that were followed clinically were not present at the 1-year follow-up, and the majority (70%) were not present at the 5-year follow-up.

Conclusions.—In the current study, the authors quantified the malignant potential of clinically diagnosed AKs for both SCC and BCC, although many did not persist, and the results suggested that AKs may play a greater role in the overall burden of keratinocyte carcinomas than previously documented.

▶ The objectives of this study are to quantify the risk of progression of actinic keratoses (AKs) on the face and ears to squamous cell carcinoma (SCC) or basal cell carcinoma (BCC) in a high-risk population and quantify the rate of spontaneous regression of AK without treatment. A total of 7784 AKs were identified on the face and ears of 169 participants. Results of this study show a low risk of progression of AK to SCC. However, it was shown that a majority of SCC (65%) and a significant percentage of BCC (36%) arose from AKs. This study also showed most AKs (55%) that were present at baseline and followed clinically were not present at the 1-year follow-up, and most AKs (70%) were not present at the 5-year follow-up.

The data from this study both supports and refutes the idea of early eradication of AKs. However, this study demonstrated a low rate of progression of AKs to carcinomas and a high rate of spontaneous regression at 1 and 5 years, suggesting that AKs may not require early treatment. However, on the other hand, this study showed a majority of SCC, and a significant percentage of BCC, arose in previously present AKs, which implies the need for AKs to be treated early. Despite stating the economic burden of treating AKs and implying the potential to use the above data to change the way we currently manage and treat AKs, the authors of this study make no suggestion of how their final results should influence the clinical management and treatment of AKs. It is the opinion of the reviewers that AKs be treated early with ablative and field therapies as it is not possible to predict which AKs will progress to carcinoma.

Many of the limitations of this study are clearly presented by the authors. These limitations include the difficulty in consistently diagnosing AKs by clinical and histologic criteria, the potential for ambiguity in determining marked locations in serial photographs, the participants used sunscreen which can suppress actinic neoplasia, the study participants were 95% men and considered high risk for the development of AKs, the AKs that were present at the start of the study could have been present for any length of time before enrollment, and a substantial number of AKs were identified later as BCC at follow-up either representing misdiagnoses or transformation.

J. Levin, DO
J. Q. Del Rosso, DO

Predicting Risk of Nonmelanoma Skin Cancer and Premalignant Skin Lesions in Renal Transplant Recipients
Urwin HR, Jones PW, Harden PN, et al (Keele Univ, Staffordshire, UK; Churchill Hosp, Oxford; et al)
Transplantation 87:1667-1671, 2009

Background.—Nonmelanoma skin cancer (NMSC) and associated premalignant lesions represent a major complication after transplantation, particularly in areas with high ultraviolet radiation (UVR) exposure. The American Society of Transplantation has proposed annual NMSC screening for all renal transplant recipients. The aim of this study was to develop a predictive index (PI) that could be used in targeted screening.

Methods.—Data on patient demographics, UVR exposure, and other clinical parameters were collected on 398 adult recipients recruited from the Princess Alexandra Hospital, Brisbane. Structured interview, skin examination, biopsy of lesions, and review of medical/pathologic records were performed. Time to presentation with the first NMSC was assessed using Coxg's regression models and Kaplan-Meier estimates used to assess detection of NMSC during screening.

Results.—Stepwise selection identified age, outdoor UVR exposure, living in a hot climate, pretransplant NMSC, childhood sunburning, and skin type as predictors. The PI generated was used to allocate patients into three screening groups (6 months, 2 years, and 5 years). The survival curves of these groups were significantly different ($P<0.0001$). Jack-knife validation correctly allocated all patients into the appropriate group.

Conclusion.—We have developed a simple PI to enable development of targeted NMSC surveillance strategies.

▶ The current recommendation is for annual screening of nonmelanoma skin cancer (NMSC) in renal transplant recipients (RTR), according to the American Society of Transplantation. Yet, this can result in significant costs. Thus, a predictive index (PI) to separate patients by risk category and frequency as this article attempts to formulate would be very useful.

The strengths of this article lie in the detailed manner in which the risk factors for developing NMSCs were extracted and analyzed to give rise to a specific equation, the PI. Some pitfalls to this article are the retrospective nature of the study, especially with regard to the potential underestimation of previous NMSCs in RTRs; the lack of data on melanoma and failure to address the risk of previous melanoma in RTRs; the subjective nature of risk factor recall in RTRs (ie, pretransplant squamous cell carcinomas [SCCs], pretransplant NMSC, history of childhood sunburns, etc); the unfamiliarity of skin typing by nondermatologists necessary for the calculation of PI; and lack of data on pretransplant immunosuppression. Despite these weaknesses, however, the article was well written and, if the PI is used to encourage RTRs with increased risk to visit a dermatologist sooner than 1-year posttransplantation, we would expect that their management should be facilitated, and the morbidity associated with multiple NMSCs in these patients should be reduced. As the authors themselves state, prospective testing of this model would be useful, and we eagerly await such a study.

N. Mehr, MD

A. Torres, MD, JD

Presence of beta human papillomaviruses in nonmelanoma skin cancer from organ transplant recipients and immunocompetent patients in the West of Scotland

MacKintosh LJ, de Koning MNC, Quint WGV, et al (Univ of Glasgow, UK; DDL Diagnostic Laboratory, Voorburg, The Netherlands)
Br J Dermatol 161:56-62, 2009

Background.—Nonmelanoma skin cancer (NMSC) has been linked to cutaneous human papillomaviruses of the genus beta (betaPV).

Objectives.—We sought to assess the presence of betaPV in NMSC biopsies from a group of Scottish skin cancer patients, both immunocompetent (IC) patients and immunosuppressed (IS) organ transplant recipients.

Methods.—One hundred and twenty-one paraffin-embedded skin tumours (27 actinic keratosis, 41 intraepidermal carcinoma, 53 squamous cell carcinoma) and 11 normal skin samples were analysed for the presence of betaPV by a polymerase chain reaction–reverse hybridization assay designed to detect the presence of the 25 known betaPV genotypes.

Results.—In IC patients, betaPV was detected in 30 of 59 (51%) tumours and two of 11 (18%) normal skin samples ($P = 0.046$). In IS patients, betaPV was found in 27 of 62 (44%) tumours; no normal skin samples were available for comparison. The most frequently found genotypes were HPV-24, HPV-15 and HPV-38. Of those tumours infected with betaPV, 28 of 57 (49%) were infected with more than one genotype (range 2–8). Tumours from IS patients were from a younger age group (mean age 57·4 years) than IC patients (mean age 73·8 years). Multiple infections were more common in tumours from IC patients (21 of 30; 70%) compared with those from IS patients (seven of 27; 26%) ($P < 0.001$). In the IC group, age did not appear to influence the distribution of single and multiple infections whereas in IS patients the proportion of multiple infections to single infections increased with age. There were no multiple infections in normal skin.

Conclusions.—A wide spectrum of betaPV types was detected in our samples. Further characterization of betaPV in vivo is needed in order to determine the mechanisms by which the virus contributes to cutaneous carcinogenesis.

▶ Several important components of the study need to be considered, including the mean age of each study group—73 in the immunocompetent (IC) group versus 57 in the immunosuppressed (IS) group—as well as the small number of patients and samples that were studied. One finding of note is the number of different human papillomaviruses (HPV) subtypes expressed in tumors and the lack of correlation to the common HPV strains found in common warts (eg, 1, 2, or 4) or those linked to cervical dysplasia (16 and 18). In addition, beta PV DNA was found to be just as common in the biopsies taken in the IC patient group. Given the small patient group studied, more data would be necessary to make conclusions about the role of HPV as carcinogens in cutaneous tumors.

N. Bhatia, MD

Patient Satisfaction After Treatment of Nonmelanoma Skin Cancer
Asgari MM, Bertenthal D, Sen S, et al (Kaiser Permanente Northern California, Oakland; San Francisco Veterans Affairs Med Ctr, CA)
Dermatol Surg 35:1041-1049, 2009

Background.—Patient satisfaction is an important aspect of patient-centered care but has not been systematically studied after treatment of nonmelanoma skin cancer (NMSC), the most prevalent cancer.

Objective.—To compare patient satisfaction after treatment for NMSC and to determine factors associated with better satisfaction.

Methods.—We prospectively measured patient, tumor, and care characteristics in 834 consecutive patients at two centers before and after destruction, excision, and Mohs surgery. We evaluated factors associated with short-term and long-term satisfaction.

Results.—In all treatment groups, patients were more satisfied with the interpersonal manners of the staff, communication, and financial aspects of their care than with the technical quality, time with the clinician, and accessibility of their care ($p < .05$). Short-term satisfaction did not differ across treatment groups. In multivariable regression models adjusting for patient, tumor, and care characteristics, higher long-term satisfaction was independently associated with younger age, better pretreatment mental health and skin-related quality of life, and treatment with Mohs surgery ($p < .05$).

Conclusions.—Long-term patient satisfaction after treatment of NMSC is related to pretreatment patient characteristics (mental health, skin-related quality of life) and treatment type (Mohs) but not tumor characteristics. These results can guide informed decision-making for treatment of NMSC.

▶ There are many different treatments of nonmelanoma skin cancer (NMSC). It has also been recognized that patient satisfaction is an important outcome measure and has been known to be associated with health care status, quality of life, and compliance. This is a prospective cohort study assessing patient short-term and long-term satisfaction after treatment of NMSC at Veterans Affairs Medical Center (VAMC). This study measured patient, tumor, and care characteristics in 834 consecutive patients. The authors evaluated these factors before and after treatment, which included destruction using electrodesiccation and curettage (19%), excision (40%), and Mohs micrographic surgery (MMS) (41%). Socioeconomic characteristics, comorbid illnesses, tumor-related quality of life, and health status were measured before therapy from a mailed survey. Patients were also asked about scar and concerns with treatment. Patients in the 3 treatment categories were similar in age, physical and mental health status, and comorbidity index but differed in education income, baseline quality of life, and tumor characteristics. In all treatment groups, patients were satisfied with the interpersonal manners of the staff, communication, and financial aspects of their care than the technical quality, time with clinician, and accessibility of their care ($P < .05$). Long-term satisfaction was assessed at 1 year after therapy with 571 (68%) individuals responding high satisfaction regardless of treatment. Long-term satisfaction was independently associated with younger age, better pretreatment mental health, skin-related quality of life, and treatment with MMS ($P < .05$). Limitations to this study included recall bias especially with long-term satisfaction. Another limitation is that questionnaires did not inquire about other key factors such as environment, nursing care, and time spent in the waiting room. In conclusion, the authors found that long-term patient satisfaction is related to pretreatment characteristics and treatment choice with NMSC.

G. K. Kim, DO

J. Q. Del Rosso, DO

Tumorigenic Effect of Some Commonly Used Moisturizing Creams when Applied Topically to UVB-Pretreated High-Risk Mice
Lu Y-P, Lou Y-R, Xie J-G, et al (The State Univ of New Jersey, Piscataway; et al)
J Invest Dermatol 129:468-475, 2009

Irradiation of SKH-1 mice with UVB ($30 \, \text{mJ} \, \text{cm}^{-2}$) twice a week for 20 weeks resulted in mice with a high risk of developing skin tumors over the next several months in the absence of further irradiation with UVB (high-risk mice). Topical applications of 100 mg of Dermabase, Dermovan, Eucerin Original Moisturizing Cream (Eucerin), or Vanicream once a day, 5 days a week for 17 weeks to these high-risk mice increased significantly the rate of formation of tumors and the rate of increase in tumor size per mouse. Additional studies indicated that treatment of high-risk mice with Dermabase, Dermovan, Eucerin, or Vanicream for 17 weeks increased the total number of histologically characterized tumors by 69% (average of two experiments; $P < 0.0001$ in each experiment), 95% ($P < 0.0001$), 24% ($P < 0.01$), and 58% ($P < 0.0001$), respectively. Topical applications of a specially designed Custom Blend cream to high-risk mice was not tumorigenic. The results indicate that several commercially available moisturizing creams increase the rate of formation and number of tumors when applied topically to UVB-pretreated high-risk mice. Further studies are needed to determine the effects of topical applications of moisturizing creams on sunlight-induced skin cancer in humans.

▶ Moisturizing creams and ointments used for the prevention and treatment of dry skin are generally tested for safety by determining the irritant activity as well as their effects on sensitization, but skin care regimens are generally not tested for carcinogenic activity.

This study found that application of 4 commercially available and widely used moisturizing creams to chronically exposed UVB SKH-1 mice for 5 days a week for 17 weeks increased the rate of tumor formation per mouse and tumor volume per mouse when compared with control. The controls tested in this study consisted of both UVB exposure without application of any cream and UVB exposure with application of water instead of cream.

The mechanism of the tumorigenic effects of moisturizing creams in UVB-pretreated mice is not known; further studies on possible mechanisms are needed. During the course of the study, the authors developed a custom blend cream that excluded the ingredients sodium lauryl sulfate (SLS) and mineral oil. This custom blend formula was the only cream applied to the UVB-exposed mice that did not show increase in the rate of tumor formation or tumor volume. It should be noted that not all of the 4 commercially available creams tested that showed tumorigenic activity had SLS and mineral oil in their formulary, and, in fact, one cream did not contain SLS or mineral oil and still showed tumorigenic activity.

The results of this study are preliminary and based on testing in a murine model, so application of this information to human skin is highly speculative at this time. However, such information could lead to significant change in the way cosmetic and over-the-counter (OTC) products are tested before coming to market. Currently, the industry standard is to complete allergy and stability testing before coming to market. Taking the results of this study into account, it may be necessary to include carcinogenic studies of cosmetic and OTC formulas before coming to market. Further studies are needed in this area.

Although mouse skin in widely used in carcinogenicity studies, it should also be noted that SKH-1 mouse skin is much thinner and more permeable than human skin. Additionally, this particular type of mouse is albino and hairless. So far, the tumorigenic effect of moisturizing creams has only been tested in hairless SHK-1 mice, and therefore the clinical significance of widespread use of moisturizing creams on sunlight exposed human skin has not been established.

J. Levin, DO
J. Q. Del Rosso, DO

The role of surgery and radiotherapy in treatment of soft tissue sarcomas of the head and neck region: Review of 30 cases

Fayda M, Aksu G, Yaman Agaoglu F, et al (Kocaeli Univ, Turkey; Istanbul Univ, Turkey)
J Cranio-Maxillofac Surg 37:42-48, 2009

Background.—Thirty adult patients with head and neck soft tissue sarcoma (HNSTS) treated between 1987 and 2000 were retrospectively analysed.

Patients and Methods.—The most frequent histopathological subtypes were chondrosarcomas (27%) and malignant fibrous histiocytoma (20%). The surgical resection was performed in 25 of the 30 patients (83%). Twenty-three patients in the surgical resection arm received postoperative radiotherapy.

Results.—Five-year local control rates for patients with negative surgical margins ($n = 9$), microscopically positive disease ($n = 10$), gross residual disease ($n = 6$) and inoperable cases ($n = 5$) were 64, 70, 20 and 0%, respectively. However, there was no significant difference in local control between patients with negative or microscopically positive disease who received postoperative radiotherapy (71 vs. 70%). The patients who received doses ≥ 60 Gy had significantly higher local control rates than the ones who received doses lower than 60 Gy ($p = 0.048$). The local control rates were lower in patients with grade 2–3 tumours when compared with grade 1 tumours (44 vs. 83%). The median overall survival of whole group was 31 months. Median survivals of patients receiving both surgery and radiotherapy with negative and microscopically positive margins were significantly better than patients who were not treated with surgery (34.8 and 36 vs. 13.3 months).

Conclusion.—Our results confirm that the optimal treatment of HNSTSs is complete surgical excision, and that postoperative adjuvant radiotherapy clearly improves local control.

▶ The goal of this article was to review treatment options, including surgery and radiotherapy, in treatment of soft tissue sarcomas of the head and neck region. The article meets its goal and is well written and well referenced. Complete excision is the most optimal treatment. Postoperatively, radiation may be important in reducing the risk of local recurrence. Sarcomas are rare and thus the study size of 30 patients is relatively large in this setting. High radiotherapy doses are more effective than lower doses in local control, but recurrences are still high. However, the recurrence is higher with surgical excision without use of postoperative radiation. An important point to note is that the most common presentation of soft tissue sarcomas of the head and neck is a painless mass, which may be subcutaneous and misdiagnosed clinically as a lipoma or cyst.

S. Bhambri, DO
J. Q. Del Rosso, DO

Vulvar basal cell carcinoma in China: a 13-year review
Lui PCW, Fan YS, Lau PPL, et al (the Chinese Univ of Hong Kong, China; Queen Mary Hosp, Hong Kong, China; Queen Elizabeth Hosp, Hong Kong, China; et al)
Am J Obstet Gynecol 200:514.e1-514.e5, 2009

Objective.—We conducted a 12-year retrospective review of vulvar basal cell carcinoma (BCC) in a Chinese population.

Study Design.—Medical records and histopathologic reports were examined from 5 major Hospitals in Hong Kong to list all patients diagnosed with vulvar BCC. Clinical data and histologic materials were reviewed.

Results.—Sixteen vulvar BCCs were diagnosed. Most of them were pigmented. They were removed by simple excision or wide local excision. All the carcinomas were identified in the reticular dermis. The predominant histologic pattern was nodular, which may be mistaken as adenoid cystic carcinoma.

Conclusion.—The high proportion of pigmented vulvar BCCs suggested that biopsy should be performed for any pigmented lesion in a Chinese patient. The BCCs are superficial and tissue-preserving treatment approach is recommended. The tumor depth estimation is difficult and intraoperative frozen section consultation may be helpful. Formal histopathologic assessment should be used to reach an objective diagnosis.

▶ Although ultraviolet (UV) light and inadequate sun protection have been linked to an increased risk for development of basal cell carcinoma (BCC), other anatomic sites that receive negligible UV exposure, such as the vulvar region, can be affected. This is a 12-year retrospective review from 1995-2007 of 16 patients diagnosed with vulvar BCC in the Chinese population, evaluating medical records and histopathologic reports from 5 major hospitals in Hong Kong. This study sought to assess the features of vulvar BCC in the Chinese population. Clinical data included gross morphology, size, depth of invasion, histologic type, treatment, length of recurrence, and BCC in other anatomic sites. This study suggests that the occurrence of vulvar BCC in the Chinese population is comparable with the incidences seen in fair-skinned individuals. The incidence of vulvar BCC among all BCCs in the Chinese population was found to be 0.92%. The authors also found that the mean age of presentation was also similar in both the Caucasian and the Chinese populations, with a propensity for the elderly. Most of the vulvar BCCs were pigmented (81%) and were histologically the nodular type. This is different from the Caucasian population, whose incidence of pigmented BCC is approximately 3%. With these findings in mind, the authors suggested that more biopsies of pigmented lesions in the vulvar area are needed. They also found no direct correlation between tumor width and depth of invasion.

G. K. Kim, DO
J. Q. Del Rosso, DO

Atypical and malignant hidradenomas: a histological and immunohistochemical study

Nazarian RM, Kapur P, Rakheja D, et al (Massachusetts General Hosp and Harvard Med School, Boston; Univ of Texas Southwestern Med Ctr, Dallas; et al)

Mod Pathol 22:600-610, 2009

The histological features of atypical hidradenoma are worrisome for increased risk of recurrence and possible malignant potential; however, earlier studies with immunohistochemistry or patient follow-up have not been reported. In addition, immunohistochemical analysis of hidradeno-carcinoma exists in the literature mainly as case reports and as a single series of six cases. We compare the histological features and Ki-67, phosphorylated histone H3, epidermal growth factor receptor, and Her2/neu expression profiles of 15 atypical and 15 malignant hidradenomas with those of benign hidradenoma and metastasizing adnexal carcinomas. Infiltrative growth pattern, deep extension, necrosis, nuclear pleomorphism, and ≥ 4 mitoses per 10 high-power fields are specific features of hidradenocarcinomas. Significant difference in mean Ki-67% was observed between benign and malignant hidradenomas ($P < 0.001$), benign and metastasizing adnexal carcinomas (0.002), atypical and malignant hidradenomas ($P < 0.001$), and between atypical hidradenomas and metastasizing adnexal carcinomas (0.002). Significant difference in mean phosphorylated histone H3% was observed between benign and malignant hidradenomas ($P < 0.001$), benign and metastasizing adnexal carcinomas (0.003), atypical and malignant hidradenomas ($P < 0.001$), and between atypical hidradenomas and metastasizing adnexal carcinomas ($P < 0.001$). Mean epidermal growth factor receptor total score was significantly different in benign and atypical hidradenoma when compared with that in metastasizing adnexal carcinoma ($P = 0.014$ and 0.019, respectively). Equivocal or 2+ Her2/neu positivity was observed in one hidradenocarcinoma and in two metastasizing adnexal carcinomas. Receiver operating characteristic curve analysis for Ki-67 and phosphorylated histone H3% positivity reveals statistically significant criterion values of >11.425 and >0.7, respectively, for distinguishing malignant hidradenomas from atypical hidradenomas. Despite the presence of some worrisome histological features, the significantly different immunoprofile from the malignant counterpart suggests that atypical hidradenomas are likely to recur but are unlikely to metastasize. A tumor with Ki-67 > 11% and/or phosphorylated histone H3 > 0.7% would likely be a malignant rather than an atypical hidradenoma. The infrequent Her2/neu overexpression in hidradenocarcinoma suggests its limited therapeutic role.

▶ In the case of rare tumors and the differentiation between benign and malignant variants, the histological and immunohistochemical findings help the clinician manage the patient more than any other tool. For example, the summary of findings comparing the tumors as demonstrated in Tables 3 and 4 in the original article defines how integral histologic markers are to determining how to manage these patients.

Although only a small population of tumors ($n = 30$) was studied, this article helps support this concept, and although this tumor is less common than other adnexal neoplasms seen in daily practice, the malignant variants left undiagnosed will have similar untoward consequences to the patient.

The authors clarify that the tumors were completely excised for this study and the identification by staining patterns is only part of the evaluation, along with histological findings and patient demographics. Nevertheless, this article represents a good overview of the use of immunohistochemistry in the objective evaluation of rare but potentially significant cutaneous tumors.

N. Bhatia, MD

Incidence of nonmelanoma skin cancer in a cohort of patients with vitiligo

Hexsel CL, Eide MJ, Johnson CC, et al (Multicultural Dermatology Ctr, Detroit, MI; Henry Ford Hosp, Detroit, MI)
J Am Acad Dermatol 60:929-933, 2008

Background.—Nonmelanoma skin cancer (NMSC) incidence in patients with vitiligo has not been studied.

Objective.—We sought to quantify the incidence of NMSC in patients with vitiligo.

Methods.—A cohort of 477 patients with vitiligo and no history of NMSC seen in an outpatient academic center between January 2001 and December 2006 was established. All charts for patients with vitiligo were reviewed for incident NMSC, and histopathology verified. Age-adjusted (2000 US Standard Million) incidence rates were calculated and compared to US rates.

Results.—Six patients with NMSC were identified; all were Caucasian (>61 years). Age-adjusted incidence rates were: basal cell carcinoma, male 1382/100,000; basal cell carcinoma, female 0; squamous cell carcinoma, male 465/100,000; squamous cell carcinoma, female 156/100,000. Except for basal cell carcinoma in females, all rates were higher than US rates but not statistically significant.

Limitations.—Comparison incidence rates from the general patient population during the same time period were unavailable.

Conclusion.—Health care providers should be aware of the possible risk of NMSC in Caucasian patients with vitiligo.

▶ Vitiligo is a well-known condition characterized by immune mediated idiopathic destruction of melanocytes resulting in hypopigmented patches. Monitored exposure to ultraviolet (UV) radiation is a treatment option. Previous studies have not shown a strong correlation with nonmelanoma skin cancer (NMSC) in patients with vitiligo, which seems counterintuitive with the loss of protective melanin. This is a cohort study of 477 patients with vitiligo, with no history of NMSC, with comparisons of incidence rates of NMSC in patients with vitiligo to incidence rates in the United States during the years of 2001-2006. The authors also look at demographic characteristics of these patients based on race, age, gender, and type of skin cancer. They also note whether NMSC sites were of vitiliginous skin or normal skin and a history of UV treatment. The results revealed that NMSC was found on sun-exposed sites of Caucasian patients with vitiligo in both vitiligo-affected and unaffected skin. Compared with estimates of NMSC rates in 2 general United States Caucasian populations, incidence rates of skin cancer in patients with vitiligo appear to be higher, but the results were not statistically significant. Although this is a study with a large sample size, the confidence interval is wide and patients are followed only for a time span of 5 years. In addition, the annual incidence rates refer to people with NMSC and not the number of tumors, with patients having more than one skin cancer being counted once. In addition, the authors were unable to comment on skin cancer in non-Caucasian races, even with a diverse group of patients. Although the study might not represent the overall vitiligo United States population, it opens up discussion on the possibility of epidemiologic risk factors of patients with vitiligo and the notion that these patients could have equal or higher incidence rates of NMSC compared with the normal population.

G. K. Kim, DO

J. Q. Del Rosso, DO

Quality of life in the actinic neoplasia syndrome: The VA Topical Tretinoin Chemoprevention (VATTC) Trial

Weinstock MA, Lee KC, Chren M-M, et al (VA Med Ctr, Providence, RI; Univ of California, San Francisco)

J Am Acad Dermatol 61:207-215, 2009

Background.—Keratinocyte carcinomas (KCs) are the most common malignancies of the skin. As lesions have a low mortality rate, understanding quality-of-life (QoL) factors is necessary in their management.

Objective.—To assess QoL and associated patient characteristics in those with a history of keratinocyte carcinomas.

Methods.—We conducted a cross-sectional study of veterans with a history of KCs enrolled in a randomized controlled trial for chemoprevention of keratinocyte carcinomas. Study dermatologists counted actinic keratoses (AKs) and assessed for skin photodamage. QoL was assessed using Skindex-29 and KC-specific questions. Demographics were self-reported.

Results.—Participants (n = 931) enrolled at 5 clinical sites had worse QoL on all subscales (emotions, functioning, and symptoms) compared to a reference group of patients without skin disease. Univariate analysis demonstrated worse QoL associated with higher AK count, past 5-fluorouracil (5-FU) use, and greater sun sensitivity. Multivariate analysis demonstrated that higher AK count and past 5-FU use were independently related to diminished

QoL. Higher comorbidities showed modest associations on the symptoms and functioning subscales. Number of previous KCs was not independently associated with any QoL differences.

Limitations.—Study population may not be generalizable to the general population. Counting of AKs is of limited reliability. Previous 5-FU use is self reported.

Conclusions.—A history of ever use of 5-FU and present AKs was strongly associated with worse QoL. We find it more useful to consider these patients as having the chronic condition "actinic neoplasia syndrome," whose burden may be best measured by factors other than their history of KCs.

▶ Keratinocyte carcinomas (KC) include basal and squamous cell carcinoma, which are generally not fatal. However, assessing morbidity is critical to understanding the burden of disease for KCs because treatment may lead to severe disfigurement and related complications. This is a cross-sectional study assessing the quality of life (QoL) associated with 931 patients with a history of KC, all part of the Veterans Affairs Topical Tretinoin Chemoprevention Trial (VATTC) across multiple centers in the United States. QoL was measured by using the Skindex-29, which is a self-administered questionnaire measuring the effects of skin conditions on QoL. This consists of 29 items, reported on 3 scale-emotions, symptoms, and function. In addition, patients responded to size KC specific items—scars, appearance, persistence of actinic damage, worry from skin condition, and treatment. Also, patient's education level, marital status, previous 5-FU, and sun-sensitivity indicators were collected using the self-response surveys. Worse QoL on all 3 subscales and the KC-specific items was associated with higher actinic keratosis (AK) counts, past 5-FU use, and greater sun sensitivity. Female gender, higher education level, and being unmarried were all independently associated with worse symptoms. Number of previous KCs was not independently associated with any QoL differences. Researchers labeled those living with sun damage, having many AKs, and a history of skin cancers as a chronic condition known as actinic neoplasia syndrome (ANS). Findings suggest that KCs are not primarily responsible for the QoL impact, but other aspects of this syndrome. Being married had a strong association with improved QoL in the symptoms domain. There was a slight association of higher comorbidities with worse QoL in the symptoms and functioning domain, findings that agree with previous studies. Greater visible photodamage was not related to QoL with univariate or multivariate associations. Additional means of specific Skindex items referring to appearance suggest that the elderly male population is not particularly concerned with physical appearances. Limitations of this study were that all patients were part of the chemoprevention trial with at least 2 KCs in the 5 years before enrollment. All subjects were veterans, predominantly Caucasian, male and elderly. Also, the counting of AKs has been known to be subject to error despite evaluation by a dermatologist because they are based on clinical examination. The history of 5-FU use was obtained by self-report only without medical record verification. To add, the assessment of photodamage was of unknown reliability.

The strengths of this study were the large sample size and access to previous medical records used for measurement of comorbidities. In conclusion, authors suggest that ANS is a chronic illness as opposed to a series of cancer episodes having a significant impact on the QoL of individuals.

G. K. Kim, DO

J. Q. Del Rosso, DO

Skin cancer trends among Asians living in Singapore from 1968 to 2006
Sng J, Koh D, Siong WC, et al (Natl Univ of Singapore; Ctr for Molecular Epidemiology)
J Am Acad Dermatol 61:426-432, 2009

Background.—The incidence rates of skin cancers in Caucasian populations are increasing. There is little information on skin cancer trends in Asians, who have distinctly different skin types.

Objective.—We sought to study skin cancer incidence rates and time trends among the 3 Asian ethnic groups in Singapore.

Methods.—We analyzed skin cancer data from the Singapore Cancer Registry from 1968 to 2006 using the Poisson regression model.

Results.—There were 4044 reported cases of basal cell carcinoma, 2064 of squamous cell carcinoma, and 415 of melanoma. Overall skin cancer incidence rates increased from 2.9/100,000 in 1968 to 1972 to 8.4/100,000 in 1998 to 2002, declining to 7.4/100,000 in 2003 to 2006. Among older persons ($\geq$60 years), basal cell carcinoma rates increased the most, by 18.9/100,000 in Chinese, 6.0/100,000 in Malays, and 4.1/100,000 in Indians from 1968 to 1972 to 2003 to 2006. Squamous cell carcinoma rates among those aged 60 years and older increased by 2.3/100,000 in Chinese and by 1/100,000 in Malays and Indians. Melanoma rates were constant for all 3 races. Skin cancer rates among the fairer-skinned Chinese were approximately 3 times higher than in Malays and Indians, who generally have darker complexions.

Limitations.—Although appropriate population denominators were used, lack of data from 2007 could have affected the results for the last time period, which comprised 4 instead of 5 years.

Conclusion.—Incidence rates of skin cancer in Singapore increased from 1968 to 2006, especially among older Chinese.

▶ In the past, it has been suggested that Asians have an inherent protection from skin cancer due to their darker pigmented skin. However, other studies have suggested that skin cancer rates are underestimated in the Asian population. This is a study of skin cancer trends using a cancer registry in 3 different Asian ethnic groups living in Singapore from 1968 to 2006. Singapore is a multiethnic nation with 77% Chinese, 14% Malays, 8% Indians, and 1% of other ethnicities. This study included 4044 reported cases of basal cell carcinoma (BCC), 2064 cases of squamous cell carcinoma (SCC), and 414 cases of melanoma (M). Investigators concluded that among older persons (>60 years), BCC rates have increased by 18.9/100 000 in Chinese, 6.0/100 000 in Malays, and 4.1/100 000 in Indians between 1968-1972 and 2003-2006. Melanoma rates have remained constant for all 3 races during this time period. Skin cancer rates among fairer skinned Chinese patients were approximately 3 times higher than in darker skinned Malays and Indians. BCC was the most common skin cancer in Singapore followed by SCC then melanoma. The incidence rates of BCC, SCC, and M were relatively stable over time in all persons younger than 60 years of age regardless of ethnicity. The conclusion of this study was that incidence rates of skin cancer in Singapore have increased during 1968-2006 especially among patients older than 60 years of age. This study revealed that different ethnicities within Asian populations can have significantly different skin cancer rates. A limitation to this study was that data from 2007 and beyond were not included in this study, which could have affected the data. The sites of skin cancer occurrence were not noted in this article, which is an important factor when considering possible correlation with solar ultraviolet exposure and in identifying risk factors. There is also a possibility that a significant number of skin cancers were prophylactic excised by primary care clinics without histological confirmation, which could have underestimated rates. In addition, this study did not mention treatment modalities in Singapore, which could have also been interesting to note. Although this study concluded that skin cancer rates are on the rise among Asians in Singapore, the rising rates can be attributed to better detection methods. In conclusion, this study revealed that skin cancer rates can differ among Asian groups within the same region.

G. K. Kim, DO

J. Q. Del Rosso, DO

Short incubation with methyl aminolevulinate for photodynamic therapy of actinic keratoses

Braathen LR, Paredes BE, Saksela O, et al (Univ Clinic for Dermatology, Bern, Switzerland; Helsinki Univ Central Hosp, Finland; et al)
J Eur Acad Dermatol Venereol 23:550-555, 2009

Background.—Photodynamic therapy (PDT) using methyl aminolevulinate (MAL) is an effective first-line treatment for actinic keratoses. A reduced incubation period may have practical advantages.

Objective.—This study aims to evaluate the effect of incubation time (1 vs. 3 h), MAL concentration (160 mg/g vs. 80 mg/g) and lesion preparation in the setting of MAL-PDT for treatment of actinic keratosis (AK).

Design.—Open, randomized, parallel-group multicentre study.

Setting.—Outpatient dermatology clinics.

Subjects.—One hundred and twelve patients with 384 previously untreated AK. Most lesions (87%) were located on the face and scalp and were thin (55%) or moderately thick (34%).

Methods.—Lesions were debrided, and MAL cream (160 mg/g or 80 mg/g) was applied before illumination with red light (570–670 nm; light dose, 75 J/cm^2). Patients were followed up at 2 and 3 months. Sixty patients (54%) were re-treated and assessed at 6 months.

Main Outcome.—Complete lesion response rates 3 and 12 months after last treatment.

Results.—For lesions on the face/scalp, lesion complete response rates were 78% for thin AK and 74% for moderately thick AK lesions after 1 h vs. 96% and 87% after 3 h incubation with MAL 160 mg/g. Lesion recurrence rates at 12 months after two treatments were similar [19% (3 of 16) with 1 h vs. 17% (3 of 18) with 3 h 160 mg/kg MAL-PDT] and lower than for 80 mg/g MAL-PDT (44–45%).

Conclusion.—MAL-PDT using a 1-h incubation may be sufficient for successful treatment of selected AK lesions.

▶ The objective of this article was to evaluate the efficacy of a shortened drug incubation time for the use of methyl aminolevulinate (MAL) photodynamic therapy (PDT) in the treatment of actinic keratoses (AKs). For the past several years, we have learned from our European colleagues that the use of MAL-PDT and a red light source was a useful modality for the treatment of AKs and for nonmelanoma skin cancers, especially basal cell carcinomas. Clinical trials have borne out that MAL-PDT using a red light source is safe and effective and yields long-term clinical results. Recently, MAL-PDT has received Food and Drug Administration (FDA) clearance for the treatment of AKs, but not for basal cell carcinomas. The European and United States recommended therapy involves lesion preparation with curettage debridement, drug incubation for 3 hours, and treatment with a red light source. Two treatments 1 week apart have been shown the most effective.

In the United States, most using 5-aminolevulinic acid (ALA)-PDT have used a shortened drug incubation time, based on clinical trials that have shown its effectiveness at treating AKs, as compared with longer drug incubation times, with increasing comorbidities. This multicenter European study examined using a shorter drug incubation time from 3 to 1 hour, and also looked at a decreased dose of MAL, all with the hopes of addressing improved patient compliances and outcomes, as has been witnessed in the United States with ALA.

Patients were randomized to either a 1- or 3-hour drug incubation period after lesion preparation (most) as well as having the dose of MAL randomized to either 160 mg/g or 80 mg/g. This study examined these effects on 383 previously untreated AKs, randomized according to a randomized system put in place by the Clinical Research Organization in charge of the study. Patients were followed at 2 to 3 months following their initial treatment and if there was not a complete response, the lesions were treated for a second time. This was required in 54%. Complete lesion responses were evaluated at 3 and 12 months following the last treatment. For AKs on the face and scalp, a 1-hour drug incubation yielded complete responses in 74% (thin) and 78% (thick) AK lesions compared with 96% (thin) and 87% (thick) after a 3-hour drug incubation.

Lesion recurrence rates were similar in both treatment groups. The 160 mg/g group yielded better results than the lower concentration of MAL. The overall cosmetic improvement in the skin was seen in both treatment groups.

Adverse events were seen in almost every patient, most commonly including redness, which lasted several weeks in the majority of the patients. Other adverse events, such as skin burning and pain were also commonly reported.

The authors concluded that short-term drug incubation may be a more tolerable and satisfactory option for AK patients having PDT therapy. This study demonstrates the United States belief that shorter drug incubation times are helpful in addressing patient compliance issues and the associated potential adverse events seen with traditional PDT therapy. This study also demonstrated that short contact MAL-PDT can induce acceptable results with PDT, and that it is useful in considering in patients undergoing PDT, especially for thinner AK lesions on the face and scalp.

M. H. Gold, MD

16 Nevi and Melanoma

The Use of Imiquimod to Minimize the Surgical Defect When Excising Invasive Malignant Melanoma Surrounded by Extensive Melanoma In Situ, Lentiginous Type
Missall TA, Fosko SW (Saint Louis Univ School of Medicine, MO)
Dermatol Surg 35:868-874, 2009

Malignant melanoma in situ, lentiginous type (LM), is a precursor lesion for malignant melanoma, lentiginous type (LMM). LM is characterized as an irregular, pigmented patch that is most commonly found on chronically sun-exposed skin, including the head and neck. LM is shown to be increasing in incidence and is the most prevalent subtype of in situ melanoma. Although LM constitutes only 4% to 15% of all melanomas, it is the most common type of head and neck melanoma. The progression of LM to its invasive form, LMM, is estimated to occur after 10 to 15 years. During this time, there is a protracted radial growth phase that is unique to LM among the in situ melanomas. Local recurrence of LMM is reported to account for 37% of all locally recurrent melanomas, which is most likely influenced by the clinical and histopathologic challenge of defining tumor margins in the context of chronically sun exposed skin. Although the recommended surgical margin for melanoma in situ is 5 mm, it has been well documented that, for the LM subtype, this is often inadequate and most likely contributes to local recurrence. The formation of LM, as well as its progression to LMM, is thought to involve the decrease in cell-mediated immunity in sun-damaged skin. Although first-line recommended treatment for LM is surgical excision, noninvasive therapies may be considered in certain clinical situations. Imiquimod is a topical immune-modulator acting on Toll-like receptors and has been shown to be a potent enhancer of innate and acquired immune responses. Various small open-label studies have reported treatment of LM with 5% imiquimod cream. The current study reports the use of this topical drug as an adjunct to surgical excision when treating extensive LM with focal invasive malignant melanoma.

▶ The use of topical imiquimod to minimize surgical defects in melanoma in situ, lentiginous type, or lentigo maligna (LM), as illustrated in this case report, is a valid consideration especially when approached with cases where a considerable defect is anticipated. Difficulty in histologic clearance of LM warrants consideration of adjunctive topical therapy if such a therapy is helpful in reducing lateral extension of atypical melanocytic proliferation. Topical imiquimod may provide such benefit; however, large studies confirming its benefit for LM are lacking.[1,2] Minimizing the surgical defect is not only cosmetically desirable, but also is associated with decreases in surgical complications and length of recovery. It is also hopeful that use of imiquimod would result in a lower risk of recurrence, especially at the periphery of the surgical site. Larger controlled studies with longer follow-up periods are necessary to fully evaluate the effectiveness of imiquimod as adjunctive treatment with surgical excision in LM.

J. Q. Del Rosso, DO
S. Bellew, DO

References

1. Ahmed I, Berth-Jones J. Imiquimod: a novel treatment for lentigo maligna. *Br J Dermatol.* 2000;143:843-845.
2. Naylor MF, Crowson N, Kuwahara R, et al. Treatment of lentigo maligna with topical imiquimod. *Br J Dermatol.* 2003;149:66-70.

Early Cure Rates with Narrow-Margin Slow-Mohs Surgery for Periocular Malignant Melanoma
Then S-Y, Malhotra R, Barlow R, et al (Queen Victoria Hosp, East Grinstead, UK; St. Thomas' Hosp, London, UK; et al)
Dermatol Surg 35:17-23, 2009

Background.—Staged excision with rush-processed paraffin-embedded tissue sections (Slow-Mohs) is an effective treatment for periocular melanoma. Although there is no consensus on initial margins of excision, narrower margins in the eyelids have the functionally and cosmetically important consequence of smaller postoperative wounds.

Objectives.—To report early cure rates for periocular melanoma using Slow-Mohs surgery with en-face margin sectioning.

Methods.—Retrospective, multicenter, noncomparative case series. Slow-Mohs surgery in 14 patients with periocular melanoma from 2000 to 2006.

Results.—Fourteen patients underwent 14 Slow-Mohs procedures for eight lentigo maligna, one nodular, and one superficial spreading melanoma, and four lentigo maligna, 12 primary, and two recurrent tumors. The most common site was the lower eyelid (8/14, 57.1%). Breslow thickness ranged from 0.27 to 1.70 mm, with four cases less than 0.76 mm and one case greater than 1.5 mm. Five cases were a Clark level II or greater. Complete excision was achieved with one level (6 cases) or two or three levels (8 cases), with 2- to 3-mm margins at each level in all but one case. With median follow-up of 36 months, there were two local recurrences (2/14, 14.3%).

Conclusion.—Slow-Mohs with en-face sections achieves similar early cure rates to previously published margin-controlled excision techniques.

Narrow margins of excision can optimize tissue preservation without compromising outcome.

▶ "Slow-Mohs" is used in certain cases such as treating periocular melanoma. The aim of the study was to look at cure rates in patients treated with Slow-Mohs. The study size was small but appropriate given the relative rarity of periocular melanoma and then choosing those patients who are felt to be candidates for the Slow-Mohs technique. Most lesions were lentigo maligna (LM) and lentigo malignant melanoma (LMM) and were excised with 2 to 3 mm margins in 1 to 2 stages. Two cases of recurrent LM and LMM were effectively treated with Slow-Mohs with no recurrence after a median follow-up of 36 months. This article portrays that smaller postoperative defects can be achieved successfully by performing Slow-Mohs technique using narrow margins. Conserving tissue can be critical, especially in the periocular region. Zitelli demonstrated preservation of 1.8 cm of normal skin when compared with excision. The limitations are as suggested by the authors, that is, the retrospective nature of the report and short follow-up period.

S. Bhambri, DO

J. Q. Del Rosso, DO

Evaluation of a Program for the Automatic Dermoscopic Diagnosis of Melanoma in a General Dermatology Setting

Fueyo-Casado A, Váquez-López F, Sanchez-Martin J, et al (Univ of Oviedo, Spain)
Dermatol Surg 35:257-262, 2009

The accuracy of automated programs for the computerized, dermoscopic diagnosis of melanoma has been found to be similar or superior to that of expert clinicians, even in evidence-based meta-analysis. Most of this research has been performed in pigmented skin lesion (PSL) units, where the number of diagnostically challenging PSLs is high. We consider it of interest to expand the investigation in a different setting. Our aim was to evaluate the usefulness of a commercially available program for the dermoscopic diagnosis of melanoma. The study was mainly focused on the detection of obvious melanoma at the first examination of patients, in the daily routine practice of a general dermatology consultancy, where it has been suggested that the value of these programs would be great.

▶ The detection of melanoma has long been a diagnostic challenge even for experienced dermatologists. Dermoscopy, as well as other diagnostic aids, is becoming increasingly used. It remains to be seen, however, if newer technologies will become a part of routine dermatologic care. Several approaches exist to this end and have been reviewed in previous studies.[1]

This is one of the first studies to evaluate the use of computer-assisted diagnostics in a general dermatologic practice. Their findings support recent evidence that the degree of sensitivity and specificity may not be as high as originally thought. The ideal use of such technology in a general dermatologic practice would be for evaluation of clinically subtle melanomas. To do so, the reliability of a negative result must be very high, as false negatives have an unacceptable outcome.

More studies will be needed to evaluate programs such as the Fotofind in routine dermatologic practice, and this is an honest and well-intentioned first step in this process. Although highly sensitive and specific computer-based programs could theoretically decrease medical costs by limiting the number of unnecessary biopsies performed by dermatologists, it remains to be seen how such programs will affect clinical practice. Further studies are needed to determine the practicality and cost-effectiveness of this exciting new technology.

R. I. Ceilley, MD

Reference

1. Patel JK, Konda S, Perez OA, Amini S, Elgart G, Berman B. Newer technologies/techniques and tools in the diagnosis of melanoma. *Eur J Dermatol.* 2008;18: 617-631.

Clinical features of 36 cases of amelanotic melanomas and considerations about the relationship between histologic subtypes and diagnostic delay
Gualandri L, Betti R, Crosti C (Università degli Studi di Milano, Italy; Università di Milano, Italy)
J Eur Acad Dermatol Venereol 23:283-287, 2009

Background.—Amelanotic melanomas (AM) are a difficult diagnostic challenge for clinicians.

Objective.—To consider the clinical presentation of AM, the histologic subtypes involved, the relationship with the diagnostic delay and the possible involvement in overall prognosis.

Patients/Methods.—Patients who were observed in our department to be affected by cutaneous melanomas were recorded. Sex, age, the clinical features, the site of presentation, the suspected diagnosis, the clinical course, the histological type, the Clark level and the Breslow thickness were recorded. AM were divided in three main clinical types: an erythematous macule or patch on sun-exposed skin, a dermal plaque or nodule without a particular epidermal change, an exophytic nodule. Only pure AM were considered. Histological subtypes considered were superficial spreading melanoma, nodular melanoma, and lentigo maligna melanoma. Diagnostic delay considered from when the patients first noticed the lesion on the site where the melanoma was diagnosed and when the physician or the patient first proposed the removal was recorded. The chi-squared test was used for statistical evaluation with $P < 0.05$ as level of significance.

Results.—Thirty-six cases of AM out of a total of 500 melanomas (7.2%) were collected. The most frequent morphology of clinical presentation was the papulo-nodular form, followed by the plaque form. Mean Breslow thickness of AM was 1.72 mm compared to 0.61 mm of pigmented cases. Nodular histotype was highly represented in AM (30.5% of cases) with respect to pigmented nodular melanomas (2.9%). The diagnostic delay did not differ between amelanotic and pigmented melanomas, nor between nodular AM and nodular pigmented melanomas.

Conclusion.—The great prevalence of clinical and histological nodular cases, the higher mean Breslow thickness (considered as the most important factor of prognosis) of AM compared with a not significant greater diagnostic delay may point out that a good percentage of AM have an intrinsic faster speed of growth with a worse prognosis irrespectively of the diagnostic performance. The importance of educational campaign for patient and physicians is stressed.

▶ Amelanotic melanoma (AM) continues to be a very difficult diagnostic challenge for all clinicians, including dermatologists. These growths often mimic dermal nevi, pyogenic granuloma, dermatofibroma, and warts. It is certainly logical to assume that patients would seek medical attention for a growing pigmented lesion more readily than a growing nonpigmented lesion. This is the first study to document (based on patient recall) for their population of patients that there was no difference in diagnostic delay between pigmented melanomas and AMs. Many previous articles state that AMs tend to have a deeper Breslow depth and therefore have poorer prognosis because of delay in diagnosis. Based on this study we must seriously consider the possibility that AMs are simply more aggressive from the onset.

This population of patients had more than twice (7.2%) the incidence of AM compared with most previous series (2%-3%). Subungual melanoma, while commonly amelanotic, were not represented in this series of 500 patients. Public awareness programs often neglect to mention this type of malignant melanoma. Adding the "E" to the ABCD-E rules applied to skin lesions seems more important than ever because AMs would be suspicious because they would be an evolving lesion. At this point, these evolving AMs appear to be the most critical to diagnose early.

R. I. Ceilley, MD
A. K. Bean, MD

Subclassification of desmoplastic melanoma: pure and mixed variants have significantly different capacities for lymph node metastasis

George E, McClain SE, Slingluff CL, et al (Univ of Washington, Seattle; Univ of Maryland, Baltimore; Univ of Virginia Med Ctr, Charlottesville; et al)

J Cutan Pathol 36:425-432, 2009

Background.—There is disagreement about the behavior and optimal management of desmoplastic melanoma (DM), particularly regarding the incidence of lymph node (LN) involvement. Recently, investigators have noted the frequently heterogenous histologic composition of DM and have found significant differences between pure desmoplastic melanoma (PDM) (≥90% comprised of histologically typical DM) and mixed desmoplastic melanoma (MDM) [≥10% DM and > 10% conventional melanoma (CM)].

Method.—We reviewed 87 cases of DM comparing the histologic and clinical features of PDM (n = 44) to MDM (n = 43).

Results.—At surgical staging, there were LN metastases in 5 of 23 (22%) MDM patients, whereas all 17 PDM patients had negative LN biopsies (0%) (p = 0.04). PDM was less often clinically pigmented (36% vs. 67%) and had a lower mean mitotic index (1.3 vs. 3.0).

Conclusions.—There are differences between PDM and MDM, the most important of which is the incidence of LN involvement. Our findings support the clinical utility of classifying DM into pure and mixed subtypes because the negligible rate of nodal involvement in PDM does not support the routine performance of sentinel LN biopsy in this subgroup of melanoma patients. In contrast, the incidence of LN involvement in MDM is comparable to that of CM.

▶ The article is well written, well organized, and clearly states the differences between the pure desmoplastic melanoma (PDM) and mixed desmoplastic melanoma (MDM) variants of desmoplastic melanoma. They convincingly point out the importance of the subclassification because the negligible rate of nodal metastasis does not support routine sentinel lymph node biopsy in this group.

Their methods are sound and appear valid, given the limitation of the study size, and are not based on case reports. Some of the definitions are rather vague, and they didn't go far enough into histologic/immunophenotyping studies. Perhaps this will be reported in a future publication by the authors. If the tissue blocks are still available, it may be useful to have the immunoperoxidase results for modern reagents all performed in the same laboratory for all of these cases.

The article is probably more important for dermatopathologists than for dermatologists except for highlighting the distinction between desmoplastic and spindle cell diagnoses. This is a good reminder of the importance of the dermatologists working closely with their consultant dermatopathologists to provide optimal care for their patients.

R. I. Ceilley, MD

Use of Photographs Illustrating ABCDE Criteria in Skin Self-examination
Robinson JK, Ortiz S
Arch Dermatol 145:332-333, 2009

Dermatologists support public education campaigns using photographic references of nevi and melanoma, and they distribute brochures with these images to their patients in the belief that such images teach people to self-detect changing nevi and melanomas. Photographic images of melanomas optimize people's spontaneous image recognition. After the initial review, it is unclear how reference materials are used. We explored the use of educational material by people at risk to develop melanoma.

▶ An important goal of melanoma detection by patients is to create a paradigm between normal and abnormal features of a pigmented lesion in order that a patient should know when to be concerned. As many patients have not seen a melanoma previously, creating this construct can be difficult. Active learning involving patients in their own care may be one way to increase compliance with self examinations and aid in creating a model for abnormal changes.

However, the question remains as to whether active patient-involved intervention will lead to increased detection of melanoma, and it would be interesting to see long-term follow-up data. Application to a general practice, where many patients do not routinely monitor their pigmented lesions due to inconsistent patient education, may not be as relevant. Selection bias in such a study would be inherent, as participants are likely to be more highly motivated and compliant with monitoring.

This report emphasizes the importance of educating and using a consistent partner in examination. Advising patients to keep their cards in a bathroom or bedroom for quick and easy access is advisable. Also, it is not uncommon for patients to come into our office for evaluation after seeing the asymmetry, border irregularity, color variegation, diameter ≥ 6 mm, and evolution (ABCDE) photos in brochures or magazines.

On a cost-benefit basis for patient resource allocation, it can be argued that nearly 50% of recipients *never* using the resource supports that this is not the most appropriate allocation of a physician's funds. The participants in the study had already been diagnosed with a melanoma; therefore, other learning methods most likely had a much greater impact on the patients, and directing funds to this patient base was not purposeful.

A much broader study looking into the overall population in general dermatology practices, and the response of these patients to the ABCDE card would be of much greater importance for the clinician. ABCDE card usage and subsequent behavioral changes in patients without a history of melanoma or other skin cancers would provide the clinician with much more usable feedback.

R. I. Ceilley, MD

Factors Related to the Presentation of Thin and Thick Nodular Melanoma From a Population-based Cancer Registry in Queensland Australia

Geller AC, Elwood M, Swetter SM, et al (Harvard School of Public Health, Boston, MA; British Columbia Cancer Agency, Vancouver, Canada; Veterans Affairs Palo Alto Health Care System, CA; et al)

Cancer 115:1318-1327, 2009

Background.—Worldwide, the incidence of thick melanoma has not declined, and the nodular melanoma (NM) subtype accounts for nearly 40% of newly diagnosed thick melanoma. To assess differences between patients with thin (≤2.00 mm) and thick (≥2.01 mm) nodular melanoma, the authors evaluated factors such as demographics, melanoma detection patterns, tumor visibility, and physician screening for NM alone and compared clinical presentation and anatomic location of NM with superficial spreading melanoma (SSM).

Methods.—The authors used data from a large population-based study of Queensland (Australia) residents diagnosed with melanoma. Queensland residents aged 20 to 75 years with histologically confirmed first primary invasive cutaneous melanoma were eligible for the study, and all questionnaires were conducted by telephone (response rate, 77.9%).

Results.—During this 4-year period, 369 patients with nodular melanoma were interviewed, of whom 56.7% were diagnosed with tumors ≤2.00 mm. Men, older individuals, and those who had not been screened by a physician in the past 3 years were more likely to have nodular tumors of greater thickness. Thickest nodular melanoma (4 mm+) was also most common in persons who had not been screened by a physician within the past 3 years (odds ratio, 3.75; 95% confidence interval, 1.47-9.59). Forty-six percent of patients with thin nodular melanoma (≥2.00 mm) reported a change in color, compared with 64% of patients with thin SSM and 26% of patients with thick nodular melanoma (>2.00 mm).

Conclusions.—Awareness of factors related to earlier detection of potentially fatal nodular melanomas, including the benefits of a physician examination, should be useful in enhancing public and professional education strategies. Particular awareness of clinical warning signs associated with thin nodular melanoma should allow for more prompt diagnosis and treatment of this subtype.

▶ Melanoma is a major concern in Australia, where the incidence of this skin cancer is very high. The statistical evidence from the Cancer Registry in Queensland, Australia, and its subsequent analysis clearly point out that the general population needs to be made aware of the need for self-examination. It has been shown that early detection of nodular melanoma can reduce the fatality rate of this disease. Melanoma thickness is strongly related to survival. There has been a decrease in median tumor thickness, but the incidence rate of thick melanomas has not decreased. In this study, nodular melanomas were mostly self detected, and only 11% were detected by physicians. Only 28% of patients had received a whole or nearly whole body exam in the past

3 years, and only 15% had performed self examinations in the 3 years before their nodular melanoma was diagnosed. Patients 60 to 75 years of age were 3 times more likely to have a T4 nodular melanoma than a T1 nodular melanoma compared with 40- to 59-year-old patients. Those who did not have a clinical skin exam were 4 times more likely to have a T4 nodular melanoma than a T1. Those patients with nodular melanoma revealed by self diagnosis were 5 times more likely to have a T4 rather than a T1. There also needs to be a greater awareness by the general practitioner of the need to complete a dermatological survey during a patient's general physical. More frequent physician clinical exams and self exams can provide earlier diagnosis and can reduce a thick or thin rapidly growing melanoma.

L. Cleaver, DO

Health Care System and Socioeconomic Factors Associated With Variance in Use of Sentinel Lymph Node Biopsy for Melanoma in the United States
Bilimoria KY, Balch CM, Wayne JD, et al (Northwestern Univ, Chicago, IL; Johns Hopkins School of Medicine, Baltimore, MD; Bloomberg School of Public Health, Baltimore, MD)
J Clin Oncol 27:1857-1863, 2009

Purpose.—Guidelines recommend sentinel lymph node biopsy (SLNB) for patients with clinical stage IB/II melanomas, but not clinical stage IA melanoma. This study examines factors associated with SLNB use for clinically node-negative melanoma.

Methods.—Patients diagnosed with clinically node-negative invasive melanoma in 2004 and 2005 were identified from the National Cancer Data Base. Regression models were developed to assess the association of clinicopathologic (sex, age, race/ethnicity, comorbidities, T stage), socioeconomic (insurance status, educational level, income), and hospital (hospital type, geographic area) factors with SLNB use.

Results.—A total of 16,598 patients were identified: 8,073 patients with clinical stage IA and 8,525 patients with clinical stage IB/II melanoma. For clinical stage IB/II melanoma, SLNB use was reported in 48.7% of patients. Patients with clinical stage IB/II melanoma were less likely to undergo SLNB if they were older than 75 years; had T1b tumors, no tumor ulceration, or head/neck or truncal lesions; were covered by Medicaid or Medicare; or lived in the Northeast, South, or West census regions. SLNB use was reported in 13.3% of patients with clinical stage IA melanoma and was more likely in patients who were younger than 56 years or lived in the Mountain or Pacific census regions. Patients treated at National Comprehensive Cancer Network–or National Cancer Institute–designated hospitals were most likely to undergo SLNB in adherence with national consensus guidelines.

Conclusion.—SLNB use was associated with clinicopathologic factors but also with health system factors, including type of insurance, geographic area, and hospital type. These findings have implications for provider education and health policy.

▶ The usefulness of sentinel lymph node biopsy (SLNB) for melanoma is a hotly debated issue with experts from many specialties on both sides of the debate. The article clearly points out that no study to date has demonstrated a survival benefit of the procedure, but the authors of this study imply that SLNB is, or should be, the standard of care. Although some benefit has been observed related to prognosis and staging, no benefit related to morbidity and mortality can be found. However, the literature does establish that it is an expensive procedure, that it is technically difficult for both the surgeon and the pathologist, as well as assuming a lymphatic mode of metastasis without ability to assess metastasis through a direct hematologic route.

The authors conclude that socioeconomic and health system factors dictate the use of SLNB. They also state that patients in lower socioeconomic strata and with access to different health care settings are not receiving access to this procedure. This point is a red herring to the topic of effectiveness of SLNB. As the authors state, "It is unknown whether such individuals will have poorer overall survival, but at the very least, they will live with greater uncertainty in their prognosis and can be expected to be at higher risk of regional nodal recurrence."

This conclusion sums up exactly why SLNB should not be considered as the "standard of care." As concluded in *Clinical Trials in Oncology*, some readers may feel disheartened to learn the truth that many, probably most, promising therapies prove, once aptly tested, worthless, and some may feel in some fuzzy way that to accept this reality is cruelly to deny hope to those who need it badly.[1] On the contrary, to offer false hope is the ultimate cruelty.

A recent review points out that SLNB followed with completion lymph node dissection (CLND) for melanoma is not the standard of care; rather, performance of SLNB/CLND for risk stratification and combination therapy in an experimental protocol would be appropriate.[2] Is SLNB experimental or is it standard of care?

As Tsai concluded, "There is no systemic adjunctive therapy for melanoma that confers a statistically significant long-term overall survival benefit."[3]

Clearly, SLNB/CLND is a modality that generates no discernable positive survivability outcomes. A hypothetical question was raised by Coldiron et al that clinicians must encourage their patients to ask the hard questions of their surgeon or oncologist.[2] Is there any overall survival benefit from SLNB/CLND? If not, why do they perform/advocate the procedure? In the absence of survival benefit, it seems inappropriate to promote this as standard of care to all patients, hospitals, and locations.

R. I. Ceilley, MD
A. K. Bean, MD

References

1. Green S, Benedetti J, Crowley J. *Clinical Trials in Oncology.* 2nd ed. Boca Raton, FL: CRC Press; 2003.

2. Coldiron BM, Dinehart S, Rogers HW. Sentinel lymph node biopsy and completion lymph node dissection for malignant melanoma are not standard of care. *Clin Dermatol.* 2009;27:350-354.
3. Tsai KY. Systemic adjuvant therapy for patients with high-risk melanoma. *Arch Dermatol.* 2007;143:779-782.

Factors Associated With Physician Discovery of Early Melanoma in Middle-aged and Older Men

Geller AC, Johnson TM, Miller DR, et al (Boston Univ, MA; Univ of Michigan Med School, Ann Arbor; Veterans Affairs Med Ctr, Bedford, MA; et al)
Arch Dermatol 145:409-414, 2009

Objective.—To determine factors associated with physician discovery of early melanoma in middle-aged and older men.

Design.—Survey.

Setting.—Three institutional melanoma clinics.

Participants.—A total of 227 male participants (aged ≥40 years) with invasive melanoma who completed surveys within 3 months of diagnosis.

Intervention.—Survey.

Main Outcome Measures.—Factors associated with physician-detected thin melanoma.

Results.—Patients with physician-detected melanoma were older, 57% were 65 years or older compared with 34% for other-detected (odds ratio [OR], 2.57; 95% confidence interval [CI], 1.19-5.55) and 42% for patient-detected melanoma ($P = .07$). Physician-detected melanoma in the oldest patients (aged ≥65 years) had tumor thickness equal to that of self-detected melanoma or melanoma detected by other means in younger patients. Back lesions composed 46% of all physician-detected melanoma, 57% of those detected by other means, and 16% of self-detected lesions (physician- vs self-detected: OR, 4.25; 95% CI, 1.96-9.23). Ninety-two percent of all physician-detected back-of-the-body melanomas were smaller than 2 mm compared with 63% of self-detected lesions ($P = .004$) and 76% of lesions detected by other means ($P = .07$).

Conclusions.—Skin screenings of at-risk middle-aged and older American men can be integrated into the routine physical examination, with particular emphasis on hard-to-see areas, such as the back of the body. "Watch your back" professional education campaigns should be promoted by skin cancer advocacy organizations.

▶ Given the many controversies about preventative medicine, this article would be a good source of enlightenment for those who set protocols for skin screening and melanoma detection. Many would agree that men aged 35 to 50 are the most resistant to seeking medical care, let alone preventative health screenings, and unfortunately the consequences can be serious. This article gives us a good example of that dilemma where melanomas found by physicians compared with self-examination by the patients were often more advanced, derived from previously benign nevi, or not reported. The observation that men with atypical nevi at baseline developed thin melanomas, compared with those without atypical nevi who reported melanoma later on, emphasizes the need for routine screening of patients after age 40 similar to hypertension, hyperlipidemia, and prostate disease. The finding that melanomas on the back were most reported cases should emphasize the need for high-risk patients and men over 40 years of age to have a regular screening to reduce the potential morbidity of melanoma, given the risks of those not screened as presented here.

N. Bhatia, MD

Risk Factors in Elderly People for Lentigo Maligna Compared With Other Melanomas: A Double Case-Control Study

Gaudy-Marqueste C, Madjlessi N, Guillot B, et al (Hôpital Sainte Marguerite, Marseille, France; Hôpital Saint-Eloi, Montpellier, France; et al)
Arch Dermatol 145:418-423, 2009

Objective.—To assess lentigo maligna (LM) as an epidemiological entity separate from other melanomas (OMs) in elderly people.

Design.—Double age- and sex-matched case-control study to compare the risk factors for LMs and OMs.

Setting.—General community.

Patients.—A total of 76 patients with LM were paired by age and sex with 76 patients with OMs and 152 controls.

Main Outcome Measures.—The association of melanoma risk with the following potential risk factors: sun exposure history by 10-year periods, frequency of sunburns, phenotypic traits, density of freckles and sun sensitivity at age 20 years, counts of nevi larger than 2 mm in diameter on the face and forearm, skin aging features (as assessed using a photographic scale), and history of basal and/or squamous cell carcinomas.

Results.—Risk of LMs and OMs were similarly associated with history of sunburns, light skin type, and freckling. Cumulative chronic outdoor and occupational sun exposures were not risk factors in any of the 2 groups of melanomas. Lentigo maligna differed from OMs by the absence of a detectable association with the number of nevi and a greater association with nonmelanoma skin cancers.

Conclusions.—Although chronically sun-exposed skin is a prerequisite for LM, risk of LM does not increase with the cumulative dose of sun exposure, but LM is associated with sunburn history, like all other types of melanomas. The main epidemiological characteristic of LM is the absence of an apparent relation with the genetic propensity to develop nevi. This epidemiological profile is in accordance with recent molecular findings and may also account for the histoclinical and evolutive characteristics of LM.

▶ Lentigo maligna (LM) is considered a subtype of melanoma that is predominantly seen in older people, grows slowly, and is associated with cumulative ultraviolet (UV) exposure on sun-exposed sites such as the head and neck region. This is a double age and sex matched case-control study conducted in patients older than 65 to assess risk factors in 3 French hospitals comparing LMs and other melanomas (OM)—superficial spreading (SSM) and nodular (NM) subtypes. All cases, controls, and pathology reports were examined by one dermatologist. Patients were asked standardized questionnaires that required them to recall their phenotypic traits when they were 20 years old, about their skin and hair color using a photographic scale, density of freckles, cumulative lifetime sun exposure, and history of sunburns. Those who had a memory disorder, had previous melanoma, were taking immunosuppressive drugs, and those with any chronic disease over the last 50 years were not included. Findings suggest that patients with OMs had significantly more nevi larger than 2 mm in diameter on the forearms compared with controls and LM patients, suggesting that there may be a link between the number of nevi and the risk of OMs but not necessarily with the risk of LMs. This study found that LMs had a higher rate of occurrence on the face (89% as compared with OMs on the face, which reported as 13%). LMs were also linked with an increase of sunburns but not with chronic sun exposure. LMs reported having more nonmelanoma skin cancer (NMSC) removed in the past versus OMs. Predictors of LMs were previous history of NMSC, frequency of sunburns during first 20 years of life, and guttate hypomelanosis. In contrast, OM and the number of nevi on the forearm and history of NMSC, pale skin, and previous history of having other skin lesions being removed was a risk factor. This study directed attention to sun exposure from birth to diagnosis with the degree of exposure, cumulative daily ambient exposure, occupational exposure, and even leisurely exposure being part of the questionnaire. Memory seemed to be the most problematic area in this study, with individuals being asked to recall an estimate of the number of nevi at the age of 20. Furthermore, it would have also been interesting to include the geographic location where these patients received the most amount of sun exposure, because UV intensity also varies between geographic locations. In addition, when asked if patients had NMSC or other skin lesions removed, analysis of data was based purely on recall, whereas reviewing past medical records could have yielded more accurate results. The authors also used history of other skin lesions removed as a risk factor variable, yet they failed to define what these other skin lesions were. This study helps to differentiate risk factors for LMs and OMs and suggests that there may be less genetic propensity than with OM, or less of a link with dysplastic nevi, associated with the pathogenesis to LMs. This article also proposes that there may be nevus-prone individuals who develop melanoma after intense sun exposure. In conclusion, the authors suggest that LMs may result after a history of sunburns, with an acquired mutation as an additional promoting factor, raising the interesting possibilities of LMs having unique pathogenic factors and a different molecular profile compared with OMs.

G. K. Kim, DO
J. Q. Del Rosso, DO

Acral Lentiginous Melanoma: Incidence and Survival Patterns in the United States, 1986-2005
Bradford PT, Goldstein AM, McMaster ML, et al (Natl Insts of Health, Bethesda, MD)
Arch Dermatol 145:427-434, 2009

Objective.—To examine incidence and survival patterns of acral lentiginous melanoma (ALM) in the United States.

Design.—Population-based registry study. We used the Surveillance, Epidemiology, and End Results (SEER) Program of the National Cancer Institute to evaluate data from 17 population-based cancer registries from 1986 to 2005.

Participants.—A total 1413 subjects with histologically confirmed cases of ALM.

Main Outcome Measure.—Incidence and survival patterns of patients with ALM.

Results.—The age-adjusted incidence rate of ALM overall was 1.8 per million person-years. The proportion of ALM among all melanoma subtypes was greatest in blacks (36%). Acral lentiginous melanoma had 5- and 10-year melanoma-specific survival rates of 80.3% and 67.5%, respectively, which were less than those for all cutaneous malignant melanomas overall (91.3% and 87.5%, respectively; $P < .001$). The ALM 5- and 10-year melanomaspecific survival rates were highest in non-Hispanic whites (82.6% and 69.4%), intermediate in blacks (77.2% and 71.5%), and lowest in Hispanic whites (72.8% and 57.3%) and Asian/Pacific Islanders (70.2% and 54.1%). Acral lentiginous melanoma thickness and stage correlated with survival according to sex and in the different racial groups.

Conclusions.—Population-based data showed that ALM is a rare melanoma subtype, although its proportion among all melanomas is higher in people of color. It is associated with a worse prognosis than cutaneous malignant melanoma overall. Hispanic whites and Asian/Pacific Islanders have worse survival rates than other groups, and factors such as increased tumor thickness and more advanced stage at presentation are the most likely explanations.

▶ Acral lentiginous melanoma (ALM) is rare comprising of less than 3% of all melanomas. The authors started out with an objective of examining the incidence and survival patterns of ALM. I believe they have met this objective. The study size was large given the rarity of ALMs. ALM was found to be most common in blacks followed by Asian/Pacific Islanders followed by Hispanic whites. The mean age of diagnosis of ALM is slightly higher than that of cutaneous melanoma (62.8 years vs 58.5 years). The survival rates were highest in non-Hispanic whites. The article is well written, and the study was thorough and well coordinated. Several limitations exist and as the authors recognized, most melanoma cases in the Surveillance, Epidemiology, and End Results (SEER) registry were histologically specified as "not otherwise specified" (NOS). Also, there were tumors that were labeled as ALM but were located on locations other than upper or lower extremities.

S. Bhambri, DO

J. Q. Del Rosso, DO

Head and Neck Malignant Melanoma: Margin Status and Immediate Reconstruction

Sullivan SR, Scott JR, Cole JK, et al (Univ of Washington, Seattle; et al)
Ann Plast Surg 62:144-148, 2009

Head and neck melanoma often approaches critical structures. Therefore, excision is often limited, leading to positive margins, and increased local recurrence. Immediate reconstruction carries concern for rearrangement or concealment of cancerous tissues. Therefore, reconstruction is often delayed until confirming negative margins on permanent pathology. Our purpose is to identify variables associated with a positive margin and establish criteria for reconstruction timing. We reviewed 117 consecutive patients who underwent wide local excision of head and neck melanoma. Reconstruction was immediate for 107 and delayed for 10. Six percent of patients had a positive margin after wide local excision with no difference in incidence between immediate and delayed reconstruction ($P = 0.11$). Tumor characteristics associated with a positive margin were locally recurrent, ulcerated, and T4 tumors ($P < 0.05$); and delayed reconstruction should be considered in these circumstances. Immediate reconstruction is safe for the majority of head and neck melanoma and should be based on knowledge of tumor characteristics.

▶ This study reviews the clinical and tumor characteristics associated with a histologically positive margin after wide local excision (WLE) and the subsequent reconstruction timing in 117 consecutive patients. The conclusions drawn from this study are that immediate reconstruction is safe for most of the head and neck (HN) melanomas, but clinical characteristics associated with positive margins after WLE of HN melanomas need to be established to determine which cases are suitable for immediate reconstruction. The study found patients with locally recurrent melanoma, patients with T4 tumors, and those with ulceration to have a significantly higher risk of having positive margins after WLE. In such cases, it may be best to delay reconstruction until pathology is reviewed and margins are deemed to be clear. Only 7 of the 117 patients had positive margins; therefore, this is a small sample size. This article also mentions that larger studies inclusive of a higher incidence of positive margins are needed to determine other factors known to be associated with recurrence.

S. B. Momin, DO

J. Q. Del Rosso, DO

Sentinel Node Tumor Burden According to the Rotterdam Criteria Is the Most Important Prognostic Factor for Survival in Melanoma Patients: A Multicenter Study in 388 Patients With Positive Sentinel Nodes

van Akkooi ACJ, Nowecki ZI, Voit C, et al (Erasmus Univ Med Ctr – Daniel den Hoed Cancer Ctr, The Netherlands; EORTC Melanoma Group, Brussels, Belgium)

Ann Surg 248:949-955, 2008

Summary Background Data.—The more intensive sentinel node (SN) pathologic workup, the higher the SN-positivity rate. This is characterized by an increased detection of cases with minimal tumor burden (SUB-micrometastasis <0.1 mm), which represents different biology.

Methods.—The slides of positive SN from 3 major centers within the European Organization of Research and Treatment of Cancer (EORTC) Melanoma Group were reviewed and classified according to the Rotterdam Classification of SN Tumor Burden (<0.1 mm; 0.1–1 mm; >1 mm) maximum diameter of the largest metastasis. The predictive value for additional nodal metastases in the completion lymph node dissection (CLND) and disease outcome as disease- free survival (DFS) and overall survival (OS) was calculated.

Results.—In 388 SN positive patients, with primary melanoma, median Breslow thickness was 4.00 mm; ulceration was present in 56%. Forty patients (10%) had metastases <0.1 mm. Additional nodal positivity was found in only 1 of 40 patients (3%). At a mean follow-up of 41 months, estimated OS at 5 years was 91% for metastasis <0.1 mm, 61% for 0.1 to 1.0 mm, and 51% for >1.0 mm ($P < 0.001$). SN tumor burden increased significantly with tumor thickness. When the cut-off value for SUB-micrometastases was taken at <0.2 mm (such as in breast cancer), the survival was 89%, and 10% had additional non-SN nodal positivity.

Conclusion.—This large multicenter dataset establishes that patients with SUB-micrometastases <0.1 mm have the same prognosis as SN negative patients and can be spared a CLND. A <0.2 mm cut-off for SUB-micrometastases does not seem correct for melanoma, as 10% additional nodal positivity is found.

▶ Sentinel node biopsy (SN) is gaining popularity after several studies have supported prognostic benefit. It has been proposed that SN biopsy would identify those patients that could possibly benefit from the removal of all regional lymph nodes leading to a survival benefit. The aim of this study was to analyze the occurrence rate of minimal SN tumor burden in different centers and to correlate this to Breslow thickness, pathologic work-up of the SN, and to evaluate the survival rate of minimal SN tumor burden. In this study, there were 3 centers that were used to evaluate information on primary tumor information, follow-up, and all pathology slides were reviewed again. All patients were previously diagnosed with melanoma with a minimum Breslow thickness of 1.00 mm or Clark IV/V. The work-up of the SN was the same for all 3 participating centers. SN tumor burden was measured according to the Rotterdam criteria. The median Breslow thickness of all patients was 4.00 mm. Median Breslow thickness of the 3 centers was Rotterdam, 2.9 mm, Berline, 3.4 mm, and Warsaw, 4.0 mm. The mean/median duration of follow-up was 41/36 months. Ulceration was present in 56% of patients, and 40 (10%) patients had metastasis (0.1 mm). Nodal positivity was found in 1 of 40 patients (3%). This study confirms that patients with SUB-micrometastases (maximum diameter <0.1 mm) had an excellent 5-year overall survival rate of 91%. The overall survival at 5-year was 91% for metastasis <0.1 mm, 61% for 0.1 mm and 1.0 mm, and 51% for >1.9 mm (*P* < .001). The amount of SN tumor burden increased significantly with the increase in primary tumor stage. Authors have suggested that 0.2 mm should be the cut-off for SUB-microscopic SN tumor burden in melanoma patients. Overall survival rate for <0.2 mm SUB-micrometastases seems very promising with an estimated 5-year overall survival rate of 89%, which is very similar to SN negative patients. In conclusion, SN tumor burden according to the Rotterdam criteria was found to be the most important prognostic factor for overall survival in this large multicenter study. This study validates the previous observation that patients with SUB-micrometastases (defined as <0.1 mm in maximum diameter) have an excellent estimated 5-year overall survival rate. The cut-off value for melanoma SUB-micrometastases appears to be <0.1 mm rather than <0.2 mm. SUB-micrometastases (<0.1 mm) may also be considered as biologically false positive SN similar to negative SN, and a complete lymph node dissection (CLND) is not warranted. In conclusion, data from this large multicenter study suggest that patients with SN-SUB-micrometastases, according to the Rotterdam criteria (<0.1 mm), have the same survival rate as SN negative patients with a low risk to develop nodal recurrence.

J. Q. Del Rosso, DO

G. K. Kim, DO

Management of Primary Cutaneous Melanoma of the Hands and Feet: A Clinicoprognostic Study

Rex J, Paradelo C, Mangas C, et al (Universitat Autònoma de Barcelona, Badalona, Spain)
Dermatol Surg 35:1505-1513, 2009

Background.—Although acral lentiginous melanoma is the most common subtype of malignant melanoma in acral locations, the term acral melanoma (AM) has to be differentiated from the histopathologic description.

Objectives.—To characterize the clinical and pathologic features of patients with a primary AM and to elucidate whether the prognosis of patients with AM differs from that of those with melanoma at other sites (nonacral melanoma; NAM).

Patients and Method.—Over a 20-year period, a series of 822 consecutive patients with melanoma were recorded in the database. Clinical and follow-up data were retrieved from the melanoma register and prospectively analyzed.

Results.—Eighty-nine patients had a malignant melanoma located on the acral sites of extremities. Breslow thickness and Clark level were found to be related to specific and disease-free survival. Breslow thickness greater than 4mm was associated with greater risk of recurrence, and amelanosis and age of 60 and older were significantly associated with greater risk of death. Comparison of survival of patients with AM with that of those with NAM clearly showed that disease-free survival and overall survival were significantly lower in the former.

Conclusion.—Survival differences between patients with AM and NAM are due to differences in already known prognostic factors, probably as a consequence of a delay in the diagnosis in these locations.

▶ The perennial debate regarding the prognosis of acral melanoma versus non-acral melanoma arising is re-examined. This article examines a series of 822 consecutive patients with melanoma identified over a 20-year period. Eighty-nine of these patients had melanoma of acral skin (10.8%), a percentage that compares favorably with that reported by other institutions. Interestingly, these authors from Spain report a foot to hand ratio of 4:1, whereas in other literature this ratio has varied from 7:1 to 34:1.

The authors attribute this to improved surveillance (and implicitly), removal of precursor lesions, second to the regional, but widespread, practice of wearing sandals.

This explanation is interesting, because it necessitates acceptance of a concept that melanoma, in particular acral melanoma, arises in pre-existing atypical nevi; hence, removal of precursor lesions lessens the disease burden. Certainly, a rather vocal faction of American dermatologists will find this distressing.

Ultimately, the authors find that prognostic data for acral melanoma did not differ in a meaningful way from the normal prognostic data for melanoma occurring upon nonacral skin. They further assert that any difference in survival within their cohorts was second to a difference in depth of invasion (2.8 mm vs 1.57 mm). Similarly, for acral melanoma, recurrence locally preceded distant recurrence, a pattern also common to melanoma occurring upon nonacral skin. In sum, they conclude that the histological subtype of melanoma does not influence biological behavior, and that as depth is always the key predictor of outcome, early detection is key.

A meritorious consideration not addressed by this article is the substantial genetic distinctions researchers have observed when studying various subtypes of melanoma. Rather recently, Curtin et al[1] used array-based comparative genomic hybridization, DNA sequencing, and immunohistochemical techniques to search for various mutations in melanomas predivided into 4 classes: (1) mucosal lesions, (2) acral lesions, (3) chronically sun-exposed skin, and (4) intermittently sun-exposed skin. Remarkably, Curtin et al were able to subclassify, with up to 89% accuracy, melanomas using genetic observations common to these categories.

Therefore, one might contend that even while the classic subcategories of melanoma, which were based upon clinicopathological factors (superficial spreading, nodular, lentigo maligna, acral lentiginous) fall by the wayside, the genetic classification of melanoma is just beginning, with resultant prognostic and even therapeutic implications.

W. A. High, MD, JD, MEng

Reference

1. Curtin JA, Fridlyand J, Kageshita T, et al. Distinct sets of genetic alterations in melanoma. *N Engl J Med.* 2005;353:2135-2147.

Completeness of Histopathology Reporting of Melanoma in a High-Incidence Geographical Region
Thompson B, Austin R, Coory M, et al (Viertel Centre for Res in Cancer Control, Spring Hill, Queensland, Australia; Univ of Queensland, Herston, Australia; et al)
Dermatology 218:7-14, 2009

Background.—Appropriate histopathology reporting helps to ensure effective therapy and prognosis.

Objective.—To examine compliance with clinical practice guidelines for histopathology reports of melanomas.

Methods.—A sample of melanoma histopathology reports in Queensland was audited for inclusion of recommended information. The quality of documentation was constructed and multivariate analysis used to determine factors affecting the quality of reporting practices.

Results.—Documentation of the most important features of melanoma was high: clear diagnosis (99.8%; 95% CI 98.6–100), thickness (99.8%; 95% CI 98.6–100), comment on adequacy of excision (87.9%; 95% CI 84.9–91.0) and measurement of margins (91.9%; 95% CI 88.8–91.4). Overall reporting of ulceration and regression was of lesser completeness (83.0 and 77.8%, respectively) and these features were more likely to be reported by high-volume laboratories ($p < 0.001$ and $p = 0.037$, respectively). This trend was not apparent for other features. Fewer than 50% of reports documented mitotic rate per square millimetre, predominant cell type, microsatellites, growth phase and desmoplasia.

Conclusion.—Awareness of current reporting practices and identification of areas in which insufficiencies exist enable the revision of systems and potential improvements to the transfer of information to treating clinicians.

▶ The article demonstrates how the level of awareness of melanoma in Queensland, Australia, sets a standard in pathology reports as well as prevention and clinical management. Pathologists have established uniform reporting methods and protocols for specimens, which allow for easy translation among colleagues. This standardization for conveying potential severity of melanoma is a significant advantage given the prevalence of the disease there, but it should also be accepted in other parts of the world where melanoma may be dealt with less often but at the same level of severity. Dermatologists are aware of the prognosis when evaluating Breslow's depth and Clark's level, but a uniform evaluation of mitotic figures, histological subtype, ulceration, and radial and/or vertical phase changes that is standardized may assist clinicians to further assess a patient's therapy and prognosis.

N. Bhatia, MD

The Role of Surveillance Chest X-Rays in the Follow-up of High-Risk Melanoma Patients

Morton RL, Craig JC, Thompson JF (The Univ of Sydney, Australia; Melanoma Inst Australia, Sydney; et al)
Ann Surg Oncol 16:571-577, 2009

We sought to evaluate the accuracy of detecting asymptomatic pulmonary metastases by surveillance chest X-rays (CXRs) in melanoma patients with a positive sentinel node biopsy. Sentinel node–positive patients treated at the Sydney Melanoma Unit between 1994 and 2003 were prospectively enrolled onto a monitoring schedule of 6 monthly CXRs for 5 years, then annual CXRs for another 5 years. The reference standard for pulmonary metastasis was a positive histopathology diagnosis from a lung biopsy. A total of 108 patients were followed for a median of 52.5 months. A total of 21% (23 of 108) developed pulmonary metastases, which were detected in 48% (11 of 23) by surveillance CXR (sensitivity, 48%; 95% confidence interval [95% CI], .27–.68), leading to resection in 13% (3 of 23). CXRs were abnormal in 19 additional patients but not due to recurrence (specificity, 78%; 95% CI, .77–.79). Additional metastatic disease was apparent in 18% of CXR-detected versus 76% of non-CXR-detected patients ($p < .05$), but median time to diagnosis of pulmonary metastases was 24 months (95% CI, 12–41) versus 16 months (95% CI, 10–30, $p = .30$ log rank) and median survival of 42 months (95% CI, 24–84) versus 36 months (95% CI, 18–46, $p = .53$ log rank) were not significantly different. The 6 to 12 monthly surveillance CXRs detected only half of pulmonary metastases, infrequently identified patients for potentially curative surgery, and did not lead to earlier detection of pulmonary metastases. Further, they may cause unnecessary patient anxiety, given the high rate of false-positive findings.

▶ The aim of this study is to evaluate the accuracy of detecting asymptomatic pulmonary metastasis by surveillance chest X-ray (CXR) in melanoma patients with a positive sentinel lymph node biopsy. The value of pulmonary radiologic surveillance in melanoma follow-up for the early detection of disease spread is unclear. Limited published data exist on the role of surveillance CXR in the sentinel node positive patient population. Previous studies simply report the frequency of pulmonary metastasis detected by surveillance CXRs.

The results of this study suggest that 6 to 12 monthly CXRs in patients with sentinel lymph node positive melanoma may not be a beneficial screening tool to detect pulmonary metastases. Serial CXRs only detected approximately one half of pulmonary metastases present, rarely identified patients for potential curative surgery, and did not lead to earlier detection of pulmonary metastases. In addition, the authors feel that frequent CXRs may cause unnecessary patient anxiety, given the high rate of false positive findings.

The data in this study showed the sensitivity for detecting pulmonary metastases by CXR to be 48% and the specificity to be 78%, demonstrating a relatively high rate of false positive findings. Such a low sensitivity for detecting pulmonary metastasis draws the conclusion that CXR may not be a good screening tool for pulmonary metastasis, just as CXRs are not universally considered good screening tools for primary pulmonary tumors.

The limitations of this study include the limited sample size of patients and the lack of a comparison control group. However, a randomized controlled trial comparing surveillance CXR with no CXR is unlikely to be undertaken in high-risk melanoma population.

J. Levin, DO

J. Q. Del Rosso, DO

Method of Detection of Initial Recurrence of Stage II/III Cutaneous Melanoma: Analysis of the Utility of Follow-Up Staging
Meyers MO, Yeh JJ, Frank J, et al (Univ of North Carolina at Chapel Hill)
Ann Surg Oncol 16:941-947, 2009

Background.—The follow-up of patients with cutaneous melanoma is controversial. Current recommendations suggest routine history and physical examination every 3 to 6 months for the first 3 years and correlate studies including laboratory tests and radiographic imaging. However, the utility of these recommendations are unclear. The purpose of this study was to determine the impact of routine imaging on the method of detection of first recurrence in patients with stage II and sentinel lymph node-positive stage III melanoma.

Methods.—We analyzed a prospective database of all cutaneous melanoma patients treated at our institution from 1997 to 2005 who had at least 2 years of follow-up. The method of detection of initial recurrence was analyzed.

Results.—One hundred eighteen patients with stage II ($n = 83$) or III ($n = 35$) melanoma who were followed for at least 2 years were identified. Forty-three of these patients developed recurrence (median time to recurrence, 14 months). Site of first recurrence was as follows: 4 local, 17 in transit, 7 regional lymph node, and 15 distant. Twenty-nine recurrences (67%) were either patient detected or symptomatic. Eleven (26%) were detected by the physician at routine follow-up. Only three (7%) were identified by imaging (two chest X-ray and one brain magnetic resonance imaging) in an otherwise asymptomatic patient.

Conclusions.—Two-thirds of all initial recurrences of cutaneous melanoma were either detected by a patient or were symptomatic, with most of the remainder detected during routine physical examination. Routine imaging added little value in the detection of initial recurrence.

▶ The methodology of follow-up of patients with melanoma has long been debated and still remains controversial. Currently, there is no international consensus on the optimal follow-up schedule or the added value of diagnostic tests. In addition, past reports have demonstrated that most recurrences were detected by patients or partners. This is a prospective study of 118 patients with stage II ($n = 83$) or III ($n = 35$) melanoma followed for 2 years to evaluate methods of first time recurrence and evaluate the use of routine imaging. Authors sought to evaluate if the use of full body CT scans, combined positron emission tomography (PET)/CT scans, or brain MRI had any impact on detection of first time recurrence. Forty-three of these patients developed recurrence with a median time of 14 months. Twenty-nine recurrences (67%) were either patient detected or symptomatic. Eleven (26%) were detected by the physician at routine follow-up and only 3 (7%) were identified by imaging (2 chest X-ray and 1 magnetic resonance imaging). Most recurrences in this study were locoregional with only 35% of patients having distant recurrences. Of those, 75% of recurrences were identified by either the patient or a partner or were detected during routine physical examination by the physician. In this study, routine imaging is unlikely to be very helpful in improving early detection of regional recurrence. It was concluded that routine physician follow-up visits remain a relatively cost-effective means of following the patients with stage II/III melanoma. This study also revealed the importance of patient education with local recurrence being detected by the patient or a partner. Limitations to this study included a small sample size and short follow-up period of 2 years. There may also be benefits to routine imaging with those that have a high risk for recurrence, which would be of interest in future studies. Follow-up care for patients offers many benefits and can optimize early detection of recurrence and improve survival rates for melanoma.

G. K. Kim, DO

J. Q. Del Rosso, DO

Solitary Dermal Melanoma: Beginning or End of the Metastatic Process?
Lee CC, Faries MB, Ye X, et al (John Wayne Cancer Inst at Saint John's Health Ctr, Santa Monica, CA)
Ann Surg Oncol 16:578-584, 2009

Background.—Solitary dermal melanoma (SDM) is confined to the dermal and/or subcutaneous tissue without an epidermal component. It is unclear whether this lesion is a subtype of primary melanoma or distant cutaneous metastasis from an unknown primary. We evaluated our large experience to determine the prognosis and optimal management of SDM.

Methods.—Our melanoma referral center's database of prospectively acquired records was used for identification and clinicopathologic analysis of patients presenting with SDM between 1971 and 2005.

Results.—Of 12,817 database patients seen during a 34-year period, 101 (0.8%) had SDM. Of 92 patients free of distant metastasis on initial presentation, 55 (60%) were observed and 37 (40%) underwent surgical nodal staging: regional metastases were identified in 7 (19%). Nodal recurrence occurred in 1 of 30 patients (3.3%) with histopathology-negative nodes compared with 13 of 55 patients (24%) who underwent nodal observation instead of nodal staging. Thus, 21 of 92 patients (23%) had nodal metastasis identified during surgical nodal staging or postoperative nodal observation. At a median follow-up of 68 months, estimated 5-year overall survival rate was 73% for 71 patients with localized disease versus 67% for 21 patients with regional disease ($P = 0.25$) versus 22% for 9 patients with distant disease ($P = 0.009$, regional versus distant disease).

Conclusions.—SDM resembles intermediate-thickness primary cutaneous melanoma with respect to prognostic characteristics and clinical evolution, but its rate of distant metastasis justifies radiographic staging and its high rate of regional node metastasis justifies wide excision and sentinel node biopsy.

▶ Solitary dermal melanoma (SDM) is a current topic of debate. Some argue that SDM is an epidermal primary melanoma with regression, and others state that it is likely a metastatic melanoma. This is a retrospective study of 12 817 patients diagnosed with melanoma and 101 having SDM by histological evidence. All patients had a cutaneous examination, radiographic studies, including brain and body imaging to search for distant metastases. Diagnosis was confirmed by excisional biopsy with some patients undergoing nodal evaluation. The original slides and tissues were not available in all cases. In addition, the histopathologic characteristics of these lesions were not considered in this study. To make a stronger argument for a true diagnosis of SDM in this study histological evaluation would best be completed by one pathologist, or a team working together to assure agreement, and the specimens should have been reanalyzed. The diagnosis of SDM could have been based on areas of regression from a primary melanoma, which could have been missed by the pathologist. This study concluded that SDMs have a prognosis similar to primary dermal melanoma or primary melanoma with regressed epidermal component. In addition, prognosis of patients with nodal involvement matched those seen in primary melanoma. Some have argued that a primary dermal melanoma may arise from nonepidermal melanocytes or intradermal nevi; however, this study did not reveal clinical characteristics of each biopsied lesion, and there was also no record of previously preexisting residual nevus mentioned or explored, which would have also been helpful.

G. K. Kim, DO

J. Q. Del Rosso, DO

An Increased Number of Sentinel Lymph Nodes Is Associated with Advanced Breslow Depth and Lymphovascular Invasion in Patients with Primary Melanoma
Schmidt CR, Panageas KS, Coit DG, et al (Memorial Sloan-Kettering Cancer Ctr, NY)
Ann Surg Oncol 16:948-952, 2009

Background.—The pathologic status of the sentinel lymph node (SLN) is a powerful prognostic factor for patients with intermediate thickness melanoma. We hypothesize that a high number of SLNs identified may be associated with poor outcome.

Methods.—We evaluated the impact of number of SLNs removed in patients undergoing SLN mapping for cutaneous melanoma at our institution between 1996 and 2006. We excluded patients with multiple primary or synchronous primary lesions ($n = 144$) to eliminate any chance of erroneous association between a SLN and the wrong primary melanoma. We also excluded patients with in-transit disease ($n = 37$) and one patient in whom no SLN was identified, leaving 970 patients. We evaluated factors associated with the number of SLNs removed by multivariate Poisson regression and determined whether an increased number of SLNs was associated with poorer overall (OS) or recurrence-free survival (RFS).

Results.—Clinical factors independently associated with increased number of SLNs were younger age and head and neck primary site. Pathologic factors associated with an increased number of SLNs were lymphovascular invasion and increased Breslow thickness. There was no association between number of SLNs removed and OS or RFS in all patients or in patients with negative SLNs ($n = 803$).

Conclusions.—The number of SLNs identified during staging of the regional nodal basin for primary melanoma is not an independent prognostic factor. Drainage to multiple SLNs is more common in the setting of an increased Breslow depth and lymphovascular invasion suggesting that tumors with these adverse features may enhance peritumoral lymphangiogenesis.

▶ The purpose of this study was to look at whether increased sentinel lymph nodes (SLNs) correlate with poor outcomes and whether higher numbers of sentinel nodes are associated with other clinical or pathologic factors in patients with primary melanoma. The study size was adequate with 970 patients. The study was thorough and well conducted. Increased number of SLNs correlated with clinical factors of younger age and primary tumor site of head and neck.

Increased SLN was also associated with increased Breslow depth and lympho-vascular invasion while not adversely affecting outcome.

S. Bhambri, DO

J. Q. Del Rosso, DO

Microscopic Satellitosis in Patients with Primary Cutaneous Melanoma: Implications for Nodal Basin Staging

Kimsey TF, Cohen T, Patel A, et al (Memorial Sloan-Kettering Cancer Ctr, NY; et al)

Ann Surg Oncol 16:1176-1183, 2009

Background.—Microscopic satellitosis in melanoma is uncommon. The role of regional basin staging/therapy in patients with this high-risk feature has not been well defined.

Methods.—Patients presenting from 1996 to 2005 with clinically local-ized melanoma containing microscopic satellitosis were identified from a prospective, single-institution database. Multiple factors were analyzed to determine their predictive value for recurrence. The management of the draining nodal basin was evaluated to determine its impact on recurrence and survival.

Results.—Thirty-eight patients presented to our institution during this time period with clinically localized melanoma containing microscopic satellitosis. The 5-year overall and disease-free survivals in these patients were 34% and 18%, respectively. Sixty-eight percent had pathologically involved regional nodal metastases. With median follow-up of 21 months, 68% recurred, with a median time to recurrence of 9 months. Lymphovas-cular invasion (LVI) ($p = 0.01$), tumor regression ($p = 0.04$), and positive regional lymph nodes ($p = 0.02$) were associated with an increased risk of recurrence. Of the 31 patients who underwent sentinel lymph node (SLN) biopsy, 22 had metastasis in the SLN (71%). Fifteen of these patients underwent completion lymphadenectomy (CLND) and seven were observed. There was no difference in disease-free survival (DFS), disease-specific survival (DSS), or overall survival (OS) between these groups ($p = 0.42$).

Conclusions.—Pathological lymph node metastases were more preva-lent (68%) than in any group previously defined. Regional nodal status predicted recurrence but not nodal recurrence. In SLN-positive patients, CLND did not improve DFS, DSS, or OS, although the number of patients was small. Further studies are needed to determine the utility of regional nodal staging/therapy in these high-risk patients.

▶ In patients with melanoma and microscopic satellitosis, the prognosis is very grim with a 5-year disease-free (DFS) survival of only 36%. This is most likely due to the aggressive underlying tumor biology. These patients also have a high incidence of regional lymph node metastasis. This likely represents a continuum from microscopic satellitosis to intransit metastases to regional nodal metastases. Given the data showing completion lymphadenectomy (CLND) did not improve DFS, disease-specific survival (DSS), or overall survival (OS), routine sentinel lymph node (SLN) biopsy may not be beneficial in these patients.

Routine serial selecting of melanoma specimens would be ideal but perhaps not a practical approach to diagnosis and staging.

J. Q. Del Rosso, DO

In Vivo Confocal Microscopic and Histopathologic Correlations of Dermoscopic Features in 202 Melanocytic Lesions

Pellacani G, Longo C, Malvehy J, et al (Univ of Modena and Reggio Emilia, Italy; Melanoma Unit, Hosp Clínico, Barcelona, Spain)
Arch Dermatol 144:1597-1608, 2008

Objectives.—To identify in vivo microscopic substrates of the dermoscopic patterns of melanocytic lesions and to correlate them with histopathologic features.

Design.—Before excision, lesion areas that showed characteristic dermoscopic patterns were imaged by dermoscopy and confocal microscopy and directly correlated with histopathologic features.

Setting.—Departments of Dermatology of the University of Modena and Reggio Emilia and Hospital Clínico of Barcelona, between July 2006 and March 2007.

Patients.—Patients with 202 melanocytic lesions, corresponding to 76 melanomas, 114 nevi, and 12 Spitz or Reed nevi.

Main Outcome Measures.—Correlation of dermoscopic patterns in melanocytic lesions with confocal microscopic findings and conventional histopathologic findings.

Results.—Characteristic architectural and cytologic substrates were identified in vivo with the use of confocal microscopy and correlated with histopathologic features. Pigment network atypia was evidenced through confocal microscopy as a disarrangement of dermoepidermal junction architecture and cellular atypia. Pigmented globules consisted of cell clusters, corresponding to melanocytic nests identified on histopathologic analysis. Black dots correlated with intraepidermal reflective spots or with large pagetoid cells in nevi and melanoma, respectively. Blue structures usually consisted of numerous pleomorphic cells, corresponding to malignant melanocytes and inflammatory cells in melanomas, whereas plump bright cells, corresponding to melanophages on histopathologic analysis, characterized benign lesions. Within regression, a retiform distribution of collagen fibers, which sometimes intermingled with melanophages and rarely with nucleated cells, was observable.

Conclusions.—The knowledge of the cytologic and architectural aspects of the different dermoscopic patterns, as they appear by in vivo confocal microscopy, may guide the user to the identification of specific substrates in melanocytic lesions and consequently the interpretation of the dermo-scopic features.

▶ Dermoscopy as a tool for the noninvasive diagnosis of high-risk lesions for melanoma has made enormous strides in the past few years. However, the specificity needed to rule out malignant neoplasms has not yet reached the level needed to avoid unnecessary biopsies of numerous benign nevi. Reflectance confocal microscopy (RCM) paired with dermoscopy offers the promise of minimizing this issue. This study aimed to systematically explore the RCM substrates of the dermoscopic features of melanocytic lesions and correlate them with conventional histopathologic features. One strength of this article is that the quality of the images and explanations allow the newcomer to either appreciate RCM or dermoscopy to gain a better understanding of the histopathological correlations and basic concepts in the 2 areas. The overall analysis in this study showed the capability of this technique in improving diagnostic specificity for malignant melanoma if the RCM focuses on specific dermoscopic features such as dark pigmentation, pigment blotches, or blue structures. This may be helpful since currently the labor, time, and learning curve for performing RCM limits its use as a screening tool. Yet, if we can instead focus on selected lesions to improve the effectiveness of the effort expended, it should make RCM a more useful modality. This study is a good start at refining the use of this tool, but as the authors themselves state, larger studies are needed.

S. K. McCarty, MD

A. Torres, MD, JD

Study of Nevi in Children (SONIC): Baseline Findings and Predictors of Nevus Count
Oliveria SA, Satagopan JM, Geller AC, et al (Memorial Sloan-Kettering Cancer Ctr, NY; Boston Univ, MA; et al)
Am J Epidemiol 169:41-53, 2009

The authors report baseline findings and predictors of nevus count (log total nevi) at the completion of year 1 (2004) of the first known population-based, prospective study of nevi in a US cohort of children. Overall, 64% ($n = 443/691$) of grade 5 students and their parents in Framingham, Massachusetts, completed surveys and underwent digital photography. Total nevus count was associated with skin and hair color and tendency to burn, as measured by a sun sensitivity index. In multivariate analyses, male gender (rate ratio (RR) = 1.38, 95% confidence interval (CI): 1.22, 1.55; $P < 0.0001$), spending 5–6 weekly hours outdoors between 10 AM and 4 PM (RR = 1.13, 95% CI: 1.00, 1.28; $P = 0.051$), getting a painful sunburn once (RR = 1.24, 95% CI: 0.98, 1.57; $P = 0.073$) and at least twice (RR = 1.34, 95% CI: 0.99, 1.82; $P = 0.061$), and wearing a shirt at the beach or pool rarely (RR = 1.29, 95% CI: 1.08, 1.54; $P = 0.005$), sometimes (RR = 1.26, 95% CI: 1.01, 1.57; $P = 0.041$), and often and always (RR = 1.32, 95% CI: 1.13, 1.54; $P = 0.001$) were associated with increased number of nevi. Identifying factors that predict the development of nevi will improve primary prevention efforts during early life.

▶ Increased number of nevi is an important risk factor in the development of cutaneous melanoma. Therefore, researchers continue to examine the potential predictors of nevus count. Studies conducted from Australia suggest that 68% of nevus density is determined by genetic factors and the remainder attributed to environmental factors.[1] Through a population based, longitudinal study of United States children in Framingham, Massachusetts, investigators concluded that total nevus count is closely associated with color of skin and hair as well as the tendency to burn. In other words, children with lighter hair and lighter skin color with an increased tendency to burn were found to have greater total nevus count. As a portion of the study is dependent on fifth grade students and their parents to complete self-administered surveys, it may be subject to responder bias. In addition, there was a contradictory result where the sun protective behavior of wearing a shirt or hat was associated with increased number of nevi. This may be attributed to confounding errors.

S. Bellew, DO

J. Q. Del Rosso, DO

Reference

1. Harrison SL, MacLennan R, Buettner PG. Sunexposure and the incidence of melanocytic nevi in young Australian children. *Cancer Epidemiol Biomarkers Prev.* 2008;17:2318-2324.

The prevalence of melanocytic nevi on the soles in the Japanese population
Kogushi-Nishi H, Kawasaki J, Kageshita T, et al (Kumamoto Univ, Japan)
J Am Acad Dermatol 60:767-771, 2009

Background.—Acral lentiginous melanoma (ALM) is the most common type of melanoma in Japan. The association between ALM and acral nevus has not been elucidated.

Objective.—To investigate the prevalence and dermatoscopic patterns of plantar melanocytic nevi on the soles in the Japanese and to evaluate the relationship between acral nevi and ALM.

Methods.—All outpatients (N = 1697) and melanoma patients (N = 104) were included. We examined the number, size, and dermatoscopic images of nevi.

Results.—In the control group, the prevalence of plantar nevi was 10.9%, and the mean size was 3.8 ± 2.4 mm. The prevalence of nevi in patients with ALM and melanoma in situ on the soles was 8.6% and that of patients with melanoma on other sites was 14.5%. The main dermatoscopic pattern was "parallel furrow" in both groups.

Limitations.—This was a clinical observational study only.

Conclusion.—The number, size, and dermatoscopic patterns of nevi on the soles of patients with ALM and melanoma in situ on the soles did not differ from those of the control group.

▶ In some minority populations, primary melanoma occurs in more unusual sites, including palms and soles when compared with the Caucasian population. More specifically, acral lentiginous melanoma (ALM) is a common type in Asians, as compared with Caucasians. As there is an overall rise in melanoma and the United States Census Bureau projects further increases in the Asian population in the United States, it becomes more important to be well informed on melanoma in this minority population. Keep in mind that information specific to Japan may not be generalized to Asian Americans living in the United States. One clinically interesting finding that supports previous studies is that authors found no difference in prevalence of plantar melanocytic nevi between the acral melanoma group and the control group. Hence, increases in melanocytic nevi may not be a risk factor in acral melanoma. Given the poor survival rates in ALM and its unusual locations, clinicians should maintain a high index of suspicion in Asian populations.

S. Bellew, DO
J. Q. Del Rosso, DO

Imiquimod and lentigo maligna: a search for prognostic features in a clinicopathological study with long-term follow-up
Powell AM, Robson AM, Russell-Jones R, et al (St John's Inst of Dermatology, London, UK)
Br J Dermatol 160:994-998, 2009

Background.—Melanoma *in situ*/lentigo maligna (LM) is a potential precursor of LM melanoma. It occurs most commonly in elderly individuals on sun-exposed skin of the head and neck. Although surgical excision is the treatment of choice, this may not be desirable or feasible for large lesions at functionally or cosmetically important sites. Imiquimod is a topical immunomodulator which can generate a local cytotoxic response with potentially antiviral and antitumour effects.

Objectives.—To present our experience of LM treated with imiquimod.

Methods.—A retrospective review was performed of all patients with facial LM treated in our unit with topical imiquimod between January 2001 and December 2006. Pretreatment diagnostic biopsies were also reviewed and histologically graded.

Results.—Forty-eight patients were treated with imiquimod. There were 37 responders and 11 treatment failures (of whom two were 'partial responders'). Of the 37 responders, 31 showed a clinical inflammatory response to imiquimod. One patient in whom treatment failed subsequently developed invasive disease. The mean follow-up duration was 49 months. We could not identify histological features of prognostic significance. However, the ability to develop an inflammatory reaction to imiquimod was a strong predictor of therapeutic benefit.

Conclusions.—We consider imiquimod to have a role in the treatment of LM in patients in whom surgery may be contraindicated or for those in whom the cosmetic or functional consequences may be considerable. Until better characterized, its use should probably be confined to centres with experience in the detection and treatment of LM and melanoma.

▶ Lentigo maligna (LM) is seen frequently in elderly patients on sun-exposed areas. Surgical treatment has been the mainstay of therapy. Topical therapies are emerging, and this article looks at treating LM with topical imiquimod. The study size was inclusive of only 48 patients; however, the follow-up period was reasonable at approximately 4 years (49 months). It was reported that 77% of patients responded favorably to topical imiquimod therapy with no evidence of LM on subsequent biopsies. However, a failure rate of 23% is high given the capability of LM to invade and become lentigo maligna melanoma (LMM). Treatment of LM with topical imiquimod should be conducted in selected cases and by clinicians experienced with use of topical imiquimod for this off-label indication. It is important that patients be followed closely even if clinical clearance of LM is suspected by visible inspection and biopsy sample posttreatment. Interestingly, 6 of 37 patients who responded to topical imiquimod had no visible inflammatory reaction during treatment. Also, clinical persistence of pigmentation at completion of therapy was observed in 8 of 37 responders. The major disadvantage, as stated by authors, is the lack of tissue for histological examination of margins. Furthermore, randomly performed post-treatment biopsies may miss foci of the residual lesion, if present. The article reviews use of topical imiquimod for LM, which can serve in selected cases as an alternative treatment when surgery is not an option.

S. Bhambri, DO
J. Q. Del Rosso, DO

Does Shave Biopsy Accurately Predict the Final Breslow Depth of Primary Cutaneous Melanoma?
Moore P, Hundley J, Hundley J, et al (Wake Forest Univ School of Medicine, Winston-Salem, NC)
Am Surg 75:369-373, 2009

Shave biopsy (SB) is used for the diagnosis of suspicious skin lesions, including melanoma. Its accuracy for melanoma has not been confirmed. We examined our experience with SB to determine its ability to predict true Breslow depth (BD). We performed a retrospective review of the tumor registry for all patients diagnosed with melanoma by SB from 1995 to 2004. Site and depth of lesion, tumor stage, correlation of BD between SB and wide local excision (WLE), and changes in surgical management due to discordance were examined. Melanoma-in-situ was defined as a depth of 0 for this analysis. One hundred thirty-nine patients were diagnosed with melanoma by SB. Pathology after WLE were as follows: 54 (39%) patients had no residual disease, 67 (48%) had a BD equal to or less than the SB, and 18 (13%) had a thicker BD compared with the SB. For these 18 patients, the median BD by SB and WLE was 1.1 mm (range 0–6.5) and 3.5 mm (range 0.5–20.5), respectively ($P = 0.0017$). Upstaging of final BD from SB to WLE was significantly associated with increasing tumor depth and higher stage of melanoma ($P < 0.0001$). Only seven of the 139 patients (5%) required further surgery because of the increased depth of the WLE. SB underestimated the final BD of melanoma in 13 per cent of patients, but changed the management of few patients. SB is a valuable tool for practitioners in the diagnosis of melanoma. Nevertheless, patients diagnosed with melanoma by SB should be counseled about the rare need for additional surgery.

▶ This study demonstrates many factors that a clinician needs to consider to determine which type of biopsy is appropriate for the pigmented lesion, either superficial shave biopsy (SB), deep SB (referred to as saucerization biopsy in our practice), or excisional biopsy (EB). It would have been interesting to see the initial Breslow depth (BD) of all 139 patients after SB, including its clinical description, location and if superficial or deep SB was done, and the BD after wide local excision (WLE). It is important to keep in mind the location of the lesion to determine whether superficial or deep SB was done (dermal thickness of eyelid vs back). In our practice, we recommend EB if the lesion looks like a melanoma or if the pigmented lesion is associated with signs and symptoms of melanoma, including ulceration, pain, bleeding, and itching. There is always a risk of transecting the lesion during the SB, especially in this group of lesions; therefore, it may be difficult to determine the accurate BD after WLE. Also, when possible, always try to do a deep SB or EB of the entire lesion. When presented with a very large lesion, always biopsy the thickest portion of the lesion. Although the management changed in only a small percentage (13%) of patients in this study, this may vary among clinicians who are technically skilled and experienced versus those who are not. Also, as physicians, we would like to see this percentage be as close to zero as possible. In conclusion, deep shave biopsies can accurately predict the final Breslow depth of primary cutaneous melanomas if the lesions are biopsied earlier in the course of their progression (superficial or thin).

S. B. Momin, DO
J. Q. Del Rosso, DO

The Cost-Effectiveness of Sentinel Node Biopsy in Patients with Intermediate Thickness Primary Cutaneous Melanoma

Morton RL, Howard K, Thompson JF (Univ of Sydney, Australia)
Ann Surg Oncol 16:929-940, 2009

Background.—The aim of this study was to determine the cost-effectiveness of wide excision (WEX) + sentinel node biopsy (SNB) compared with WEX only in patients with primary melanomas ≥ 1 mm in thickness.

Methods.—A Markov model was populated with probabilities of disease progression and survival from the published literature. Costs were obtained from diagnostic-related group weightings and health outcomes were measured in quality-adjusted life years (QALYs).

Results.—Base case analyses suggested that, over a 20–year timeframe, the mean total cost per patient receiving WEX only was AU $23,182 with 10.45 life years (LY) and 9.90 QALYs. The mean cost per patient for WEX + SNB was AU $24,045 with 10.77 LY and 10.34 QALYs. The incremental cost effectiveness ratio for WEX + SNB was AU $2,770 per LY and AU $1,983 per QALY.

Conclusion.—WEX + SNB appears to offer an improvement in health outcomes (in both LYs and QALYs) with only a slight increase in cost.

▶ This article claims to be the first study that addresses the cost-effectiveness of sentinel node biopsy (SNB) plus wide excision (WEX) in intermediate thickness melanoma compared with WEX alone. Most of the articles used in the study were published outside the United States, and most of the guidelines were those of the United Kingdom and Europe, but these numbers are similar and can be extrapolated to the United States. The results were calculated using a Markov model for economic evaluation. Markov models are used to evaluate random processes such as health care interventions of chronic diseases. The model can also evaluate costs and outcomes. The one limitation this type of model has stems from the well-known Markov memory-less assumption. This means that while calculating the data, there is no effect of previous history with each cycle transition, therefore, there is an assumed constant probability, as in this case, a constant probability for melanoma disease progression from 1 year to the next. As may well be known, there can be no constants in relation to melanoma as all persons are different and may have other factors that may play a role in disease progression or remission.

We found that the tables and figures, although very detailed and multiple, could have been clearer and more straightforward. Some were not explained during the article, often only referred to for review. Clarification of some of the values (ie, how they were obtained, what they infer) would make them more useful.

This article does do a good job overall in making the point that SNB and WEX performed together in patients with primary melanoma greater than or equal to 1 mm in Breslow thickness may result in only a small increase in cost, but a solid evidence-based benefit for the health improvement is still pending further data, and it's not clear if the cost of surgical morbidity associated with SNB, though small, may further increase the cost.

M. J. Messina, MD

A. Torres, MD, JD

Spitz Nevus: Follow-Up Study of 8 Cases of Childhood Starburst Type and Proposal for Management

Nino M, Brunetti B, Delfino S, et al (Univ Federico II of Naples, Italy; S. Maria delle Speranze Hosp, Salerno, Italy; Univ Campus Bio-Medico, Rome, Italy)
Dermatology 218:48-51, 2009

Spitz nevus is an uncommon, benign melanocytic neoplasm that shares many clinical and histological features with melanoma. It presents clinical ambiguity that makes the diagnosis and management of the patient difficult. We present our experience in the management of Spitz nevus by rigorous dermoscopic long-term follow-up of 8 Spitz nevi in patients younger than 12 years. Dermoscopic images, acquired every 6 months, show evolution and modifications of these lesions. The aim of this paper is to better understand the long-term modifications of nevi with starburst pattern to avoid surgical excision of these lesions in the pediatric age group.

▶ The results of this long-term follow-up of 8 patients with Spitz nevi with starburst pattern in patients under 12 years of age are that all the patients presented a dermoscopic transition from the starburst to the reticular pattern. The transition was observed at the first follow-up in 3 of the cases and in the second year of follow-up in 5 cases. The authors propose follow-ups every 6 months for the first 2 or 3 years, and then every year for the management of dermoscopically starburst type nevi in children under 12 years of age. The article's limitation is the study size. In further large studies, not only should there be long-term follow-up of patients clinically and dermoscopically in the pediatric group, but there should also be a follow-up of evolution of lesions from pediatric cases into adulthood and lesions presenting in adulthood. Also, histopathological differences should be assessed and compared within each group.

S. B. Momin, DO

J. Q. Del Rosso, DO

Management of Congenital Nevi at a Dermatologic Surgical Paediatric Outpatient Clinic: Consequences of an Audit Survey 1990–1997

Mérigou D, Prey S, Niamba P, et al (Natl Reference Ctr for Rare Skin Disorders, Bordeaux, France; et al)
Dermatology 218:126-133, 2009

Background.—Since 1987 we have run a Dermatologic Surgical Paediatric Outpatient Clinic (DSPOC) within the Children's Hospital in Bordeaux.

Objective.—We analyse the consequences of an audit survey concerning the management of patients with congenital nevi (CN) seen at this clinic.

Methods.—We reviewed the cases of 192 children examined and photographed at the DSPOC during the period January 1990–December 1997. Patients were contacted for a reassessment of their status. The management options chosen at the DSPOC were reviewed as well as the satisfaction of the patients or parents of young children.

Results.—Of 192 children prerecruited, 56 girls and 52 boys could be included in the survey. They were mostly European whites and 67% were <6 months of age at the first DSPOC visit. 65/108 (61%) had been operated following the first DSPOC visit. The mean follow-up based on the 1997–1998 survey was 33 months (8 months to 10 years). The size of the nevus, independently of location, influenced decision for early surgery. Another important factor was the estimated disfigurement risk (15% of decisions) mostly related to CN of the face. There was a significant risk of pigmentary recurrence around the scar in children operated before the age of 2, but long-term follow-up indicated a spontaneously regressive course.

Conclusions.—Nevus recurrence in cases operated early suggests a time-dependent phenomenon in nevogenesis. Early counselling is important. Early surgery seems associated with a better scar quality. Explanations concerning risks and outcome are best given with the cooperation of a surgeon and a dermatologist.

▶ This article provides observations, more so than conclusive evidence, about the surgical findings, outcomes, and management of patients with congenital nevi. The motivation for this article appears to be the lack of consensus for optimal management of congenital nevi and makes observations on how the authors have modified their management after the audit survey was performed. The survey was based on the patients seen at their outpatient clinic. A few points of interest included the finding that a better aesthetic outcome was achieved with early surgery, although it was also associated with an increased risk of pigmentation around the scar, especially in children less than 2 years of age. This finding was thought to be possibly due, in part, to skin nevogenesis not being complete until the second year of life. Additional helpful considerations were related to the type of surgical technique that provided better results, the resolution of pigment recurrence, and observations regarding the reasons for delaying surgery. Other more general points discussed were common practice pointers that may already be used by dermatologists, including consent issues and discussions regarding risk and outcomes with both the surgeon and dermatologist. Overall, the article provides interesting information to consider in handling a patient with a congenital nevus, but lacks certainty in its conclusions to provide an overall consensus on management. A review of the article makes it apparent that follow-up studies are needed in hopes of a future consensus on the issue of the management of congenital nevi.

B. D. Michaels, DO

J. Q. Del Rosso, DO

Dermoscopic patterns and subclinical melanocytic nests in normal-appearing skin
Scope A, for the SONIC Study Group (Memorial Sloan-Kettering Cancer Ctr, NY; et al)
Br J Dermatol 160:1318-1321, 2009

Background.—Dermoscopic patterns of normal-appearing skin have received little scrutiny. We have recently completed an analysis of dermoscopic patterns of naevi in children.

Objectives.—To describe dermoscopic patterns in the normal-appearing skin surrounding naevi and to explore histological features of patterned background skin.

Methods.—Dermoscopic images of back naevi were obtained from a population-based sample of fifth grade students. The dermoscopic pattern of the background skin around the naevi was analysed. We examined histopathological features of background skin patterns in a convenience sample of seven specimens from six adult patients.

Results.—We observed a dermoscopic pattern in the background of normal-appearing skin in 41% of 1192 dermoscopic images from the backs of the 443 children. The background skin pattern was less frequent in individuals with a fair skin (P < 0·001). A globular pattern was observed in 201 images (17%) and a reticular pattern was seen in 287 images (24%), of which 112 images also showed globules. Inter-rater reliability between the two observers for a random sample of 100 images was excellent ($\kappa = 0·77$). In four specimens with a globular background pattern, microscopic melanocytic nests were observed in the normal-appearing skin. No subclinical naevus nests were observed in three reticular pattern specimens.

Conclusions.—Dermoscopically recognized patterns are commonly present in clinically normal skin of children. Microscopic melanocytic nests may be observed in normal-appearing skin with a globular skin pattern.

▶ Dermoscopic patterns have been developed for recognizing several cutaneous lesions. However, this article sought to determine if a dermoscopic pattern exists in normal-appearing skin surrounding nevi and then to determine the histological features of the normal skin. To this end, the study partially achieved its objective. The study was comprised of 1192 dermoscopic images on the backs 443 healthy children. In approximately 40% of the samples, either a globular pattern or a reticular pattern existed, which was somewhat dependent on skin color. The globular pattern may display subclinical melanocytic nests on histopathology and thus it was hypothesized that they may be the "seeds" that give rise to the clinically apparent acquired nevi with a globular pattern. The difficulty with this study is that there were no such findings in most patients—approximately 59%. Furthermore, as acknowledged, the study was comprised of healthy skin on the backs of children and therefore, it is unlikely that findings can be extrapolated to the adult population. Also, may these findings change in different areas of body that may not be as exposed to sunlight? The study is an interesting starting point and leaves the door open for further studies on this subject.

B. D. Michaels, DO

J. Q. Del Rosso, DO

Accuracy of teledermatology for nonpigmented neoplasms
Warshaw EM, Lederle FA, Grill JP, et al (Minneapolis Veterans Affairs Med Ctr, MN; et al)
J Am Acad Dermatol 60:579-588, 2009

Background.—Studies of teledermatology utilizing the standard reference of histopathology are lacking.

Objective.—To compare accuracy of store-and-forward teledermatology for non-pigmented neoplasms with in-person dermatology.

Methods.—This study was a repeated-measures equivalence trial involving veterans with non-pigmented skin neoplasms. Each lesion was evaluated by an in-person dermatologist and a teledermatologist; both generated a primary diagnosis, up to two differential diagnoses, and management plan. The primary outcome was aggregated diagnostic accuracy (percent correct matches of any chosen diagnosis with histopathology). Secondary outcomes included management plan accuracy (percent correct matches with expert panel management plan). Additional analyses included evaluation of the incremental effect of using polarized light dermatoscopy in addition to standard macro images, and evaluating benign and malignant lesion subgroups separately.

Results.—Most of the 728 participants were male (97.8%) and Caucasian (98.9%). The aggregated diagnostic accuracy (primary outcome) of teledermatology (macro images) was not equivalent (95% confidence interval [CI] for difference within +/−10%) and was inferior (95% CI lower bound <10%) to in-person dermatology for all lesions and the subgroups of benign and malignant lesions. However, management plan accuracy was equivalent. Teledermatology aggregated diagnostic accuracy using polarized light dermatoscopy was significantly better than for macro images alone ($P = .0017$). The addition of polarized light dermatoscopy showed the same pattern for malignant lesions, but not for benign lesions. Most interestingly, for malignant lesions, the addition of polarized light dermatoscopy yielded equivalent aggregated diagnostic accuracy rates.

Limitations.—Non-diverse study population.

Conclusions.—Using macro images, the diagnostic accuracy of teledermatology was inferior to in-person dermatology, but accuracy of management plans was equivalent. The addition of polarized light dermatoscopy yielded significantly better aggregated diagnostic accuracy, but management plan accuracy was not significantly improved. For the important subgroup of malignant lesions, the addition of polarized light dermatoscopy yielded equivalent diagnostic accuracy between teledermatologists and clinic dermatologists.

▶ Teledermatology holds great allure as a means to offer affordable and wide-reaching dermatologic care, particularly in an era of budget constraints and health care reform. Store-and-forward (SAF) technology, where stored clinical images are reviewed remotely by a practitioner at a time of convenience, has proven more economical than live video teleconferencing formats, and this has been true since I, myself, performed investigations in the realm nearly a decade ago.[1]

Still, as one might intuitively expect, it seems some entities, particularly inflammatory conditions, are better suited to teledermatology than are some neoplastic processes. In this study, these authors combined not only classic SAF teledermatology but also incorporated dermatoscopy images and examined nonpigmented neoplastic processes within the Veterans Administration health care system.

Not surprisingly, teledermatology proved inferior to in-person dermatology with regard to diagnosis, but with respect to management plans (which were frequently: remove, biopsy, destroy, observe, reassure, etc) the 2 means of rendering care were equivalent and did not result in discrepancies that would have resulted in clinically relevant differences in care.

For example, for the patients with Merkel cell carcinoma, proven by histological examination, none of the dermatologists, examining in-person or by teledermatology, were correct in making the diagnosis, but no clinically relevant discrepancy resulted as all parties indicated a need to "remove/biopsy," and hence the ultimate diagnosis and disposition were reassured.

One interesting factor worth mentioning as teledermatology and teledermatoscopy merge, is that the inclusion of the latter technology with the consultation did improve the diagnostic accuracy of the teledermatologists, brought them on par with in-person examination for malignant processes, but not for benign processes. Therefore, where teledermatology is pursued as viable means of providing care, the addition of teledermatoscopy may prove wise, particularly as malignant diagnoses pose the greatest risk, both to the patient and to the practitioner, from the perspective of medical malpractice, if they are underdiagnosed and underappreciated.

W. A. High, MD, JD, MEng

Reference

1. High WA, Houston MS, Calobrisi SD, Drage LA, McEvoy MT. Assessment of the accuracy of low-cost store-and-forward teledermatology consultation. *J Am Acad Dermatol.* 2000;42:776-783.

17 Lymphoproliferative Disorders

Subcutaneous Panniculitis-like T-cell Lymphoma: A Clinicopathologic, Immunophenotypic, and Molecular Study of 22 Asian Cases According to WHO-EORTC Classification

Kong Y-Y, Dai B, Kong J-C, et al (Fudan Univ, Shanghai, PR China; Shanghai Jiaotong Univ, PR China)

Am J Surg Pathol 32:1495-1502, 2008

Subcutaneous panniculitis-like T-cell lymphoma (SPTL) is defined as a rare cytotoxic α/β T-cell lymphoma characterized by primary involvement of subcutaneous tissue mimicking panniculitis and a predominant CD3$^+$/CD4$^-$/CD8$^+$ phenotype in 2005 World Health Organization-European Organization for Research and Treatment of Cancer (WHO-EORTC) classification for cutaneous lymphomas. We presented a detailed study of SPTL, describing clinicopathologic, immunophenotypic, and molecular features of 22 cases in China. Strict diagnostic criteria according to the WHO-EORTC definition were applied to the diagnosis of all SPTL cases. Besides the common features described before, unusual CD4$^+$/CD8$^-$ and CD4$^-$/CD8$^-$ T-cell phenotypes were noted in 2 of our cases, respectively. CD30 was negative in all cases and CD56 was focally positive in 2 cases. Mortality in cases with angioinvasion (75%) was significantly higher than that in cases without angioinvasion (14.3%). Epstein-Barr virus (EBV) infection was detected in 1 immunocompetent patient by in situ hybridization. The frequency of rearranged TCRB, TCRG, and TCRD genes detected by BIOMED-2 multiplex polymerase chain reaction tubes was 80%, 67%, and 13%, respectively, with a total clonality detection rate of 100%. Clinical follow-up was available in 18 patients, ranging from 6 to 80 months. Most patients obtained complete or partial remission after therapy including one accompanied with EBV infection; 5 patients died: 3 of disease progression, 1 of severe infection, and 1 of complications caused by diabetes and hypertension. We conclude that SPTL as a cytotoxic lymphoma derived from α/β T cell has a predominant CD4$^-$/CD8$^+$ phenotype, but unusual CD4$^+$/CD8$^-$ and CD4$^-$/CD8$^-$ phenotypes do exist. Owing to its indolent clinical course and relatively high survival rate, SPTL should be differentiated from cutaneous γ/δ T-cell lymphoma. EBV is generally absent in SPTL but can rarely be detected especially in Asian population. Angioinvasion is a poor prognostic factor in SPTL.

▶ A retrospective analysis was performed on 22 cases of subcutaneous panniculitis-like T-cell lymphoma (SPTL) in China. SPTL is a cytotoxic α/β T-cell lymphoma involving subcutaneous tissue with a relatively indolent course, and predominantly a CD4⁻/CD8⁺ phenotype. Due to its favorable clinical outcome, authors suggest to separate SPTL from other more aggressive cutaneous T-cell lymphomas. Clinical features more commonly include multiple subcutaneous nodules and/or indurated, erythematous plaques, although solitary lesions may exist. Common sites of involvement in descending order are lower extremities, trunk, upper extremities, and face. Other associated symptoms may consist of fever, leukocytopenia, or hepatosplenomegaly. Histopathologically, lobular panniculitis is seen with pleomorphic, hyperchromatic, irregular T cells rimming individual fat cells. However, the rimming of adipocytes is useful but not specific for SPTL. Fat necrosis is seen in some and numerous mitotic figures. Further confirmation for the clonal T-cell origin of SPTL can be made with TCRB combined with TCRG gene rearrangement. Limitations of the study include the small number of patients studied and those known to be inherent to retrospective analysis. The study population was limited to patients in China and therefore may not be applicable to other populations.

S. Bellew, DO

J. Q. Del Rosso, DO

Use of oral glucocorticoids and risk of skin cancer and non-Hodgkin's lymphoma: a population-based case–control study

Jensen AØ, Thomsen HF, Engebjerg MC, et al (Aarhus Univ Hosp, Denmark; et al)
Br J Cancer 100:200-205, 2009

In North Jutland County, Denmark, we investigated whether use of oral glucocorticoids was associated with an increased risk of developing basal cell carcinoma (BCC), squamous cell carcinoma (SCC), malignant melanoma (MM), and non-Hodgkin's lymphoma (NHL). From the Danish Cancer Registry we identified 5422 BCC, 935 SCC, 983 MM, and 481 NHL cases during 1989–2003. Using risk-set sampling we selected four age- and gender-matched population controls for each case from the Civil Registration System. Prescriptions for oral glucocorticoids before diagnosis were obtained from the Prescription Database of North Jutland County on the basis of National Health Service data. We used conditional logistic regression to estimate incidence rate ratios (IRRs), adjusting for chronic medical diseases (information about these were obtained from the National Patient Registry) and use of other immunosuppressants. We found slightly elevated risk estimates for BCC (IRR, 1.15 (95% CI:

1.07–1.25)), SCC (IRR, 1.14 (95% CI: 0.94–1.39)), MM (IRR, 1.15 (95% CI: 0.94–1.41), and NHL (IRR, 1.11 (95% CI: 0.85–1.46)) among users of oral glucocorticoids. Our study supports an overall association between glucocorticoid use and risk of BCC that cannot be explained by the presence of chronic diseases or concomitant use of other immunosuppressants.

▶ At first glance this article should be quite important. The risk of squamous cell carcinoma and non-Hodgkin's lymphoma in transplant patients on multiple immunosuppressive agents is well known. The increased incidence rate ratios in this study are only modest, however, with 10% to 15% increases in basal cell carcinoma, squamous cell carcinoma, melanoma, and non-Hodgkin's lymphoma. For non-Hodgkin's lymphoma this study reports a linear increase in risk with the amount of corticosteroids prescribed. There was an incidence rate ratio risk increase of 2.26 per 10 000 mg of steroid. Similarly, there was a statistically significant increased risk of squamous cell carcinoma with increasing corticosteroids with a cumulative incidence ratio per 10 000 mg of 7.4. Basal cell carcinoma risk and malignant melanoma risk do not appear to increase with increasing doses of corticosteroids. The risk of basal cell carcinoma did increase with longer duration of use, however.

The study has flaws that are inherent to any study based on a cancer registry for a prescription database. Compliance is always a problem so that prescription data do not necessarily reflect use of the drugs. Nondermatologists often overlook nonmelanoma skin cancer, and diagnosis of nonmelanoma skin cancer is therefore often underestimated in cancer registries. The data also don't provide information about skin type or sunbathing habits. Certainly, the diseases that require treatment with corticosteroids may impact on the likelihood of patients' sunbathing. And some of the diseases treated with corticosteroids, such as rheumatoid arthritis, have been associated with an increase in non-Hodgkin's lymphoma. Despite these unavoidable flaws in this study, the data presented are important for practicing physicians.

M. Lebwohl, MD

Bexarotene therapy for mycosis fungoides and Sézary syndrome
Abbott RA, Whittaker SJ, Morris SL, et al (St John's Inst of Dermatology, London, UK)
Br J Dermatol 160:1299-1307, 2009

Background.—Bexarotene (Targretin®) is a synthetic retinoid which is licensed for the treatment of advanced refractory cutaneous T-cell lymphoma (CTCL).

Objectives.—To summarize our experience with bexarotene for patients with CTCL with the aim of assessing efficacy and safety.

Methods.—A retrospective study of 66 patients (44 male, 22 female) with mycosis fungoides (40 patients) or Sézary syndrome (26 patients) who were commenced on bexarotene prior to August 2007 was carried out. Nineteen patients had early-stage (IB–IIA) refractory mycosis fungoides and 47 patients had advanced-stage CTCL (IIB–IVB).

Results.—Fifty-two out of 66 (79%) patients completed over 1 month of therapy with an intention-to-treat response rate of 44% (29/66). Of the patients, six (9%) had a complete response, 23 (35%) had a partial response, 15 (23%) had stable disease and eight (12%) had progressive disease. Median time to maximal response was 3 months (1–9 months). Median response duration was 8 months (1 to > 48 months). Median time to progression was 9 months (3–44 months). Fourteen patients (21%) did not complete a month of bexarotene therapy. Adverse effects of the whole group included central hypothyroidism in 100% (all grade II and managed with thyroid replacement) and hyperlipidaemia in 100% (all managed with lipid-lowering therapy ± dose reduction). Responses were seen in all stages and were higher in advanced stages: 26% (five of 19) with early-stage and 51% (24/47) of advanced-stage disease. Responses were seen in skin, blood and lymph nodes. Twenty-eight out of 66 patients were treated with bexarotene monotherapy and the remainder were on one or more additional anti-CTCL therapies.

Conclusions.—Our data demonstrate that bexarotene is well tolerated in most patients and responses are seen in almost half of patients with all disease stages. However partial responses were not graded and would include any improvement seen in the skin, blood and lymph node.

▶ This article provides a detailed summary of clinical experience for treating cutaneous T-cell lymphoma (CTCL) with oral bexarotene. Their aim was to assess the efficacy and safety of this therapy and give guidance to other prescribers.

The most significant of all of the findings was the higher response seen in advanced stages of CTCL and in patients with Sézary syndrome (SS). Patients with SS had an intention-to-treat response of 78% (7 of 9) while on monotherapy bexarotene. The response rate in SS may be higher than other forms of CTCL because Sézary cells express cutaneous lymphocyte antigen and chemokine receptor-4. In vitro studies have shown that bexarotene may inhibit malignant Sézary cells trafficking to the skin by suppressing chemokine receptor-4 expression.

Additionally, the authors provided excellent guidance for the management of the side effects of bexarotene therapy. While the side effects of oral retinoids can be extensive, only a small percentage of patients in this cohort discontinued therapy due to major side effects of the medication. Most notably, while 100% of cases demonstrated hypothyroidism and hyperlipidemia, no patient discontinued bexarotene therapy due to dysthyroidism, and only 4 patients stopped bexarotene therapy due to hyperlipidemia. It is noteworthy that a pre-existing hyperlipidemia may be an exclusion criteria for using bexarotene therapy to treat CTCL. The 9 other patients that discontinued bexarotene therapy did so for nonlife-threatening side effects such as diarrhea, constipation, and lethargy.

The major limitations of this study include the lack of comparison of response rates versus other CTCL therapies and the lack of dose-response analysis, as many patients had dose escalations or reductions during this study.

J. Levin, DO

J. Q. Del Rosso, DO

Granulomatous Mycosis Fungoides and Granulomatous Slack Skin: A Multicenter Study of the Cutaneous Lymphoma Histopathology Task Force Group of the European Organization for Research and Treatment of Cancer (EORTC)

Kempf W, Ostheeren-Michaelis S, Paulli M, et al (Univ Hosp, Zürich, Switzerland; Univ of Pavia, Italy; et al)
Arch Dermatol 144:1609-1617, 2008

Background.—Granulomatous cutaneous T-cell lymphomas (CTCLs) are rare and represent a diagnostic challenge. Only limited data on the clinicopathological and prognostic features of granulomatous CTCLs are available. We studied 19 patients with granulomatous CTCLs to further characterize the clinicopathological, therapeutic, and prognostic features.

Observations.—The group included 15 patients with granulomatous mycosis fungoides (GMF) and 4 with granulomatous slack skin (GSS) defined according to the World Health Organization–European Organization for Research and Treatment of Cancer classification for cutaneous lymphomas. Patients with GMF and GSS displayed overlapping histologic features and differed only clinically by the development of bulky skin folds in GSS. Histologically, epidermotropism of lymphocytes was not a prominent feature and was absent in 9 of 19 cases (47%). Stable or progressive disease was observed in most patients despite various treatment modalities. Extracutaneous spread occurred in 5 of 19 patients (26%), second lymphoid neoplasms developed in 4 of 19 patients (21%), and 6 of 19 patients (32%) died of their disease. Disease-specific 5-year survival rate in GMF was 66%.

Conclusions.—There are clinical differences between GMF and GSS, but they show overlapping histologic findings and therefore cannot be discriminated by histologic examination alone. Development of hanging skin folds is restricted to the intertriginous body regions. Granulomatous CTCLs show a therapy-resistant, slowly progressive course. The prognosis of GMF appears worse than that of classic nongranulomatous mycosis fungoides.

▶ This multicenter study helps expand our understanding of granulomatous cutaneous T-cell lymphoma (CTCL), a rare subtype includes granulomatous mycosis fungoides (GMF) and granulomatous slack skin (GSS). As a result of the low incidence of these conditions and the care of the authors to only include patients that met World Health Organization-European Organization for Research and Treatment of Cancer criteria for GMF and GSS, patient numbers are limited with only 15 patients in the GMF and 4 in the GSS groups. The article highlights the delay often seen in diagnosing GMF with a median of 11 years between clinical presentation and diagnosis. Histologically, the lack of epidermotropism did not exclude the diagnosis of granulomatous CTCL. Importantly, T-cell gene rearrangement studies were positive in 17/18 patients. Unfortunately, the study did not include any discussion regarding how pathologic specimens were evaluated. It is not clear if one or multiple clinicians were responsible for evaluating the pathologic specimens and how disagreements between pathologists or dermatopathologists were resolved. Clinically significant, both conditions show an increased risk of a second lymphoid neoplasia with 21% of the patients developing a second lymphoma, most commonly Hodgkin's lymphoma. Overall, GSS was shown to treatment resistant, but not fatal, whereas GMF was progressive and fatal in 40% of the cases despite various treatment regimens. These variants are both rare and challenging to diagnose and require a high level of suspicion and comprehensive clinical-pathologic collaboration. Differentiating between the 2 is critically important for proper management.

R. I. Ceilley, MD
D. M. MacAlpine, MD

Quality of life and psychological distress in patients with cutaneous lymphoma

Sampogna F, Frontani M, Baliva G, et al (Istituto Dermopatico dell'Immacolata, Rome)
Br J Dermatol 160:815-822, 2009

Background.—Cutaneous lymphomas may have a profound impact on patients' health-related quality of life (HRQoL) and psychological well-being.

Objectives.—To evaluate HRQoL and psychological distress in patients with cutaneous lymphoma, and to evaluate them in relation to personal and clinical characteristics.

Methods.—Patients with cutaneous T-cell lymphoma or cutaneous B-cell lymphoma (CBCL) were consecutively recruited in a dermatological hospital. Data on HRQoL were collected using a dermatology-specific questionnaire, the Skindex-29, and an oncology-specific questionnaire, the EORTC QLQ-C30.

Results.—Of 95 patients, there were 24 with CBCL, 59 with mycosis fungoides (MF) and 12 with Sézary syndrome (SS). The most frequent items reported in Skindex-29 were itching and sensitive skin, being annoyed by the disease, worry that it could get worse, affected interactions, and impairment in sexual life. The most frequent problems appearing from the EORTC QLQ-C30 analysis were fatigue, pain and

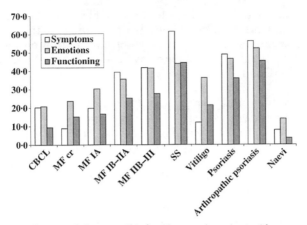

FIGURE 1.—Bar diagram of the mean Skindex-29 scores in patients with cutaneous lymphomas compared with vitiligo, psoriasis and naevi. Higher scores indicate lower health-related quality of life. CBCL, cutaneous B-cell lymphoma; MF, mycosis fungoides; MF cr, mycosis fungoides in complete remission; SS, Sézary syndrome. (Reprinted from Sampogna F, Frontani M, Baliva G, et al. Quality of life and psychological distress in patients with cutaneous lymphoma. *Br J Dermatol.* 2009;160:815-822, with permission from the British Association of Dermatologists.)

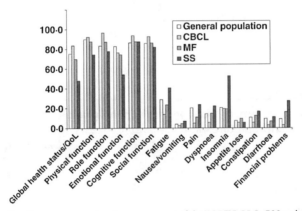

FIGURE 2.—Bar diagram representing the mean scores of the EORTC QLQ-C30 scales in 95 patients with cutaneous lymphoma, separately for cutaneous B-cell lymphoma (CBCL), mycosis fungoides (MF) and Sézary syndrome (SS). The general population is represented by 1965 Norwegian people sampled at random from the general population. Higher scores indicate a better health-related quality of life (HRQoL) in the scales from global health status to social function, and worse HRQoL in the remaining scales. (Reprinted from Sampogna F, Frontani M, Baliva G, et al. Quality of life and psychological distress in patients with cutaneous lymphoma. *Br J Dermatol.* 2009;160:815-822, with permission from the British Association of Dermatologists.)

insomnia. A worse HRQoL was observed for all the scales in patients with SS, followed by MF, and CBCL. HRQoL impairment in all histotypes was higher in women than in men, in patients with probable anxiety or depression, and when the disease worsened. The highest prevalence of probable anxiety or depression was observed in patients treated with systemic steroids (60%) and interferon (50%).

Conclusions.—The detailed evaluation of HRQoL and psychological problems in patients with cutaneous lymphomas, and their relationship with clinical variables, may give important information on the burden of the disease for patients, and thus improve communication and satisfaction with care (Figs 1 and 2).

▶ Patients with cutaneous lymphomas suffer not only from the disease process, the itching and sensitivity of the skin, but also the grave concerns of the disease progressing. These do cause a profound effect psychologically and have a negative impact on the quality of life. The article and its statistical analysis point out the negative effect in the patients' quality of life with regard to cutaneous lymphoma. This negative effect in life quality is noted in numerous patients with a disease process where there is no cure available. When treating this disease, a physician must remain vigilant to the possible presence of depression or anxiety in these patients. Physicians should be prepared to offer supportive help and realize that some therapeutic modalities such as systemic steroids and interferon may also have a negative psychological effect. The use of quality of life assessment tools will enable clinicians to better identify patient difficulties and in turn help the patient improve their life quality status. Tools used included Dermatology Quality of Life Skindex-29, cancer quality of life instrument EORTC-QLQ-C30, and a general health survey General Health Questionnaire (GHQ-12). The lymphomas were given a global severity on a 5-point scale of very mild to very severe. The study compared the severity of the disease with these psychological and quality of life parameters.

L. Cleaver, DO

Cutaneous lymphomas showing prominent granulomatous component: clinicopathological features in a series of 16 cases
Gallardo F, García-Muret MP, Servitje O, et al (Catalonian Cutaneous Lymphoma Network; et al)
J Eur Acad Dermatol Venereol 23:639-647, 2009

Background.—The presence of a prominent granulomatous tissue reaction in skin biopsies from primary cutaneous or systemic malignant lymphomas with secondary cutaneous involvement is a rare but well-known phenomenon.

Objective.—This paper aims to characterize and study a series of cutaneous lymphomas showing a prominent granulomatous component.

Patients and Methods.—The clinical, histopathological and evolutive features of granulomatous variants of mycosis fungoides (5 patients, 2 of them associating 'granulomatous slack skin' features), Sézary syndrome (1 patient), CD30+ cutaneous T-cell lymphoma (2 patients), CD4+ small/medium pleomorphic cutaneous T-cell lymphoma (1 patient), primary cutaneous B-cell lymphoma (3 patients) and peripheral T-cell lymphoma with secondary epithelioid granulomatous cutaneous involvement (4 patients) were reviewed.

Results.—The observed features were clinically non-distinctive. Only those cases presenting with granulomatous slack skin features were clinically suspected (2 patients). Non-necrotizing granulomata (11 patients) and granuloma annulare-like (4 patients) were the most frequently observed histopathological patterns. In five cases, no diagnostic lymphomatous involvement was initially observed. From our series, no definite conclusions regarding prognosis could be established.

Conclusion.—The diagnosis of cutaneous lymphoma may be difficult when a prominent cutaneous granulomatous inflammatory infiltrate obscures the true neoplastic nature of the condition. However, the presence of concomitant lymphoid atypia may help to suspect the diagnosis. In doubtful cases, the clinical evolution and the demonstration of a monoclonal lymphoid B- or T-cell population may lead to a definite diagnosis.

▶ The importance of this article lies in reminding dermatologists, and particularly dermatopathologists, that lurking within a granulomatous infiltrate could always be a lymphoproliferative disorder. Certainly, this does not mean to say that every case of an acral, annular, asymptomatic lesions, which clinically and histologically appears to be granuloma annulare, requires a dozen immunohistochemical stains and gene rearrangement studies, but certainly, on occasion, when the clinical situation merits it, or when the histology reveals cytological atypia to the mononuclear infiltrate, it is appropriate to consider the possibility that a granulomatous process obscures a lymphoproliferative condition.

In this series, after considering 987 cutaneous lymphomas in a central registry, the authors report an incidence (but apparently actually more of a prevalence, as no time period was defined) of 1.6% was found for specimens with a granulomatous component. This granulomatous component was defined as the presence of more than 25% of the inflammatory infiltrate corresponding to a histiocytic/granulomatous inflammation at least in 2 different biopsy specimens. Using this definition the authors found examples of both T-cell and B-cell disorders with this degree of granulomatous inflammation, either as a nonspecific manifestation of underlying disease, or as a true granulomatous cutaneous lymphoma.

Therefore, it would always behoove the dermatologist and dermatopathologist to consider the possibility of a lymphoproliferative disorder when confronted with a granulomatous process that is not well explained as a simple inflammatory or infectious condition.

W. A. High, MD, JD, MEng

Treatment of Early Stages of Mycosis Fungoides with Narrowband Ultraviolet B: A Clinical, Histological and Molecular Evaluation of Results
Dereure O, Picot E, Comte C, et al (Univ of Montpellier I, France)
Dermatology 218:1-6, 2009

Background.—Narrowband ultraviolet B (UVB) phototherapy is increasingly used in mycosis fungoides (MF).

Objective.—We report on the results obtained in a prospective series of early MF patients receiving this therapeutic regimen.

Methods.—In total, 22 patients were treated. Therapeutic results were evaluated on clinical, histological and molecular levels. Patients were then submitted to a clinical follow-up.

Results.—The cumulative number of treatments ranged from 22 to 48 (mean: 29). A complete clinical remission (CCR) was obtained in 18/22 patients, and a partial clinical remission in 4 cases. Complete or partial histological responses were achieved in 9/15 (all in CCR) and 4/15 patients, respectively. The molecular response was evaluated in 12 patients, and a disappearance of the dominant T cell clone in the skin was obtained in only 3 cases. After 4–48 months of follow-up (mean 20.1 months), 7/18 patients in CCR (39%) relapsed.

Conclusion.—Narrowband UVB phototherapy is a well-tolerated treatment of early-stage MF, and its efficiency is maximal in very early stages (Ia). Even though clinical results seem very similar to PUVA through indirect and tentative comparisons with historical series, relapses tend to occur earlier than with PUVA, especially when an incomplete histological or molecular response was achieved.

▶ This study credentials the use of narrow band therapy for early-stage mycosis fungoides. Histological and molecular markers were used to correlate therapy and response. The remissions induced by this therapy alone were substantial and relatively long lived. Where long-term intermittent therapy is needed, this type of therapy might have advantages over psoralen and ultraviolet A (PUVA).

E. A. Tanghetti, MD

18 Miscellaneous Topics in Dermatologic Surgery and Cutaneous Oncology

---

Dermatofibrosarcoma protuberans in children
Reddy C, Hayward P, Thompson P, et al (The Children's Hosp at Westmead, Sydney, Australia)
J Plast Reconstr Aesthet Surg 62:819-823, 2009

Dermatofibrosarcoma protuberans (DFSP) is a relatively rare neoplasm affecting the skin. It is an infiltrative tumour of intermediate malignancy, with a limited potential for metastasis but a high rate of recurrence. The incidence in children is even less frequent, although a proportion of those identified in adulthood may reflect a delay in diagnosis of childhood DFSP. We report the experience of DFSP seen at The Children's Hospital at Westmead (Sydney, Australia). Three children aged 5, 10 and 11 years of age underwent surgical excision of their lesions. Recurrence was evident in one child whose initial histopathology was not definitive for DFSP, and whose initial surgery had not involved wide local excision. All three children were male, and all had lesions affecting their trunk. One child whose lesion was thought to have been evident since birth may have represented congenital DFSP.

▶ This article details the presentation of 3 pediatric cases of dermatofibrosarcoma protuberans (DFSP) and provides an excellent review of the epidemiology, clinical presentation, diagnostic methods, treatment options, and recurrence rates for DFSP in children and adults. One of the main points of the article is to remind physicians to consider DFSP in children with persistently growing indurated lesions. Delays in diagnoses of DFSP can be devastating, including for children, as if the lesion continues to grow, especially subcutaneously, more extensive and disfiguring surgery is likely to be needed.

J. Levin, DO

J. Q. Del Rosso, DO

Pseudocyst of pinna: a recurrence-free approach

Kanotra SP, Lateef M (Government Med College, Srinagar, J and K, India)
Am J Otolaryngol 30:73-79, 2009

Objective.—The aims of the article were to study the epidemiological profile of pseudocyst of pinna in non-Chinese population, to propose a hormonal basis of pseudocyst formation, and to compare 2 commonly used treatment modalities of incision drainage with compression and deroofing with compression, so as to ascertain the definitive treatment of this frequently recurring condition.

Material and Methods.—Twenty-nine patients were diagnosed with pseudocyst of the auricle between June 2005 and December 2006 in a medical college hospital. All the patients were initially subjected to aspiration with contour dressing. Of the 29 patients, 28 showed recurrence with in 1 week. These 28 patients were divided into 2 groups—13 patients underwent incision and drainage with curettage followed by buttoning, whereas 15 underwent surgical deroofing of the cyst along with buttoning.

Results.—All the 29 patients were males with a mean age of 32.6 ± 4.3 years. Sixteen (55.17%) patients had a right-sided lesion, whereas 13 (44.82%) patients had a left-sided lesion. No case of bilateral pseudocyst was seen. The pseudocyst was most commonly located in the concha. After aspiration with contour dressing, 28 (96.55%) patients showed recurrence within 1 week. Of the 13 patients who underwent incision drainage with buttoning, 5 (38.46%) showed recurrence. Of the 13 patients who underwent incision drainage, 3 (23.07%) showed permanent thickening of the auricular cartilage. The 5 cases that recurred then underwent deroofing with buttoning along with 15 patients. Thus, a total of 20 patients underwent surgical deroofing. No recurrence was seen with this technique. The patients were followed up for 1 month. No complication was noted, and the results were cosmetically acceptable.

Conclusion.—Pseudocyst of the pinna is an uncommon condition of the auricle presenting as a painless swelling in young adult males. The epidemiological profile of this condition is similar in Chinese and non-Chinese (Indian) population. A hormonal influence modulating the inflammatory process explains the marked male predominance of this condition. Surgical deroofing followed by buttoning is the definitive treatment of this entity as it is associated with no recurrence and gives a cosmetically acceptable result.

▶ Pseudocyst of the pinna is an uncommon condition that can frequently recur after treatment. The definitive treatment still remains controversial because of the high recurrence rate. This study compares 2 treatments using incision and drainage with compression and deroofing with compression. This is a study of 29 male patients with pseudocyst of pinna with a mean age of 32.4 years and a slight predominance for right-sided lesions. The follow-up period post-treatment was 1 month. The etiology of pseudocysts is still not well understood. Some have suggested a hormonal component in the pathogenesis of the disease. It was found that aspiration followed by pressure dressing is an ineffective method of treating pseudocyst. Incision and drainage followed by buttoning considerably decreased the rate of recurrence (38.46%). The buttoning offers a better more constant compression compared with contour dressings. Patients who had incision and drainage developed thickening of the auricular cartilage. In contrast, deroofing of the cavity followed by buttoning was associated with 0% recurrence and offered a cosmetically better result with no complications. Surgical deroofing removes the degenerated cartilage and effectively reduces any chance of recollection of fluid.

G. K. Kim, DO

J. Q. Del Rosso, DO

Phenol peels as a novel therapeutic approach for actinic keratosis and Bowen disease: Prospective pilot trial with assessment of clinical, histologic, and immunohistochemical correlations
Kaminaka C, Yamamoto Y, Yonei N, et al (Wakayama Med Univ)
J Am Acad Dermatol 60:615-625, 2009

Background.—Although chemical peels may be used for precancerous lesions, no histologic or immunohistochemical studies have been performed to validate clinical impressions and/or outcome.

Objective.—Our purpose was to investigate the efficacy and prognostic relevance of phenol peels in Japanese patients with actinic keratosis and Bowen disease using clinical and histologic criteria.

Methods.—A total of 46 patients were treated with phenol peels, and followed up for at least 1 year after treatment. Biopsy specimens were taken before and after treatment. Cases of complete response were classified by the number of treatment sessions. We evaluated parameters for epidermal thickness, proliferation, dysplasia, and apoptosis, and clinical characteristics to correlate phenol peels with assessments of efficacy, patient-selection criteria, and risk for transformation to cutaneous squamous cell carcinoma.

Results.—There were 39 (84.8%) patients with a complete response after one to 8 treatment sessions. Statistically, differences in clinical improvement with peels and the number of treatment sessions correlated with histology, personal history of skin cancer, tumor thickness, and cyclin A expression.

Limitations.—This study was a prospective pilot trial. Blinded, placebo-controlled, randomized studies would be ideal.

Conclusion.—We conclude that phenol peels are very effective for treating precancerous lesions of actinic keratosis and Bowen disease. In addition, our study clearly demonstrates that tumor thickness and cyclin A could be specific and useful markers as adjunctive diagnostic tools to predict the efficacy of phenol treatment of these lesions.

▶ Numerous destruction treatments for actinic keratosis (AK) and Bowen's disease are available: cryosurgery, laser surgery, photodynamic therapy, curetting, electrodessication, dermabrasion, and chemical peeling. Dermabrasion as a treatment for AK is an option, but with the noted high recurrence rate it is not an effective modality overall. This report of repeated monthly phenol peeling (up to 8 peels) is intriguing. Because of better full thickness epidermal destruction with phenol peeling, this may be a better approach than some other peeling methods. The histopathologic and immunohistochemical findings shown in this report seem to confirm this clinical consideration. The incidence of adverse skin reactions was not reported. Reasonable concerns include scarring and dyspigmentation (hyper or hypopigmentation). Long-term follow-up studies will be needed to determine the efficacy and true therapeutic value of this modality.

R. I. Ceilley, MD

Ultrasound for initial evaluation and triage of clinically suspicious soft-tissue masses
Lakkaraju A, Sinha R, Garikipati R, et al (Leeds Teaching Hosps, UK)
Clin Radiol 64:615-621, 2009

Aim.—To evaluate the efficacy of ultrasound as a first-line investigation in patients with a clinical soft-tissue mass.

Methods.—Three hundred and fifty-eight consecutive patients (155 male, 203 female, mean age 48 years) referred from primary and secondary care with soft-tissue masses underwent ultrasound evaluation. Five radiologists performed ultrasound using a 10–15 MHz linear transducer and recorded the referrer diagnosis, history, lesion size, anatomical location and depth, internal echogenicity, external margins (well-defined rim or infiltrative), and vascularity on power Doppler (absent or present, if present the pattern was listed as either linear or disorganized). A provisional ultrasound diagnosis was made using one of eight categories. Benign categories (categories 1–5) were referred back to a non-sarcoma specialist or original referrer for observation. Indeterminate or possible sarcomas (categories 6–8) were referred for magnetic resonance imaging (MRI) within 14 days. Additionally category 8 lesions were referred to the regional sarcoma service. Institutional and regional database follow-up was performed.

Results.—Two hundred and eighty-four of the 358 (79%) lesions were classified as benign (categories 1–5). On follow-up 15 of the 284 patients were re-referred but none (284/284) had a malignancy on follow-up (24–30 months). Overall at ultrasound 33 lesions were larger than 5 cm, 42 lesions were deep to deep fascia with 20 showing both features.

In this subgroup of 95 patients there were six malignant tumours with the rest benign. Seventy-three of the 358 patients underwent MRI; the results of which indicated that there were 60 benign or non-tumours, 10 possible sarcomas, and three indeterminate lesions. Overall six of 12 (6/358, 1.68% of total patients) lesions deemed to represent possible sarcomas on imaging were sarcomas.

Conclusion.—Ultrasound is an effective diagnostic triage tool for the evaluation of soft-tissue masses referred from primary care.

▶ Soft tissue sarcomas constitute less than 1% of all malignant tumors. Most soft tissue masses are benign; however, many of these appendicular and truncal soft tissue masses warrant an evaluation by some form of imaging. The imaging options include computed tomography (CT), magnetic resonance imaging (MRI), or ultrasound. Ultrasound was used in this study as the initial imaging assessment and was able to diagnose 79% of the lesions as benign immediately. This proportion was increased further using MRI for suspicious or indeterminate ultrasound findings with less than 2% of lesions subsequently found to be histologically malignant at surgery. Therefore, ultrasound is an effective diagnostic triage tool for the evaluation of soft tissue masses referred from primary care. This provides for an efficient pathway for more rapid diagnosis in this patient group.

R. I. Ceilley, MD

Recent Changes in the Workforce and Practice of Dermatologic Surgery
Tierney EP, Hanke CW, Kimball AB (Henry Ford Health System, Detroit, MI; Laser and Skin Surgery Ctr of Indiana, Carmel; Harvard Med School, Boston, MA)
Dermatol Surg 35:413-419, 2009

Background.—The increasing number of American College of Mohs Surgery (ACMS) fellowship positions over the last decade has resulted in a greater number of fellowship-trained surgeons in dermatologic surgery.

Methods.—Mohs micrographic fellowship-trained surgeons (MMFTSs) and non-Mohs fellowship-trained surgeons performing Mohs micrographic surgery (NMMFTSs) were compared using the American Academy of Dermatology Practice Profile Survey (2002/05). An analysis of recent Mohs fellowship classes was also performed.

Results.—In 2005, there was an equivalent proportion of MMFTSs and NMMFTSs in the workforce (ratio MMFTS:NMMFTS = 0.9) but, in 2005, there was a shift in the youngest age cohort (29–39) to a greater proportion of MMFTSs (MMFTS:NMMFTS = 1.55). In 2005, the youngest MMFTSs (29–39) were more likely to be female (47.1%) than of MMFTSs overall (24%). MMFTSs were 5 times as likely to be in full-time academic positions and performed 2 to 3 times as many Mohs cases per week as NMMFTSs.

Conclusions.—Consistent with demographic shifts in dermatology, differences have emerged in the demographics, surgical volumes, and settings of MMFTSs and NMMFTSs. Recent increases in the ACMS fellowship positions have resulted in a greater proportion of MMFTSs among younger dermatologic surgeons. It will be important to follow how this increase in fellowship trainees affects the dermatologic surgery workforce.

▶ Mohs micrographic surgery (MMS) is becoming increasingly important and used in dermatology. Fortunately, there has been an increasing number of fellowship-trained dermatologists entering into academic practice or academic affiliation. This parallels the rapid rise in research and publications relating to dermatologic surgery, MMS, and cutaneous oncology. Because of the well-established high cure rates of MMS for nonmelanoma skin cancers treated by MMS, dermatologists are more inclined to use this technique.

A debate is currently raging over the proper use and potential overuse of this modality. Outcome and cost-effective studies are needed to determine if the procedure is used for appropriate lesions and is properly performed. This increasing number of fellowship-trained dermatologists in excellent private practice settings and academic centers will continue to improve this important modality. Although the title of this article states "practice of dermatologic surgery," the article focuses primarily on MMS. There has also been a parallel increase in the use of other dermatologic procedures such as lasers, light-based therapies, liposuction, fillers, relaxants, hair transplantations, and other cosmetic procedures. It would be helpful to compare the percentage of MMS cases with other dermatologic surgery procedures by dermatologists in the categories of age, gender, academic, and nonacademic practices. Because a MMS fellowship also provides a major source of training in these other procedures, many residents are drawn to surgery through such fellowships. Because some programs give residents significant exposure to MMS, this likely encourages them to use this modality in their practice without further training.

R. I. Ceilley, MD

The role of the plain radiograph in the characterisation of soft tissue tumours

Gartner L, Pearce CJ, Saifuddin A (RNOH Stanmore, Middlesex, UK; Kingston Hosp, UK)
Skeletal Radiol 38:549-558, 2009

A radiograph is often the first investigation to be requested when a patient presents with limb pain or a mass. Whilst we do not advocate that this is the only investigation to be employed in the evaluation of such patients, a working knowledge of the variety of abnormal findings that can present in the soft tissues on radiographs remains useful. We reviewed the radiographic findings of soft tissue masses from a prospectively compiled database of all such lesions presenting to a specialist orthopaedic oncology service over the past 8 years. Of the cohort of 1,058 individuals with a proven soft tissue tumour, 454 had had a radiograph taken of the affected area. Of these, 281 (62%) patients had a positive radiographic finding. The most common findings were a visible soft tissue mass ($n = 141$), the presence of calcification ($n = 76$), fat ($n = 32$) and evidence of bone involvement ($n = 62$). More than one finding was sometimes present in the same patient. These findings were present in both benign and malignant tumours. This review article describes the incidence and diagnostic relevance of these plain film findings for suspected soft tissue tumours.

▶ Soft tissue (ST) tumors are rare and most of them are benign. The most common symptom is a painless mass. Plain radiographs are simple, fast, and can provide a cost-effective way to evaluate these lesions. Plain radiographs revealed a positive radiographic finding in 62% of patients who had a radiograph taken of the affected area. A visible ST mass was the most common finding on a positive radiograph followed by the presence of calcification or fat. Furthermore, the location of visible mass may provide information on the mass being benign or malignant. As the authors suggest, "If a radiographically visible ST mass was present in the thigh, calf or arm, it was more likely to be malignant, with sarcoma being, by far, the most common pathology." MRI is a superior modality, but plain radiographs are valuable when evaluation by MRI is not available, and may be clinically relevant if a radiographic abnormality is noted. However, a negative radiograph does not definitively exclude presence of a ST tumor. Additionally, the question of a benign versus a malignant ST tumor warrants histologic evaluation.

S. Bhambri, DO

J. Q. Del Rosso, DO

The efficacy of a smoking cessation programme in patients undergoing elective surgery – a randomised clinical trial
Sadr Azodi O, Lindström D, Adami J, et al (Karolinska Inst, Stockholm, Sweden; et al)
Anaesthesia 64:259-265, 2009

It is known that smokers constitute an important risk group of patients undergoing surgery. It is unknown how smoking cessation intervention initiated 4 weeks prior to elective surgery affects the probability of permanent cessation. We randomly assigned 117 patients, scheduled to undergo elective orthopaedic and general surgery, to smoking cessation intervention and control group. The intervention group underwent a programme initiated, on average, 4 weeks prior to surgery with weekly meetings or telephone counselling and were provided with free nicotine replacement therapy (NRT). The control group received standard care. As a result,

20/55 (36%) patients the intervention group vs 1/62 (2%) in the control group became completely abstinent throughout the peri-operative period (p < 0.001). After 1 year, those in the intervention group was most likely to be abstinent (18/55 (33%) vs 9/62 (15%) of the controls (p = 0.03). Level of nicotine dependence and obesity seemed to be a predictor of long-term abstinence (p = 0.02).

▶ Smoking has a variety of adverse effects on the skin. Survival of grafts and flaps and healing of some wound closures are adversely affected. Any effort to enhance smoking cessation is laudable as part of general health recommendations by physicians. A standardized effective approach that can be effectively and practically incorporated in dermatology practices that would be helpful in getting more patients to cease smoking is welcome. Patients who will be undergoing dermatologic surgical procedures, especially flaps, grafts, and complex procedures, may be encouraged to initiate cessation of smoking around the time of their procedure, with the hopes that cessation of smoking may persist. This may be the first time many of them have been offered a formal try at smoking cessation.

R. I. Ceilley, MD

Cutaneous Cysts of the Head and Neck

Al-Khateeb TH, Al-Masri NM, Al-Zoubi F (Jordan Univ of Science and Technology and King Abdullah Univ Hosp, Irbid, Jordan)
J Oral Maxillofac Surg 67:52-57, 2009

Purpose.—A retrospective study on the features of cutaneous cysts of the head and neck as seen in a North Jordanian population.

Patients and Methods.—The records of the Department of Pathology at Jordan University of Science and Technology were reviewed for patients with cutaneous cysts of the head and neck during the 12-year period extending between 1991 and 2002. Applicable records were retrieved, reviewed, and analyzed. Primary analysis outcome measures included patient age, gender, location of the cyst, type, clinical presentation, and treatment. The records of 488 patients were available for analysis.

Results.—Epidermoid cyst was the most frequent lesion (49%) followed by pilar cysts (27%), and dermoid cysts (22%). The site affected most frequently was the scalp (34%), predominantly with pilar cysts (96%). Epidermoid cyst was the most frequent lesion in the neck (68%), cheeks (77%), periauricular area (70%), and the nasal area (55%). Dermoid cyst was the most frequent lesion in the periorbital area (52%). Females represented 51% of the patients and males accounted for 49%. The peak of age distribution for patients with dermoid cysts was at the first decade, and both of epidermoid and pilar cysts peaked at the third decade. Infection presented in 2.5% of cases. All cysts were enucleated surgically.

Conclusion.—Maxillofacial surgeons often encounter cutaneous cysts of the head and neck, and they must be familiar with the clinicopathologic characteristics of these lesions.

▶ This retrospective review of 488 patients presenting with cystic neoplasms involving the head and neck region did not necessarily reveal any surprising information other than the consideration of a diagnosis of a dermoid cyst when the periorbital area is involved. Surprisingly, dermoid cysts represented approximately half of the periorbital lesions in this analysis, and were seen most commonly in the first decade of life. As anticipated, most scalp lesions were pilar cysts (96% of scalp cyst lesions). Epidermoid cysts were seen in 49% of cases overall, representing the most common form of cystic neoplasm on the neck, cheeks, periauricular area, and nasal region. Regardless of these tendencies related to anatomic location, histologic confirmation of diagnosis is needed. Importantly, infection was uncommon among these cystic lesions (2.5%), emphasizing that oral antibiotic therapy is likely not needed overall when treating cytstic lesions of the head and neck with surgical excision.

J. Q. Del Rosso, DO

Comparison of Mohs Micrographic Surgery and Wide Excision for Extramammary Paget's Disease: Korean Experience

Lee K-Y, Roh MR, Chung WG, et al (Yonsei Univ College of Medicine, Seoul, Korea)
Dermatol Surg 35:34-40, 2009

Background.—Extramammary Paget's disease (EMPD) is an uncommon tumor that usually occurs on the genitalia. It almost always extends beyond clinically apparent margins and has a high rate of recurrence.

Objective.—To establish treatment guidelines for EMPD in Asian patients.

Methods.—A retrospective review was done on pertinent demographic data, tumor data, treatment characteristics, and follow-up data of 35 patients between 1996 and 2006. Review of literature for treatment modalities and recurrence rates of EMPD was also performed.

Results.—Thirty-four of the 35 patients (30 men and 5 women) had lesions in the genital area and one patient in the axilla. Mean follow-up duration was 62.7 months (8–156 months) and two of 11 (18.2%) recurred after Mohs micrographic surgery (MMS), compared with eight recurrences of 22 (36.4%) after standard wide excision. Two patients treated with nonsurgical modalities did not achieve complete remission. Estimated 5-year tumor-free rate using Kaplan-Meier graph was 69.7% in all patients, with a rate of 81.8% for MMS and 63.6% for wide excision.

Conclusions.—MMS is more effective, with lower recurrence rate than wide excision, and should be regarded as the first-line treatment for nonmetastatic EMPD.

▶ The objective of this retrospective study was to establish treatment guidelines for extramammary Paget's disease in Asian patients. In particular, Mohs micrographic surgery (MMS) was shown to have less recurrence and a greater 5-year disease-free interval rate when compared with wide surgical excision. It is important to note, however, that the mean follow-up duration was 15.5 months less in patients treated with MMS than wide excision. The authors bring to light a critical feature of extramammary Paget's disease and that is the marked tendency of the disease to exhibit subclinical histologic extension beyond the clinically visible lesion borders, thus supporting the use of MMS as treatment of choice. A larger prospective study with longer duration of follow-up for patients treated with MMS compared with wide excision would be beneficial for future study. Currently, the treatment of choice for local extramammary Paget's disease remains surgical excision; however, in experienced hands, MMS is a viable option.

S. Bellew, DO
J. Q. Del Rosso, DO

Assessment of Lifetime Cumulative Sun Exposure Using a Self-Administered Questionnaire: Reliability of Two Approaches
Yu C-L, Li Y, Freedman DM, et al (NIH, Rockville, MD; et al)
Cancer Epidemiol Biomarkers Prev 18:464-471, 2009

Few studies have evaluated the reliability of lifetime sun exposure estimated from inquiring about the number of hours people spent outdoors in a given period on a typical weekday or weekend day (the time-based approach). Some investigations have suggested that women have a particularly difficult task in estimating time outdoors in adulthood due to their family and occupational roles. We hypothesized that people might gain additional memory cues and estimate lifetime hours spent outdoors more reliably if asked about time spent outdoors according to specific activities (an activity-based approach). Using self-administered, mailed questionnaires, test-retest responses to time-based and to activity-based approaches were evaluated in 124 volunteer radiologic technologist participants from the United States: 64 females and 60 males 48 to 80 years of age. Intraclass correlation coefficients (ICC) were used to evaluate the test-retest reliability of average number of hours spent outdoors in the summer estimated for each approach. We tested the differences between the two ICCs, corresponding to each approach, using a t test with the variance of the difference estimated by the jackknife method. During childhood and adolescence, the two approaches gave similar ICCs for average numbers of hours spent outdoors in the summer. By contrast, compared with the time-based approach, the activity-based approach showed significantly higher ICCs during adult ages (0.69 versus 0.43, $P = 0.003$) and over the lifetime (0.69 versus 0.52, $P = 0.05$); the higher ICCs for the activity-based questionnaire were primarily derived from the results for females. Research is needed to further improve the activity-based questionnaire approach for long-term sun exposure assessment.

▶ Dermatologists account for a patient's cumulative exposure to the sun, history of sunburns, and routine use of sunscreen in daily evaluation to stratify any potential risk of skin cancer. Unfortunately, there is no clear objective index for placing a patient at a risk level aside from documenting years of living in warm climates, skin type, or history of outdoor activities. Patients also tend to underestimate both the time spent outdoors as well as how significant some activities resulted in unprotected solar exposure.

This study is based on the authors attempt to establish an objective measure for historical photo exposure, accounting for the differences in gender, activities, and geography among the 300 patients studied, in an attempt to create a standard measure for historical calculation of the amount of hours spent exposed to ultraviolet (UV) radiation. They refer to the intraclass correlation coefficients (ICC) as a basis for measuring cumulative solar exposure involving questionnaires to patients based on either time spent outdoors or activities that were performed during prime sunshine hours.

The study results suggest that the activity-based survey provided a more accurate history of solar exposure, which might be of value to the dermatologist taking into account a patient's risk for skin cancer. For example, the assessment of a construction worker or a farmer may have as much importance as the history of excessive use of tanning beds from an activity standpoint even though the cumulative time spent by these patients may vary and not have the same impact. Although the results may be difficult to reproduce, the model posed by the authors may provide some evidence for a template for taking a history and determining relative risk.

N. Bhatia, MD

Sources of sensitization, cross-reactions, and occupational sensitization to topical anaesthetics among general dermatology patients
Jussi L, Lammintausta K (Turku Univ Central Hosp, Finland)
Contact Dermatitis 60:150-154, 2009

Background.—Contact sensitization to local anaesthetics is often from topical medicaments. Occupational sensitization to topical anaesthetics may occur in certain occupations.

Objectives.—The aim of the study was to analyse the occurrence of contact sensitization to topical anaesthetics in general dermatology patients.

Patients and Methods.—Patch testing with topical anaesthetics was carried out in 620 patients. Possible sources of sensitization and the clinical histories of the patients are analysed.

Results.—Positive patch test reactions to one or more topical anaesthetics were seen in 25/620 patients. Dibucaine reactions were most common (20/25), and lidocaine sensitization was seen in two patients. Six patients had reactions to ester-type and/or amide-type anaesthetics concurrently. Local preparations for perianal conditions were the most common sensitizers. One patient had developed occupational sensitization to procaine with multiple cross-reactions and with concurrent penicillin sensitization from procaine penicillin.

Conclusions.—Dibucaine-containing perianal medicaments are the major source of contact sensitization to topical anaesthetics. Although sensitization to multiple anaesthetics can be seen, cross-reactions are possible. Contact sensitization to lidocaine is not common, and possible cross-reactions should be determined when reactions to lidocaine are seen. Occupational procaine sensitization from veterinary medicaments is a risk among animal workers.

▶ Topical anesthesia is an integral component of dermatological surgery and cosmetic surgery, but is often underused in conditions requiring maintenance such as eczematous dermatosis. When therapy is limited by contact dermatosis to one of the agents in a specific chemical class, there needs to be awareness of sensitization to other combination agents to avoid potential hypersensitivity responses.

N. Bhatia, MD

Surgical Treatment of Lip Cancer: Our Experience With 106 Cases

Salgarelli AC, Sartorelli F, Cangiano A, et al (Modena and Reggio Emilia Univ, Italy; Carlo Poma Hosp, Mantova, Italy)
J Oral Maxillofac Surg 67:840-845, 2009

Purpose.—To report our experience with 106 cases of lip cancer.

Patients and Methods.—We treated 106 patients with stages T1, T2, or T3 lip cancer (76, 22, and 8 cases, respectively). For the 34 T1 lesions up to 1 cm in diameter, we used a V or W excision. In the 42 T1 lesions greater than 1 cm and the 20 T2 lesions, we used the staircase technique. In 2 T2 cases, the carcinoma was located on the labial commissure and was treated with the Fries technique. For the 8 T3 cases, we used the Bernard-Freeman-Fries technique. In 28 patients, a lip shave was performed and tumor was removed. The 7 patients who were N+ at diagnosis underwent modified radical neck dissection and radiotherapy.

Results.—Ten patients died during the follow-up period of 11 to 65 months: 8 of unrelated causes and 2 of new upper aerodigestive tract carcinoma. None of the patients died of their lip cancer.

Conclusions.—Lip cancer is a frequent disease of the oral cavity. Although general agreement has been reached concerning stage T and N+ surgical treatment, unresolved questions remain with regard to N0 treatment. We present our experience and suggestions.

▶ Cutaneous malignancies on the lip are frequently encountered by dermatologists and dermatologic surgeons. Squamous cell carcinoma (SCC) involving the lip has an overall higher risk of metastasis, as compared with most other anatomic sites. Surgery, among other treatment modalities, is probably the most used modality for the treatment of lip cancers. The approach to surgical treatment varies depending on the size and the site of the malignancy. In this article, the author reviewed 106 cases treated with different surgical methods depending on the stage of lip cancer. One drawback or weakness of the article is that the staging system is not stated and the reader is left to look up the staging system. Patients with nodal involvement were treated with unilateral modified radical neck dissection and were given postoperative radiotherapy. The article reviews various surgical techniques such as V or a W resection for smaller tumors, staircase technique for tumors involving up to 60% of the lip, and Bernard-Freeman-Fries technique for tumors involving 60% of the lip. Dermatologic surgeons should be aware of these techniques as they can be used when reconstructing the lip. However, margin control is critical before planning reconstruction, with Mohs micrographic surgery, or careful frozen section control, optimal in assuring clearance of tumor. Otherwise, it is recommended overall that at least 4 mm surgical margins be used for low-risk SCC lesions and 6 mm for more higher risk lesions if routine histologic evaluation is being used with frozen section control.

S. Bhambri, DO
J. Q. Del Rosso, DO

Prevalence of Methicillin-Resistant *Staphylococcus aureus* in the Setting of Dermatologic Surgery
Sica RS, Spencer JM (Nova Southeastern Univ, Largo, FL; Mt. Sinai School of Medicine, NY)
Dermatol Surg 35:420-424, 2009

Background.—The prevalence of methicillin-resistant *Staphylococcus aureus* (MRSA) in the postoperative setting of dermatologic surgery is unknown. Such data could influence the empirical treatment of suspected infections.

Objective.—To examine the period prevalence of MRSA infections in the postoperative setting of dermatologic surgery.

Methods.—We performed chart reviews of 70 patients who had bacterial cultures taken from January 2007 to December 2007. In the 21 postsurgical cases, we analyzed age, risk factors, sites of predilection, method of repair, and pathogen of growth.

Results.—The mean age of the overall study population was 57, with the mean age of postsurgical MRSA-positive cases being 75.5. Of the 21 postsurgical cultures taken, 16 cultures grew pathogen, and two of the 16 (13%) pathogen-positive cultures grew MRSA.

Limitations.—This is a retrospective chart review of a relatively small sample size in one geographic location. Our patient population is known to contain a large number of retirees.

Conclusion.—The increasing prevalence of MRSA skin and soft tissue infections and recommendation to modify empirical antibiotic therapy have been well documented in particular patient populations, but we caution against the empirical use of MRSA-sensitive antibiotics in the postoperative setting of dermatologic surgery. We advocate culturing all infectious lesions upon presentation and reserve empirical use of MRSA-sensitive antibiotics for high-risk patients or locations.

▶ The greatest strength of this study is that it presents dermatology-specific data. This alone makes it of interest to dermatologists. The weaknesses, readily acknowledged by the authors, include the small numbers of patients studied, the low rate of pathogen recovery, and the fact that the study presents data from only a single practice and geographic site. Only 70 patients were screened, and only 16 cultures grew a pathogen. Still the results are reassuring, and should discourage the routine use of methicillin-resistant *Staphylococcus aureus* (MRSA) antibiotics as a prophylactic measure.

It should be noted that the infection rate in routine dermatologic surgery remains quite low (less than 2%). Previous data suggest that the postoperative use of white petrolatum (rather than bacitracin) reduces the risk of contact allergy, is associated with a negligible increase in infection rate, and most infections that do occur are easily treated with an oral cephalosporin. In patients with a higher risk of perioperative infection, reasonable approaches to prophylaxis include a single preoperative dose of antibiotic or the addition of clindamycin to the local anesthetic.

D. M. Elston, MD

The Importance of Reviewing Pathology Specimens Before Mohs Surgery
Butler ST, Youker S, Mandrell J, et al (Saint Louis Univ, MO)
Dermatol Surg 35:407-412, 2009

Background.—The review of outside biopsy slides before performing surgery is the standard of care in many surgical specialties. Previous studies have shown high discrepancy rates between the original and second-opinion diagnoses. The frequency with which this practice changes the diagnosis and management of patients undergoing Mohs surgery is undocumented in the literature. It is standard practice at our institution to review all outside biopsy slides before Mohs surgery.

Objective.—To investigate how often review of outside biopsies by an internal dermatopathologist changes patients' initial referral diagnosis and subsequent management.

Methods & Materials.—This is a retrospective review of all patients referred to Mohs surgery from January 2003 through March 2007. The number of cases in which the diagnosis changed and how this change affected management were recorded.

Results.—Seventy-four of 3,345 (2.2%) cases were identified in which the diagnosis changed after review of the biopsy slides. Management was affected in the majority (61%) of cases. Board-certified dermatopathologists originally read nearly half of the biopsies.

Conclusion.—Review of outside biopsy slides before surgery can change the diagnosis in a large proportion of patients, with a resulting change in management. This quality-assurance practice may improve patient care.

▶ This article emphasizes the importance of reviewing slides before performing Mohs surgery. A total of 3345 cases were reviewed, and 2.2% of cases had their diagnosis changed. The authors suggest having slides reviewed by a dermatopathologist for a second opinion. Having each slide reviewed by a dermatopathologist is a good theoretical concept but has little practical value in majority of Mohs surgical practices. The most common change noted was from one malignant tumor to another, followed by change from malignant to benign. The change in diagnosis can change treatment options and potentially have a cost saving role. Most of the misdiagnosed cases were read by nondermatopathologists (53%) so a second opinion may be more practical in those cases originally read by someone other than a board-certified dermatopathologist. An important point here is that Mohs surgeons should be routinely reviewing his or her own slides before surgery at a minimum.

S. Bhambri, DO

J. Q. Del Rosso, DO

Dose-effect relationships for recurrence of keloid and pterygium after surgery and radiotherapy
Kal HB, Veen RE, Jürgenliemk-Schulz IM (Univ Med Ctr Utrecht, The Netherlands)
Int J Radiat Oncol Biol Phys 74:245-251, 2009

Purpose.—To show radiation dose–response relationships for recurrence of keloid and pterygium after radiotherapy following surgery.

Methods and Materials.—Using PubMed, we performed a retrospective review of articles reporting incidences and/or dose–response relationships for recurrence of keloid and pterygium after radiotherapy following surgery. The irradiation regimens identified were normalized by use of the linear–quadratic model; biologically effective doses (BEDs) were calculated.

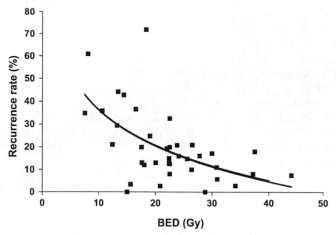

FIGURE 1.—Keloid recurrence after surgery and radiotherapy as a function of the biologically effective dose (BED). The data points were fitted with a logarithmic function. (Reprinted from Kal HB, Veen RE, Jürgenliemk-Schulz IM. Dose-effect relationships for recurrence of keloid and pterygium after surgery and radiotherapy. *Int J Radiat Oncol Biol Phys.* 2009;74:245-251, with permission from Elsevier.)

Results.—For keloid recurrence after radiotherapy following keloid removal, with either teletherapy or brachytherapy, the recurrence rate after having delivered a BED greater than 30 Gy is less than 10%. For pterygium recurrence after bare sclera surgery and ^{90}Sr β-irradiation, a BED of about 30 Gy seems to be sufficient also to reduce the recurrence rate to less than 10%.

Conclusions.—Most of the doses in the radiotherapy schemes used for prevention of keloid recurrence after surgery are too low. In contrast, the doses applied in most regimens to prevent pterygium recurrence are too high. A scheme with a BED of 30 to 40 Gy seems to be sufficient to prevent recurrences of keloid as well as pterygiums.

▶ This article is very useful in treating keloid scars in combination with surgery. The radiation dosage is quite variable in past literature. This reviews multiple studies in the literature for radiation dosage, techniques, and recurrence for both keloids and pterygiums. The data for keloids demonstrate a high recurrence rate of 60% to 80% with low doses of radiation. In keloids treated with the higher biologically effective doses (BED) greater than 30 Gy, the rate is less than 10%.

Table 1 reviews dosage and recurrence rates of 27 reported keloid radiation studies, and Fig 1 shows that doses above 30 Gy have an improved rate of reoccurrence. This article also comments on good safety of radiation of this benign condition. This should be a reference for treating keloids.

L. Cleaver, DO

TABLE 1.—Recurrence Rate, Treatment Scheme, and BED of Radiotherapy for Prevention of Keloids After Surgery

Reference	No. of Keloids	Recurrence Rate (%)	Dosage and Type of Radiation	Overall Treatment Time (d)	BED (Gy)
Cosman and Wolff (2)	76	36	2 × 4 Gy 4 × 2 Gy* X-rays (assumed to be 100 kV)	14	Mean, 10.6*
Edsmyr *et al.* (14)	53	11	1,200 R‡ 45- and 100-kV X-rays	1	30.8
Levy *et al.* (15)	35	12	5 × 3 Gys 6 × 3 Gy 100-kV X-rays	12–14	Mean, 18*
Malaker *et al.* (16)	31	19.4	20 Gy ^{192}Ir LDR	1	22
Ollstein *et al.* (17)	68	21	3 × 5 Gy 100-kV X-rays	<6	26.5
Sallstrom *et al.* (18)	124	8	3 × 600 R‡ 50-kV X-rays	3	37.2
Bertiere *et al.* (19)	38	13	16 Gy LDR	<2	17.6
Lo *et al.* (20)	14	43	8 Gy	5	14.4
	77	13	10 Gy	5	20
	41	10	12 Gy	5	26.4
	17	18	15 Gy 1.5- to 3.5-MeV electrons	5	37.5
	41	61	3 × 2 Gy	3–10	8.05
Doornbos *et al.* (21)	71	29.6	3 × 3 Gy		13.2
	12	25	3 × 4 Gy		19
	27	14.8	3 × 5 Gy 120-kV X-rays		25.6
	20	20	4 × 5 Gy	12	17.5*
Supe *et al.* (22)	44	35	4 × 5 Gy ^{90}Sr beta rays	26	7.5*
Meythiaz *et al.* (23)	54	7.5	10 × 300 R 50-kV X-rays	10	44*
Clavere *et al.* (24)	38	36.8	12–15 Gy LDR	1	16.5
Chaudhry *et al.* (25)	36	2.8	3 × 6 Gy 100-kV X-rays	<6	34.1
Maalej *et al.* (26)	114	13	20.4 Gy ^{192}Ir LDR	1	22.4
Guix *et al.* (27)	147	3.4	4 × 3 Gy HDR	1	15.6
Caccialanza *et al.* (28)	88	5.7	6 × 5 Gy	33	30.9*
	31	16.1	5 × 5 Gy 50-kV X-rays	26	27.8*
Ogawa *et al.* (29)	147	32.7	3 × 5 Gy 4-MeV electrons	4	22.5
Ragoowansi *et al.* (30)	80	16	10 Gy 100-kV X-rays	1	24.1
Malaker *et al.* (31)	47	12.8	4 × 4 Gy ^{60}Co	4	22.4
Narkwong and Thirakhupt (32)	16	12.5	3 × 5 Gy ^{192}Ir	2	22.5
Ogawa *et al.* (33)	28	0	2 × 5 Gy	1	15
	35	22.5	3 × 5 Gy	2	22.5

(Continued)

TABLE 1. (*continued*)

Reference	No. of Keloids	Recurrence Rate (%)	Dosage and Type of Radiation	Overall Treatment Time (d)	BED (Gy)
	58	30	4 × 5 Gy 4-MeV electrons	3	30
Akita *et al.* (34)	38	21.1	6 × 3 Gy, linear accelerator	18	12.4*
Bischof *et al.* (35)	60	15	4 × 4 Gy 6-MeV electrons	4	22.4
Van de Kar *et al.* (36)	32	71.9	3 × 4 Gy/4 × 3 Gy, X ray	3–4	18.3
Veen and Kal (37)	9	44.4	1 × 4 + 2 × 3 Gy	1	13.4
	18†	0	3 × 6 Gy	1	28.8
	38	2.6	1 × 6 + 2 × 4 Gy ¹⁹²Ir HDR	1	20.8
De Lorenzi *et al.* (38)	30	20.9	2 × 7 Gy ¹⁹²Ir HDR	1	23.8
Arneja *et al.* (39)	25	8	3 × 5 Gy ¹⁹²Ir HDR	2	22.5

Editor's Note: please check the original article for the full reference.
Abbreviations: BED = biologically effective dose; LDR = low dose rate; HDR = high dose rate.
*Corrected for overall treatment time.
†Updated results.
‡For BED calculation, we applied 1 R = 0.96 cGy.

More Than 2 Decades of Treating Atypical Fibroxanthoma at Mayo Clinic: What Have We Learned From 91 Patients?
Ang GC, Roenigk RK, Otley CC, et al (Mayo Clinic, Rochester, MN)
Dermatol Surg 35:765-772, 2009

Background.—Atypical fibroxanthoma (AFX) typically occurs on the head and neck of elderly white men. Usually considered a malignancy, it is treated with wide local excision (WLE) or total margin control using Mohs micrographic surgery (MMS).

Objective.—To determine the most appropriate treatment for this tumor based on a review of cases treated at Mayo Clinic.

Methods.—We reviewed the medical records of patients with AFX treated at Mayo Clinic from 1980 to 2004.

Results.—We identified 91 patients with 93 tumors. Treatment information was available for 88 tumors (59 treated with MMS, 23 with WLE, and 6 by other means). There were no recurrences in the patients treated with MMS, with a median follow-up of 4.5 years (range 1.0–16.1 years). Two patients treated with WLE had single recurrences, with a median follow-up of 8.7 years (range 1.5–26.3 years).

Conclusions.—Total microscopic margin control using MMS was the most effective means of treating AFX.

► This retrospective review of 91 patients sought to find the most effective treatment modality for atypical fibroxanthoma (AFX). AFX is more commonly considered a malignancy that is treated with either wide local excision (WLE) or Mohs micrographic surgery (MMS). The authors sought to find the most effective method and concluded that MMS is superior to WLE in the management of AFX. Review of records indicate that no patients experienced recurrence when treated with MMS at median follow-up of 4.5 years compared with 2 patients with local recurrence using WLE. Limitations of this study include those that are inherent to retrospective analysis, including results relying on the accuracy of previous written records, and difficulty controlling bias or confounders (ie, not blinded or randomized). Clinicians should respect the aggressive potential of this tumor, and follow-up visits with careful examination of the surgical site as well as regional lymph nodes should be performed for at minimum 2 years.

S. Bellew, DO

J. Q. Del Rosso, DO

Botulinum Toxin: A Treatment for Compensatory Hyperhidrosis in the Trunk

Kim WO, Kil HK, Yoon KB, et al (Anesthesia and Pain Res Inst, Seoul, South Korea)

Dermatol Surg 35:833-838, 2009

Background.—Severe compensatory hyperhidrosis (CH) in the trunk occurs after sympathectomy in some patients. Limited treatment options for these cases have been proposed, and the overall results have been disappointing, but injection of botulinum toxin-A (BTX-A) is an emerging, reliable treatment method for focal hyperhidrosis.

Objective.—To demonstrate the efficacy, longevity, and safety of BTX-A injection for severe truncal sweating in CH patients who were refractory to conventional treatment.

Methods.—Seventeen patients were injected with 100 to 500 U of BTX-A in the truncal area. After the follow-up period, the Hyperhidrosis Disease Severity Scale (HDSS) for efficacy and the Dermatology Life Quality Index (DLQI) were measured for improvement in patients' quality of life.

Results.—The baseline mean HDSS score ± standard deviation was 3.6 ± 0.5, and the sweating resolved within 5 days. The effect was sustained for 2 to 8 months (4.1 ± 1.5 months) and the baseline DLQI score of 9.4 ± 2.0 fell to 2.8 ± 1.0. No serious side effects or adverse events resulted from the treatment.

Conclusions.—BTX-A injection was a well-tolerated, effective, and safe method for treating severe truncal CH, although the considerable cost and limited duration of the treatment effects were major disadvantages.

▶ The objective of this article was to report a series of patients who developed severe and oftentimes disabling compensatory hyperhidrosis (CH) following T2, T3, or T2 to 3 sympathectomy for the treatment of their palmar hyperhidrosis. In the 17 patients retrospectively reported in this series, the patients had failed traditional therapy for their palmar hyperhidrosis and had their sympathectomies to induce a clinical cure. Instead, they developed what is known as compensatory hyperhidrosis (CH), an often disabling adverse event which has been reported in as many as 89% of patients undergoing this surgical procedure. And upwards of 35% of these patients report serious CH, which affects the quality of their daily living.

Treatment options for CH have been disappointing at best. This group used intradermal injections of botulinum toxin-A as a treatment of CH, and the results were nothing but impressive. They injected from 100 to 500 units of botulinum toxin-A to the most affected areas and followed their patients through telephone follow-ups and found that all of the patients improved significantly. The mean Hyperhidrosis Disease Severity Scale (HDSS) at baseline was 3.6 ± 0.5, and the botulinum affect occurred within 5 days. The decreased sweating effects lasted from 2 to 8 months, with an average of 4.1 ± 1.5 months. All the patients had at least a 2-point drop in the HDSS scale. And the Dermatology Life Quality Index (DLQI) scale saw an improvement from 9.4 ± 2.0 to 2.8 ± 1.0 during the course of the study. No serious adverse events were noted, and the patients were pleased with their results.

This is an important retrospective analysis of what many in dermatology know little about. We routinely inject botulinum toxin-A for the treatment of palmar hyperhidrosis, and we usually do not follow patients who turn to sympathectomy for their treatment course. We must be aware of the associated risks from this procedure and counsel patients that the risk for CH is real, and we must keep in mind that we can treat these patients with botulinum toxin-A, at least improving their quality of life for the duration of the botulinum effect.

M. H. Gold, MD

Cutaneous Surgery in Patients on Warfarin Therapy
Nelms JK, Wooten AI, Heckler F (Allegheny General Hosp, Pittsburgh, PA)
Ann Plast Surg 62:275-277, 2009

Warfarin is a commonly used anticoagulant for patients with prosthetic heart valves, atrial fibrillation, stroke, deep vein thrombosis, or pulmonary emboli to prevent thromboembolic events. There is no clear consensus regarding the perioperative management of warfarin therapy for plastic surgery procedures. Our objective is to evaluate the safety and quantify any increased morbidity in patients on warfarin therapy, undergoing soft tissue surgery.

In a retrospective chart review of prospectively collected data, patients undergoing cutaneous surgery on warfarin therapy from 2000 to 2006 were identified. Perioperative complications were evaluated, including major hemorrhage, incisional bleeding, hematoma, wound or flap complications, graft success, and cosmetic surgical outcome. A total of 26 anticoagulated patients who underwent 56 procedures were included. Intraoperative bleeding was controlled in all cases without difficulty. Minor postoperative bleeding was noted in 1 patient, and this was easily controlled with gentle pressure. All wounds healed without complication, including 2 split thickness skin grafts. The cosmesis of all scars was acceptable.

Anticoagulation with warfarin can be safely continued in patients undergoing minor soft tissue procedures, thereby avoiding the risk of potentially devastating thromboembolic events.

▶ Warfarin is one of the most commonly prescribed anticoagulants for the prevention and treatment of thromboembolism. The perioperative cessation of warfarin can carry an increased risk for thromboembolic events. However, no clear consensus exists in literature regarding perioperative management of patients on warfarin, however, continuation is commonly recommended if the international normalized ratio (INR) value is < 3.5. This is a retrospective cohort study conducted at Allegheny General Hospital in Pittsburg, PA during 2000-2006. Twenty-six patients undergoing 56 procedures were identified, and data concerning the procedure performed, type of lesion, area of excision, method of closure, and complications were noted. All patients were continued on their normal dosage of warfarin from their primary care physician's orders. Prothrombin times and bleeding times were not evaluated preoperatively. Indications for surgery included basal cell carcinoma ($n = 28$), squamous cell carcinoma ($n = 19$), melanoma ($n = 1$), dysplastic nevi ($n = 2$), and keratoacanthomas ($n = 1$). Patients were then evaluated for hemorrhagic complications, immediately postoperatively and after 1 week. One patient (1.8%) experienced a minor complication involving oozing from the surgical site at 1-week postoperatively. Most researchers agree that for minor surgeries an INR < 3.5 is relatively safe and an INR > 5.0 could have substantially devastating risks. One limitation to this study was that there was no control group in which to compare results. To add, prothrombin times and bleeding times of patients were not monitored preoperatively and therefore hemorrhagic complications could not be definitively linked to elevated INRs. To draw more definitive conclusions, larger, prospective, randomized controlled trials will be necessary in the future. In conclusion, this study illustrates that anticoagulation can be continued, especially for minor superficial soft tissue surgery.

G. K. Kim, DO

J. Q. Del Rosso, DO

Low-Dose Methotrexate Enhances Aminolevulinate-Based Photodynamic Therapy in Skin Carcinoma Cells *In Vitro* and *In Vivo*
Anand S, Honari G, Hasan T, et al (Lerner Res Inst, Cleveland Clinic, OH; Harvard Med School, Boston, MA)
Clin Cancer Res 15:3333-3343, 2009

Purpose.—To improve treatment efficacy and tumor cell selectivity of δ-aminolevulinic acid (ALA)-based photodynamic therapy (PDT) via

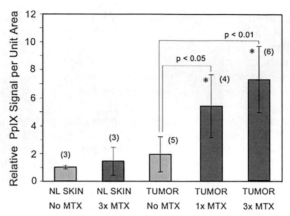

FIGURE 5.—D, quantitation of the PpIX signal from digital confocal images, from tumors preconditioned with no methotrexate, 1 d of methotrexate, or 3 d of methotrexate before harvest. Mean ± SD of images from at least three independent tumors (numbers in parentheses). (Reprinted from Anand S, Honari G, Hasan T, et al. Low-dose methotrexate enhances aminolevulinate-based photodynamic therapy in skin carcinoma cells in vitro and in vivo. *Clin Cancer Res.* 2009;15:3333-3343, with permission from American Association for Cancer Research, Inc.)

pretreatment of cells and tumors with methotrexate to enhance intracellular photosensitizer levels.

Experimental Design.—Skin carcinoma cells, *in vitro* and *in vivo*, served as the model system. Cultured human SCC13 and HEK1 cells, normal keratinocytes, and *in vivo* skin tumor models were preconditioned with methotrexate for 72 h and then incubated with ALA for 4 h. Changes in protoporphyrin IX (PpIX) levels and cell survival after light exposure were assessed.

Results.—Methotrexate preconditioning of monolayer cultures preferentially increased intracellular PpIX levels 2- to 4-fold in carcinoma cells versus normal keratinocytes. Photodynamic killing was synergistically enhanced by the combined therapy compared with PDT alone. Methotrexate enhancement of PpIX levels was achieved over a broad methotrexate concentration range (0.0003-1.0 mg/L; 0.6 nmol/L-2 mmol/L). PpIX enhancement correlated with changes in protein expression of key porphyrin pathway enzymes, ~4-fold increase in coproporphyrinogen oxidase and stable or slightly decreased expression of ferrochelatase. Differentiation markers (E-cadherin, involucrin, and filaggrin) were also selectively induced by methotrexate in carcinoma cells. *In vivo* relevance was established by showing that methotrexate preconditioning enhances PpIX accumulation in three models: (*a*) organotypic cultures of immortalized keratinocytes, (*b*) chemically induced skin tumors in mice; and (*c*) human A431 squamous cell tumors implanted subcutaneously in mice.

Conclusion.—Combination therapy using short-term exposure to low-dose methotrexate followed by ALA-PDT should be further investigated as a new combination modality to enhance efficacy and selectivity of PDT for epithelial carcinomas (Fig 5).

▶ This article might not seem relevant to those of us that use δ-aminolevulinic acid photodynamic therapy (ALA-PDT) for field therapy of actinic keratosis. However, this very interesting article suggests that protoporphyrin IX levels can be induced in precancerous and cancerous cell lines and that there are inducible intracellular systems, which enhance this response when given with a low dose of methotrexate. This has been examined in cell culture lines and in vivo animal models. The doses of methotrexate used are in the order of those used for the treatment of psoriasis and rheumatoid arthritis. It is not practical to use this drug in this manner to treat actinic keratosis, but we commonly use 5-FU in the treatment of actinic keratosis. It appears that 5-FU and methotrexate have a similar mechanism of action and pretreatment with 5-FU might result in a similar enhanced response. In my clinical practice we pretreat all of our ALA-PDT patients with 6 days of topical 5-FU followed by ALA-PDT with a 1.5- to 2-hour incubation period. This has resulted in a substantially better clinical response in the order of that seen with 2 to 3 weeks of topical 5-FU or ALA-PDT with a 14- to 18-hour incubation period. This certainly deserves a well-designed clinical study.

E. A. Tanghetti, MD

The influence of a Eutectic Mixture of Lidocaine and Prilocaine on Minor Surgical Procedures: A Randomized Controlled Double-Blind Trial
Shaikh FM, Naqvi SA, Grace PA (Mid-Western Regional Hosp, Limerick, Ireland; Univ of Limerick, Ireland)
Dermatol Surg 35:948-951, 2009

Background.—A eutectic mixture of lidocaine and prilocaine (EMLA) has been shown to be effective in reducing pain from needle sticks, including those associated with blood sampling and intravenous insertion.

Objective.—To evaluate the effectiveness of EMLA cream applied before needle puncture for local anesthetic administration before minor surgical procedures in this double-blind, randomized, controlled, parallel-group study.

Materials and Methods.—Patients were randomly assigned to receive EMLA or placebo cream (Aqueous) applied under an occlusive dressing. After the procedure, patients were asked to rate the needle prick and procedure pain on a visual analog scale (0 = no pain; 10 = maximum pain).

Results.—A total of 94 minor surgical procedures (49 in EMLA and 45 in control) were performed. The mean needle-stick pain score in the EMLA group was significantly lower than in the control group (2.7 vs. 5.7, $p < .001$, Mann-Whitney U-test). There was also significantly lower procedure pain in the EMLA group than in the control group

(0.83 vs. 1.86, $p = .009$). There were no complications associated with the use of EMLA.

Conclusion.—EMLA effectively reduces the preprocedural needle-stick pain and procedural pain associated with minor surgical procedures.

▶ The objective of this clinical trial was to determine the effectiveness of a combination of lidocaine and prilocaine versus a placebo in reducing the pain associated with infiltration of local anesthesia and from the surgical procedure itself. Patients ($n = 36$ in each group) were randomized to receive either the active combination or a placebo. Ninety-four minor surgical procedures were performed in this clinical trial. There was a statistically significant reduction in local anesthesia pain (2.7 vs 5.7, $P < .001$) and a reduction in procedure pain (0.83 vs 1.86, $P = .009$) during this study.

This is an important article that once again showed the effects of this eutectic mixture of lidocaine and prilocaine. This medication has been available for quite some time, and many are familiar with its benefits. One important ingredient missing from this clinical trial would have been to also break down the eutectic mixture into its component parts having a lidocaine arm and also a prilocaine arm and complete these individual comparisons with the eutectic mixture and to the placebo, and then one would have had all the conclusive evidence of its effects versus placebo and versus its individual components.

This study confirms that a combination of anesthetics works better than placebo.

M. H. Gold, MD

Trichloroacetic Acid Matricectomy in the Treatment of Ingrowing Toenails

Kim S-H, Ko H-C, Oh C-K, et al (Pusan Natl Univ, Busan, Korea)
Dermatol Surg 35:973-979, 2009

Background.—Ingrowing toenails can be treated with conservative therapy or surgery, but frequent relapse can be a problem in conservative therapy and surgical therapy without matricectomy. Thus, permanent nail ablation by partial matricectomy is now accepted as the treatment of choice.

Objective.—To evaluate the efficacy and safety of trichloroacetic acid (TCA) matricectomy in the treatment of ingrowing nail.

Materials and Methods.—Forty ingrowing toenail edges in 25 patients were enrolled. TCA matricectomy with 100% trichloroacetic acid after partial nail avulsion was performed. For a few weeks after surgery, postoperative complications such as pain, discharge, and infection were assessed. After a mean follow-up period of 22.9 months, recurrence rate and cosmetic outcomes were investigated to evaluate the effects of the surgery.

Results.—The wounds almost always healed within 2 weeks without prolonged exudative discharge. Pain was mild and transient. A case of secondary infection occurred. Recurrence was found in only two nails of one patient, and the success rate was 95%, with good cosmetic results.

Conclusion.—TCA matricectomy showed a low recurrence rate with minimal side effects and was easy to perform in outpatient clinic. Therefore, it may be a good alternative treatment of ingrowing toenails.

▶ Ingrowing toenail is a common nail complaint that causes erythema and tenderness of the lateral nail fold. Surgical management is considered when the symptoms progress to involve drainage, infection, and nail fold hypertrophy. While nonselective surgical techniques such as nail avulsion and cryotherapy are generally tolerated well by patients, they are associated with an increased risk of recurrence. Selective matricectomy and chemical matricectomy have a much lesser risk of recurrence, but have significant adverse effects such as prolonged healing time and poor cosmetic outcome. Kim et al proposed a previously unreported technique using trichloroacetic acid (TCA) to destroy the nail matrix after partial nail avulsion, with the intention to prevent recurrence of the problem while minimizing healing time and maximizing cosmetic outcome. The authors found this technique to have only a 5% recurrence rate, which was noted to be equivalent to published recurrence rates of phenol and sodium hydroxide based therapies. The apparent benefit of the TCA technique over other chemicals is a reduced severity and duration of postoperative pain, drainage, and infection. Furthermore no adverse cosmetic outcomes were observed in this trial. A larger study with direct comparison of this technique with other chemical and nonselective surgical methods may clarify whether the TCA technique is truly superior to other therapies, or simply an alternate option.

J. Moore, MD

P. Rich, MD

Patient satisfaction with receiving skin cancer diagnosis by letter: comparison with face-to-face consultation
Karri V, Bragg TWH, Jones A, et al (St George's Hosp, Tooting, UK; Kingston Hosp, Kingston-upon-Thames, UK)
J Plast Reconstr Aesthetic Surg 62:1059-1062, 2009

Providing patients with clear and concise information is central to modern medical practice. Patients diagnosed with skin cancer are traditionally told their result by face-to-face consultation in the outpatient clinic. Previous studies have shown poor patient satisfaction with the traditional outpatient consultation.

The skin oncology service at Kingston Hospital uses two different methods to inform selected patients of their skin cancer diagnosis. Those diagnosed with thin melanoma (MM) or squamous cell carcinoma (<2 cm) (SCC) are informed by letter (with an accompanying information leaflet), or seen in outpatient clinic for a face-to-face consultation. However, it is unclear which of these methods patients prefer.

We performed a retrospective postal questionnaire survey to elicit the views of patients that had been informed of their skin cancer by these two methods. Patients had been diagnosed with either MM or SCC between February 2005 and March 2006. Demographic details and patient satisfaction using five-point Likert scales were determined.

Of the eligible 118 patients, 90 (76%) completed the questionnaire. Questionnaires from five respondents were incorrectly completed and excluded from further analysis. Of the final 85 patients, 41 (48%) were told their diagnosis via face-to-face consultation (clinic) and 44 (52%) by letter. The demographic profile of both groups was similar ($P > 0.05$).

Patients of both groups had a similar expectation of being told a skin cancer diagnosis ($P > 0.05$). A high level of satisfaction was expressed for both methods of communication, with no difference between the groups ($P > 0.05$).

In the letter group, patients placed more value on convenience than preference to seeing a doctor ($P < 0.001$). The option of contacting a support nurse was also cited as a reassuring feature.

The findings of this study suggest disclosure of skin cancer diagnosis by letter has high satisfaction, for selected patients. Using this method of communication may ultimately lessen the burden on outpatient service.

▶ Traditionally, patients with skin cancer are often told their results by face-to-face consultation, allowing for information to be conveyed and questions to be answered in the clinic. However, previous studies have shown that retention of new information is limited after verbal consultation alone. This is a retrospective study done by the oncology department at Kingston hospital using 2 different methods to inform selected patients of their skin cancer diagnosis with thin melanoma (size not verified) or squamous cell carcinoma (< 2 cm) informed by letter or seen in the outpatient clinic. Of the 118 patients, 90 patients (76%) completed the questionnaires. Forty-one patients (52%) were told their diagnosis by face-to-face consultation, and 44 (52%) were told by letter. Eighty percent of the patients stated that they preferred the convenience of a letter. In addition to satisfaction, previous history of skin cancer, contact with support nurse, and demographic details were also included in the study. Feedback from patients suggests receiving their diagnosis by letter has a number of perceived benefits. Comparison of the 2 groups showed there was no statistically significant differences ($P > .05$) in regard to satisfaction. However, there was a statistical significance ($P < .001$) with convenience in the group with patients informed by letter compared with face-to-face contact. The authors suggest that a letter can act as an aide-mémoire, allowing patients to comprehend information at their own pace, read to the family, and assist in communication. It is well recognized that patients can have poor recall following outpatient consultation. Anxiety, time constraints, and poor communication are all contributing factors. It is the belief of the authors that any written information should be well presented, concise, and jargon free. One weakness of this study was that not all patients replied to the questionnaires, and it is unknown whether the patients followed up after their diagnosis of skin cancer or simply chose not to reply. The downside to diagnosis by letter is that the clinician does not know for sure if patients received their diagnosis, if they understand the information, and if they will follow-up for treatment. When a call is made, documentation of who was called and when they were called are much more definitive. With a letter, it is unknown if the patients received their diagnosis until a follow-up appointment if no call is placed. Due to both medical and legal issues, a follow-up call should always be done if patients do not return, especially in cases of melanoma, regardless of depth of invasion, which is an issue not discussed in this article. Letters should also emphasize the importance of treatment and follow-up to enhance patient compliance. In addition, a sample letter would have also been useful to assess which elements were included in the study and how much information the authors felt was just enough information for the patient.

G. K. Kim, DO

J. Q. Del Rosso, DO

Ultrasound Assessment of Deep Tissue Injury in Pressure Ulcers: Possible Prediction of Pressure Ulcer Progression
Aoi N, Yoshimura K, Kadono T, et al (Univ of Tokyo Graduate School of Medicine, Japan)
Plast Reconstr Surg 124:540-550, 2009

Background.—The concept of deep tissue injury under intact skin helps us understand the pathogenesis of pressure ulcers, but the best method for detecting and evaluating deep tissue injury remains to be established.

Methods.—Intermediate-frequency (10-MHz) ultrasonography was performed to evaluate deep tissue injury. The authors analyzed 12 patients (nine male patients and three female patients aged 16 to 92 years) who showed deep tissue injury–related abnormal findings on ultrasonography at the first examination and were followed up until the pressure ulcer reached a final stage.

Results.—The stage of ulcer worsened in six of 12 cases compared with baseline, and healed in the remaining six patients. The authors recognized four types of abnormal signs unique to deep tissue damage in ultrasonography: unclear layered structure, hypoechoic lesion, discontinuous fascia, and heterogeneous hypoechoic area. Unclear layered structure, hypoechoic lesion, discontinuous fascia, and heterogeneous hypoechoic area were detected at the first examination in 12, 10, seven, and five patients, respectively. Unclear layered structure and hypoechoic lesion were more commonly seen in pressure ulcers in deep tissue injury than the other features, but the follow-up study suggested that discontinuous fascia and heterogeneous hypoechoic area are more reliable predictors of future progression of pressure ulcers.

Conclusions.—The use of intermediate-frequency ultrasound reliably identified deep tissue injury and was believed to contribute to prevention and treatment of pressure-related ulcers. The results suggest that specific ultrasonographic characteristics may predict which pressure ulcers will progress.

▶ There is growing evidence suggesting that most pressure ulcers are the result of deep tissue injury supporting the "bottom-up theory." In addition, there may be both internal and external factors contributing to the pathogenesis of deep tissue ulcers. The importance of diagnosing deep tissue injury in the early stages and evaluating the prognosis of ulcers is well recognized. This is a survey of 12 patients (ages 16-92 years) using intermediate-frequency (10 MHz) ultrasonography to evaluate deep tissue injury and following them to their final stages. Ultrasonography (US) is a safe, economical, noninvasive method that can be easily and repeatedly performed at bedside. All patients were seen at the University of Tokyo Hospital between the years of 2006-2007. There were 4 findings unique to deep tissue damage that were recognized: unclear layered structure, hypoechoic lesions, discontinuous fascia, and heterogeneous hypoechoic area. Unclear layered structure and hypoechoic lesions were observed in 12 and 10 patients respectively. These features were more common in deep tissue pressure ulcers but were not reliable predictors of progression of ulcers. Discontinuous fascia was detected in 7 cases. Six of the 7 primary discontinuous fascia progressed to stage IV, making it a reliable predictor of advancement of the ulcers. Heterogeneous hypoechoic areas were detected in 5 patients with all 5 patients progressive to stage IV. Discontinuous fascia may be from inflammatory changes, ischemia, or anatomical disruption of the fascia and may be nonspecific. Limitations of this study included small sample size and nonrandomized patients with no controls provided. Another limitation to the study was that 1 of 3 investigators reading the US was nonblinded, which could have affected the data. Future limitations to the study include variations in US results depending who reads and evaluates the images. In conclusion, the authors emphasize the importance of early identification of deep tissue injury and the use of intermediate-frequency ultrasonography with prediction of ulcer progression.

G. K. Kim, DO
J. Q. Del Rosso, DO

Comparison of superior eyelid incision and directly over the lesion incision to brow dermoid cyst excision
Köse R, Okur MI (Harran Univ Hosp, Sanliurfa, Turkey; Firat Univ Hosp, Elazig, Turkey)
Eur J Plast Surg 32:83-85, 2009

A superior eyelid incision and a directly over the lesion incision to access lateral brow dermoid cysts were compared in terms of cosmetic results, operating time, complication, recurrence, and cyst rupture. From February 2004 to March 2008, 27 patients underwent excision of lateral brow dermoid cyst lesions. Dermoid cyst excision was performed using a directly over the lesion incision in 14 patients and 13 patients via a superior eyelid incision. Both incision scars were very good in adult patients, but the aesthetic results of the superior eyelid incision were judged to be better in children. The parents were satisfied in both groups. We suggest the using of the upper eyelid crease incision in children.

▶ Dermoid cysts are common in the periorbital location. The authors looked at incisions placed over the lesion, versus incisions placed on the superior eyelid, and compared various factors, such as cosmetic result, operating time, complications, recurrence, and cyst rupture. It is an interesting concept as both options are used by surgeons treating cysts on a daily basis. The study size was small with 27 patients. The satisfaction score in both groups were comparable and with no significant differences observed. Operating time was similar in both groups, 20 minutes in directly over the lesion incision and 24 minutes in superior eyelid incision. It was noted that directly over the lesion incisions produce a scar that is more prominent in childhood, and that scars are better or less prominent when an excision was performed via an upper eyelid crease incision.

S. Bhambri, DO

J. Q. Del Rosso, DO

Facial skin sensibility in a young healthy chinese population
Hung J, Samman N (Univ of Hong Kong)
Oral Surg Oral Med Oral Pathol Oral Radiol Endod 107:776-781, 2009

Objective.—To quantify normal neurosensory facial sensibility in a young healthy Chinese population for use as a reference when evaluating postoperative nerve damage.

Study Design.—One hundred consecutive eligible normal young Chinese individuals were included. Each subject underwent objective neurosensory testing (static light touch, 2-point static, and pain detection thresholds) at 8 facial sites within the distribution of the trigeminal nerve. Data were calculated into means and standard deviations, and paired t tests were used to compare values between the left and right sides and quadrants; unpaired t test was used to compare the values between genders. A P value of $\leq.05$ was considered to be significant.

Results.—The chin region was least sensitive to light touch detection, and the normal thresholds ranged from 1.72 to 1.80. The infraorbital areas were least sensitive for 2-point discrimination, and the normal values for this modality ranged from 7.04 mm to 11.87 mm. Infraorbital areas were also most resistant to pain, and normal values ranged from 13.17 g to 20.30 g. There was no statistically significant difference between facial sides or quadrants. Male subjects were found to have a higher pain detection threshold, especially in the chin and the right infraorbital areas.

Conclusion.—Reference values for normal facial sensibility in the form of objective neurosensory testing scores have been documented for a healthy Chinese population. These results provide baseline data for future surgical studies in this and similar populations.

▶ Nerve dysfunction or degree of severity of nerve damage is always a concern when performing cutaneous surgical procedures. As the authors state, postsurgical sequelae are usually sensory in nature, which may often be concerning to patients. This article documents normal facial sensibilities in the Chinese population, using neurosensory testing in order to provide baseline data for facial sensations. Neurosensory testing measures subtle changes in the function of peripheral nerves—the nerves that transmit information from the brain and the spinal cord to the rest of the body. These results may be beneficial when evaluating Chinese or other patients of Asian decent; however, the same may not be applicable to other ethnicities. The main points of the article: chin is least sensitive to light touch, infraorbital areas are least sensitive to 2-point discrimination, and men have higher pain detection threshold.

S. Bellew, DO

J. Q. Del Rosso, DO

Nerve blocks enable adequate pain relief during topical photodynamic therapy of field cancerization on the forehead and scalp

Halldin CB, Paoli J, Sandberg C, et al (Göteborg Univ, Sweden)

Br J Dermatol 160:795-800, 2009

Background.—Topical photodynamic therapy (PDT) is an effective method when treating extensive areas of sun-damaged skin with multiple actinic keratoses (AKs) (field cancerization) on areas such as the forehead and scalp, and offers excellent cosmetic outcome. The major side-effect of PDT is the pain experienced during treatment.

Objectives.—To investigate whether nerve blocks could provide adequate pain relief during PDT of AKs on the forehead and scalp.

Methods.—Ten men with symmetrically distributed and extensive AKs on the forehead and scalp were included in the study. Prior to PDT one side of the forehead and scalp was anaesthetized by nerve blocks while the other side served as control.

Results.—The mean visual analogue scale (VAS) score on the anaesthetized side was 1 compared with 6·4 on the nonanaesthetized side during PDT. This difference was significant ($P < 0·0001$), implying that nerve blocks reduce VAS scores during PDT.

Conclusions.—The results of the study support the use of nerve blocks as pain relief during PDT of field cancerization on the forehead and scalp, although individual considerations must be taken into account to find the most adequate pain-relieving method for each patient.

▶ Halldin et al performed a small ($N = 10$) but informative study to support the use of nerve blocks in patients undergoing photodynamic therapy (PDT) of actinic keratosis (AK) on the scalp and forehead. Previous methods of pain relief have proven largely ineffective. The strength of the study was in the finding that when providing nerve blocks to the greater and lesser occipital nerves in combination with frontal nerve blocks to the supraorbital and supratrochlear nerves, there was a statistically significant decrease in the pain experienced by patients versus the nonanesthetized portion of the scalp and forehead. This implies that nerve blocks are effective in reducing pain in PDT treatment for AK. In addition, it was also found that patients had reduced pain at 6 to 8 hours after treatment. A limitation is the small study population. Ten patients is a small number and may not entirely account for enough variability in the pain tolerance of all patients. Moreover, although no adverse effects were reported in this study (such as hematomas, paresis, and systemic toxicity), further investigation in a larger patient population is warranted. Further, all patients in the study had methyl aminolevulinate (MAL) applied as a photosensitizer instead of aminolevulinic acid (ALA). The article noted previous studies finding MAL-PDT to be less painful than ALA-PDT. Thus, would the same results have been obtained in patients using ALA-PDT as a photosensitizer? Ultimately, the article is persuasive on a pilot basis, and it provides an effective alternative method for increasing patient comfort in PDT therapy for AK.

B. D. Michaels, DO
J. Q. Del Rosso, DO

19 Miscellaneous Topics in Cosmetic and Laser Surgery

Treatment of Angiokeratoma of Fordyce with Long-Pulse Neodymium-Doped Yttrium Aluminium Garnet Laser

Özdemir M, Baysal I, Engin B, et al (Selçuk Univ, Konya, Turkey; et al)

Dermatol Surg 35:92-97, 2009

Background.—Angiokeratomas are typically asymptomatic, blue-to-red papules with a scaly surface located on the scrotum, shaft of penis, labia majora, inner thigh, or lower abdomen. The treatment of angiokeratomas may be necessary if they bleed and lead to patient anxiety.

Objective.—To determine the safety and effectiveness of long-pulse 1,064 neodymium-doped yttrium aluminium garnet (Nd:YAG) laser for the treatment of angiokeratomas of Fordyce.

Materials and Methods.—Ten consecutive patients with angiokeratoma of Fordyce were treated with long-pulse Nd:YAG laser in two to six sessions. The three authors independently assessed improvement of the lesion based on digital photographs taken before the treatment and 2 months after the end of the treatment.

Results.—Significant (> 75%, < 100%) and moderate (> 50%, < 75%) improvement was seen in six and two patients, respectively. Complete improvement was achieved in one patient. Transient swelling, purpura, bleeding, and some pain in the treated area were noted in all patients as short-term side effects. There were no permanent side effects.

Conclusion.—The long-pulse Nd:YAG laser is a highly effective and safe treatment for angiokeratoma of Fordyce.

▶ The long-pulsed neodynium-doped yttrium aluminum garnet (Nd:YAG) laser can be used effectively, as described in this study, to treat angiokeratomas in the groin area. A major limitation of this device is the occurrence of scarring, which in the groin area may not be as significant an issue. However, when using this device in other more visible areas, the unwanted thermal damage and scarring that can be seen with this device limits its cosmetic use.

E. A. Tanghetti, MD

Pulsed dye laser vs. intense pulsed light for port-wine stains: a randomized side-by-side trial with blinded response evaluation

Faurschou A, Togsverd-Bo K, Zachariae C, et al (Univ of Copenhagen, Denmark)
Br J Dermatol 160:359-364, 2009

Background.—Pulsed dye lasers (PDLs) are considered the treatment of choice for port-wine stains (PWS). Studies have suggested broadband intense pulsed light (IPL) to be efficient as well. So far, no studies have directly compared the PDL with IPL in a randomized clinical trial.

Objectives.—To compare efficacy and adverse events of PDL and IPL in an intraindividual randomized clinical trial.

Methods.—Twenty patients with PWS (face, trunk, extremities; pink, red and purple colours; skin types I–III) received one side-by-side treatment with PDL (V-beam Perfecta, 595 nm, 0·45–1·5 ms; Candela Laser Corporation, Wayland, MA, U.S.A.) and IPL (StarLux, Lux G prototype handpiece, 500–670 and 870–1400 nm, 5–10 ms; Palomar Medical Technologies, Burlington, MA, U.S.A.). Settings depended on the preoperative lesional colour. Treatment outcome was evaluated by blinded, clinical evaluations and by skin reflectance measurements.

Results.—Both PDL and IPL lightened PWS. Median clinical improvements were significantly better for PDL (65%) than IPL (30%) (P = 0·0004). A higher proportion of patients obtained good or excellent clearance rates with the PDL (75%) compared with IPL (30%) (P = 0·0104). Skin reflectance also documented better results after PDL (33% lightening) than IPL (12% lightening) (P = 0·002). Eighteen of 20 patients preferred to receive continued treatments with PDL (P = 0·0004). No adverse events were observed with PDL or IPL.

Conclusions.—Both the specific PDL and IPL types of equipment used in this study lightened PWS and both were safe with no adverse events. However, the PDL conveyed the advantages of better efficacy and higher patient preference.

▶ This study effectively compares the clinical response of one treatment with a pulsed dye laser (PDL) and intense pulsed light (IPL) for patients with port-wine stains (PWS). The results illustrate a significant improvement with the PDL versus the IPL after one treatment as evaluated by a blinded third party evaluation, objective skin reflectance measurements, and patient self-evaluation.

The authors of this study astutely limited interindividual variation and experimental bias by using a side by side intraindividual comparison of PDL and IPL treatments, using both third party, objective, and patient evaluation of the treatment results. Additionally, the study incorporated the manufacturer-specified settings to treat patients accordingly, and lastly, used one operator to deliver all the laser treatments.

However, there are still several limitations to this study, the first being that the patients were only treated once, which is in contrast to the clinical setting where patients are usually treated several times. PDL has been shown to have the greatest effect in the first 5 treatments, therefore, it is possible that after 5 treatments the results of the IPL and PDL may be equivalent. In other words, there is a possibility that after 5 treatments the IPL could have achieved similar results to the PDL. Further research needs to be done with a larger group of patients. In addition, there needs to be a comparison of PDL and IPL results in PWS patients after more than one treatment.

However, given the results of this study it seems reasonable for physicians to consider PDL as first line for the treatment of PWS given that it produces the maximal result after one treatment, and patients may be limited in the number of therapeutic sessions they can complete.

J. Levin, DO

J. Q. Del Rosso, DO

Intense Pulsed Light for Skin Rejuvenation, Hair Removal, and Vascular Lesions: A Patient Satisfaction Study and Review of the Literature
Fodor L, Carmi N, Fodor A, et al (Technion-Israel Inst of Technology, Haifa; Tel Hai Academic College, Upper Galilee, Israel)
Ann Plast Surg 62:345-349, 2009

There are very few studies in the English literature that evaluate the patient satisfaction after treatment using intense pulsed light (IPL) and there is no reported study comparing the results of the three major IPL applications: rejuvenation, hair removal, and treatment of small vascular lesions. This study was designed to compare results after IPL treatment for skin rejuvenation, hair removal, and vascular lesions. Three groups of 30 consecutive patients having skin rejuvenation, hair removal, and small vascular lesions were selected and treated with the same IPL system. The evaluation was performed 1 year after the last treatment for the following parameters: age, sex, skin type, satisfaction, willingness to continue the treatment, willingness to recommend the treatment, and complications. Most of the minor complications occurred in the rejuvenation group (86.6%). No complications were recorded for 67% of patients having hair removal and for 75% having vascular lesion treatment. There was no significant difference in the level of satisfaction between the 3 groups (Kruskal Wallis test; $P = 0.257$). No difference regarding satisfaction was recorded in this study, but complications were more frequently encountered after rejuvenation. The findings of this study are useful when discussing IPL treatments with patients considering IPL procedures.

▶ This article provides insight into a relatively focused topic involving cosmetic procedures. The purpose of the article was to compare such concepts as patient complications, patient satisfaction, willingness to continue therapy, and willingness to recommend treatment with intense pulsed light (IPL) among 3 specific treatment areas: skin rejuvenation, hair removal, and leg veins. In comparing these 3 particular areas, the article achieved its objective. Ultimately, there was little statistical difference between patient satisfaction, and patient willingness to continue or recommend treatment involving use of IPL for skin rejuvenation, hair removal, and small vascular lesions. The article also points out that there was a relatively low major complication rate among these treatment areas, and despite a higher minor complication rate among IPL for skin rejuvenation, the satisfaction level was comparable with IPL for these 3 areas. The article also provides useful clinical suggestions for improvement in patient satisfaction involving these treatment areas and comparing the results of this study with other IPL patient satisfaction studies. Although not necessarily an objective of the study, there was little numerical data provided on the willingness of patients to continue with IPL treatment or the recommendation of the treatment, noting mainly that there was little significant difference in these factors among the 3 treatment areas. Information as to the percentage of patients who would actually continue with IPL therapy or would recommend IPL therapy as it related to this study would have provided further substantative perspective into the effectiveness of IPL treatment. In the end, however, the article is useful to the practicing cosmetic clinician in providing further detailed information on the application of IPL treatments and providing useful information to patients considering IPL therapy.

B. D. Michaels, DO

J. Q. Del Rosso, DO

Comparative Efficacy of Nonpurpuragenic Pulsed Dye Laser and Intense Pulsed Light for Erythematotelangiectatic Rosacea
Neuhaus IM, Zane LT, Tope WD (Univ of California at San Francisco)
Dermatol Surg 35:920-928, 2009

Background.—Erythematotelangiectatic (ET) rosacea is commonly treated with a variety of laser and light-based systems. Although many have been used successfully, there are a limited number of comparative efficacy studies.

Objective.—To compare nonpurpuragenic pulsed dye laser (PDL) with intense pulsed light (IPL) treatment in the ability to reduce erythema, telangiectasia, and symptoms in patients with moderate facial ET rosacea.

Methods.—Twenty-nine patients were enrolled in a randomized, controlled, single-blind, split-face trial with nonpurpuragenic treatment with PDL and IPL and untreated control. Three monthly treatment sessions were performed with initial PDL settings of 10-mm spot size, 7 J/cm², 6-ms pulse duration and cryogen cooling, and initial IPL settings of 560-nm filter, a pulse train of 2.4 and 6.0 ms in duration separated by a 15-ms delay, and a starting fluence of 25 J/cm². Evaluation measures included spectrophotometric erythema scores, blinded investigator grading, and patient assessment of severity and associated symptoms.

Results.—PDL and IPL resulted in significant reduction in cutaneous erythema, telangiectasia, and patientreported associated symptoms. No significant difference was noted between PDL and IPL treatment.

Conclusion.—A series of nonpurpuragenic PDL and IPL treatments in ET rosacea was performed with similar efficacy and safety, and both modalities seem to be reasonable choices for the treatment of ET rosacea.

▶ This article provides evidence supporting laser treatment for erythematote-langiectatic rosacea (ETR) comparing the performance of both nonpurpuragenic pulsed dye laser (PDL) and intense pulse light (IPL) in the reduction of erythema, telangiectasia, and associated symptoms. Although the study was limited in the enrolled number of patients (30 patients enrolled, 29 completed the study), there is ultimately no statistical significance in the outcomes of patients with ETR treated with either PDL or IPL. The only question remaining is whether the outcomes can be projected to all dermatologists using PDL and IPL, as the results with either PDL or IPL are likely operator dependent. In other words, would a physician who is better adapted to using PDL rather than IPL obtain the same results for treating ETR if IPL was used? Altogether, the information gleaned from this well-designed study is clinically relevant.

B. D. Michaels, DO

J. Q. Del Rosso, DO

Increased Insulin Sensitivity by Metformin Enhances Intense-Pulsed-Light-Assisted Hair Removal in Patients with Polycystic Ovary Syndrome
Rezvanian H, Adibi N, Siavash M, et al (Isfahan Endocrine and Metabolism Res Ctr, Iran; Isfahan Univ of Med Sciences, Iran; et al)
Dermatology 218:231-236, 2009

Background.—Polycystic ovary syndrome (PCOS) is an insulin-resistant state with hirsutism as a common manifestation.

Objective.—We hypothesized that treatment with metformin would improve the cosmetic effects of intense pulsed light (IPL) therapy for hair removal in PCOS patients.

Methods.—In a prospective randomized controlled trial, 70 PCOS patients randomly received metformin (1,500 mg daily) + IPL therapy or IPL therapy alone for 5 IPL sessions during a 6-month period, followed by an additional 6 months of observation. Hirsutism score, homeostasis model assessment for insulin resistance (HOMA-IR), free androgen index (FAI) and patient satisfaction were evaluated at every visit.

Results.—Fifty-two patients finished the study. Hirsutism was significantly better controlled in the metformin group (p = 0.009). Patient satisfaction was significantly better in the metformin group at the end of the observation period (52.9 vs. 34.1%, p = 0.019). HOMA-IR and FAI scores improved after metformin + IPL treatment (p < 0.05).

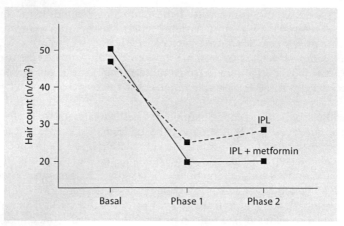

FIGURE 1.—Mean hair count in the two groups during the study. (Courtesy of Rezvanian H, Adibi N, Siavash M, et al. Increased insulin sensitivity by metformin enhances intense-pulsed-light- assisted hair removal in patients with polycystic ovary syndrome. *Dermatology.* 2009;218:231-236.)

Conclusion.—Adding metformin to IPL in women with PCOS results in a significant improvement in insulin sensitivity and hirsutism (Fig 1).

▶ This well-done study addresses adjunctive therapy for patients who have polycystic ovary syndrome and hirsutism. Laser and light-based hair removal is an effective treatment for unwanted hair; however, in some patients with an underlying hormonal abnormality, the problem is more difficult to treat and often persists. This study uses metformin as an adjunct to light-based hair removal with success. The exact mechanism of action of metformin in this situation is not entirely clear, but it does appear to offer efficacy in this population of patients.

E. A. Tanghetti, MD

Comparison of a 585-nm pulsed dye laser and a 1064-nm Nd:YAG laser for the treatment of acne scars: A randomized split-face clinical study
Lee DH, Choi YS, Min SU, et al (Seoul Natl Univ College of Medicine, Korea)
J Am Acad Dermatol 60:801-807, 2009

Background.—No studies have reported a comparison of the pulsed dye laser (PDL) and the 1064-nm long-pulsed neodymium:yttrium-aluminum-garnet (Nd:YAG) laser treatment of acne scars in the same patient.

Objective.—To compare the efficacies of these two lasers in the treatment of acne scars.

Methods.—Eighteen patients received 4 sessions of PDL or Nd:YAG laser at 2-week intervals in a randomized split-face manner.

Results.—Both lasers induced notable and comparable improvement in the appearance of acne scars, particularly superficial scars, with significant reductions in the scores associated with the clinical evaluation scale for acne scarring (ECCA). Histologic evaluations revealed significant increases in collagen production and deposition following both lasers. Patient satisfaction scores concurred with these improvements. Ice-pick scars and boxcar scars tended to respond better to PDL and Nd:YAG lasers, respectively.

Limitations.—The number of subjects was small.

Conclusions.—Both lasers are effective modalities for the treatment of acne scars. Optimal outcomes might be achieved considering scar types and responses to a specific laser.

▶ This article describes treatment of 18 patients with scarring acne using the neodymium:yttrium-aluminum-garnet (Nd:YAG) or pulsed dye laser (PDL). Four sessions of split-face treatment separated at 2-week intervals were performed. Graders were blinded and scars were judged using a clinical scale. There was no untreated control group. The lack of a control is a common problem with laser studies, which is a shame, because it makes the data hard to interpret.

One pair of photographs is presented. What impressed me more than the changes in scarring was the improvement in redness and inflammatory acne as a result of laser treatment.

I have reservations about clinical grading of acne scars, which are often little things whose color and lighting can change their apparent severity. The authors made a good effort, but I'd find this study much more persuasive if image analysis had been used to judge scar response. It isn't too late for that as high quality digitized photographs were taken.

G. Webster, MD

Skin Rejuvenation with 1,064-nm Q-switched Nd:YAG laser in Asian Patients

Lee M-C, Hu S, Chen M-C, et al (Chang Gung Memorial Hosp, Taipei and Taoyan, Taiwan; Chang Gung Univ, Taiwan)
Dermatol Surg 35:929-932, 2009

Background.—In recent years, using the 1,064-nm Q-switched neodymium-doped yttrium aluminium garnet (Nd:YAG) laser (QSNYL) with or without exogenous topical carbon solution application for facial skin rejuvenation has become popular in Southeast Asia, but there has not been any published clinical report discussing the rejuvenation effect of QSNYL for Asian patients.

Objective.—To evaluate the efficacy of QSNYL in improvement of pore size, sebaceous secretion, skin texture, and skin tone of Asian patients.

We also observed whether there is any enhancement of application of topical carbon solution before the therapy.

Methods.—Twenty-four female patients completed four sessions of treatments at 4-week intervals. The assessment was evaluated by the patients, two independent physicians, and Canfield VISIA Complexion Analysis. In addition, we conducted a split-face study such that, in each case, topical carbon solution was applied to the right side of the face before the laser treatment.

Results.—All evaluations showed significant improvement in rejuvenation effect. There was no difference in improvement in skin texture even after the application of topical carbon solution in our split-face study.

Conclusion.—The QSNYL is a safe and effective rejuvenation modality in Asian patients. Topical carbon solution application did not enhance laser efficacy.

▶ Nonablative laser skin resurfacing has increased in popularity due to fewer side effects experienced by the patient, with the convenience of minimal recovery time. Investigators used the MedLite C6TM Q-switched neodymium-doped yttrium aluminum garnet (Nd:YAG) laser (QSNYL) to examine its efficacy in skin rejuvenation. In addition, the application of topical carbon solution, reportedly thought to enhance the effects of QSNYL, was also studied using split-face evaluations. Authors indicate positive results using QSNYL as evidenced by subjective and objective reports of decrease in pore size, less sebum secretion, and reduction in uneven skin pigmentation. Results also indicate no difference in the additional use of topical carbon; however, the small sample size limits the broad interpretation of this finding. There are additional limitations to this study, including short duration for treatment and follow-up. Also, results may not be generalized to other ethnicities or population groups as subjects were limited to Asian patients in Taiwan. Future histological evaluation would be beneficial to support investigative findings of this study.

S. Bellew, DO

J. Q. Del Rosso, DO

Treatment of Melasma Using Variable Square Pulse Er: Yag Laser Resurfacing
Wanitphakdeedecha R, Manuskiatti W, Siriphukpong S, et al (Mahidol Univ, Bangkok, Thailand)
Dermatol Surg 35:475-482, 2009

Background.—Treatment of melasma remains a challenge. Laser treatments show limited efficacy, with a high rate of recurrence and side effects. Recently, variable-pulsed erbium:yttrium aluminum garnet (Er:YAG) lasers have shown favorable results in skin resurfacing, with minimal downtime and adverse effects.

Objective.—To determine the efficacy and side effects of variable square pulsed (VSP) Er:YAG laser resurfacing for treatment of epidermal type melasma.

Methods.—Twenty Thai women with epidermal-type melasma were treated with two passes of VSP Er:YAG laser resurfacing using a 7-mm spot size, pulse duration of 300 µs, and a fluence of 0.4 J/cm^2. Two treatments were given 1 month apart. Visual analog scale (VAS), Melasma Area and Severity Index (MASI) score and melanin index (MI) were measured at baseline and 1, 2, and 4 months after treatment.

Results.—There was a significant improvement in VAS from baseline at 1-, 2-, and 4-month follow-up visits ($p < .001$). Significant improvement in MASI score at the 2-month visit from baseline ($p = .004$) was also observed. The average MI measured using melanin reflectance spectrometry measurements corresponded to MASI score rating.

Conclusions.—VSP Er:YAG laser resurfacing effectively but temporarily improved epidermal-type melasma. Recurrence was observed after the treatment was discontinued.

▶ The variable square pulse (VSP) erbium:yttrium aluminum garnet (Er:YAG) laser appears to effectively but temporarily improve epidermal-type melasma. The real question is the expense and morbidity worth this type of short-lived improvement to the patient. The topical combination of hydroquinone, topical retinoid, and a low strength topical corticosteroid appears to provide for many patients this type of improvement without the higher cost or down time associated with laser treatment. Ultimately, we have to develop a better treatment approach that addresses the etiology of this abnormal pigmentation and provides a more sustained therapeutic benefit.

E. A. Tanghetti, MD

Clinical Trial of Dual Treatment with an Ablative Fractional Laser and a Nonablative Laser for the Treatment of Acne Scars in Asian Patients

Kim S, Cho K-H (Yonsei-Zium Skin Laser Clinic, Seoul, Korea; Armed Forces Daegu Hosp, Gyeongbuk, Korea)
Dermatol Surg 35:1089-1098, 2009

Background.—Many methods have been proposed for the treatment of acne scars, with variable cosmetic results. Nonablative skin resurfacing is one method that has been proposed. Because of a need for more noticeable clinical improvements, the ablative fractional laser was recently introduced.

Objective.—To reduce complications and improve the results of ablative fractional laser resurfacing by combining this treatment of acne scars with nonablative lasers.

Methods.—A series of 20 patients (skin phototypes IV–V) with atrophic facial acne scars were randomly divided into two groups that received three successive monthly treatments with an ablative fractional laser using high (group A) and low (group B) energy on one facial half and an ablative fractional laser with low energy plus a nonablative resurfacing laser on the other facial half. Patients were evaluated using digital photography at each treatment visit and at 3 months postoperatively. Clinical assessment scores were determined at each treatment session and follow-up visit.

Results.—Although the use of the ablative fractional laser with high energy resulted in an improvement in patients' acne scars, the combination of ablative fractional laser resurfacing and nonablative laser resurfacing yielded the best results, as assessed in photographs as well as by the overall appearance of the acne scars. With the combination method, fewer complications were observed.

▶ Acne scars can range from being a cosmetic nuisance to being severely disfiguring for the patient. In fact, scars are many times the number one concern expressed by acne patients. It is difficult to predict who will scar and who will not, as sometimes mild acne can lead to pitted scarring. Fortunately, there are several treatment modalities available today to help mitigate scarring including lasers, dermabrasion, chemical peels, fillers, surgical techniques, and topical retinoid therapy. Treatment modalities depend upon the type and severity of scarring present. This article focuses on laser therapy, specifically using a combination of nonablative laser resurfacing (long pulse 1064-nm Nd:YAG laser) followed by a low-energy ablative fractional resurfacing (AFR) carbon dioxide laser for atrophic scars. This combination therapy was shown to have greater clinical efficacy than using high-energy AFR alone. The most common side effect was postinflammatory hyperpigmentation, which resolved sooner with dual treatment than with high-energy AFR alone. It is important to mention that the patients were all of Korean decent, therefore results may not be generalized to other ethnic groups. Furthermore, the small number of patients ($N = 20$) involved in the study is a major limitation as this number is too small to assess statistically, and clinical extrapolation warrants evaluation in a larger number of patients.

S. Bellew, DO

J. Q. Del Rosso, DO

5-Fluorouracil Treatment of Problematic Scars
Haurani MJ, Foreman K, Yang JJ, et al (Henry Ford Hosp, Detroit, MI; Alabama Surgical Associates, Huntsville)
Plast Reconstr Surg 123:139-148, 2009

Background.—Keloids and hypertrophic scars can be uncomfortable, disfiguring, and aesthetically undesirable. Anecdotal reports suggest that low-dose intralesional fluorouracil can be used to treat these undesirable scars.

Methods.—Using a prospective case series protocol, both keloid and hypertrophic scar patients were included. Keloid patients underwent excision followed by a series of treatments with intralesional 5-fluorouracil into the healing scar to prevent recurrence ($n = 32$). The hypertrophic scar patients were treated with the same series of injections without scar excision to both control symptoms and improve scar appearance ($n = 21$). The primary outcome measures were scar volume and a symptom questionnaire. Patients were followed for 1 year after completing the injection treatments.

Results.—In the keloid group, the recurrence rate was 19 percent at 1-year follow-up for this group of patients who had failed previous corticosteroid injection therapy. In the hypertrophic scar group, 14 percent did not respond to the series of injections. In this group, there was a median volume decrease of 50 percent maintained for 1 year after injection therapy was terminated.

Conclusions.—Intralesional fluorouracil is a safe and effective means of controlling problem scars in terms of both recurrence and symptom control. Benefits were maintained for at least 1 year after completion of therapy. Intralesional 5-fluorouracil should be considered another option for patients suffering from problematic scars.

▶ 5-fluorouracil (5FU) is a fluorinated pyrimidine that acts as an antimetabolic agent that inhibits RNA synthesis thereby blunting rapidly proliferating cells. There is recent evidence to suggest that 5FU may selectively block collagen synthesis and augment scar formation. This is a prospective cohort study of patients with both keloid and hypertrophic scars treated with intralesional 5FU at the Henry Ford Hospital, Detroit, Michigan. The authors sought to examine the effects of intralesional 5FU on the recurrence rates and long-term formation of keloid and hypertrophic scars. All patients included in the study had failed corticosteroid therapy and other conventional treatments. All patients in the keloid group underwent excision before treatment with 5FU. In the keloid group, 32 of the 35 enrolled patients completed treatment and the 1-year follow-up. All patients had received previous intralesional corticosteroid injections, and 71% had undergone previous excision. The hypertrophic scar patients did not undergo excision or debulking of the scar before the initiation of therapy. Symptoms of scars and side effects of 5FU were noted. Scar volume was measured with polyvinyl molds before beginning treatment, at the completion of treatment (11 months), and 1-year follow-up after therapy. There were no treatment related complications in both groups. In the keloid group, there was no significant difference in volumes between baseline and posttreatment values or between baseline and 1-year follow-up values ($P > .05$ for both). There was a 65% reduction after treatment and a 40% reduction at 1-year follow-up in this group. Although no scars recurred during the course of 5FU treatment, there were 6 recurrences in the keloid group at 1-year posttreatment. In the hypertrophic scar group, the volume changes after treatment and at 1-year follow-up compared with baseline values were statistically significant ($P < .001$ for both). Keloid and hypertrophic scars groups were compared. Patients in the hypertrophic group experienced 86% improvement in their lesions. The keloid group were younger ($P < .001$) in age and had a higher percentage of scars on the face compared with the hypertrophic scar group ($P < .001$). There was no evidence of long-term sequelae due to injection of 5FU. With a success rate of 81%, 5FU may be a more favorable treatment compared with excision alone and corticosteroid injections. One limitation to this study was the short follow-up period of 1 year. To add, patients with keloid scars can experience recurrence long after a year and therefore a longer follow-up period is needed for this group to assess the efficacy of 5FU. In addition, excision alone in the keloid group could have prevented new recurrence in some individuals. Another limitation was the lack of a control group. The investigators concluded that 5FU is a safe and effective method for both keloid and hypertrophic scars, especially in those that have failed multiple treatment modalities.

G. K. Kim, DO

J. Q. Del Rosso, DO

Treatment of Surgical Scars with Nonablative Fractional Laser Versus Pulsed Dye Laser: A Randomized Controlled Trial
Tierney E, Mahmoud BH, Srivastava D, et al (Laser and Skin Surgery Ctr, Carmel, IN; Henry Ford Health System, Detroit, MI)
Dermatol Surg 35:1172-1180, 2009

Objective.—Comparison of the efficacy of nonablative fractional laser (NAFL) and the V-beam pulsed dye laser (PDL) for improvement of surgical scars.

Methods.—A randomized blinded split-scar study. Fifteen scars in 12 patients were treated a minimum of 2 months after Mohs surgery. Patients were treated on half of the scar with a 1,550-nm NAFL and on the contralateral half with the 595nm PDL.

Main Outcome Measure(S).—A nontreating physician investigator evaluated the outcome of the scar in terms of scar dyspigmentation, thickness, texture, and overall cosmetic appearance (5-point grading scale).

Results.—After a series of four treatments at 2-week intervals, greater improvements were noted in the portion of surgical scars treated with NAFL (overall mean improvement 75.6%, range 60–100%, vs. PDL, 53.9%, range 20–80%; $p < .001$).

Conclusion.—These data support the use of NAFL as a highly effective treatment modality for surgical scars, with greater improvement in scar appearance than with PDL. It is likely that the greater depth of penetration and focal microthermal zones of injury with NAFL, inducing neocollagenesis and collagenolysis, account for its greater improvement in scar

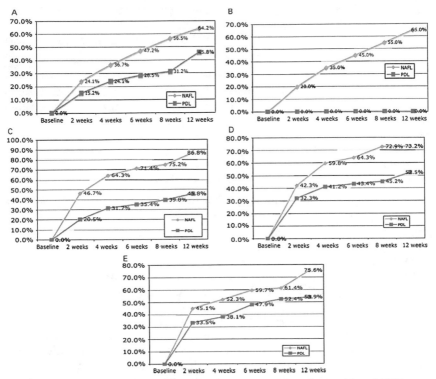

FIGURE 1.—(A) Improvement in scar dyspigmentation: non-ablative fractional laser (NAFL) versus pulsed dye laser (PDL). (B) Improvement in scar hypopigmentation: NAFL vs. PDL. (C) Improvement in scar thickness: NAFL vs. PDL. (D) Improvement in scar texture: NAFL vs. PDL. (E) Overall cosmetic improvement: NAFL vs. PDL. (Reprinted from Tierney E, Mahmoud BH, Srivastava D, et al. Treatment of surgical scars with nonablative fractional laser versus pulsed dye laser: a randomized controlled trial. *Dermatol Surg.* 2009;35:1172-1180, with permission from Blackwell Publishing.)

remodeling. These encouraging results lead us to recommend that NAFL be added to the current treatment armamentarium for surgical scars (Fig 1).

▶ This article suggests that fractional nonablative treatments are effective for the treatment of surgical scars. In this blinded randomized comparative split scar trial, both the pulse dye laser (PDL) and a fractional 1550 erbium-doped laser produced improvement in scar outcomes. It appeared that the 1550 device had superior results. Unfortunately, there were a number of issues that lead to more questions. An evaluation of these scars 1 month after the final treatment is not long enough to adequately access the ultimate effect of these 2 devices on these scars. The pulse duration of the PDL was not the 0.5 msec that had been reported in the past. The energy for the nonablative device produced an injury that was fairly deep. There have been some recent data that suggest lower energy treatments would produce a similar clinical effect for photodamaged and aged skin. Perhaps less might be better. Finally, it would have been ideal to have a nontreated control to compare the natural healing process of these surgical wounds. It appears that the fractional nonablative devices do have a place in the treatment of surgical scars.

E. A. Tanghetti, MD

Glycolic Acid Peels Versus Salicylic–Mandelic Acid Peels in Active Acne Vulgaris and Post-Acne Scarring and Hyperpigmentation: A Comparative Study
Garg VK, Sinha S, Sarkar R (Maulana Azad Med College and Associated Lok Nayak Hosp, New Delhi, India)
Dermatol Surg 35:59-65, 2009

Background.—Many clinicians have used glycolic acid (GA) peels for facial acne, scarring, and hyperpigmentation, mainly in lighter skin types. Salicylic–mandelic acid combination peels (SMPs) are a newer modality, and there have been no well-controlled studies comparing them with other conventional agents.

Objective.—To compare the therapeutic efficacy and tolerability of 35% GA peels and 20% salicylic–10% mandelic acid peels in active acne and post-acne scarring and hyperpigmentation.

Methods and Materials.—Forty-four patients with facial acne and post-acne scarring and hyperpigmentation were divided into two groups, with one receiving GA peels and the other SMPs at fortnightly intervals for six sessions. The treating physician performed objective evaluation of treatment outcomes. The patients, the treating physician, and an independent observer made subjective assessments. Side effects of both agents were also noted.

Results.—Both the agents were effective, but SMPs had a higher efficacy for most active acne lesions ($p < .001$) and hyperpigmentation ($p < .001$). Side effects were also lesser with SMPs.

Conclusion.—Both the agents were effective and safe in Indian patients, with SMPs being better for active acne and post-acne hyperpigmentation.

▶ Alpha hydroxy acids (AHAs) and beta hydroxy acids (BHAs) are common chemical peels used for a variety of different indications, including acne vulgaris. Peeling with either 35% glycolic acid (GA) or 20% salicylic acid-10% mandelic acid (SMA) have been used as components of acne therapy, including for superficial scarring and postinflammatory dyschromia. Mandelic acid penetrates the epidermis slowly and uniformly due to its large size while the salicylic acid exhibits desmolytic and antiinflammatory properties and penetrates the epidermis quickly. Twenty-two patients in group A received GA peels, and 22 patients in group B received SMA peels, with a total of 6 sessions 2 weeks apart. Both agents were effective in reduction of comedones, papules, and pustules, but significant improvement was seen earlier in group B patients treated with salicylic-mandelic acid peel (SMP). No significant improvement in nodules and cysts was seen with either agent. Also, neither agent led to significant improvement of icepick, boxcar, and rolling acne scars. Sixty-one percent of patients in group A and 76% of patients in group B did not develop any significant side effects. Approximately 9% of the GA peel group had visible desquamation while no patient experienced it in the SMA group, although dryness was more often seen with SMA peels. Both agents were effective for postacne hyperpigmentation with SMA showing a greater response.

S. B. Momin, DO

J. Q. Del Rosso, DO

Excellent Clinical Results with a New Preparation for Chemical Peeling in Acne: 30% Salicylic Acid in Polyethylene Glycol Vehicle
Dainichi T, Ueda S, Imayama S, et al (Kyushu Univ, Fukuoka, Japan; Ueda-Setsuko Clinic, Fukuoka, Japan; Kyushu Med Ctr, Fukuoka, Japan)
Dermatol Surg 34:891-899, 2008

Background.—Chemical peeling by salicylic acid in ethanol or another vehicle may be accompanied bystinging and burning followed by post-inflammatory hyperpigmentation in the treated area, or salicylism. We have developed a new formulation: 30% salicylic acid in polyethylene glycol (SA-PEG). A topical application of SA-PEG remodels photodamaged skin in mice and humans, without systemic absorption.

Objective.—The objective was to evaluate the safety and efficacy of SA-PEG for clinical use in the treatment of acne.

Materials and Methods.—We evaluated the effects of the preparation histologically in mice and its safety and efficacy in 44 volunteers with normally aged skin and in 436 patients with acne.

Results.—Histologic studies in animals showed no inflammatory changes in the skin following topical application of SA-PEG. Volunteers noted an improved skin texture. In the acne patients, the comedones and papules disappeared, resulting in an excellent outcome. There was a notable absence of stinging and burning, edema, bleeding, or crusting in the treated area.

Conclusion.—The SA-PEG preparation appeared to be safe and effective, with minimal associated inflammation or adverse effects, even in Asian patients who tend to develop hyperpigmentation or keloids. This preparation is thus ideal for chemical peeling.

▶ Salicylic acid (SA) peels have the potential to penetrate the skin, which may lead to salicylism systemically. Also, SA may cause significant cutaneous irritation and inflammation, which may lead to hyperpigmentation in some patients. The authors of this study have successfully formulated a SA peel that they report maximizes the benefits and minimizes the side effects by using a polyethylene glycol vehicle. We compliment the authors of this article in their study design and their diverse and extensive testing in animals, healthy human skin, and in a large number of acne patients ($N = 436$). In addition, the use of split face application as a control minimized interindividual variation.

The major limitation of this study is the lack of comparison of this newly formulated peel with other previously used formulations and therapies. Further studies are needed to compare this new peel with old formulations and possibly even to new methodologies for treating both acne and the signs of photoaging.

J. Levin, DO

J. Q. Del Rosso, DO

A Four-Month Randomized, Double-Blind Evaluation of the Efficacy of Botulinum Toxin Type A for the Treatment of Glabellar Lines in Women with Skin Types V and VI

Grimes PE, Shabazz D (Vitiligo and Pigmentation Inst of Southern California, Los Angeles; Dermatology Associates of Northern Virginia, Sterling)
Dermatol Surg 35:429-436, 2009

Background.—Histologic differences (e.g., dermal thickness, collagen fibers) between Caucasian and other racial and ethnic groups may affect wrinkle formation and influence responses to treatment with botulinum toxin type A (BoNT-A).

Objective.—To evaluate the degree and duration of efficacy of 20 and 30 U of BoNT-A for the treatment of glabellar lines in African-American women with skin types V and VI.

Materials & Methods.—Women aged 18 to 65 with a glabellar rhytid score of 2 or more at maximum frown on an investigator-rated 4-point facial wrinkle scale (FWS; $0 =$ none, $3 =$ severe) were eligible for this study. Patients were randomly assigned to receive 20 U or 30 U of BoNT-A in the glabellar region. Evaluations were conducted at baseline and days 30, 60, 90, and 120 postinjection. The investigator and patient graded the severity of wrinkles at maximum frown and repose on the same 4-point FWS. BoNT-A was administered at the assigned dose, divided between five equal intramuscular injections into the procerus muscle, each corrugator muscle, and a site above the midpupillary line on each side.

Results.—The percentage of responders at maximum frown did not differ significantly between the two groups. Although not statistically significant, the effect lasted somewhat longer in the subjects receiving the 30U dose. No differences were evident between groups at repose through day 120. Adverse events were mild and transient and did not differ between the groups.

Conclusion.—These results indicate that doses of 20 and 30 U of BoNT-A demonstrate efficacy and safety in African-American women with skin types V and VI.

▶ The objective of this study was to determine whether there was a difference in therapeutic effect of 2 dosing treatment schemes of botulinum toxin type A (BoTN-A) in the treatment of glabellar lines in women of color, specifically those with skin types V and VI. Skin of color makes up a much higher percentage of patients seeking cosmetic treatments than ever before, and our literature is scant with descriptions of the effects of varying procedures and therapeutic outcomes in this group of individuals. As more recognize the importance of including this group in newer clinical studies, most pharmaceutical companies studying cosmetic treatments include a certain percentage of skin of color in their original trial designs; this was not the case when BoTN-A made its debut.

This study examined 2 dosing regimens—20 U or 30 U of BoTN-A in 31 black females in this phase IV clinical trial. Patients were randomized as to the dosing schema they received. Patients were followed at 30, 60, 90, and 120 days following their initial injection in the glabellar region. The injection process was the same as previous clinical trials. The primary efficacy outcome was the investigator's assessment on the facial wrinkle scale (FWS) at maximum frown and at repose. Responder rates at maximum frown were defined as the percentage of subjects with a score of none (0) or mild (1) on the FWS as compared with their entry, which was required to be a 2 or a 3. Secondary outcomes included the patient's assessment of rhytid severity at maximum frown and repose, patient satisfaction, and the incidence of adverse events.

The results showed that the percentage of responders at maximum frown was not different between those receiving 20 U or 30 U of BoTN-A. There was a trend toward longer duration of effect for those receiving 30 U of BoTN-A, although it was not found to be significant. There was no difference noted between the 2 groups at repose at day 120. Adverse events were mild and similar in both groups.

The results here are significant and an important contribution to our medical literature. Patients of color are making up more of our cosmetic and aesthetic practices, and we need to have them included in the clinical trials to assess whether there are interracial differences that could suggest differences in doses of medicines or in injection techniques. This article helps clarify the effectiveness of BoTN-A in women of color and in doses comparable with what is commonly used in whites.

M. H. Gold, MD

Comparative Physical Properties of Hyaluronic Acid Dermal Fillers
Kablik J, Monheit GD, Yu L, et al (Genzyme Corporation, Cambridge, MA; Total Skin and Beauty Dermatology Ctr, P.C., Birmingham, AL; et al)
Dermatol Surg 35:302-312, 2009

Background.—Hyaluronic acid (HA) fillers are becoming the material of choice for use in cosmetic soft tissue and dermal correction. HA fillers appear to be similar, but their physical characteristics can be quite different. These differences have the potential to affect the ability of the physician to provide the patient with a natural and enduring result.

Objective.—The objective of this article is to discuss the key physical properties and methods used in characterizing dermal fillers. These methods were then used to analyze several well-known commercially available fillers.

Methods and Materials.—Analytical methods were employed to generate data on the properties of various fillers. The measured physical properties were concentration, gel-to-fluid ratio, HA gel concentration, degree of HA modification, percentage of cross-linking, swelling, modulus, and particle size.

Results.—The results demonstrated that commercial fillers exhibit a wide variety of properties.

Conclusion.—Combining the objective factors that influence filler performance with clinical experience will provide the patient with the optimal product for achieving the best cosmetic result. A careful review of these gel characteristics is essential in determining filler selection, performance, and patient expectations.

▶ The objective of this article is to look at the various hyaluronic acid (HA) fillers available in the United States and to review the main physical properties and characteristics, which help to define the different HA fillers. This was a well-written, well-conceived article that answered some of the more difficult questions many have when trying to compare and contrast the HA fillers we use in our everyday clinical practices. This is a review article per se, and we also need to keep in mind that all but one of the authors are employed by a company that had one of the first HA fillers on the market, now no longer available, but with plans to launch its latest HA dermal filler later in 2009 or in early 2010.

The article reviews some of the important differences between HA fillers, like the cross-linking of HAs and what specific cross-linkers are being used in the current HA formulations and the degree of cross-linking for the HA fillers, which has a significant impact on the hardness or stiffness of the product. The article reviews the concentrations of HAs found in each filler, taking into account the amount of free or uncross linked HA versus cross-linked HA. The elastic modulus (G′) helps describe the firmness of the HA gel, or the amount of stress required to deform the gel. Next described is the swelling properties of the HA—whether the HA has reached its own equilibrium for bound water. The swelling capacity varies from product to product and is dependent upon concentration, cross-link density, and the process used to hydrate the gel. Fully hydrated HAs will not swell upon injection into the skin, whereas nonequilibrium gels will swell upon injection. Also important and reviewed in the article is the HA particle size and the extrusion force upon injection. The HA fillers are small enough to be able to be injected with small-bore needles and based on their modulus will have an extrusion force unique to each individual filler. The remainder of the article reviewed some of the currently available HA fillers.

I would strongly recommend this article to anyone interested in better understanding the biology and chemistry behind HA dermal fillers. We often take science at its word, and we are too busy to ask the questions that make products similar, yet different. We must constantly seek out the answers, and many for HA fillers are given here.

M. H. Gold, MD

A Prospective Study of Fractional Scanned Nonsequential Carbon Dioxide Laser Resurfacing: A Clinical and Histopathologic Evaluation
Berlin AL, Hussain M, Phelps R, et al (Skin Laser and Surgery Specialists of NY and NJ; Mount Sinai School of Medicine, NY)
Dermatol Surg 35:222-228, 2009

Background.—Although unparalleled in its efficacy, carbon dioxide (CO_2) laser resurfacing has a high risk:benefit ratio. A modified device uses a novel handpiece and software to deliver nonsequential fractional ablative CO_2 laser exposures.

Objective.—To evaluate the safety and efficacy of this fractional ablative, scanned, nonsequential CO_2 laser in the treatment of photo-damaged skin and to evaluate histologic and ultrastructural changes after the treatment.

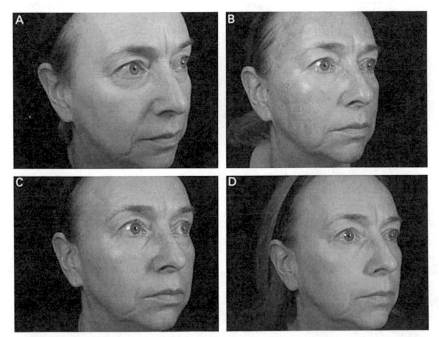

FIGURE 1.—Fifty-five-year-old woman before (A) and 1 week (B), 2 weeks (C), and 24 weeks (D) after the treatment. (Reprinted from Berlin AL, Hussain M, Phelps R, et al. A prospective study of fractional scanned nonsequential carbon dioxide laser resurfacing: a clinical and histopathologic evaluation. *Dermatol Surg.* 2009;35:222-228, with permission from Blackwell Publishing.)

Materials and Methods.—Ten subjects with Fitzpatrick skin types I to III with photo-damaged facial skin underwent a single CO_2 ablative laser treatment using a scanning handpiece in a nonsequential fractional mode. Clinical improvement and histologic and ultrastructrural changes were assessed.

Results.—All subjects completed the study with no serious or long-term complications. Blinded evaluator and subject assessment documented improvement in cutaneous photoaging. Light microscopy revealed changes consistent with a wound repair mechanism, and electron microscopy confirmed evidence of new collagen deposition.

Conclusion.—Nonsequential scanned fractional CO_2 laser resurfacing can lead to improvement in photo-damaged skin, accompanied by histologic and ultrastructural evidence of wound repair and subsequent new collagen formation (Fig 1).

▶ This thoughtful but small study describes one of the many fractional ablative carbon dioxide (CO_2) lasers used for cutaneous resurfacing. This study demonstrates mild to moderate efficacy with significantly less down time when compared with the standard ablative CO_2. The textural change as noted in the improvement of solar elastosis is significant. An intriguing observation is the slightly better improvement in those receiving the lower setting than those receiving the higher density setting. Recent data presented at the 2009 ASLMS meeting with nonablative devices also reported a similar observation. Perhaps a mild wounding process is just as efficacious as a more aggressive treatment? Hopefully, there will be more to follow.

E. A. Tanghetti, MD

The Long-Term Efficacy and Safety of a Subcutaneously Injected Large-Particle Stabilized Hyaluronic Acid–Based Gel of NonAnimal Origin in Esthetic Facial Contouring
DeLorenzi C, Weinberg M, Solish N, et al (The DeLorenzi Clinic, Ontario, Canada; Mississauga Cosmetic Surgery Centre, Ontario, Canada; Cosmetic Care and Laser Surgery Centre, Ontario, Canada; et al)
Dermatol Surg 35:313-321, 2009

Background.—Nonanimal stabilized hyaluronic acid (NASHA) offers longer-lasting correction than many other injectable products and is associated with low risk of immunogenic and hypersensitivity reactions. A new large-particle stabilized hyaluronic acid-based gel has been developed to restore facial volume and define facial contours.

Objective.—This study was conducted to assess the long-term efficacy and safety of a large-particle stabilized hyaluronic acid–based gel in patients seeking facial contouring.

Methods.—Fifty-seven adult patients seeking esthetic cheek or chin augmentation or both received subcutaneous or supraperiosteal injections or both of large-particle stabilized hyaluronic acid–based gel (20 mg/mL). Efficacy was assessed subjectively using the Global Aesthetic Improvement Scale at intervals up to 12 months after treatment.

Results.—After treatment, patients and investigators independently considered treatment sites to be at least somewhat improved in 91% and 96% (6 months), 68% and 77% (9 months), and 58% and 52% (12 months) of cases, respectively. Patient- and investigator-assessed treatment response rates (the proportion of patients showing at least moderate improvement) were 72% and 81% (6 months), 42% and 40% (9 months), and 21% and 15% (12 months), respectively. Most commonly reported adverse events were local injection-site reactions, skin induration, and implant mobility.

Conclusion.—This large-particle stabilized hyaluronic acid–based gel is well tolerated and provides relatively long-lasting esthetic correction of the cheeks and chin after subcutaneous or supraperiosteal injection.

▶ The objective of this prospective, open-label study was to evaluate a larger sized nonanimal stabilized hyaluronic acid (NASHA) for the purpose of volume enhancement in patients requiring soft-tissue augmentation of the cheeks and/or chin.

NASHA, commonly known as the brand Restylane, has been used for the treatment of fine lines, wrinkles, and lip enhancement for many years. It has a predictable duration of effect, and various forms or particle sizes have been evaluated. A new form, known under the brand name of Restylane SubQ, has been formulated for volume enhancement. It contains 1000 gel particles per 1 mL of product versus 100 000 particles per 1 mL as in the original Restylane product. It has been developed for injection in the subcutaneous and supraperiosteal facial planes to replace lost volume and to create more defined facial contours; thus, its clinical applicability differs from the original Restylane product. The material is approved for use in the European Union (EU), Australia, Brazil, Canada, Columbia, Iran, Israel, Korea, Phillipines, and Russia. It is not approved by the United States Food & Drug Administration at this time.

Fifty-nine patients were screened at 4 clinical research sites. Fifty-seven patients satisfied inclusion and exclusion criteria and were treated with Restylane SubQ. Forty-four patients completed the 12-month clinical evaluation. Ninety-eight cheeks and 16 chins were treated with small microdroplet injections of Restylane SubQ. The mean volumes injected into the cheeks were 2.2 mL (range 0.7-5.0 mL) and 2.1 mL in the chin (range 0.6-5.5 mL). The mean total volume injected into each patient was 4.3 mL (range 1.3-9.0 mL). Thirteen patients (23%) received a touch-up injection at 20 treatment sites at 4 weeks.

This study raises some interesting questions, especially with concerns about the injection technique, where skin incisions and large bore cannulas are used. Whether these injection techniques will be commonly used by injectors remains to be seen. Also, other injectable materials have been developed which are being evaluated for volume enhancement, which may not require these special injection techniques. But in skilled and experienced hands, Restylane SubQ may prove a valuable injectable material for volume enhancement.

M. H. Gold, MD

Topical Fluorouracil for Actinic Keratoses and Photoaging: A Clinical and Molecular Analysis

Sachs DL, Kang S, Hammerberg C, et al (Univ of Michigan, Ann Arbor; Johns Hopkins Univ, Baltimore)

Arch Dermatol 145:659-666, 2009

Objective.—To examine clinical and molecular changes after topical fluorouracil treatment of photodamaged human facial skin for actinic keratoses.

Design.—Nonrandomized, open-label 2-week treatment with fluorouracil cream, 5%, followed by clinical and molecular evaluation.

Setting.—Academic referral center.

Patients.—Twenty-one healthy volunteers, 56 to 85 years old, with actinic keratoses and photodamage.

Interventions.—Twice-daily application of fluorouracil cream for 2 weeks and biopsies and clinical evaluation at baseline and periodically after treatment.

Main Outcome Measures.—Gene and protein expression of molecular effectors of epidermal injury, inflammation, and extracellular matrix remodeling 24 hours after fluorouracil treatment; clinical improvement measured by evaluators, photography, and patient questionnaires.

Results.—One day after the final fluorouracil treatment, gene expression of the effectors of epidermal injury (keratin 16), inflammation (interleukin 1β), and extracellular matrix degradation (matrix metalloproteinases 1 and 3) was significantly increased. Types I and III procollagen messenger RNA were induced at week 4 (7-fold and 3-fold, respectively). Type I procollagen protein levels were increased 2-fold at week 24. Actinic keratoses and photoaging were statistically significantly improved. Most patients rated photoaging as improved and were willing to undergo the therapy again.

Conclusions.—Topical fluorouracil causes epidermal injury, which stimulates wound healing and dermal remodeling resulting in improved appearance. The mechanism of topical fluorouracil in photoaged skin follows a predictable wound healing pattern of events reminiscent of that seen with laser treatment of photoaging.

▶ Topical 5% fluorouracil (5FU) has been widely used over several years for the treatment of actinic keratosis (AK). Some clinicians have also observed a marked reduction in photodamage changes after treatment, including wrinkling, resulting in an excellent cosmetic and therapeutic response. This is a non-randomized open-label 2-week study of treatment with topical 5FU 5% cream involving 21 patients incorporating both clinical and molecular evaluation. Those that were included had moderate to severe photoaging judged by the presence of rhytids, dyspigmentation, poikiloderma, lentigines, skin thinning, and/or telangiectasias. Patients also underwent clinical photography of the face, and baseline punch biopsies were performed. The study measured tumor necrosis factor (TNF), interleukins 1β (IL-1β), keratin 16, matrix metalloproteinases (MMPs), and type I and III procollagen. Patients also completed questionnaires concerning overall appearance of their skin. Wrinkling, tactile roughness, lentigines, hyperpigmentation, and sallowness were rated on a scale of 0 to 9 by dermatologists. Results revealed that AKs were significantly reduced, which was as predicted. Results also concluded that keratin 16, TNF, IL-1β, MMPs, and procollagen became elevated at certain treatment points. The biochemical changes simulated wound healing and dermal remodeling similar to those observed in, but not as dramatic as with, carbon dioxide laser resurfacing of photodamaged skin. This study opens up new possibilities for cosmetic use of topical 5FU in photodamaged skin. This medication may be more cost-effective for those who cannot afford laser resurfacing but due to its relatively long treatment course may not be ideal for those who do not want such a visible and symptomatic reaction for many weeks.

G. K. Kim, DO

J. Q. Del Rosso, DO

Lip augmentation with a new filler (agarose gel): a 3-year follow-up study
Scarano A, Carinci F, Piattelli A (Univ of Chieti-Pescara, Italy; Univ of Ferrara, Italy)
Oral Surg Oral Med Oral Pathol Oral Radiol Endod 108:e11-e15, 2009

Background.—Many fillers have been used to augment lips. Agarose gel is a new and absorbable filler indicated for the correction of soft tissues and lip.

Objective.—This article reviews the results of 68 cases that have undergone lip augmentation with this new filler in the last 3 years.

Study Design.—A total of 68 patients received agarose gel for treatment for lip augmentation in a 3-year period from 2005 to 2008. Each of the patients signed an informed consent form. The patients were between 35 and 70 years of age. Three patients were male, and 65 were female. A volume of 0.5-1.0 mL of agarose gel was sufficient for each lip. A bigger volume may result in a dense mass and pain. All patients were successfully treated with injections of agarose gel.

Results.—Clinical improvement was noted immediately, and only mild bruising was recorded. All of the patients returned to the clinic 10 days after treatment for follow-up, and all felt that an excellent cosmetic result was obtained. The patients were told to return after an additional month for follow-up and possible reinjection. The results lasted approximately 5 months with a gradual decline to baseline. The agarose gel was very well tolerated with only a few mild adverse reactions that resolved spontaneously.

Conclusion.—During 3 years of clinical use, agarose gel proved to be a reliable and predictable treatment for lip augmentation.

▶ This study examines a new agarose gel filler. It apparently has a longevity similar to the hyaluronic acid fillers used in the lip. However, no comments are made about the histology or repeated use of this drug over many years. While I was recently visiting Los Angeles, I could not help but notice the duck billed appearance of many of the women waiting for flights. It is apparent that many patients are overfilled, but also are poorly filled with our current array of volumizing agents. A closer look at these lips reveal a distortion of the normal sharp blurring of the mucosal portion to the cutaneous aspect. It has been shown that stimulation of collagen production by hyaluronic acid fillers occurs. Could it be that this new filler as well as the hyaluronic acid fillers cause a fibro-blastic reaction that is long-lived and far outlasts the dermal life of these fillers? It appears that repeated use of these products in the vermillion border of the lip compounds this reaction and results in an unnatural appearing lip.[1] It is impor-tant that we be aware of this potential problem.

E. A. Tanghetti, MD

Reference

1. Wang F, Garza LA, Kang S, et al. In vivo stimulation of de novo collagen produc-tion caused by cross-linked hyaluronic acid dermal filler injections in photodam-aged human skin. *Arch Dermatol.* 2007;143:155-163.

The Tear Trough and Lid/Cheek Junction: Anatomy and Implications for Surgical Correction
Haddock NT, Saadeh PB, Boutros S, et al (New York Univ School of Medicine)
Plast Reconstr Surg 123:1332-1340, 2009

Background.—The tear trough and the lid/cheek junction become more visible with age. These landmarks are adjacent, forming in some patients a continuous indentation or groove below the infraorbital rim. Numerous, often conflicting procedures have been described to improve the appear-ance of the region. The purpose of this study was to evaluate the anatomy underlying the tear trough and the lid/cheek junction and to evaluate the procedures designed to correct them.

Methods.—Twelve fresh cadaver lower lid and midface dissections were performed (six heads). The orbital regions were dissected in layers, and medical photography was performed.

Results.—In the subcutaneous plane, the tear trough and lid/cheek junction overlie the junction of the palpebral and orbital portions of the orbicularis oculi muscle and the cephalic border of the malar fat pad. In the submuscular plane, these landmarks differ. Along the tear trough, the orbicularis muscle is attached directly to the bone. Along the lid/cheek junction, the attachment is ligamentous by means of the orbicularis retain-ing ligament.

Conclusions.—The tear trough and lid/cheek junction are primarily explained by superficial (subcutaneous) anatomical features. Atrophy of skin and fat is the most likely explanation for age-related visibility of these landmarks. "Descent" of this region with age is unlikely (the structures are fixed to bone). Bulging orbital fat accentuates these landmarks. Interventions must extend significantly below the infraorbital rim. Fat or synthetic filler may be best placed in the intraorbicularis plane (tear trough) and in the suborbicularis plane (lid/cheek junction).

▶ This is a good article demonstrating the anatomy of the tear trough and lid/cheek junction. This study concludes that there is no age-related descent of the structures because they are fixed to the bone, and that atrophy of the skin and underlying subcutaneous fat is likely the reason for increasing visibility with age. This article also demonstrates why any surgical intervention for correction of the tear trough and lid/cheek junction must extend significantly below the infraorbital rim because the deformities extend approximately 4 mm or more below the arcus marginalis at the rim. The study suggests that based on these findings, treatment may be best if directed to the suborbicularis plane in the case of the lid/cheek junction and intraorbicularis plane in the case of the tear trough.

S. B. Momin, DO
J. Q. Del Rosso, DO

Palmar Hyperhidrosis: Long-Term Follow-up of Nine Children and Adolescents Treated with Botulinum Toxin Type A
Coutinho dos Santos LH, Gomes AM, Giraldi S, et al (Federal Univ of Paraná, Brazil)
Pediatr Dermatol 26:439-444, 2009

Primary palmar hyperhidrosis in children and adolescents may be severe enough to affect school and physical activities, causing emotional problems, stress in the patient's life, and a compromised quality of life. Nine patients with palmar hyperhidrosis underwent treatment with botulinum A. Before the session, and in the 1-, 3-, 6-, 9-, and 12-month post-session follow-ups, the patients were administered the Minor test, gravimetry, the Scales of Frequency and Severity, and the Questionnaire of Quality of Life. The mean age was 11 years, with seven girls and two boys. Each patient was administered at least one treatment of botulinum toxin in the palm of the hands (75–150 U for palm), with the mean number of sessions 2.2 (range: 1–4). All sessions in the patients resulted in drying of the hands, with a mean duration of effect of 7 months. Botulinum toxin A controls excessive sweat in the palms of children and adolescents who have primary palmar hyperhidrosis, with an improvement in the quality of life. The therapy is safe and effective in this pediatric group and can be considered before surgical interventions.

▶ Primary palmar hyperhidrosis in children can be a debilitating disease affecting quality of life. This is a study of 9 patients diagnosed with palmar hyperhidrosis treated with botulinum toxin A (BTA) with a mean age of

11 years. Patients were seen at 1, 3, 6, 9, and 12 months after follow-up. At each appointment, patients were administered the minor starch iodine test, gravimetry, and classified according to the Scale of Frequency and Scale of Severity. Patients also answered the Questionnaire of Quality of Life composed of 14 subjects administered to the patients at each evaluation. Each patient was administered at least one treatment of botulinum toxin in the palm of the hands (75-150 U in palm), with the mean number of 2.2 sessions (range: 1-4). The effects ranged from 3 to 16 months (average 7 months) with the first session demonstrating better results than subsequent ones, with an improvement in the quality of life. Of the 9 patients, 2 patients were administered 4 sessions, 1 patient with 3 sessions, 3 patients with 2 sessions, and 3 patients with 1 session. The study included patients who had up to 3 treatment sessions and follow-ups ranged from 1 to 2.5 years. Side effects observed in the study were localized injection pain and difficulty in fine handling up to 3 days after the session that lasted approximately 1 week with no loss of muscular force. There were no reports of compensatory hyperhidrosis or paresthesias. The advantages of botulinum toxin therapy are its effectiveness, fast action, ease of use, and safety profile. The disadvantages are the aforementioned temporary side effects and costs. All patients had clinical improvement after 1 treatment with BTA. Some patients were free of symptoms longer than others. Emotional factors could have been a varying factor for patients who needed more sessions compared with others. Self-esteem also showed a large impact at the beginning of the treatment sessions. Although the children in this study experienced minimal side effects, administration of BTA to a child is still not well accepted by the public due to its respiratory effects at high doses. The ability of hyperhidrosis to interfere with a child's daily life should be thoroughly evaluated before starting treatment. In conclusion, BTA therapy is effective for children and adolescents with palmar hyperhidrosis and should be considered before any aggressive surgical interventions are considered.

G. K. Kim, DO

J. Q. Del Rosso, DO

Treatment of Punched-Out Atrophic and Rolling Acne Scars in Skin Phototypes III, IV, and V with Variable Square Pulse Erbium:Yttrium-Aluminum-Garnet Laser Resurfacing
Wanitphakdeedecha R, Manuskiatti W, Siriphukpong S, et al (Mahidol Univ, Bangkok, Thailand, et al)
Dermatol Surg 35:1376-1383, 2009

Background.—Treatment of acne scars remains a challenge, especially in dark-skinned individuals. Treatment parameters may be optimized by selecting appropriate pulse width and laser energy that enhance tissue thermal response with limited morbidity.

Objective.—To determine the efficacy and side effects of variable square pulse (VSP) erbium:yttrium-aluminum-garnet (Er:YAG) laser resurfacing for treatment of punched-out atrophic and rolling acne scars.

Methods.—Twenty-four subjects with acne scars were treated monthly for 2 months with four passes of VSP Er:YAG laser resurfacing using a 7-mm spot size and a fluence of 0.4 J/cm^2. Subjects were divided into two groups and treated with two different pulse widths: 300 μs (short pulse, SP) and 1,500 μs (extralong pulse, XLP). Objective and subjective assessments were obtained at baseline and 1, 2, and 4 months after treatment.

Results.—In the SP group, skin smoothness improved significantly ($p < .01$); in the XLP group, skin smoothness ($p < .05$) and scar volume ($p < .05$) improved significantly from baseline. Adverse effects consisted of transient postinflammatory hyperpigmentation (18%) and acneiform eruption (9%).

Conclusions.—Low-fluence VSP Er:YAG laser resurfacing is a promising treatment option for acne scars, with minimal risk of side effects. Laser pulse width and energy determine the efficacy and the risk of side effects.

▶ The destruction of connective tissue during the inflammatory process can occur as a consequence of severe acneiform episodes resulting in punched out atrophic and rolling acne scars. This is a study that determines the efficacy and side effects of variable square pulse (VSP) erbium:yttrium-aluminum-garnet (Er:YAG) laser resurfacing for treatment of acne scars. This is a study of 24 Thai subjects with phototypes III-V with moderate to severe acne scars treated monthly for 2 months separated into 2 groups: 300 μs (short pulse, SP) and 1500 μs (extra long pulse, XLP). Objective and subjective assessments were obtained by both clinicians and patients at baseline and at 1, 2, and 4 months posttreatment. Skin smoothness ($P < .01$) improved significantly in the SP group. In the XLP group, skin smoothness ($P < .05$) and scar volume ($P < .05$) improved significantly from baseline. There was no significant difference in the volume of acne scars between the SP and XLP groups at baseline and at 1, 2, and 4 months after treatment ($P > .05$). Side effects were mild. There was postinflammatory hyperpigmentation in 18% of patients with skin phototypes III-V that resolved within 2 weeks. One subject had a mild acneiform eruption. Authors concluded that VSP Er:YAG improved acne scars with minimal down time and side effects. Limitations to this study included small sample size and nonrandomized patients. A more diverse group of Asians should be used in future studies to fully assess the benefits and side effects of VSP Er:YAG. In addition, objective assessments of improved scars were done by photographic documentation by 2 blinded dermatologists, which could have affected the data due to alterations in lighting and imaging quality.

G. K. Kim, DO

J. Q. Del Rosso, DO

Carbon dioxide laser treatment of rhinophyma: a review of 124 patients
Madan V, Ferguson JE, August PJ (Salford Royal Hosps Found Trust, United Kingdom)
Br J Dermatol 161:814-818, 2009

Background.—Rhinophyma is a progressive, localized or generalized nasal deformity resulting from hypertrophy of sebaceous and connective tissue. The CO_2 laser has been used for treatment of rhinophyma, but the long-term efficacy of the treatment is unknown.

Objectives.—To review the outcome of 124 patients with rhinophyma treated with the CO_2 laser between 1996 and 2008 in our centre.

Patients and Methods.—Exuberant sebaceous tissue was ablated using the Sharplan 40C CO_2 laser (Sharplan Lasers UK Ltd, London, U.K.) under local anaesthesia. The technique varied with the severity of rhinophyma; the laser was used in a continuous mode to debulk the larger rhinophymas, and in a resurfacing mode (Silk Touch® scanner; Sharplan, 4–7-mm spot at 20–40 W) or continuous mode (10–20 W using a defocused 2–3-mm beam) to reshape the nasal contours. Outcomes were determined by case notes, clinical review and questionnaire.

Results.—Laser treatment was completed in a single session in 115 of 124 patients. All patients were reviewed 3 months post-treatment. Results were classified as good to excellent in 118 and poor in six patients. All patients were sent a satisfaction questionnaire in 2008 and 52 patients replied. Patients reported high levels of satisfaction following treatment. The post-treatment response at 3-month review was maintained long term. The main complications were pain associated with injection of local anaesthetic, scarring and hypopigmentation (four patients) and open pores (two patients).

Conclusions.—The CO_2 laser is an effective and durable treatment for rhinophyma. Treatment carries a low risk of side-effects and is associated with high patient acceptability and satisfaction.

▶ Rhinophyma is a vexing outgrowth of the rosacea process in a few unfortunate patients. Rarely seen in women, the process has been unfairly associated with alcoholism and debauchery and carries an unfair stigma. The mechanism underlying the disease remains a mystery. In the earlier stages rhinophyma will respond to isotretinoin (off-label), but once fibrosis has developed a surgical approach is required. The traditional method is hot loop cautery, but more recently CO_2 laser ablation has been widely adopted. In this large series, the authors demonstrate the safety and satisfactory outcomes from this more advanced technique.

G. Webster, MD

Treatment of Melasma in Asian Skin Using a Fractional 1,550-nm Laser: An Open Clinical Study

Lee HS, Won CH, Lee DH, et al (Gowoonsesang Dermatology Clinic, Seoul, Korea; Univ of Ulsan; Seoul Natl Univ Hosp, Korea; et al)
Dermatol Surg 35:1499-1504, 2009

Background.—Melasma is a common hyperpigmentation disorder that can cause refractory cosmetic disfigurement, especially in Asians. Fractional photothermolysis (FP) has been reported to be effective for the treatment of melasma, despite small study populations and short follow-up periods.

Objective.—To evaluate the efficacy and safety of FP for the treatment of melasma in Asians.

Patients and Methods.—Twenty-five patients with melasma received four monthly FP sessions and were followed up to 24 weeks after treatment completion. Efficacy was evaluated using objective and subjective ratings, Melasma Area and Severity Index (MASI), melanin index tracking, and skin elasticity measurements.

Results.—Investigators observed clinical improvements in 60% and patients in 44% at 4 weeks after treatment, but the figures decreased to 52% and 35%, respectively, at 24 weeks after treatment. Mean MASI scores decreased significantly from 7.6 to 6.2. Mean melanin index decreased significantly after the first two sessions, but it relapsed slightly in subsequent follow-ups. The treatment did not alter skin elasticity. Hyperpigmentation was observed in three of 23 subjects (13%).

Conclusion.—Treatment of melasma with FP led to some clinical improvements, but it was not as efficacious as previously reported at 6-month follow-up. We recommend judicious use of FP for the treatment of melasma in Asian skin because of its limited efficacy.

► Previous reports indicate that fractional photothermolysis (FP) is a successful treatment option for melasma in Asian patients. However, these reports were based on short follow-up durations and small study populations. The current investigators aimed to further evaluate the efficacy and safety of FP in a slightly larger population. Authors found noticeable improvement in the first 4 weeks of treatment, however, improvement declined thereafter. In fact, the mean melanin index showed a significant decrease from baseline to week 8, but increased after that point.

Limitations of this study still include a small number of subjects (25 patients), and patients were limited to a single institution in Korea, which make the results difficult to generalize to other populations.

It appears that FP is one of the newer treatment options for melasma; however, its efficacy seems comparable with other conventional treatments. Keep in mind that risk of postinflammatory hyperpigmentation is always an important consideration when treating darker Asian skin.

S. Bellew, DO
J. Q. Del Rosso, DO

Use of topical herbal remedies and cosmetics: a questionnaire-based investigation in dermatology out-patients
Corazza M, Borghi A, Lauriola MM, et al (Univ of Ferrara, Italy)
J Eur Acad Dermatol Venereol 23:1298-1303, 2009

Background.—Although topical remedies and cosmetics based on herbal ingredients are becoming increasingly popular with the public due to the perception that botanical compounds are safer and healthier than their synthetic counterparts, a large number of adverse cutaneous effects of plant extracts, notably contact sensitization, have been reported in medical literature.

Objective.—To evaluate the prevalence of herbal compound usage in a dermatological out-patient population and to estimate the incidence of consequent cutaneous side-effects.

Methods.—Four hundred patients were subjected to a self-administered 15-item questionnaire to assess both prevalence and type of topical botanical preparations used and occurrence of skin adverse reactions.

Results.—Two hundred forty-one patients (60.25%) reported use of natural topical products, predominantly aloe, marigold, chamomile, propolis and arnica. Females used herbal products, for both medicinal and cosmetic purposes, more frequently than males. Fifteen patients (6.22%) referred one or more adverse cutaneous reactions.

Conclusion.—Herbal preparations were widely used in the examined population, but, despite the common belief in the innocuous nature of botanical extracts, the incidence of side-effects referred by the patients confirms that they should be regarded as a potential source of adverse skin events. The lack of adequate patch testing in case of suspected contact allergic dermatitis, incomplete or misleading product labelling, and the risk of chemical adulteration may represent further concerns as regards application of botanical products.

▶ There has been an increase in demand for more cosmetic and topical herbal products in recent years. This is a study of 400 patients subjected to a self-administered 15-item questionnaire to assess the prevalence of topical botanical products used and the occurrence of adverse cutaneous reactions. This study sought to determine the most common botanical extracts, the function of these preparations, tolerance, and efficacy of herbal cosmetic products. Of the 400 patients, 241 (60.25%) used natural topical products; 184 were women (65.7% of the enrolled female population) and 57 were men (47.5% of the male population). In most cases, herbal preparations were used sporadically (51.75% of the interviewed people) while 8.5% of the studied population used botanicals on a regular basis. Fifteen patients (6.22%) described an adverse reaction with a higher prevalence in women (7.07%) compared with males (3.51%). However, women use more cosmetic products compared with males. The largest prevalence was among the 31- to 40-year-old patients, while patients 50 years and older had a lesser tendency to use these products. The highest prevalence was in the lowest age group (55.88% of 18- to 20-year-old patients), which seems to suggest a greater interest in alternative natural remedies among young adults. Herbal products were reported more frequently by women than by men (65.7% compared with 47.5%, respectively). Patients also used herbal remedies because of the perceived safety profile compared with synthetic alternatives. Dermatological creams and ointments were the most widely used topical herbal preparations, with the face being the most common area. Patient's self-reported the herbal compound's efficacy and tolerability profile through the questionnaires. A limitation to this study includes recall bias due to the nature of the study. In addition, researchers measured efficacy and cutaneous side effects of herbal products by patient's subjective responses. Further, it was unknown whether other topical products were used in combination with the herbal products, therefore a direct causal relationship with efficacy cannot be made. In addition, herbal products are not FDA regulated and active ingredients are not standardized. Also, the purity, concentration and safety profile of most herbal products may be difficult to assess due to this limitation. However, this study does reveal the younger generation's desire for more natural products, especially in females, and may reflect a target group for marketing purposes.

G. K. Kim, DO

J. Q. Del Rosso, DO

Surgical Complications in Hair Transplantation: A Series of 533 Procedures
Salanitri S, Gonçalves AJ, Helene A Jr, et al (Santa Casa de Misericórdia de São Paulo, Brazil)
Aesthet Surg J 29:72-76, 2009

Background.—Surgical complications in hair transplantation can sometimes be a serious matter. Most of the published literature on this issue deals with individual case reports rather than larger series of patients.

Objective.—The authors analyze complications in 425 consecutive patients undergoing 533 hair transplantations.

Methods.—Patients with androgenetic alopecia (407 men and 17 women), cicatricial alopecia (9 men and 8 women), and malformations (1 man and 3 women) with a mean age of 36.9 years (standard deviation, 10.4 yrs) underwent hair transplantation between 1995 and 2006 and were followed up postoperatively for at least 1 year. Data on surgical complications were retrospectively analyzed.

Results.—The overall complication rate in our series was 4.7%, including enlarged scar (1.2%), folliculitis (1.0%), necrosis in the donor area (0.8%), keloids (0.4%), bleeding (0.2%), hiccups (0.2%), infection (0.2%), and pyogenic granuloma (0.2%). The frequency of enlarged scar increased proportionally according to the number of surgical procedures.

Conclusions.—The hair transplantation complication rate in this series was 4.7%. Good communication between patient and surgeon, a complete clinical and laboratory assessment of the patient, accurate surgical technique, specific equipment, a trained surgical team, and careful postoperative attention to the patient are crucial for successful hair transplantation and for decreasing complication rates.

▶ This large retrospective study is a good article to increase awareness and frequency of complications seen in hair transplantations. Most complications were observed in scalp hair transplantation procedures. Patients who underwent only one procedure had significantly lower risk of developing complication than patients who underwent more than 1 session. Black patients presented with complications more frequently than whites or Asians. Scar enlargement was the main complication encountered in this series followed by folliculitis. There does need to be a large multicentered study, including centers from other countries to standardize evaluation of patients, surgical techniques, and postoperative evaluations. Patient education is also essential to decrease the number of complications seen following hair transplantations.

S. B. Momin, DO
J. Q. Del Rosso, DO

Eyebrow Transplantation in Asians
Laorwong K, Pathomvanich D, Bunagan K (Stough Clinic, Bangkok, Thailand)
Dermatol Surg 35:496-504, 2009

It is generally accepted that dense, wide, dark-colored eyebrows make the face look charming and attractive in men.

The shape and hair direction of the eyebrows in Asian men and women are not much different. Men appear to have wider eyebrows than women. In fact, most women often pluck or shave the lower border especially at the lateral third of their eyebrows to make them narrow and appear more aesthetically pleasing. In Chinese and Japanese male culture, bushy eyebrows are believed to be a sign of strength, power, prosperity, and charm.

The eyebrows remain an important cosmetic asset of the face; if eyebrows are absent, some individual may suffer significant distress over their appearance.

Eyebrow transplantation is performed to improve the patient's appearance and self-esteem.

Reconstruction techniques of eyebrows using micrografts of various sizes usually yield good results. Transplantation methods vary from physician to physician; some use a 19-G to 21-G needle with stick-and-place, some use implanters, and others use pre-made incisions with a tiny microblade, such as a 15° Sharpoint, and place the grafts afterwards. Many Asian patients who need eyebrow restoration have patchy or thin low-density eyebrows. Asians have less dense but coarser caliber and a higher skin–hair color contrast than Caucasians, which is the most important reason why only single hair grafts should be used to restore a natural-looking brow. Meticulous dissection of the ultraskinny single hair graft under 10 times stereomicroscope should be done to make sure that only single hairs will grow. Insertion using 23-, 24-G needle in stick-and-place fashion under three times magnification loupes improve the outcome by increasing density and matching the graft size to needle size. The success of reconstruction depends on the surgeon's knowledge of eyebrow anatomy and his or her ability to reproduce the angle and direction of single-hair grafts to achieve natural results.

▶ Eyebrows serve many important functions. Eyebrows frame the face and are crucial to facial expressions or displaying emotions. There seems to be ethnic differences in preference of eyebrow shape. In fact, authors indicate that Asians prefer them to be thicker and fuller. It could also be said that with the continued influence of western culture in Asia, that a more shapely, defined eyebrow would be more desirable. This can be observed in modern Asian media. One important point that needs to be emphasized is that eyebrow transplantation is meant mainly for reconstruction as opposed to cosmetic purposes. Patients should be carefully selected by experienced hair transplant surgeons and have reasonable expectations regarding outcome as there will never be a perfect match. Also, newly transplanted hairs will need regular trimming every 2 to 3 weeks. This is an informative article on modern follicular unit transplantation.

S. Bellew, DO
J. Q. Del Rosso, DO

Article Index

Chapter 1: Urticarial and Eczematous Disorders

Chapter 2: Psoriasis and Other Papulosquamous Disorders

Chapter 3: Bacterial and Fungal Infections

Chapter 4: Viral Infections (Excluding HIV Infection)

Chapter 5: HIV Infection

Chapter 6: Parasitic Infections, Bites, and Infestations

Chapter 7: Disorders of the Pilosebaceous Apparatus

Chapter 8: Photobiology

Chapter 9: Collagen Vascular and Related Disorders

Chapter 10: Blistering Disorders

Chapter 11: Drug Actions, Reactions, and Interactions

Chapter 12: Drug Development and Promotion

Chapter 13: Practice Management and Managed Care

Chapter 14: Miscellaneous Topics in Clinical Dermatology

Chapter 15: Nonmelanoma Skin Cancer

Chapter 16: Nevi and Melanoma

Chapter 17: Lymphoproliferative Disorders

Chapter 18: Miscellaneous Topics in Dermatologic Surgery and Cutaneous Oncology

Chapter 19: Miscellaneous Topics in Cosmetic and Laser Surgery

Author Index

Edwards Brothers Inc.
Ann Arbor MI. USA
July 19, 2011